ORTHOPEDIC

SECRETS

ORTHOPEDIC SECRETS

4th Edition (The Secrets Series®)

FOURTH EDITION

SURENA NAMDARI, MD, MSc
Assistant Professor of Orthopaedic
  Surgery
Shoulder & Elbow Surgeon
Rothman Instiitute – Thomas
  Jefferson University
Philadelphia, PA, USA

STEPHAN G. PILL, MD, MSPT
Orthopedic Surgeon
Orthopedic Specialists of the
  Carolinas
Winston-Salem, NC, USA

SAMIR MEHTA, MD
Chief, Orthopedic Trauma and
  Fracture Service
Hospital of the University of
  Pennsylvania
Assistant Professor
Department of Orthopedic Surgery
Perelman School of Medicine at the
  University of Pennsylvania
Philadelphia, PA, USA

ELSEVIER
SAUNDERS

London, New York, Oxford, Philadelphia, St Louis, Sydney, Toronto

ELSEVIER
SAUNDERS

SAUNDERS is an imprint of Elsevier Inc.

© 2015, Elsevier Inc. All rights reserved.

First edition 1994
Second edition 1999
Third edition 2004

Notices

Knowledge and best practice in this field are constantly changing. As new research and experience broaden our understanding, changes in research methods, professional practices, or medical treatment may become necessary.

Practitioners and researchers must always rely on their own experience and knowledge in evaluating and using any information, methods, compounds, or experiments described herein. In using such information or methods they should be mindful of their own safety and the safety of others, including parties for whom they have a professional responsibility.

With respect to any drug or pharmaceutical products identified, readers are advised to check the most current information provided (i) on procedures featured or (ii) by the manufacturer of each product to be administered, to verify the recommended dose or formula, the method and duration of administration, and contraindications. It is the responsibility of practitioners, relying on their own experience and knowledge of their patients, to make diagnoses, to determine dosages and the best treatment for each individual patient, and to take all appropriate safety precautions.

To the fullest extent of the law, neither the Publisher nor the authors, contributors, or editors, assume any liability for any injury and/or damage to persons or property as a matter of products liability, negligence or otherwise, or from any use or operation of any methods, products, instructions, or ideas contained in the material herein.

ISBN: 978-0-3230-7191-8
Content Strategist: James Merritt
Content Development Specialist: Nani Clansey
Content Coordinator: Trinity Hutton
Project Manager: Anne Collett
Design: Steven Stave
Illustration Manager: Amy Naylor
Illustrator: TNQ
Marketing Manager(s) (UK/USA): Melissa Darling

Printed in China
Last digit is the print number: 9   8   7   6   5   4   3   2

CONTENTS

PREFACE TO THE 4TH EDITION   vi

CONTRIBUTORS   vii

CHAPTER 1   ADULT RECONSTRUCTION   1
Pramod B. Voleti and Atul F. Kamath

CHAPTER 2   BASIC SCIENCE   23
Paul Maxwell Courtney and Jason E. Hsu

CHAPTER 3   FOOT AND ANKLE   51
J. Gabriel Horneff III and Stephan G. Pill

CHAPTER 4   HAND   81
Joshua A. Gordon and Adam Griska

CHAPTER 5   ORTHOPEDIC ONCOLOGY   125
J. Gabriel Horneff III and Stephan G. Pill

CHAPTER 6   PEDIATRIC ORTHOPEDICS   145
Eileen A. Crawford, Corinna C.D. Franklin, David A. Spiegel and Keith D. Baldwin

CHAPTER 7   REHABILITATION AND NEURO-ORTHOPEDIC SURGERY   220
Keith D. Baldwin, Alberto Esquenazi and Mary Ann Keenan

CHAPTER 8   SHOULDER AND ELBOW   244
Surena Namdari and Jason E. Hsu

CHAPTER 9   SPINE   281
Andrew H. Milby, Jonathan B. Slaughter and Nader M. Hebela

CHAPTER 10   SPORTS   328
Hassan Alosh, Kevin McHale, Laura Wiegand, Surena Namdari and Fotios P. Tjoumakaris

CHAPTER 11   ORTHOPEDIC TRAUMA   381
John A. Scolaro and Ryan M. Taylor

INDEX   443

PREFACE TO THE 4TH EDITION

We are excited by the opportunity to present the 4th edition of *Orthopedic Secrets*. The aim of this series is to continue in the tradition of the first three editions by providing an overview of orthopedics in a question-and-answer format that is the hallmark of The Secrets Series. We have attempted to present a vast amount of information in a concise format. It is important to recognize that some questions have more than one right answer, no right answer, or are controversial.

The goal of this publication is to discuss orthopedic topics that are commonly encountered in clinical practice, discussed on rounds, and found on board and in training examinations. The authors of each chapter have attempted to ask key questions and provide their best answers based on the current available literature. As we appreciated texts that included a case-based approach to teaching during our own training, in this updated edition we have asked the authors to include appropriate cases as well as descriptive images and drawings for each chapter. Each chapter in the new edition has been revised and updated, and several chapters from the 3rd edition have been merged to follow a subspecialty-specific format.

This work would not have been possible without the efforts of the editors of the 3rd edition, David E. Brown and Randall D. Neumann, or their chapter authors. We would like to thank all of the chapter authors for their contributions to the 4th edition and the leadership and staff at Elsevier for their hard work and patience in making this project possible. We hope that you, the reader, will benefit from their efforts, enjoy this book, and find it valuable.

Surena Namdari, MD, MSc

Stephan G. Pill, MD, MSPT

Samir Mehta, MD

CONTRIBUTORS

Hassan Alosh, MD
Physician Fellow
Department of Orthopedic Surgery
Rush University
Chicago, IL, USA

Keith D. Baldwin, MD, MSPT, MPH
Assistant Professor of Orthopedic Surgery
Department of Orthopedic Surgery
Children's Hospital of Pennsylvania
Hospital of the University of Pennsylvania
Philadelphia, PA, USA

Paul Maxwell Courtney, MD
Resident Physician
Department of Orthopedic Surgery
Hospital of the University of Pennsylvania
Philadelphia, PA, USA

Eileen A. Crawford, MD
Fellow Physician
Department of Orthopedic Surgery
University of Michigan
Ann Arbor, MI, USA

Alberto Esquenazi, MD
Chairman and Professor
PM&R
MossRehab/Einstein Healthcare Network
Elkins Park, PA, USA

Corinna C.D. Franklin, MD
Pediatric Orthopedic Surgeon
Shriners Hospital for Children
Philadelphia, PA, USA

Joshua A. Gordon, MD
Orthopedic Surgery Resident
Post-doctoral Research Fellow
Department of Orthopedic Surgery
Hospital of the University of
   Pennsylvania
Philadelphia, PA, USA

Adam Griska, MD
Hand Surgery Fellow
Tufts Combined Hand Surgery Fellowship
Boston, MA, USA

Nader M. Hebela, MD
Orthopedic & Spine Surgery
Neurological Institute
Cleveland Clinic Abu Dhabi
Abu Dhabi, United Arab Emirates

J. Gabriel Horneff III, MD
Resident
Department of Orthopedic Surgery
University of Pennsylvania
Philadelphia, PA, USA

Jason E. Hsu, MD
Assistant Professor
Department of Orthopedics and Sports
   Medicine
University of Washington
Seattle, WA, USA

Atul F. Kamath, MD
Attending Surgeon
Department of Orthopedic Surgery
Hospital of the University of Pennsylvania
Philadelphia, PA, USA

Mary Ann Keenan, MD
Professor of Orthopedic Surgery
Orthopedic Surgery
Hospital of the University of Pennsylvania
Philadelphia, PA, USA

Kevin McHale, MD
Department of Orthopedic Surgery
Hospital of the University of Pennsylvania
Philadelphia, PA, USA

Andrew H. Milby, MD
Resident
Department of Orthopedic Surgery
University of Pennsylvania
Philadelphia, PA, USA

Surena Namdari, MD, MSc
Assistant Professor of Orthopaedic Surgery
Shoulder & Elbow Surgeon
Rothman Institute – Thomas Jefferson
   University
Philadelphia, PA, USA

Stephan G. Pill, MD, MSPT
Orthopedic Surgeon
OrthoCarolina
Winston-Salem, NC, USA

John A. Scolaro, MD
Assistant Professor
Department of Orthopedic Surgery
University of California
Irvine Orange, CA, USA

Jonathan B. Slaughter, MD
Resident
Department of Orthopedic Surgery
University of Pennsylvania
Philadelphia, PA, USA

David A. Spiegel, MD
Assistant Professor of Orthopedic Surgery
Department of Orthopedic Surgery
Children's Hospital of Pennsylvania
Perelman School of Medicine at the
  University of Pennsylvania
Philadelphia, PA, USA

Ryan M. Taylor, MD
Resident
Department of Orthopedic Surgery
University of Pennsylvania
Philadelphia, PA, USA

Fotios P. Tjoumakaris, MD
Assistant Professor, Orthopedic
  Surgery
Jefferson Medical College
Rothman Institute Orthopedics
Egg Harbor Township, NJ, USA

Pramod B. Voleti, MD
Department of Orthopedic Surgery
Hospital of the University of
  Pennsylvania
Philadelphia, PA, USA

Laura Wiegand, MD
Attending Surgeon
Sports Medicine
Pittsburgh Bone, Joint, & Spine, Inc.
Jefferson Hills, PA, USA

CHAPTER 1

ADULT RECONSTRUCTION

Pramod B. Voleti and Atul F. Kamath

KNEE

CASE 1-1

A 65-year-old woman presents with a 2-year history of left knee pain. The pain is exacerbated by activity and improves with rest. She denies constitutional complaints, such as fever, weight loss, and fatigue.

1. **What is the differential diagnosis?**
   The differential diagnosis for this patient includes osteoarthritis, rheumatoid arthritis, crystalline arthropathies such as gout or pseudogout (calcium pyrophosphate deposition disease), spondyloarthropathies such as psoriatic arthritis and ankylosing spondylitis, and septic arthritis. Given the patient's age and clinical presentation, osteoarthritis is the most likely diagnosis.

CASE 1-1   continued

The patient is moderately obese with a Body Mass Index (BMI) of 32. Her left knee is not warm or swollen, but there is crepitus and medial joint line tenderness. Range of motion of the left knee is from 5° to 90°. Plain films of the left knee demonstrate narrowing of the medial joint space, subchondral sclerosis, and osteophyte formation (Fig. 1.1).

2. **What is the likely diagnosis?**
   Osteoarthritis (also known as OA, osteoarthrosis, degenerative joint disease) is the most common form of joint disease. Osteoarthritis is characterized by loss of articular cartilage, which results in damage to the underlying bone. The process results in pain, stiffness, and loss of joint mobility. The pain is typically worse with use of the joint and improves with rest. Loss of the smooth articulating surface accounts for the finding of crepitus when the joint is moved. The most common joints affected are the hips, knees, and proximal and distal interphalangeal joints (Bouchard's and Heberden's nodes, respectively), with the knee being the most commonly involved joint. Radiographs of the affected joint typically show joint space narrowing, subchondral sclerosis, osteophyte formation, and subchondral cysts. The patient's symptoms, physical exam findings, and radiographs are most consistent with osteoarthritis.

3. **What is the pathogenesis of osteoarthritis?**
   Osteoarthritis is characterized by degeneration of articular cartilage and often is associated with overuse or trauma to the joint. Chondrocytes produce and maintain type II collagen, which is the primary component of articular cartilage. Osteoarthritis is thought to be a result of a failed attempt of chondrocytes to repair damaged articular cartilage. When the articular cartilage is not properly maintained, the joint space narrows, and the bones in the diarthrodial knee joint may come into direct contact with one another. The resulting wear and tear leads to bony proliferation, with formation of subchondral sclerosis and osteophytes. Subchondral cysts arise secondary to microfractures and may contain amorphous gelatinous material.

4. **What changes occur in the cartilage of osteoarthritic joints?**
   Osteoarthritic cartilage is characterized by increased water content (in contrast with the decreased water content seen with aging), alterations in proteoglycans (decrease in overall content, shorter chain structure, an increase in the chondroitin/keratin sulfate ratio), and collagen abnormalities.

5. **What are the anatomic sources of the joint pain in osteoarthritis?**
   Although articular cartilage is the primary site of injury in this disease, cartilage is aneural, and, therefore, no pain is transmitted from this tissue. The pain of osteoarthritis primarily

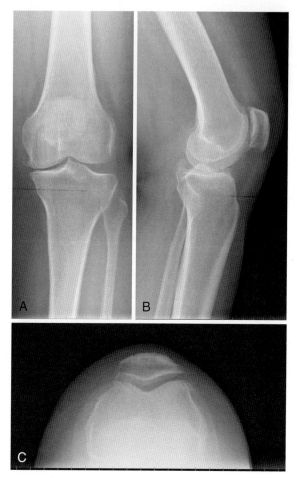

Figure 1.1. Anteroposterior (A), lateral (B), and merchant view (C) knee radiographs demonstrating medial joint space narrowing, subchondral sclerosis, and osteophyte formation, consistent with osteoarthritis.

originates from the periosteum surrounding the bone. As the articular cartilage wears away and the bones of the joint begin to rub against one another, the highly innervated periosteum becomes damaged and results in the joint pain seen in osteoarthritis. Other potential anatomic sources of osteoarthritic pain include subchondral bone, capsule, synovium, and periarticular tendons and bursae.

6. What are the risk factors associated with developing osteoarthritis?
   Obesity, joint trauma, and muscle weakness are some of the risk factors for osteoarthritis. These factors all increase the mechanical forces to which the articular cartilage is subjected. Gender, hormones, metabolic disorders, and genetics also play a role. Elderly populations are affected by this disease more frequently and more severely than younger populations. Obesity is the strongest modifiable risk factor for osteoarthritis.
   Note: Osteoarthritis can be classified as primary (idiopathic disease caused by intrinsic defect, the most common form), or secondary, with an underlying cause (e.g., trauma, infection, congenital deformity).

7. **What are the initial treatment options for osteoarthritis of the knee?**
Treatment begins with supportive measures, including weight loss and activity modification. Bracing, including compartmental unloader bracing, and/or ambulatory assistive devices may also be prescribed. Oral pain medications (such as NSAIDs), corticosteroid injections, viscosupplementation, and topical analgesics have been shown to alleviate the pain associated with osteoarthritis. While not demonstrating a clear benefit in the literature, supplements such as glucosamine and chondroitin sulfate may be tried. Moderate physical therapy may provide some symptomatic benefit, but it may only aggravate more advanced disease. Low-impact or aquatic therapy, in conjunction with stretching and isometric strengthening, may prove helpful. Other "joint protection" programs, those that cause low loads across the joint, include swimming, bicycling, walking, or tai chi; these activities increase muscle mass while protecting joints from undue stresses. Alternative therapies such as acupuncture may provide benefit in some patients, but there are no well-controlled data regarding efficacy in advanced osteoarthritis of the knee. Below is Table 1.1 summarizing the strong and moderate recommendations of the American Academy of Orthopaedic Surgeons (AAOS) with regard to treatment of knee osteoarthritis.

Table 1.1. AAOS Recommendations for Knee Osteoarthritis

STRONG RECOMMENDATIONS

We recommend patients with symptomatic osteoarthritis (OA) of the knee, who are overweight (as defined by a BMI >25), should be encouraged to lose weight (a minimum of five percent [5%] of body weight) and maintain their weight at a lower level with an appropriate program of dietary modification and exercise.

We recommend patients with symptomatic OA of the knee be encouraged to participate in low-impact aerobic fitness exercises.

We recommend glucosamine and/or chondroitin sulfate or hydrochloride not be prescribed for patients with symptomatic OA of the knee.

We recommend against performing arthroscopy with debridement or lavage in patients with a primary diagnosis of symptomatic OA of the knee.

MODERATE RECOMMENDATIONS

We suggest patients with symptomatic OA of the knee be encouraged to participate in self-management educational programs such as those conducted by the Arthritis Foundation, and incorporate activity modifications (e.g. walking instead of running; alternative activities) into their lifestyle.

We suggest quadriceps strengthening for patients with symptomatic OA of the knee.

We suggest patients with symptomatic OA of the knee use patellar taping for short-term relief of pain and improvement in function.

We suggest lateral heel wedges not be prescribed for patients with symptomatic medial compartmental OA of the knee.

We suggest patients with symptomatic OA of the knee receive one of the following analgesics for pain unless there are contraindications to this treatment: acetaminophen or NSAIDs

We suggest intra-articular corticosteroids for short-term pain relief for patients with symptomatic OA of the knee.

We suggest that needle lavage not be used for patients with symptomatic OA of the knee.

We suggest against using a free-floating interpositional device for patients with symptomatic unicompartmental OA of the knee.

CASE 1-1 continued

The patient has failed 6 months of non-operative therapy, including attempts at weight loss and activity modification, physical therapy, bracing, and pain medication. Her left knee pain has become progressively more severe and her range of motion has worsened (5° to 80°).

8. What is the next appropriate treatment option?

   Once a patient has failed multiple attempts at conservative therapy, surgical treatment options should be considered. The most common and effective treatment for end-stage degenerative joint disease of the knee is total knee arthroplasty (TKA). Other surgical treatment options include arthroscopic debridement, high tibial osteotomy (HTO) for treatment of varus deformity (Fig. 1.2), distal femoral osteotomy (DFO) for treatment of valgus deformity (Fig. 1.3), unicompartmental knee arthroplasty (UKA) (Fig. 1.4), and patellofemoral arthroplasty (PFA) (Fig. 1.5).

9. What are the major indications and contraindications for high tibial osteotomy in the treatment of degenerative joint disease of the knee?

   - Indications:
     - Isolated medial compartment arthritis demonstrated by history, physical examination, and radiographs

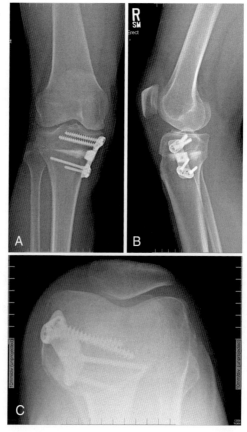

Figure 1.2. Anteroposterior (A), lateral (B), and merchant view (C) knee radiographs status post high tibial osteotomy.

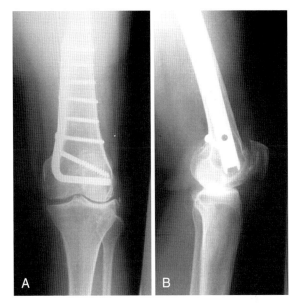

Figure 1.3. Anteroposterior (A) and lateral (B) knee radiographs status post distal femoral osteotomy.

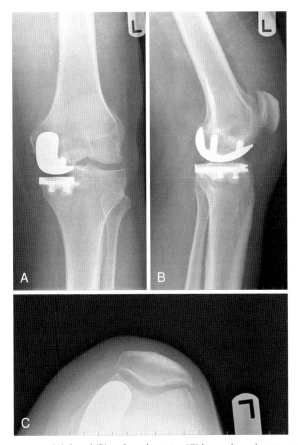

Figure 1.4. Anteroposterior (A), lateral (B), and merchant view (C) knee radiographs status post unicompartmental knee arthroplasty.

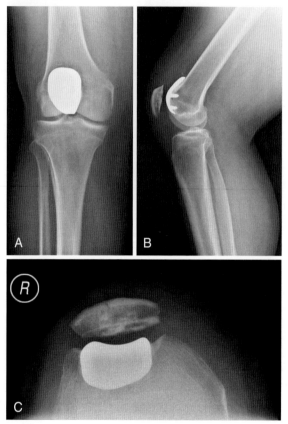

Figure 1.5. Anteroposterior (A), lateral (B), and merchant view (C) knee radiographs status post patellofemoral arthroplasty.

- Young, active patients with a strong desire to continue a vigorous lifestyle
- Fixed varus deformity <15°.
- Contraindications:
  - Range of motion <90° of flexion
  - Flexion contracture >15°
  - Fixed varus deformity >15°
  - Lateral tibial subluxation more than 1 cm
  - Inflammatory arthritis
  - ACL tear
  - Osteochondral injury with involvement of more than one-third of the condylar surface.

10. What are the major indications and contraindications for distal femoral osteotomy in the treatment of degenerative joint disease of the knee?
   The indications for distal femoral osteotomy in the treatment of degenerative joint disease of the knee are the same as the above indications for high tibial osteotomy with the following exceptions:
   - Isolated lateral compartment arthritis (rather than medial compartment arthritis)
   - Fixed valgus deformity >12–15°.

11. **What is unicompartmental knee arthroplasty and how is it different from total knee arthroplasty?**

Unicompartmental knee arthroplasty involves replacement of a single compartment of the knee, either medial or lateral, whereas total knee arthroplasty involves replacement of all three compartments of the knee: the medial and lateral compartments and the patellofemoral compartment. Both the anterior and posterior cruciate ligaments are preserved in unicompartmental knee arthroplasty. Patellofemoral joint arthroplasty is a form of unicompartmental knee arthroplasty involving replacement of just the patellofemoral articulation.

12. **What are the major indications and contraindications for unicompartmental knee arthroplasty in the treatment of degenerative joint disease of the knee?**
   - Indications:
     - Isolated compartment osteoarthritic changes
     - Arthritic pain localized to the affected compartment.
   - Contraindications:
     - Anterior cruciate ligament (ACL) deficiency
     - Fixed varus deformity that cannot be corrected on clinical examination
     - Previous meniscectomy in the opposite compartment
     - Knee flexion contracture >10°
     - Range of motion <90° of flexion
     - Inflammatory arthritis
     - Tricompartmental osteoarthritis.

13. **What are the primary goals of total knee arthroplasty (TKA)?**
   - Relief of pain
   - Restoration of function
   - Achievement of intrinsic stability
   - Creation of a durable reconstruction.

CASE 1-1   continued

Given her age, functional status, duration of symptoms, and radiographic appearance, the surgeon and patient decide that TKA is the preferred treatment option. The patient undergoes a preoperative medical workup, including a complete blood count, basic metabolic panel, type and screen, EKG, chest x-ray, urinalysis, and medicine consultation. No contraindications to surgery are identified. The patient presents on the day of surgery, and she has abstained from eating or drinking since midnight.

14. **What is the standard surgical approach for TKA? What is the rationale for its use?**

The standard surgical approach for TKA involves a straight midline skin incision, followed by a medial parapatellar arthrotomy. Despite the fact that a standard medial parapatellar (Fig. 1.6) skin incision follows Langer's lines more closely, a straight midline skin incision is used with a subsequent medial parapatellar arthrotomy so that the skin incision is not directly over the capsular incision. This slight mismatch of the capsular and skin incisions provides an overlap that allows a better seal and, therefore, effectively reduces postoperative drainage and subsequent possibility of related infection.

15. **Have any approaches other than the straight midline skin incision and the medial parapatellar capsular arthrotomy been popularized?**

The midline skin incision remains the standard approach. The skin incision may be adjusted based on prior surgical incisions/scars, as well as for particular planned procedures (e.g., unicompartmental arthroplasty). Furthermore, several alternative deep approaches/arthrotomies have been described, including the subvastus, the vastus medialis splitting (mid-vastus), the trivector, and the lateral parapatellar approaches.

16. **Describe the subvastus approach.**

The subvastus approach spares the quadriceps tendon. From the proximal to distal aspects, it involves elevation of the vastus medialis obliquus with a medial capsular arthrotomy that begins at the superior medial pole of the patella. Therefore, no incision is made into the quadriceps tendon. Advocates of this approach have noted a quicker return of quadriceps function, but no long-term advantages are seen over the more popular medial parapatellar arthrotomy.

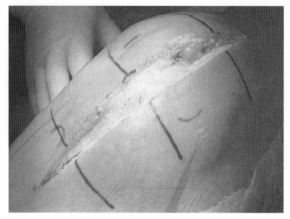

Figure 1.6. Intraoperative photograph demonstrating the midline skin incision commonly utilized for total knee arthroplasty.

17. **Describe the vastus medialis splitting approach.**

    The vastus medialis splitting approach begins with a division of the vastus medialis along its fibers at the proximal two-thirds and distal one-third junction. The muscle division ends at the superior medial pole of the patella, and the capsular arthrotomy is then carried distally along the medial aspect of the patella. It was initially reported that this approach yielded a decrease in the number of lateral retinacular releases. However, when the study was repeated in a randomized fashion, no difference in lateral retinacular release rates was noted between the medial parapatellar arthrotomy and the vastus medialis splitting approach.

18. **Describe the trivector approach.**

    The trivector approach involves an incision into the body of the vastus medialis obliquus, which begins approximately 5 cm proximal to the superior pole of the patella and extends distally along the medial aspect of the patella. Instead of splitting the quadriceps tendon, the muscle belly is divided. The term trivector arose as a result of the description of three vectors of pull on the patella: the vastus lateralis, the rectus femoris, and the vastus medialis obliquus. Proponents report that all three vectors are maintained with this approach. Original literature described early benefit with respect to the diminution of the number of lateral retinacular releases and an earlier recovery of the quadriceps function. However, a recent prospective study shows no difference between a standard medial parapatellar arthrotomy and the trivector approach.

19. **What is the indication for use of the lateral parapatellar approach?**

    A straight midline skin incision followed by a lateral parapatellar arthrotomy may be used in the exposure of a severe valgus deformity. Patients with a valgus deformity often have an associated lateral subluxation of the patella and require a lateral retinacular release at the time of surgical intervention, as well as potential significant release of the lateral structures to create a balanced TKA. Furthermore, when a surgeon performs a medial parapatellar arthrotomy and a subsequent lateral retinacular release for a valgus knee deformity, the vasculature to the patella may be somewhat compromised.

20. **What maneuvers can be performed to facilitate eversion of the patella during the standard medial parapatellar approach?**

    1. Extending the incision proximally into the quadriceps tendon
    2. Releasing adhesions in the lateral retinaculum and patellofemoral ligament
    3. Removing the peripheral osteophytes about the patella
    4. Release of tethering of the medial portion of the insertion of the patellar ligament
    5. Performing a lateral retinacular release
    6. Careful and sequential proximal medial tibial release and external rotation of the tibia.

21. **Define the mechanical axis of the knee.**
    The mechanical axis of the knee is defined as a line that intersects the center of the femoral head, the center of the knee, and the center of the ankle. The goal of TKA is to reconstruct the mechanical axis with appropriate resection of the distal femur and proximal tibia, while carefully balancing the ligamentous structures.

22. **What is the normal alignment of the distal femoral condyles with respect to the femoral axis and of the tibial plateau with respect to the tibial axis?**
    The normal alignment of the distal femoral condyles with respect to the femoral axis is approximately 9° of valgus, whereas the normal alignment of the tibial plateau with respect to the tibial axis is approximately 3° of varus. Therefore, a resultant 6° of valgus facilitates creation of the mechanical axis.

23. **How should the proximal tibia be cut with respect to the tibial axis?**
    Surgeons who follow the teaching of Insall et al. believe that the tibial resection should be created at 90° to the tibial axis in the coronal plane. They stress that varus malalignment leads to early failure. To reconstruct the mechanical axis, the distal femur must be resected at 6° of valgus. Hungerford et al., however, proposed that the proximal tibia be cut in 3° of varus and the distal femur in 9° of valgus. They argue that such resections place the joint line in the coronal plane parallel to the ground during gait. The majority of physicians, however, continue to resect the proximal tibia at 90° to the axis.

24. **What is the normal alignment of the proximal tibia in the sagittal plane?**
    In the sagittal plane, the proximal tibia generally has a posterior slope of approximately 7–10°. Therefore, two options exist in resecting the proximal tibia: (1) resection perpendicular to the axis, in which case the implant should have a posterior slope built into the articulation, and (2) resection of the proximal tibia with 5–7° of posterior slope. Reconstruction of the posterior slope is especially important in cruciate-retaining TKA.

25. **What are the palpable landmarks used to assist the placement of the extramedullary tibial alignment jigs?**
    The palpable landmarks used to place the extramedullary tibial alignment jigs are the tibial tubercle, tibial spines, and medial and lateral malleolus. The jig should be positioned over the tibial tubercle and aligned parallel with the tibial spines, while intersecting the intermalleolar distance. In this position, the jig should line up with the second ray of the foot.

26. **Describe the anatomic axes of the distal femur and proximal tibia that assist in determining rotation of the femoral component.**
    Rotation of the femoral component is determined by evaluating four distinct anatomic features of the distal femur and proximal tibia:
    1. The transepicondylar axis, which intersects the medial and lateral epicondyle.
    2. The anterior/posterior axis ("Whiteside's line") of the femur has been described as a line from the center of the trochlear groove to the center of the intercondylar notch. This axis is reported to be 90° to the transepicondylar axis.
    3. The posterior femoral condylar axis is usually 3° internally rotated relative to the transepicondylar axis. Therefore, by using a guide that references the posterior condyles with 3° of external rotation, the femoral component will be placed in line with the neutral transepicondylar axis.
    4. The tibial shaft axis has been identified as being 90° to the transepicondylar axis.
       At the time of surgical intervention, the surgeon should incorporate all four of the above anatomic references to assist in determining rotation of the femoral component.

27. **How can tightness or looseness in extension or flexion be corrected? (Table 1.2)**

28. **What structures can be released to correct a varus deformity?**
    - Osteophytes
    - Deep medial collateral ligament and meniscotibial ligament
    - Posteromedial corner with semimembranosus
    - Superficial medial collateral ligament and pes anserinus complex
    - Posterior cruciate ligament (rarely).

Table 1.2. Flexion and Extension Gap Correction in Total Knee Arthroplasty

		EXTENSION GAP		
		Tight	Normal	Loose
FLEXION GAP	Tight	Resect additional proximal tibia	Downsize femoral component OR resect additional proximal tibia and augment distal femur	Augment distal femur and either resect additional proximal tibia or downsize femoral component
	Normal	Resect additional distal femur OR perform posterior capsular release	Balanced	Augment distal femur
	Loose	Resect additional distal femur and increase polyethylene insert thickness	Upsize femoral component OR shift femoral component posteriorly	Increase polyethylene insert thickness

29. What structures can be released to correct a valgus deformity?
   - Osteophytes
   - Lateral capsule
   - Iliotibial band (if tight in extension)
   - Popliteus (if tight in flexion)
   - Lateral collateral ligament.

30. What surgical maneuvers can be performed to facilitate patellofemoral tracking?
   - Appropriate resection and resurfacing of the patella to restore preoperative thickness
   - Slight medial placement of the patellar component
   - Placement of the femoral component in neutral rotation or slight external rotation
   - Lateral translation of the femoral component
   - Appropriate rotation of the tibial component
   - Release of the patellofemoral ligament and any adhesions within the lateral retinaculum
   - Lateral retinacular release with preservation of the superior geniculate vessel
   - Advancement and reefing of the vastus medialis obliquus.

CASE 1-2

A 79-year-old man presents to clinic with a 3-month history of right knee pain. He underwent a total knee arthroplasty for the treatment of end-stage osteoarthritis 17 years ago. His postoperative course had been uncomplicated, and he had experienced immediate relief of his symptoms after surgery. Up until 3 months ago, he had been able to perform his daily activities, walk a mile, and play golf with limited pain. However, over the past 3 months, he has experienced a gradual progression of right knee pain. The pain is so severe that he is no longer able to perform his daily activities. His medical co-morbidities include hypertension and benign prostate hypertrophy, both of which are well-controlled with medication. He denies fevers, sweats, weight loss, and other constitutional symptoms. On physical exam, he has pain with right knee range of motion and tenderness over the right knee. His right knee range of motion is 3° to 85°. Radiographs of the right knee are obtained (Fig. 1.7).

31. What are the common causes of TKA failure necessitating revision?
   - Aseptic failure:
     - Component loosening
     - Polyethylene wear (osteolysis or catastrophic wear)
     - Ligament instability
     - Patellofemoral maltracking

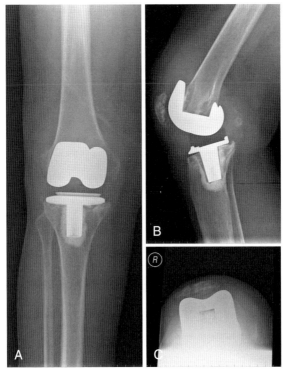

Figure 1.7. Anteroposterior (A), lateral (B), and merchant view (C) knee radiographs status post total knee arthroplasty.

- Septic failure (infection):
  - Early postoperative infection
  - Acute hematogenous infection
  - Chronic infection.

32. **What is the likely diagnosis for this patient?**
    Given the radiolucent lines surrounding the femoral and tibial components, along with the patient's clinical manifestations, this patient has experienced loosening of his total knee prosthesis. In order to differentiate between septic and aseptic failure, an infection work-up (including complete blood count (CBC) with differential, erythrocyte sedimentation rate (ESR), and C-reactive protein (CRP)) should be ordered. The presence of leukocytosis with an increased percentage of immature white blood cells on CBC and an elevated ESR and CRP are suggestive of an infectious process. If these abnormal values are detected, the right knee joint should be aspirated, and the fluid sent for cell count, gram stain, culture, and crystals.

33. **What are the expected joint fluid analysis results for an infected TKA?**
    Joint fluid analysis cell count will be elevated (depending on the study and time from surgery, >1100 cells/mm³), and the differential will show a preponderance of neutrophils. The gram stain may be positive, but it is often negative given the low sensitivity of this test. Cultures may show growth of the infecting organism.

34. **What is the incidence of periprosthetic infection following TKA?**
    The risk of periprosthetic infection following primary TKA is 1–2%. The risk of infection is greater following revision TKA is 6%.

35. Describe the main categories of prosthetic joint infection and their respective treatment options.
    - Early postoperative infection: infection within 3 weeks of the joint replacement surgery. Treatment with surgical irrigation and debridement, polyethylene component exchange, and metallic component retention is indicated. Postoperative intravenous antibiotics for a minimum of 4–6 weeks are recommended.
    - Acute hematogenous infection: the prosthetic joint is hematogenously seeded by an infection that develops at another site in the body. The treatment for an acute hematogenous infection is similar to that for an early postoperative infection. Recurrent infection requires surgical resection of the prosthetic components.
    - Late chronic infection: infection that has been present for more than 3 weeks. The persistent infection has had time to enter the boneprosthesis interface and a bacterial biofilm likely has developed over the implant (biofilm formation may be organism-dependent). Eradication of the infection requires surgical irrigation and debridement, removal of the prosthetic components usually with placement of a temporary antibiotic-impregnated spacer, and intravenous antibiotics for 4–6 weeks.
    - A fourth category is a positive intraoperative culture. Clinical suspicion of infection and consultation with an infectious disease specialist may help guide treatment.

36. What are the major goals of revision TKA?
    - Extraction of knee components with minimal bone and soft tissue destruction
    - Restoration of cavitary and segmental defects
    - Restoration of the joint line
    - Balanced knee ligaments
    - Stable knee components.

37. What are the implant choices for revision TKA?
    - Unconstrained prosthesis
    - Constrained, non-hinged prosthesis
    - Constrained, hinged prosthesis.

HIP

CASE 1-3

A 67-year-old man presents to clinic with an 18-month history of right groin pain. He has had no previous surgical procedures on his right hip. The pain is exacerbated by activity and improves with rest. He is unable to walk more than two blocks secondary to the pain, and the pain occasionally wakes him up at night. He denies constitutional complaints such as fever, weight loss, and fatigue. On physical examination, he describes pain over the right groin and hip. His right hip range of motion is limited and painful: 0–80° of flexion, abduction to 20°, adduction to 10°, internal rotation 15°, and external rotation 25°. Anteroposterior pelvis and anteroposterior and lateral right hip radiographs are obtained (Fig. 1.8). CBC, ESR, CRP, rheumatoid factor (RF), and antinuclear antibody (ANA) are all within normal limits.

38. What are the most common causes of hip arthritis in the adult patient?
    The most common causes of arthritic symptoms in the adult can be divided into two broad categories. The first is osteoarthritis, which is also called degenerative or idiopathic arthritis. This category includes the majority of patients over the age of 50 years with chronic arthritic pain in the hip. The second broad category is inflammatory arthritis, which includes rheumatoid arthritis, ankylosing spondylitis, systemic lupus erythematous, and the crystalline-induced arthritides, such as gout and pseudogout.

39. How can the types of hip arthritis be differentiated?
    The most common methods of differentiating the types of arthritis are clinical history, physical examination, and radiographic evaluation. The typical radiographic changes in the common types of arthritis are listed below (Table 1.3).

40. What is the likely diagnosis?
    The radiographs demonstrate joint space narrowing, subchondral sclerosis, and osteophyte formation, suggestive of osteoarthritis. The patient's serological work-up is negative, which is also consistent with osteoarthritis.

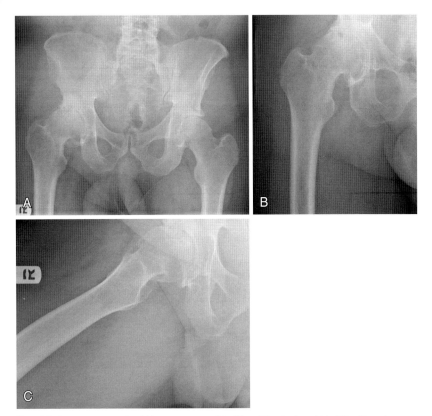

Figure 1.8. Anteroposterior pelvis (A), anteroposterior hip (B), and frog-leg lateral hip (C) radiographs demonstrating joint space narrowing, subchondral sclerosis, and osteophyte formation, consistent with osteoarthritis.

Table 1.3. Radiographic Findings with Hip Arthritis

DISEASE	TYPICAL RADIOGRAPHIC FINDINGS
Osteoarthritis	Joint space narrowing Boney sclerosis Osteophyte formation
Rheumatoid arthritis	Periarticular osteoporosis Joint erosions Loss of joint space Subluxation Ankylosis
Gout	Bony erosions
Pseudogout	Punctate linear calcification in hyaline and fibrocartilage

Infectious arthritis	Early: No change
	Late: Osteoporosis
	    Cartilage destruction
	    Erosions

41. **What are the initial treatment options for arthritis of the hip?**
Arthritis of the hip can be successfully managed by non-operative means, especially early in the course of the disease. Weight loss, activity modification, and ambulatory assistive devices may significantly reduce the patient's symptoms. NSAIDs are the most frequently prescribed pharmacologic agents for relief of symptoms. While not demonstrating a clear benefit in the literature, supplements such as glucosamine and chondroitin sulfate may be tried. Moderate physical therapy may provide some symptomatic benefit, but it may only aggravate more advanced disease. Low-impact or aquatic therapy, in conjunction with stretching and isometric strengthening, may prove helpful. Other "joint protection" programs, those that cause low loads across the joint, include swimming, bicycling, walking, or tai chi; these activities increase muscle mass while protecting joints from undue stresses.

CASE 1-3   continued

The treating physician initially recommends non-operative management, including weight loss, activity modification, a cane, and NSAIDs. The patient returns to clinic 8 months later. His pain and range of motion have not significantly improved, although the NSAIDs do alleviate some of his symptoms. He continues to have difficulties performing daily activities and has night pain.

42. **After failure of non-operative treatment options, what surgical treatments are available for arthritis of the hip?**
The most common surgical treatment for arthritis of the hip is total hip arthroplasty (THA). Hip resurfacing arthroplasty, femoral or pelvic osteotomy, arthrodesis, and Girdlestone resection are also options, although used less commonly. The patient's age, activity level, overall health, specific joint disease, other joint involvement, and radiographic presentation are considered in choosing the best surgical procedure.

43. **What are the most popular surgical approaches to the hip?**
The most popular surgical approaches to the hip for THA are posterior/posterolateral, direct lateral, anterolateral, and direct anterior approaches. The transtrochanteric approach is less common. The intervals and structures at risk for each approach are listed in the Table 1.4 below.

Table 1.4. Structures at Risk with Surgical Approach to Total Hip Arthroplasty

SURGICAL APPROACH	INTERVAL	STRUCTURES AT RISK
Posterior/ posterolateral	Gluteus maximus (inferior gluteal nerve) and gluteus medius/tensor fascia lata (superior gluteal nerve)	Sciatic nerve and inferior gluteal artery during gluteus maximus muscle split Medial femoral circumflex artery if quadratus femoris transected
Transtrochanteric	Gluteus medius (superior gluteal nerve) and vastus lateralis (femoral nerve)	Femoral nerve, artery, vein Lateral femoral circumflex artery
Anterolateral	Tensor fasciae lata (superior gluteal nerve) and gluteus medius (superior gluteal nerve)	Femoral nerve (from medial retraction) Descending branch of lateral femoral circumflex artery
Direct lateral	Tensor fasciae lata (superior gluteal nerve) and gluteus maximus (inferior gluteal nerve)	Superior gluteal nerve Femoral nerve
Direct anterior	Sartorius (femoral nerve) and tensor fasciae latae (superior gluteal nerve)	Lateral femoral cutaneous nerve Ascending branch of lateral femoral circumflex artery

44. **How is fixation of the prosthetic components achieved in THA?**
Excellent long-term fixation has been achieved using both polymethylmethacrylate (cemented) fixation and porous or bone ingrowth (non-cemented) fixation. The surgeon should consider the patient's age, activity level, and bone quality, as well as the surgeon's experience and comfort with cemented and cementless techniques, in selecting the type of fixation.

45. **Describe the generations of cement preparation technique (Table 1.5).**

Table 1.5. Cement Preparation Technique Generations	
GENERATION	**CEMENT PREPARATION TECHNIQUE**
First generation	Finger packing No canal preparation No cement plug No cement gun No pressurization Cast stem Narrow medial border on stem Sharp edges on stem
Second generation	Cement gun Pulsatile lavage Canal preparation Cement restrictor Super alloy stem Broad and round medial border Collar on stem
Third generation	Porosity reduction (vacuum) Cement pressurization Precoat stem Rough surface finish on stem Stem centralizer

46. **What is the ideal size of the cement mantle surrounding the femoral stem?**
It has been described that a minimum of 2 mm of cement thickness should be allowed between the prosthesis and bone. However, this value may be impossible to achieve in patients with narrow canals. Therefore, a more practical approach is the two-thirds rule: two-thirds of the canal is displaced by the femoral stem and the other one-third by cement.

47. **What are the advantages of cementless stems?**
Cementless stems rely on bone, a biologic interface, for fixation. This interface can react to stresses and strengthen itself over time. Cement is a non-biologic interface that can degrade with time. Theoretically, weakening of the cement–prosthesis or cement–bone interfaces could lead to loosening of a previously stable femoral stem.

48. **What design characteristics should cementless components have?**
Biologic fixation is achieved using either a porous-coated metallic surface that provides bone ingrowth fixation or a grit-blasted metallic surface that provides bone on-growth fixation. For porous-coated implants, 50–350 micron (preferably 50–150 micron) pores are created on the metallic surface. The pores allow for bone ingrowth, which secures the prosthesis to bone. The porosity of the surface should be 40–50%, thus allowing bone to fill in a significant area of the prosthesis. Greater porosity would put the porous-coated surface at risk of shearing off. Pore depth is another important characteristic: greater pore depth provides greater interface shear strength with loading. Finally, gaps between the prosthesis and bone should be less than 50 microns to allow for effective bone ingrowth. For grit-blasted implants, the metallic surface is roughened with an abrasive spray of particles

that pits the surface and creates peaks and valleys that allow for the bone to interdigitate. The surface roughness, which is defined as the average distance from the peak to the valley on the roughened surface, is directly related to an increase in interface shear strength. A newer type of cementless fixation involves the use of porous metals, which are gaining in popularity.

49. **Describe the ideal location for placement of acetabular screws.**
The key to placement of acetabular screws is to avoid neurovascular structures. A quadrant system has been developed to guide placement. The quadrants are defined by a line from the anterior superior iliac spine (ASIS) through the center of the acetabulum and a line perpendicular to that line which intersects the center of the acetabulum (Fig. 1.9). The structures at risk for each quadrant are listed in the Table 1.6 below.

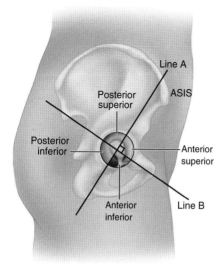

Figure 1.9. Quadrant system for acetabular screw placement during total hip arthroplasty. (*Redrawn from Wasielewski RC, Cooperstein LA, Kruger MP, et al: Acetabular anatomy and the transacetabular fixation of screws in total hip arthroplasty. J Bone Joint Surg 1990;72A:501.*)

Table 1.6. Structures at Risk with Acetabular Screw Placement

QUADRANT	STRUCTURES AT RISK
Posterior superior quadrant	Safe zone (screws less than 35 mm) Sciatic nerve Superior gluteal nerve and vessels
Posterior inferior quadrant	Safe zone (screws less than 25 mm) Sciatic nerve Inferior gluteal nerve and vessels Internal pudendal nerve and vessels
Anterior superior quadrant	External iliac vein and artery
Anterior inferior quadrant	Obturator artery and vein Anterior inferior obturator nerve

50. **What factors can lead to intraoperative femoral fractures?**
The most common factors that can lead to intraoperative femoral fractures are:
1. Failure to ream straight down the canal
2. Attempts to put too large a component down the canal

3. Attempts to impact the component down the canal too rapidly without allowing the viscoelastic nature of the bone to accept the component (bone expands with time)
4. Failure to appreciate preoperative deformities or distal tightness of the canal.

51. What are the most common nerve injuries during THA?

Nerve injury during THA may involve the sciatic nerve (80%) or the femoral nerve (20%). When the sciatic nerve is injured, the peroneal division is usually affected because it is closer to the acetabulum than the tibial division. The most common cause of sciatic nerve injury is errant retractor placement. Other potential causes of sciatic nerve palsy include hematoma and excessive leg lengthening.

52. What measures are available to decrease the incidence of thrombophlebitis after THA?

- Early mobilization
- Sequential compression stockings and venous compression devices
- Anticoagulation (e.g., warfarin, aspirin, low-molecular-weight heparin).

CASE 1-4

A 59-year-old woman presents to the emergency department 8 weeks after undergoing a right THA. She complains of severe right hip pain which began 4 hours ago while she was performing yoga. Prior to today, she did not have any pain in her right hip. On physical examination, her right lower extremity is shortened and internally rotated. An anteroposterior radiograph of the right hip demonstrates dislocation of the THA prosthesis (Fig. 1.10). This is her first episode of right hip instability.

53. How should this patient be managed?

Dislocation of a hip prosthesis should initially be managed with closed reduction under conscious sedation. Conscious sedation is necessary to achieve proper analgesia and muscle relaxation. If a closed reduction is unsuccessful in an emergency room setting, the patient should be taken to the operating room for a closed versus open reduction. If component positioning or compromise is the cause of instability, the components may be revised at the time of reduction or may be revised at a later date.

CASE 1-4   continued

The patient is sedated in the emergency room with administration of propofol. The right hip is reduced using closed techniques. An anteroposterior radiograph of the right hip demonstrates successful reduction of the right hip prosthesis (Fig. 1.11). An abduction pillow is placed between the patient's legs to maintain the reduction. The patient awakens from sedation with improvement in right hip pain and range of motion. She is discharged home with instructions for strict hip precautions.

54. What is the incidence of dislocation after THA?

The incidence of dislocation after primary THA is approximately 1–2%, but has been reported to be as high as 9.5%. Dislocation rates after revision are higher and have been reported as high as 26% in cases of multiple revisions.

55. What aspects of component design affect hip stability after THA?

- Head–neck ratio (ratio of femoral head diameter to femoral neck diameter): a larger head–neck ratio allows greater arc of motion before impingement, and skirted femoral necks reduce this ratio.
- Excursion distance (the distance the head must travel to dislocate): a greater excursion distance results in a more stable hip.
- Constrained liner: a constrained liner provides inherent stability at the cost of a reduced primary arc range and an increased risk of early loosening.

56. What soft-tissue considerations affect hip stability after THA?

Maintaining the correct tension of the abductor complex is a key to hip stability. The native femoral offset and neck length should be restored to maintain proper soft-tissue tension. Preoperative templating may assist in selecting the appropriate component sizes.

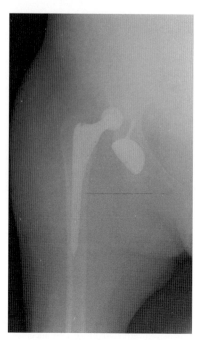

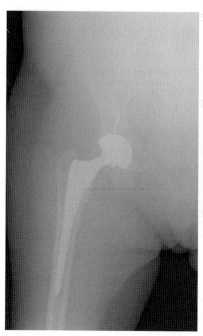

Figure 1.10. Anteroposterior hip radiograph demonstrating dislocation of the total hip arthroplasty prosthesis.

Figure 1.11. Anteroposterior hip radiograph status post closed reduction of the total hip arthroplasty prosthesis.

57. **What is heterotopic ossification and how can it be prevented in high-risk patients?**

Heterotopic ossification (HO) is the process by which bone tissue forms outside of the skeleton. Predisposing risk factors for HO after THA include hypertrophic osteoarthritis, ankylosing spondylitis, diffuse idiopathic skeletal hyperostosis (DISH), post-traumatic arthritis, prior hip arthrodesis, and a history of previous development of HO. Heterotopic ossification is seen more often in males and with the direct lateral approach to the hip (Hardinge approach). Prophylactic treatment of high-risk patients with a single dose of radiation (600 rads) within 72 hours of surgery or with NSAIDs (such as indomethacin) for 6 weeks is recommended. Meticulous soft-tissue management during surgery may also minimize trauma to the hip tissues.

58. **What is another common long-term complication after THA?**

Along with dislocation, aseptic loosening is a common long-term complication after THA. Radiographic evidence of loosening includes: (1) migration or subsidence of the component, (2) fracture of the cement, and (3) a 2 mm lucent line completely surrounding the prosthesis. Aseptic loosening is frequently associated with osteolysis, which is resorption of bone around the prosthesis mediated by collagenases, prostaglandins, and proteases. Osteolysis is thought to be the result of the body's reaction to polyethylene particulate debris that forms from polyethylene wear; it is a macrophage-mediated process. Factors that can minimize polyethylene debris include: (1) proper head size; (2) maximal polyethylene thickness (at least 6 mm); (3) alternative bearing surfaces, such as ceramics or metal; and (4) highly cross-linked polyethylene.

59. **What is the infection rate following THA? Which patients are at greatest risk for infection?**
    The prevalence of infection after THA of Medicare patients in the United States is approximately 2.3%. Patient factors associated with increased risk for infection include rheumatoid arthritis, diabetes mellitus, poor nutrition, obesity, oral steroid use, and previous surgery.

60. **What factors may decrease the incidence of infection following THA?**
    Before surgery, the patient should be in satisfactory dental health and free of infection in any other organ system. Patients should also be adequately nourished and free of any skin conditions that may provide a portal for bacterial entrance. Perioperative prophylactic antibiotics effectively reduce the incidence of deep wound infection. Laminar air flow within an enclosed area and total body exhaust-ventilated suits further decrease exogenous wound contamination. Efficient surgical technique with meticulous hemostasis and closure also contribute to uneventful wound healing.

61. **What organisms commonly cause THA infections?**
    Staphylococci bacteria are the most commonly isolated pathogens from THA infections. Among the staphylococci, *Staphylococcus epidermidis* and *Staphylococcus aureus* are the most common infecting organisms. Streptococci, enterococci, and gram-positive cocci are also frequent pathogens, while gram-negative bacteria are less common. Fungi and mycobacteria are infrequently encountered in these infections.

62. **Describe the signs and symptoms of an infected THA.**
    The clinical picture of a periprosthetic hip infection is highly variable. The majority of patients present with relatively mild signs and symptoms. Often, mild pain is the only symptom. Less frequently do these infections present as fulminant processes, with a combination of local signs such as deep throbbing pain, wound drainage, erythema, and swelling about the hip. It is not uncommon to have associated fever, chills, and generalized malaise with these overt infections.

63. **What initial diagnostic tests should be ordered for a patient with a suspected periprosthetic hip infection?**
    Plain radiographs, CBC with differential, ESR, and CRP are the initial diagnostic tests that should be ordered.

64. **What is the radiographic appearance of a periprosthetic hip infection?**
    Plain radiographs are rarely diagnostic for a total hip infection; however, they should always be obtained in suspected cases in order to rule out other causes of pain, to evaluate component positioning, and to serve as a baseline for future radiographs. One finding that may be helpful to distinguish septic from aseptic loosening is periosteal new bone formation.

65. **Describe the results of a CBC with differential, ESR, and CRP in patients with THA infections.**
    In periprosthetic infections, the CBC with differential may demonstrate the presence of leukocytosis, with an increased percentage of immature white blood cells. However, this phenomenon may not occur in indolent presentations. The ESR is an indirect indicator of a systemic response to an inflammatory process. Unfortunately, the ability of the ESR to be influenced by any inflammatory condition decreases its specificity and predictive value when used independently. For example, following uncomplicated THA, the ESR may not return to baseline levels for several months after surgery, thus making this an especially unreliable test in the early postoperative period. When used alone, the reported sensitivity and specificity of ESR in diagnosing total hip infections are 82% and 86%, respectively. CRP is also a non-specific indicator of inflammation, infections, and neoplastic processes. In contrast to the ESR, CRP levels return to baseline shortly after surgery, and normal

values have been demonstrated at an average of 3 weeks postoperatively (range, 1–8 weeks). Elevated CRP levels greater than 10 mg/L have been associated with periprosthetic infection. Although the reported sensitivity (96%) and specificity (92%) of CRP alone are superior to those reported with ESR alone, its specificity has been shown to increase to nearly 100% when used concurrently with the ESR and clinical picture.

66. **What other diagnostic studies may be used in the work-up for a suspected infected THA?**

    Hip aspiration with fluid analysis and culture and radionucleotide imaging may also be performed in the work-up for a suspected infected THA. Current recommendations discourage routine hip aspiration as a screening tool to rule out periprosthetic hip infections. When used for all THA failures, the sensitivity and specificity of hip aspiration have widely varied. Therefore, the use of hip aspiration is currently recommended only in cases that are suspicious for an infection.

67. **What are the intraoperative diagnostic studies used to confirm THA infection?**
    - *Gram stain*: This study has been fairly unreliable in the diagnosis of periprosthetic total hip infections. Sensitivities ranging from 0% to 23% (average 19%) have been reported. However, the gram stain is not to be totally abandoned as positive results could provide early information regarding the offending organism and guide initial antibiotic therapy.
    - *Cultures*: Intraoperative cultures remain the standard to which all other intraoperative diagnostic modalities are compared. As with the other diagnostic tests for this disease process, cultures are not foolproof as both significant false-positive and false-negative rates have been reported. Using proper technique, sensitivities and specificities as high as 94% and 97% have been reported respectively. To avoid inaccurate results, precise technique should be followed:
      1. Antibiotics should be withheld until specimens have been obtained in cases of suspected infection.
      2. Instruments used to obtain the culture should be prevented from touching the skin of the patient.
      3. Samples should be obtained from the environment close to the prosthesis and, if possible, from inflamed tissue.
      4. A minimum of three specimens should be sent fresh to the laboratory for immediate processing.
      5. The specimen should be obtained immediately after the pseudocapsule is opened from an area not previously cauterized and before any irrigation has been used.
    - *Frozen sections*: Intraoperative frozen sections of the prosthetic environment are used to diagnose THA infections by determining the quantity of inflammatory cells. The previous threshold of five polymorphonuclear leucocytes per high powered field (5 PMN/hpf) has been thought to be highly suggestive of infection. Sensitivities and specificities of 80% and 90%, respectively, have been reported using this 5 PMN/hpf threshold. When 10 PMN/hpf is used as the threshold, the specificity increases from 96% to 99% without decreasing the sensitivity (84%).
    - *Polymerase chain reaction*: PCR is a technique that shows promise in diagnosing infection in THA. The PCR technique involves the amplification of nucleic acid extracted from periprosthetic synovial fluid and screening it for the presence of bacterial DNA. This technique has the ability to diagnose periprosthetic infections when only a small quantity of bacteria is present. This ability to detect minute amounts of nucleic acid may result in a high false-positive rate. The hypersensitivity of PCR currently limits use of this diagnostic test, but it is anticipated that this technique will provide a useful tool in diagnosing THA infections in the future.

68. **Describe the main categories of prosthetic joint infection and their respective treatment options.**
    - Early postoperative infection: Infection within 3 weeks of the joint replacement surgery. Treatment with surgical irrigation and debridement, modular/polyethylene component exchange, and metallic component retention is indicated. Postoperative intravenous antibiotics for a minimum of 4–6 weeks are recommended. Some surgeons will consider removing cementless fixation devices that have not ingrown at this time as well.

- Acute hematogenous infection: The prosthetic joint is hematogenously seeded by an infection that develops at another site in the body. The treatment for an acute hematogenous infection is similar to that for an early postoperative infection. Recurrent infection requires surgical resection of the prosthetic components.
- Late chronic infection: Infection that has been present for more than 3 weeks. The persistent infection has had time to enter the bone–prosthesis interface and a bacterial biofilm likely has developed over the implant (biofilm formation may be organism-dependent). Eradication of the infection requires surgical irrigation and debridement, removal of the prosthetic components usually with placement of a temporary antibiotic-impregnated spacer, and intravenous antibiotics for 4–6 weeks.
- A fourth category is a positive intraoperative culture. Clinical suspicion of infection and consultation with an infectious disease specialist may help guide treatment.

69. **Describe the classification and treatment of periprosthetic femoral fractures.**
The Vancouver classification system of periprosthetic femur fractures, as modified by Duncan and Masri, along with recommended treatment options is listed in the Table 1.7 below.

Table 1.7. Modified Vancouver Classification for Periprosthetic Femur Fractures

TYPE	FRACTURE LOCATION/ CHARACTERISTICS	TREATMENT OPTIONS
Type A	Fracture located in the trochanteric region	
Type AG	Involving the greater trochanter	Symptomatic treatment with protected weight bearing and limited abduction Open reduction internal fixation (ORIF) if fracture displaced >2.5 cm or if there is pain, instability, or abductor weakness
Type AL	Involving the lesser trochanter	Symptomatic treatment with protected weight bearing Surgical treatment only if a large portion of medial cortex is attached
Type B	Fracture is located around or just distal to the femoral stem	
Type B1	Good bone stock, stem well-fixed	ORIF with fixation; may use plates, cortical strut grafts, cables, and/or cerclage wires
Type B2	Good bone stock, stem loose	Long-stem cementless revision; consider cortical strut graft to improve stability and enhance bone stock
Type B3	Poor bone stock, stem loose	Long-stem cementless revision Consider allograft-prosthetic composite in a young patient to help augment bone stock Consider proximal femur replacement in elderly or low-demand patients
Type C	Fracture is located well below the femoral stem	ORIF with blade plate, condylar screw plate, or supracondylar plate; overlap plate and stem to avoid creation of stress riser; may use cerclage wires at level of stem and screws distal to stem; newer plate options include locking screw technology Consider retrograde intramedullary nail

BIBLIOGRAPHY

1. American Academy of Orthopaedic Surgeons. Treatment of Osteoarthritis of the Knee: Evidence Based Guideline. 2013 <www.aaos.org/research/guidelines/guidelineoaknee.asp>.
2. Archibeck MJ, White RE Jr. What's new in adult reconstructive knee surgery. J Bone Joint Surg Am 2006;88:1677–86.
3. Awan O, Chen L, Resnik CS. Imaging evaluation of complications of hip arthroplasty: review of current concepts and imaging findings. Can Assoc Radiol J 2013;64:306–13.
4. Bellamy N, Campbell J, Robinson V, et al. Viscosupplementation for the treatment of osteoarthritis of the knee. Cochrane Database Syst Rev 2006;CD005321.
5. Benjamin J. Component alignment in total knee arthroplasty. Instr Course Lect 2006;55:405–12.
6. Callaghan JJ. The clinical results and basic science of total hip arthroplasty with porous-coated prostheses. J Bone Joint Surg Am 1993;75:299–310.
7. Callaghan JJ, Templeton JE, Liu SS, et al. Results of Charnley total hip arthroplasty at a minimum of thirty years. A concise follow-up of a previous report. J Bone Joint Surg Am 2004;86-A:690–5.
8. Duncan CP, Masri BA. Fractures of the femur after hip replacement. Instr Course Lect 1995;44:293–304.
9. Gupta SK, Chu A, Ranawat AS, et al. Osteolysis after total knee arthroplasty. J Arthroplasty 2007;22:787–99.
10. Hewett TE, Noyes FR, Barber-Westin SD, et al. Decrease in knee joint pain and increase in function in patients with medial compartment arthrosis: a prospective analysis of valgus bracing. Orthopedics 1998;21:131–8.
11. Koshino T, Murase T, Saito T. Medial opening-wedge high tibial osteotomy with use of porous hydroxyapatite to treat medial compartment osteoarthritis of the knee. J Bone Joint Surg Am 2003;85-A:78–85.
12. Lombardi AV Jr, Berend KR. Posterior cruciate ligament-retaining, posterior stabilized, and varus/valgus posterior stabilized constrained articulations in total knee arthroplasty. Instr Course Lect 2006;55:419–27.
13. Masri BA, Meek RM, Duncan CP. Periprosthetic fractures evaluation and treatment. Clin Orthop Relat Res 2004;80–95.
14. Mihalko WM, Manaswi A, Cui Q, et al. Diagnosis and treatment of the infected primary total knee arthroplasty. Instr Course Lect 2008;57:327–39.
15. Mont MA, Booth RE Jr, Laskin RS, et al. The spectrum of prosthesis design for primary total knee arthroplasty. Instr Course Lect 2003;52:397–407.
16. Mullins MM, Norbury W, Dowell JK, et al. Thirty-year results of a prospective study of Charnley total hip arthroplasty by the posterior approach. J Arthroplasty 2007;22:833–9.
17. Newman J, Pydisetty RV, Ackroyd C. Unicompartmental or total knee replacement: the 15-year results of a prospective randomised controlled trial. J Bone Joint Surg Br 2009;91:52–7.
18. Sharkey PF, Parvizi J. Alternative bearing surfaces in total hip arthroplasty. Instr Course Lect 2006;55:177–84.
19. Sprenger TR, Doerzbacher JF. Tibial osteotomy for the treatment of varus gonarthrosis. Survival and failure analysis to twenty-two years. J Bone Joint Surg Am 2003;85-A:469–74.
20. Toms AD, Davidson D, Masri BA, et al. The management of peri-prosthetic infection in total joint arthroplasty. J Bone Joint Surg Br 2006;88:149–55.
21. Vertullo CJ, Easley ME, Scott WN, et al. Mobile bearings in primary knee arthroplasty. J Am Acad Orthop Surg 2001;9:355–64.
22. Zhang W, Moskowitz RW, Nuki G, et al. OARSI recommendations for the management of hip and knee osteoarthritis, part I: critical appraisal of existing treatment guidelines and systematic review of current research evidence. Osteoarthritis Cartilage 2007;15:981–1000.

CHAPTER 2

BASIC SCIENCE

Paul Maxwell Courtney and Jason E. Hsu

MUSCULOSKELETAL TISSUE

BONE

1. **What is the function of bone?**

   Osseous tissue is unique in both structure and function. Its primary function is to provide mechanical stability to the body. The cellular components also regulate mineral homeostasis, while the marrow functions to produce hematopoietic cell lines.

2. **What are the anatomic differences between the different types of bones?**

   Bones can be classified histologically as *woven* or *lamellar* bone. *Woven bone* is immature or pathologic and is characterized by its weakness, flexibility, and high rate of turnover. *Lamellar bone* is stress oriented, and includes both *cortical* and *cancellous* bone. Cortical bone comprises the large majority of our skeleton and is characterized by its slow turnover rate, compactness, and low porosity. Cancellous, or trabecular bone, is softer and more elastic, making up about 20% of the skeleton. Unlike cortical bone, cancellous bone is porous and consists of a loose network of bony struts. In osteoporosis, these struts become thinned, resulting in increased macroscopic porosity.

   Anatomically, bones can be classified as long or flat. Long bones consist of the diaphysis, metaphysis, and epiphysis. The diaphysis is the shaft of the long bone responsible for load bearing and consists of a thick tube of cortical bone which surrounds a thin canal of cancellous bone that houses the marrow elements. The epiphysis is the end of a long bone which articulates with a joint and is comprised of a thin layer of cortical bone surrounding thick trabecular bone. The metaphysis functions as a transition zone from the diaphysis to the epiphysis.

3. **How do bones receive blood supply and innervation?**

   Bones receive their neurovascular supply form a series of packed osteons, or haversian systems (Fig. 2.1), each containing arterioles, venules, capillaries, and nerves. They are connected within the bone by haversian canals, which run longitudinally through the cortex, and Volkmann canals which run obliquely to the periosteum and trabecular bone. Periosteal vessels supply the *superficial third* of the cortex and are at risk of being stripped during surgical procedures. Reaming during intramedullary nailing can damage the nutrient artery, which enters the diaphysis through to the intramedullary canal and supplies the *deep two-thirds* of the cortex.

4. **What are the components to the extracellular matrix?**

   The majority of bony matrix comprises inorganic minerals, while about 20–25% of the extracellular matrix consists of organic components. The primary component of the mineral matrix is calcium hydroxyapatite, which provides the compressive strength of bone. Tricalcium phosphate, sodium, magnesium, and bicarbonate are also found. *Type I collagen* makes up 90% of the organic matrix and is responsible for the tensile strength of bone. Proteoglycans regulate tissue structure and inhibit mineralization. Other matrix proteins also play a role in bone homeostasis. *Osteocalcin* is vitamin K dependent and the most abundant non-collagenous protein. It functions to promote bone formation and mineralization and is a useful urine marker in patients with disorders of bone turnover such as Paget's disease. Adhesive proteins, growth factors, cytokines, and matricellular proteins are also found in the organic matrix.

5. **How do osteoblasts, osteoclasts, and osteocytes function in bone homeostasis?**

   Bone is a metabolically active tissue that is constantly undergoing remodeling by the biologically active cells of the bony matrix. Osteoblasts primary functions are to produce bone and regulate osteoclast activity. *Mesenchymal stem cells are stimulated to differentiate*

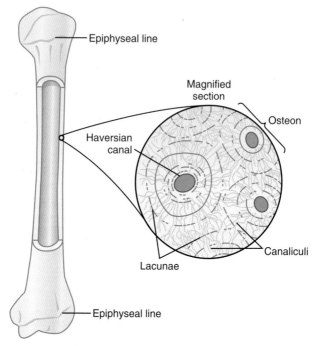

Figure 2.1. Cross-sectional diagram depicting microscopic bony anatomy. (*From Hall JE. Parathyroid Hormone, Calcitonin, Calcium and Phosphate Metabolism, Vitamin D, Bone, and Teeth. In: Guyton and Hall Textbook of Medical Physiology, 12th edn. Copyright © Saunders, Elsevier, 2011.*)

into mature osteoblasts by bone morphogenic protein (BMP), parathyroid hormone (PTH), glucocorticoids, prostaglandins, and vitamin D. Mature osteoblasts then secrete alkaline phosphatase, type I collagen, and osteocalcin to form the bone matrix. When mature osteoblasts become trapped in the bony matrix, they differentiate into osteocytes. These cells make up about 90% of the cells in the bony matrix and regulate bone homeostasis. Osteocytes are nonmitotic and produce few compounds. They are stimulated by calcitonin and inhibited by PTH.

Osteoclasts are the primary bone resorptive cells and are actually hematopoietic cells, derived from the macrophage/monocyte lineage. They reside in Howship's lacunae and attach to bone surfaces via *integrins*. By producing tartrate resistant acid phosphatase (TRAP), osteoclasts decrease the pH and increase the solubility of hydroxyapatite. The osteoclasts' ruffled border helps it bind to bone surfaces where it secretes proteases, such as *cathepsin-K*, to break down the organic matrix via proteolytic digestion. Bisphosphonates inhibit bone resorption by blocking the formation of cytoskeleton proteins in osteoclasts.

6. **What are the molecular mechanisms of bone resorption?**
   Bone resorption is primarily mediated by osteoclasts. The pathway begins with PTH stimulating osteoblasts to produce the nuclear factor ligand, *RANKL*. RANKL binds to specialized RANK receptors on osteoclast precursors, stimulating differentiation into active osteoclasts. *Osteoprotegerin (OPG) is closely related to the tumor necrosis factor family and also binds RANKL to competitively inhibit osteoclast activation* (Fig. 2.2).

7. **What are some clinical implications with errors in this pathway?**
   Several clinical conditions result when the bone resorption pathway goes awry. *Osteopetrosis is a condition caused by a lack of functional osteoclasts.* Knockout mice without the RANKL gene are found to have an osteopetrosis-like condition. Many cancers secrete PTH or parathyroid hormone related peptide (PTHrP), which stimulates RANKL production and

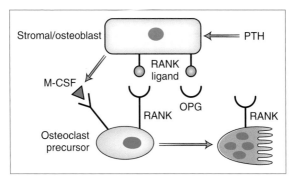

Figure 2.2. Schematic depicting bone homeostasis. Osteoblasts secrete RANK ligand which binds to the RANK receptor to stimulate osteoclast differentiation. M-CSF: macrophage colony-stimulating factor. (*From Bringhurst FR, et al. Hormones and Disorders of Mineral Metabolism. In: Melmed S, et al. [eds], Williams Textbook of Endocrinology, 12th edn. Copyright © Saunders, Elsevier Inc., 2011.*)

results in bone resorption and metastatic lytic bone lesions. Patients with multiple myeloma have high levels of interleukin-6, which also stimulates osteoclast activation. Conversely, premenopausal women have high levels of circulating estrogen, which leads to increased OPG production and less bone destruction.

8. **What changes in bone metabolism would you expect in patients with parathyroid dysfunction?**
   Hypoparathyroidism is a metabolic condition often presenting with vague nonspecific symptoms such as weakness, altered mental status, constipation, hair loss, and nausea. Low levels of PTH results in decreased osteoclastic activation and thus decreased bone resorption. As a result of less bone turnover, patients often report bone-associated pain. PTH also acts on the kidney to convert vitamin D to its active form. Laboratory findings will show *decreased levels of serum calcium with increased levels of phosphorous.* Treatment is with calcium supplementation and the active vitamin D metabolite, vitamin D3.

9. **Why do we encourage dietary calcium and vitamin D to promote bone health?**
   Bone functions as a reservoir for the body's calcium stores. While 99% of the body's calcium is stored in bone, the active 1% in plasma functions in muscle and nerve conduction as well as a cofactor in the clotting cascade. Serum calcium levels are tightly regulated by PTH and vitamin D. Adults should take at least *750 mg* of calcium per day, while those with healing fractures, postmenopausal women, and pregnant women should have a minimum of *1200 mg* of calcium in their daily diet. Supplementation of 800 IU of vitamin D is also recommended for prevention of osteoporotic fractures.
       Vitamin D is a naturally occurring steroid. UV radiation from the sun activates vitamin D from our skin into its metabolically active form. Dietary vitamin D absorbed in the intestines must be activated by both the liver and kidney before being able to act on the bone. *When calcium stores are low, PTH is increased and activates the enzyme 1-alpha hydroxylase which activates vitamin D in the kidney.* In addition to increasing calcium absorption in the small intestine, vitamin D is also an important cofactor in osteoblastic signaling and thus bone turnover.

10. **What are the clinical manifestations of vitamin D deficiency?**
    Patients with vitamin D deficiency due to inadequate dietary intake have decreased calcium absorption in the gastrointestinal tract and thus decreased serum calcium levels. A compensatory increase in PTH triggers the RANKL pathway activating osteoclasts and resulting in bone resorption. This disorder is known as *nutritional rickets.* Orthopedic manifestations of the disease include thickening of the growth plates due to decreased calcification, metaphyseal fraying, physeal cupping (metaphysis changes from a convex to a concave surface), bowing of long bones, pathologic fractures, decreased muscle tone, and stunted growth in children. Patients are unable to mineralize the bony matrix due to their lack of calcium absorption (Fig. 2.3).

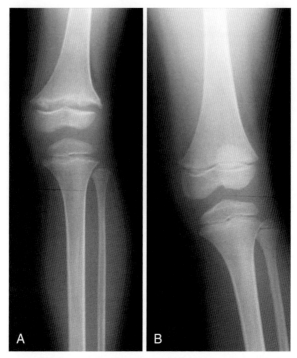

Figure 2.3. X-rays of the knees in a 7-year-old girl with distal renal tubular acidosis and rickets. (A) At initial presentation, there is widening of the growth plate and metaphysical fraying. (B) Dramatic improvement after 4 months of therapy with alkali. *(From Greenbaum LA. Rickets and Hypervitaminosis D. In: Kliegman R, Nelson WE [eds], Nelson Textbook of Pediatrics. Copyright © Saunders, Elsevier Inc., 2011.)*

11. **What are the different forms of rickets?**
    Nutritional rickets is rare in the United States due to many of our foods being fortified with vitamin D. The most common form of rickets is a genetic disease known as *familial hypophosphatemic rickets*. It is an *X-linked dominant* condition in which the proximal renal tubules have a defect in reabsorbing phosphate, thus causing a reflexive increase in PTH and bone resorption. The clinical presentation is similar to nutritional rickets. *Hereditary vitamin D dependent rickets* is another rare genetic disorder causing similar clinical symptoms due to a *defective 1-alpha hydroxylase enzyme (type I)* or a *defective vitamin D3 receptor (type II)*.

12. **Understanding the physiology of bone metabolism, what bone pathology would you expect in patients with chronic renal disease?**
    Renal rickets is common in patients with end stage kidney disease. *The kidney tubules are unable to covert vitamin D into its active form* resulting in a decrease in calcium absorption and an increase in PTH. As the failing kidney is unable to excrete phosphate, the negative ions bind to free calcium in the blood causing *hypocalcemia and secondary hyperparathyroidism*.

13. **What laboratory findings would you expect in patients with metabolic bone disease? (See Table 2.1.)**

14. **How does bone metabolism change with aging?**
    A normal person can expect to lose 0.5% to 1% of total bone mass per year as he or she ages. Bone in elderly patients loses its remodeling potential. There is decreased osteoblastic activity and decreased production of growth factors. While aging affects both cortical and

Table 2.1. Laboratory Findings in Metabolic Bone Disease

DISEASE	CALCIUM	PHOSPHATE	PTH	VITAMIN D3	ALK PHOS
Nutritional rickets	Low to normal	Low to normal	High	Low	High
Familial hypophosphatemic rickets	Normal	Low	Normal	Normal	High
Hereditary vitamin D deficient rickets (I)	Low	Low	High	Low	High
Hereditary vitamin D deficient rickets (II)	Low	Low	High	High	High
Renal osteodystrophy	High	Low	High	Low	High
Primary hypoparathyroidism	Low	High	Low	Low	Normal
Osteoporosis	Normal	Normal	Normal	Normal	Normal
Osteopetrosis	Normal	Normal	Normal	Normal	Normal to high
Paget's disease	Normal	Normal	Normal	Normal	High

trabecular bone, studies have shown that there is a *slightly greater loss of mechanical strength in trabecular bone than cortical bone*. Cortical area will decrease over time with a resultant increase in the medullary space, further decreasing mechanical strength.

15. **What is the pathophysiology of osteoporosis?**
Osteoporosis is a *quantitative* defect of bone metabolism. It results from an uncoupling of osteoblast and osteoclast signaling leading to a marked decrease in bone mass. *Type I* disease affects postmenopausal women whose decrease in estrogen levels result in a decrease in trabecular bone formation. These patients often present with distal radius or vertebral fractures. *Type II* osteoporosis can occur in men or women and more frequently in patients over the age of 75. Patients present with hip and pelvic fractures as cortical and trabecular bone is affected equally. Osteoporotic bone has thin trabeculae and decreased osteon size. Laboratory findings will be normal (Fig. 2.4).

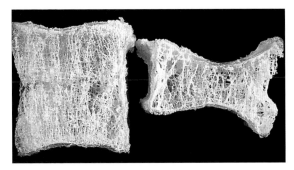

Figure 2.4. Osteoporotic vertebral body (right) shortened by compression fractures compared with a normal vertebral body. Note that the osteoporotic vertebra has a characteristic loss of horizontal trabeculae and thickened vertical trabeculae. (*From Rosenberg AE. Bones, Joints, and Soft-Tissue Tumors. In: Kumar V [ed.], Robbins and Cotran Pathologic Basis of Disease, Professional Edition. Elsevier, 2009.*)

16. **How does this mechanism compare with osteopetrosis, Paget's disease, and other metabolic disease states?**
    Paget's disease and osteopetrosis are *qualitative* defects in bone metabolism. Paget's is a disease of bone remodeling resulting from osteoclastic bone resorption followed by disordered bone formation. Osteopetrosis is characterized by defective osteoclastic bone resorption leading to dense, disorganized bone. Both of these diseases are due to a defect in biological bone cells. In contrast, osteoporotic patients have normal functioning osteoblasts and osteoclasts.

CASE 2-1

A postmenopausal 62-year-old white female presents to her primary care physician for a routine examination. Her past medical history is significant for depression, epilepsy, hypertension, and obesity. She currently takes sertraline, phenytoin, and lisinopril and smokes one pack of cigarettes per day.

17. **What risk factors place this patient at risk for developing osteoporosis?**
    Our patient has several risk factors for osteoporosis including her increasing age, female gender, and smoking history. Family history of hip fracture, heavy alcohol use, steroids, and low body weight (not obesity) also predispose one to developing osteoporosis. The patient is also taking antidepressants and anti-epileptic drugs, which are also risk factors.

18. **What laboratory and imaging studies would you order?**
    The standard for diagnosing osteoporosis is a *DEXA* (dual energy x-ray absorptiometry) scan. The World Health Organization defines the disease by a *T score of < −2.5* in the vertebrae L2–L4, meaning that the patient has the bone density of less than 2.5 standard deviations below the mean bone mass of a 25 year old. Patients with a T score of −1 to −2.5 have *osteopenia*. Radiographs are of little use in the diagnosis of osteoporosis unless severe bone loss is present. Basic chemistry, calcium, phosphorous, parathyroid, and alkaline phosphatase levels should also be ordered to rule out other types of metabolic bone disease.

19. **What is the chance that the patient develops a fracture?**
    A Caucasian, postmenopausal female with osteoporosis has approximately a 75% chance of developing a fracture. Lifetime hip fracture rates range from 15% to 20%.

20. **What therapies are available to treat osteoporosis?**
    All postmenopausal women should be counseled on adequate vitamin D and calcium intake as prophylaxis against osteoporosis. Patients diagnosed with the disease should be started on antiresorptive medication such as a bisphosphonate. The long-term use of bisphosphonates has been recently linked with a risk of insufficiency fractures, and so, the optimal duration of treatment remains an area of active investigation. Hormone replacement therapy is quite effective in reducing fracture risk in elderly women, but is rarely used because of the increased risk of breast cancer, heart attack, and stroke. Patients with severe osteoporosis or those resistant to therapy with bisphosphonates should be treated with recombinant parathyroid hormone therapy. Recombinant parathyroid hormone has an anabolic function, rather than the antiresorptive function of bisphosphonates.

CASE 2-2

A 28-year-old male was brought to the ED after being the unrestrained driver in a motor vehicle accident. He sustained an oblique fracture of his right humeral shaft and a left transverse proximal tibia fracture. His past medical history is significant for asthma and low back pain for which he takes extra strength ibuprofen. He smokes one pack of cigarettes per day and drinks a six-pack of beer daily.

21. **After closed reduction in the emergency department, he is taken to the operating room for intramedullary nailing of his left tibia. In general, what are the different types of fracture healing?**
    After a traumatic injury, bone can undergo either *primary* or *secondary* healing. *Primary fracture healing, or haversarian remodeling, requires rigid stabilization and anatomic reduction.* It is an attempt to reestablish cortical continuity by osteoblasts and osteoclasts remodeling

new bony matrix at the fracture site. There is no callus formation with primary bone healing. *Secondary bone healing is more common and involves both the periosteum and surrounding soft tissues.* Fractures undergoing secondary bone healing can repair themselves via enchondral ossification, intramembranous healing, or both.

22. **What are the steps in which this patient's fracture will heal?**
    Intramedullary nailing provides a semi-rigid construct at the fracture site causing the fracture to undergo both enchondral and intramembranous ossification. In the early stages of fracture healing, a hematoma forms around the patient's tibia fracture site, providing a source for osteoprogenitor cells. Macrophages and platelets infiltrate the site and secrete a variety of inflammatory cytokines to stimulate osteoblast and fibroblast proliferation. A primary callus will form from this hematoma within 2 weeks as chondrocytes secrete type I and II collagen to stabilize the fracture site. The amount of callus is directly proportional to the extent of motion at the fracture site. The fracture site will then remodel in accordance with *Wolff's law*, which states that bone remodels in response to mechanical stress. Hypetrophic chondrocytes undergo apoptosis while coordinated osteoblasts and osteoclasts function to form newly woven bone. Unlike scar tissue, new bone at the fracture site is histologically similar to the bone prior to injury (Fig. 2.5).

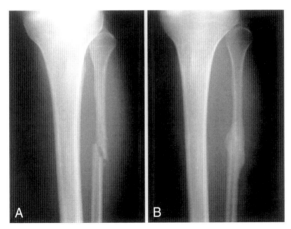

Figure 2.5. (A) Recent fracture of the fibula. (B) Marked callus formation 6 weeks later. (*Courtesy of Dr Barbara Weissman, Brigham and Women's Hospital, Boston, MA. In: Kumar V [ed.], Robbins and Cotran Pathologic Basis of Disease, Professional Edition. Elsevier, 2009.*)

23. **The next day, the patient returns to the operating room for open reduction and internal fixation of his right humerus with a compression plate. How will this patient's humerus fracture heal?**
    Compression plating offers a rigid construct for fracture healing. Due to little, to no, micromotion at the fracture site, a callus will not form and the fracture will instead undergo primary fracture healing. Osteoclasts on one cortical side of the fracture resorb bone and form a tunnel for new haversarian systems to form and allow osteoprogenitor cells to reestablish mechanical continuity with the opposing cortex.

24. **What medical and social factors in this patient will inhibit or delay fracture healing?**
    Smoking has been shown to decrease the rate of both fracture healing and callus strength. Smoking cessation counseling should be provided to all orthopedic trauma patients. Inadequate nutrition and low protein intake will also inhibit fracture healing. While controversial, there is some scientific evidence to suggest that the patient should avoid taking NSAIDs. These drugs inhibit the enzyme COX-2, which promotes fracture healing by stimulating osteoblast differentiation.

CASE 2-2 continued

Nine months later, the patient returns to your clinic still complaining of left leg pain and inability to bear weight. His right humerus fracture has healed. Radiographs of his left tibia demonstrate an atrophic nonunion.

25. **What are the types of nonunion and what are their etiologies?**
    Patients with a *hypertrophic* nonunion have adequate blood supply to the fracture site, but may have too much motion at the fracture site. *Atrophic* nonunion is frequently caused by other factors including insufficient vascular supply to the fracture site or host factors leading to poor healing. *Oligotrophic* nonunions have adequate vasculature and biologic capacity to heal, but callus formation does not occur due to displaced or distracted fracture fragments and inadequate apposition.

    Nonunions can occur for a number of reasons. First, if there is inadequate stability of the fracture site, excessive motion leads to connective tissue deposition rather than fracture healing. Second, host or patient-dependent factors, such as poor nutrition, smoking, low vitamin D levels, hypothyroidism, and hypogonadism, can lead to inadequate healing capability. Third, inadequate vascular supply to the fracture fragments and surrounding soft tissue envelope is necessary for healing. Lastly, infection at the fracture site will prevent bony union.

26. **What are your options for treating a nonunion?**
    Treatment of the nonunion is dependent on the etiology. Hypertrophic nonunions as a result of inadequate stability can be treated with revision surgery with a stiffer construct to reduce the strain and motion at the fracture site. Patients with metabolic or endocrinologic issues should be identified by laboratory values including serum calcium, phosphorus, alkaline phosphatase, 25-hydroxy-vitamin D, and thyroid-stimulating hormone levels. Patients with abnormalities should be referred to an endocrinologist for further workup and treatment. An infection workup should be performed to rule out indolent infection. This includes a blood count with differential, erythrocyte sedimentation rate (ESR), and C-reactive protein (CRP). An aspiration or open biopsy should also be considered. Management of an infected nonunion is often complex but includes debridement and antibiotics. Certain atrophic nonunions can be supplemented with various types of bone graft, including autograft, allograft, demineralized bone matrix (DBM), bone morphogenic protein (BMP), synthetic bone graft, and stem cells.

27. **What are the benefits of autograft? Allograft? Demineralized Bone Matrix Synthetics? Growth factors?**
    Bone grafts may be osteoconductive, osteoinductive, or osteogenic. *Osteogenic* bone graft provides osteoblasts and other osteoprogenitor cells which directly produce bone. Bone marrow aspirate and autograft are osteogenic. *Osteoinductive* graft materials, such as BMP, signal local factors to produce new bone. Demineralized bone matrices are examples of *osteoconductive* bone grafts, which provide a scaffold for new bone to form (Table 2.2).

28. **What are some other novel modalities to enhance bone healing?**
    Electromagnetic stimulation has been shown to aid fracture healing. Bone has a negative bioelectric potential in areas of growth or healing, which slowly progresses to neutral as the fracture site heals. *Bone is bioelectrically negative in areas of compression and positive in areas of tension.* Direct Current Electrical Stimulation (DCES) and Pulsed Electromagnetic Field (PEMF) are two modalities which make use of this physiology. Shock wave therapy is also sometimes used with mixed results. In theory, shock waves create microfractures in hypertrophic nonunions, which stimulate osteoinduction.

CARTILAGE AND MENISCUS

29. **What are the four types of cartilage?**
    Articular or hyaline cartilage is found on joint surfaces and functions to decrease friction and dissipate axial forces. *Fibrocartilage* is found at tendon and ligament insertions to bone and is also formed in response to articular cartilage injury. *Elastic* (trachea) and *fibroelastic* (the meniscus) are the other two types of cartilage.

Table 2.2. Characteristics of Bone Graft

	TYPES	OSTEOGENIC	OSTEO-INDUCTIVE	OSTEO-CONDUCTIVE	DRAWBACKS
Autograft	Cancellous (iliac crest)	Yes	Yes	Yes	Donor site morbidity
	Cortical (fibula)	Yes	Yes	Yes	Donor site morbidity
	Bone marrow aspirate	Yes	Yes	No	Not osteo-conductive
Allograft	Fresh cadaver	No	Yes	Yes	High immuno-genicity
	Fresh frozen	No	Yes	Yes	Some immuno-genicity, most common
	Freeze dried	No	Minimal	Yes	Least immunogenic, only osteo-conductive
	DBM	No	Minimal	Yes	No osteogenic cells
Synthetics	Tricalcium phosphate	No	No	Yes	Only osteo-conductive, slowly degrade
	Calcium sulfate	No	No	Yes	Only osteo-conductive, fast reabsorption
	Silicone based	No	No	Yes	Only osteo-conductive
Growth factors	BMP	No	Yes	No	Expensive

30. What is the composition of articular cartilage?

     Water makes up 65–80% of articular cartilage, and its frictional resistance and pressurization within the extracellular matrix allow the cartilage to sustain high axial loads. *Type II collagen* makes up about half of the dry weight of articular cartilage and helps provide shear and tensile strength. Compressive strength is provided by *proteoglycans*, which comprise 10–15% of articular cartilage. Glycosaminoglycans such as chondroitin sulfate and keratin sulfate bind to collagen and hyaluronic acid to reinforce the extracellular matrix. *Chondrocytes* are the only biologically active cells in articular cartilage and account for only 5% of the dry weight. They are responsible for secreting collagen, proteoglycans, and other proteins in the extracellular matrix.

31. Describe the different layers of articular cartilage.

     Articular cartilage can be divided into four zones according to depth and biochemical content. The *superficial zone* (Zone I) lies adjacent to the joint cavity. Type II collagen fibers are oriented parallel to the joint and form a smooth, gliding surface. Water and collagen content are highest in this zone. The *middle zone* (Zone II) constitutes the majority of cartilage depth and consists of obliquely oriented collagen fibers. Proteoglycan concentration increases with depth. The *deep zone* (Zone III) has the highest proteoglycan content and collagen fibers oriented perpendicular to the joint. The *tidemark* lies just deep to Zone III and separates true articular cartilage from deeper calcified cartilage. This *calcified cartilage* (Zone IV) lies adjacent to subchondral bone and consists of type X collagen, a high concentration of calcium salts, and low concentration of proteoglycans (Fig. 2.6).

32. Why do cartilage injuries have such a poor healing response?

     Cartilage is an avascular structure, as chondrocytes receive their nutrients through simple diffusion. Any superficial cartilage laceration that does not penetrate the tidemark will stimulate chondrocyte proliferation but will not heal. When a laceration through the tidemark penetrates subchondral bone, *fibrocartilaganeous healing* will occur.

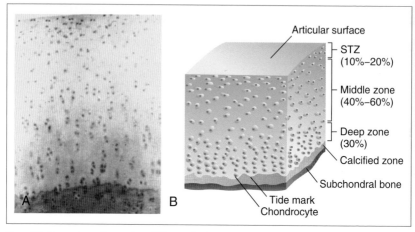

Figure 2.6. Zones of articular cartilage. STZ: superficial tangential zone. *(From Nordin M, Frankel VH. Basic Biomechanics of the Musculoskeletal System, 2nd edn. Philadelphia, Lea & Febiger, 1989, pp. 31–57. Used with permission.)*

CASE 2-3

A 68-year-old female presents with long-standing left knee pain worsening over the past few months. It is worse later in the day and relieved with acetaminophen. She has a history of diabetes and is morbidly obese. You are concerned for osteoarthritis and order radiographs of the left knee.

33. **What are the findings you would expect on her knee x-ray?**
    Typical radiographic findings of osteoarthritis include joint space narrowing, osteophyte formation, subchondral cysts, and subchondral bony sclerosis.

34. **What is the pathoanatomy of osteoarthritis?**
    Osteoarthritis is the most common disorder of the entire musculoskeletal system and is characterized by destruction of articular cartilage. The severity of the disease is directly linked with a *decrease in proteoglycan content* and an *increase in the water composition* of cartilage. Interleukin-1 (IL-1) and other cytokines disrupt cartilage homeostasis by activating proteolytic enzymes, which breakdown proteoglycan links. Although collagen levels are maintained, the extracellular matrix becomes more disorganized.

35. **How does the composition of cartilage change in patients with osteoarthritis? How does it change with normal aging?**
    Osteoarthritic articular cartilage will have an *increase in total water content, elevated levels of IL-1, increased proteolytic enzymes, and increased stiffness.* In contrast to the patient's osteoarthritic left knee, healthy, but aging articular cartilage has a *decrease in water content.* To compensate for a decrease in chondrocytes, the existing cells hypertrophy to maintain collagen and proteoglycan synthesis.

36. **What is the structure and function of synovium?**
    Synovial fluid functions to provide *lubrication and nutrients* to articular cartilage through diffusion. It is comprised of hyaluronic acid, proteinases, prostaglandins, and its key lubricant, *lubricin.* There are no blood cells or clotting factors. The surrounding synovium is vascularized connective tissue without a basement membrane, thus providing a medium for nutrient exchange between the joint and the bloodstream. Type A cells function as phagocytes, while type B cells act as fibroblasts and produce synovial fluid. Type C cells have been described, but have an unknown function and origin.

37. **What is the structure and function of the meniscus?**
    The meniscus is a unique structure that functions to *deepen the tibial surface and act as a secondary stabilizer to the knee.* It is composed mainly of *type I collagen* fibers arranged both

radially and longitudinally. This allows the meniscus to expand under a compressive force to increase the surface area of contact with the knee joint. It is both less permeable and more elastic than articular cartilage.

38. Describe the healing potential for meniscal injuries.

The peripheral 25% of the meniscus derives its blood supply from the medial and lateral inferior genicular arteries. Tears in this region will heal via fibrocartilage scar formation. The central zone, however, receives its nutrients through passive diffusion. Like articular cartilage, tears in this region have no healing ability. Meniscal tears are further discussed in the sports chapter.

INTERVERTEBRAL DISC

39. What is the structure and function of intervertebral discs?

The intervertebral disks provide mechanical stability and allow for physiologic motion of the spine. They also account for about 25% of the spinal column height. The *nucleus pulposus* comprises the center of the disk and is made primarily of water, proteoglycans, and *type II collagen*. Its high water content allows for compressibility and the even distribution of force across the end plates. The *annulus fibrosis* surrounds the nucleus pulposis. The structure's predominant *type I collagen* provides the disk with high tensile strength to prevent vertebral body subluxation, but is flexible enough to allow for spinal motion. There is no direct blood supply to the disk. Since the annulus is not porous enough, all nutrients reach the disk via diffusion through the end plates.

40. How does the composition of the disk change with aging?

As we age, disk cells produce less type II collagen leading to a *decrease in proteoglycan and water content*. The result is a decrease in disk height and ability to withstand both tensile and compressive forces. Aging does not imply pathology, however, as almost 90% of asymptomatic people over the age of 60 have some degree of disk degeneration on MRI.

41. What biomarkers are implicated in disk pathology?

Patients with herniated disks will release measurable amounts of *osteoprotegrin, interleukin-1, RANKL, and PTH*.

TENDON AND LIGAMENTS

42. What is the structure and function of tendons?

Tendons function to produce joint motion by transferring force from muscle to bone. They are made predominantly of water, *type I collagen*, and proteoglycans with fibers oriented in the direction of muscle loading, along lines of stress. Anatomically, tendons are organized in a defined hierarchical structure. Collagen bundles are arranged circumferentially into microfibrils, which combine to form subfibrils, and further organize into fibrils. Fibril units are tightly arranged in parallel to form fascicles, which combine to form the functional tendon unit.

43. How does that differ from the structure and function of ligaments?

Ligaments are composed of dense connective tissue and function to restrict joint motion and to provide joint stability. While ligaments are also comprised of water, *type I collagen*, and proteoglycans, they are shorter and wider than tendons. Ligaments have less collagen and more proteoglycans and water, but also have a highly organized structure. Unlike the tendon, ligaments are poorly vascularized and have only limited microvascularity at their insertion sites.

44. What are some of the mechanisms of tendon and ligament injury?

Some tendons, like the flexor tendons of the hand, are encased in a sheath and are often injured due to direct trauma or laceration. Early range of motion is necessary to prevent adhesions in sheathed tendon injuries. Unsheathed tendons, such as the patellar and Achilles tendons, are covered in paratenon, which provides a rich vascular supply and improved capacity for healing. These tendons usually fail due to tensile overload from trauma or an acute sports injury. Tensile overload is also the most common cause of ligamentous injuries, most often occurring at mid-substance in adults, and at the insertion site in children.

45. Describe the phases of tendon and ligament healing and repair.

Because of their similar structure and composition, tendons and ligaments undergo the same stages of healing and repair. Within minutes after injury, platelets aggregate around the site of the tear and activate the coagulation cascade. A fibrin clot forms to stabilize the torn tendon edges and create hemostasis. Over the next few days, inflammatory cells infiltrate the site of injury as macrophages debride the injured and necrotic tissue. After 1 week post injury, fibroblasts enter the wound site and begin to proliferate. They produce large amounts of type III collagen, which is weaker and more disorganized than the normal type I collagen. Finally, matrix metalloproteinases degrade the type III collagen and replace it with type I collagen, which begins to orient itself along lines of stress. This process can take several months, but even years later, tendons and ligaments often only recover up to two-thirds their original strength.

NERVE AND MUSCLE

46. What is the anatomy of a peripheral nerve?

Each neuron contains a *cell body*, which is the metabolic center of the cell. Neurons give off two types of fibers, *dendrites*, which receive sensory input from other neurons, and an *axon*, which is the primary route of conduction to tissues. Most of the larger nerve axons are myelinated with Schwann cells, which form a fatty insulating sheath to help speed conduction velocity. The *endoneurium* is a fibrous tissue surrounding the axon and is important in peripheral nerve regeneration. Surrounding the endoneurium are fasicles, which are collections of axons. The *perineurium* provides a connective tissue sheath to cover the fasicles and is the primary source of elasticity and tensile strength of the peripheral nerve. Fasicles are grouped further and covered with the *epineurium* to form the functional peripheral nerve unit. Nerve fibers can either be *afferent* (convey information to the central nervous system) or *efferent* (convey information to the periphery) (Fig. 2.7).

47. What is the most common mechanism for peripheral nerve injury?

A *stretching injury* is the most common mechanism of injury. Elongation of just 8% will disrupt blood supply and can cause a reversible conduction block. "Stingers" in football and correction of valgus deformity in knee replacement surgery are two common examples.

48. Describe the classification and prognosis of peripheral nerve injuries?

A *neuropraxia* injury results in an immediate, but reversible conduction block. The myelin sheath around the area of injury is disrupted, but the axon and endoneurium remain intact. Compression, traction, and contusions all cause neuropraxia, and prognosis for healing is quite good. *Axonotmesis* involves complete disruption of both the myelin sheath and the axon from a crushing or severe traction mechanism. The axon distal to the site of injury undergoes Wallerian degeneration as some nerve function will return as the endoneurium remains intact. *Neurotmesis* describes a complete transection of the nerve. As the endoneurium is also disrupted, no nerve function can expect to be recovered.

Like other biologic tissues affected by trauma, peripheral nerve injuries respond initially with an inflammatory response. Due to increased epineural permeability and edema, an increase in endoneural pressure often leads to compressive neuropathies after neuropraxia. If the endoneurium is disrupted, the distal segment will undergo Wallerian degeneration. Phagocytes migrate to the site of injury and degrade the damaged myelin and axon. Existing Schwann cells proliferate and migrate to the proximal and distal ends of the nerve fibers. After approximately 1 month, sprouting axons from the proximal end will grow approximately 1 mm per day.

49. When would operative treatment for nerve injuries be indicated?

The two most important factors in successful outcomes following peripheral nerve injury are *age* and *level of injury*. Young patients, those with more distal nerve injuries, and sharp lacerations (as opposed to crush injuries) tend to fare best. Any gap of more than 2.5 cm needs to be repaired with nerve graft. Delay in nerve repair often results in poor recovery as scar tissue and neuromas form in the first few days following injury. Pressure is the first sensation to return after nerve healing, followed by pain, touch, and two-point discrimination.

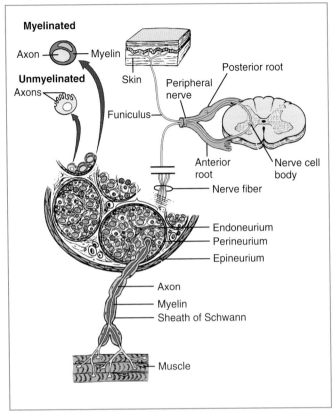

Figure 2.7. Anatomy of a peripheral nerve. (*From Canale ST, Beaty JH [eds]. Campbell's Operative Orthopaedics, 11th edn. Philadelphia, PA, Mosby Elsevier, 2007, p. 3638.*)

50. Describe the gross anatomy of skeletal muscle.
    Like the peripheral nerve, skeletal muscle fibers are highly specialized cells organized within a strict hierarchy. A *string of connected sarcomeres forms the myofibril, which represents the functional unit of contractile muscle*. Myofibrils are concentrically arranged to form a muscle fiber, which is covered in *endomysium*. A collection of muscle fibers is called a fasicle, which is covered in *perimysium*. *Epimysium* covers the group of fasicles which form the functional skeletal muscle.

51. How does muscle contract?
    The sarcomere represents the contractile element of skeletal muscle. It is composed of thick myosin filaments and thin actin filaments. As the nerve cell delivers a signal to the muscle end-plate, acetylcholine is released into the synaptic cleft and triggers depolarization of the muscle cell. Calcium is then released from the sarcoplasmic reticulum into the cytoplasm which binds to troponin on actin filaments. This process leads to a change in configuration of the filaments, exposing actin which cross-bridges to myosin. A molecule of ATP is broken down as the filaments slide past one another causing muscle contraction (Fig. 2.8).

52. What are the two types of skeletal muscle?
    Skeletal muscle is broken down into *slow twitch* (type I) and *fast twitch* (type II) muscle fibers. Slow twitch muscle fibers undergo aerobic metabolism via the Kreb's cycle and yield

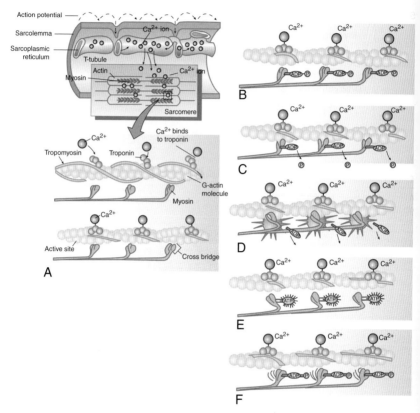

Figure 2.8. Sequence of skeletal muscle contraction: sarcolemma depolarization causes calcium release from the sarcoplasmic reticulum. (A) Calcium binds with troponin and shifts tropomyosin molecules to expose myosin-binding sites on actin. Myosin cross-bridges bind to actin, producing a "power stroke" of contraction. Adenosine triphosphate is needed to break the link and prepare for the next cycle. Cycles (B to F) continue as long as sufficient calcium is present to inhibit the troponin-tropomyosin system from blocking actin-binding sites. (*Redrawn from Seeley RR, Stephens TD, Tate P. Anatomy and Physiology, 3rd edn. St Louis, Mosby, 1995.*)

high energy. Since they require oxygen, slow twitch fibers are used in endurance running, are resistant to fatigue, and have a low strength and speed of contraction. Fast twitch fibers are primarily anaerobic and derive their energy from the ATP-creatinine system. They are used for intense exercise of less than 20 seconds, but fatigue rapidly. Creatine supplements augment this metabolic system, but have the unfortunate side effect of muscle cramping.

53. **Compare the different types of skeletal muscle contraction.**
There are four different types of skeletal muscle contraction. During *isometric contraction*, muscle length remains constant as tension increases, like pushing against an immovable wall. *Isokinetic contraction* describes muscle contracting at constant velocity. Special machines are designed to simulate this. Jumping up and down on boxes is an example of *plyometric contraction*, as muscle rapidly lengthens followed by contraction. Concentric and eccentric loading are both types of *isotonic contraction*, where muscle tension is constant. Biceps curls are an example of concentric loading, as the biceps muscle shortens during contraction. Conversely, the triceps tendon lengthens during contraction with triceps curls and is an example of eccentric loading.

54. **Which would be most likely to cause musculotendinous injury?**
    What differentiates a muscle strain from muscle soreness?
    Eccentric contraction can cause both a strain and muscle soreness, especially in unconditioned patients. The resisting load is greater than force generated by the muscle and can result in a tear (muscle strain) at the relatively weak myotendinous junction. A cellular inflammatory response occurs, causing a decreased ability to generate tension for the first week after injury, before fibroblasts begin healing the tear. Muscles that cross two joints, such as the rectus femoris and gastrocnemius are most at risk for muscle strains.

    Muscle soreness describes the inflammatory response seen 24–72 hours after intense exercise. The inflammation and edema in surrounding connective tissues results in higher intramuscular pressures causing the achy pain felt by patients.

MUSCULOSKELETAL INFECTIONS

CASE 2-4

A 28-year-old male presents to the emergency department with a 2-week history of worsening right knee pain, subjective fever, and chills. He sustained a gunshot wound to his right proximal tibia 8 months ago and was treated surgically with bullet removal and a course of oral antibiotics. He now notes purulent drainage and ulceration of his wound with marked erythema and tenderness.

55. **What is your differential diagnosis for this patient's knee pain?**
    Which radiographic or laboratory tests will you order?
    This patient's symptoms of subjective fever, erythema, and tenderness over a gunshot wound suggest an infectious etiology. Musculoskeletal infections can involve the bone, joints, or the soft tissues. In this patient, we should consider osteomyelitis, septic arthritis, surgical wound infection, and necrotizing fasciitis. After performing a physical exam, a complete blood count (CBC), ESR, and CRP should be checked, along with plain radiographs of the right knee.

CASE 2-4 continued

On exam, he is afebrile with normal vital signs. The patient is comfortable in bed and has a 1 cm wound just inferolateral to his right knee with mild focal tenderness, surrounding erythema and purulent drainage. He is neurovascularly intact, but has severe pain with active range of motion of his knee. Radiographs of the knee are normal: his WBC is 12.5×10^3/mm3, ESR is 78 mm/hr, CRP is 38.8 mg/L.

56. **What can we exclude from the differential diagnosis?**
    In the absence of a high fever or tachycardia, this patient is unlikely to have necrotizing fasciitis. Necrotizing fasciitis is an infection of the soft tissues spreading along the fascial planes and often presents with pain out of proportion to exam, hyperpyrexia, tachycardia, and other signs of sepsis. While other gram-positive and gram-negative bacteria have been implicated, Group A *Streptococcus* is the most common causal agent for necrotizing fasciitis. *Clostridium perfringens* has also been implicated in necrotizing fasciitis and causes gas gangrene. As an anaerobic bacteria it produces gas in the soft tissues apparent on radiographs and crepitus on physical exam. Necrotizing fasciitis is a serious and often fatal condition requiring immediate intravenous antibiotics and surgical debridement with a low threshold for amputation.

CASE 2-4 continued

The patient does have elevated inflammatory markers and a purulent wound. Despite the absence of fever and normal radiographs, we cannot exclude osteomyelitis or septic arthritis. Blood cultures should be taken and he should be admitted for further workup and started on intravenous antibiotics.

57. **Despite therapy with one dose of intravenous cefepime and vancomycin in the emergency department, the patient is still unable to range his knee. How can we confirm or rule out a septic knee?**
    With his subjective fevers, inability to ambulate or tolerate range of motion of his knee, hyperemia, erythema, and elevated inflammatory markers, this patient has a classic story for septic arthritis. The knee is the most commonly affected joint, followed by the hip, elbow, and ankle. Septic arthritis must be recognized and treated early, as proteolytic enzymes from neutrophils will destroy cartilage in as soon as 8 hours. It is an orthopedic surgical emergency

and the joint should be thoroughly irrigated and debrided. Common bacterial causes include *Staphylcoccus aureus*, *Staphylcoccus epidermidis*, and *Streptococcus*. Young, sexually active males are at risk for infection with *Neisserria gonorrhea*. While technetium bone scans and MRI are useful adjuncts in diagnosing septic arthritis, joint aspiration is the gold standard. Fluid should be sent for gram stain and culture, cell count, glucose, and crystal analysis.

58. The gram stain of the patient's synovial fluid is negative, culture is pending. WBC count is $27 \times 10^3/mm^3$ with 30% polymorphonuclear (PMNs) cells, and no crystals were identified. How do we interpret these findings?

    Patients with septic arthritis usually have WBC counts greater than 50 000 with over 50% neutrophils. Synovial glucose levels would be less than 60% of the serum value. While the gram stain can be negative in up to two-thirds of patients with septic arthritis, it is unlikely that a septic knee is causing our patient's symptoms. We will get an MRI of the right knee with and without gadolinium to further evaluate the patient.

59. MRI of the right knee reveals findings consistent with osteomyelitis of the proximal tibia. What would you expect to find on MRI? Why were the original radiographs negative?

    Osteomyelitis is an infection of the bone most commonly associated with a sinus tract from previous surgery, trauma, decreased vascular flow, or a wound (as in our patient). A minority of cases arise from bacteremia, however, in children hematogenous osteomyelitis is by far the most common. Like other musculoskeletal infections, patients will often present with focal pain, fever, and erythema around the site of infection. Inflammatory markers such as ESR and CRP are often elevated. MRI is the imaging modality of choice, approaching 100% sensitivity. Changes on MRI are related to an increase in *edema and water content* within the bone, so we would expect a *decrease in T1 and an increase in T2 marrow signal* in this patient's right proximal tibia. CT and technetium bone scans are useful adjuncts in patients with a contraindication to MRI. Radiographs often take 1–2 weeks to show any change and at least 30% of bone loss must be present to identify osteomyelitis on x-ray.

60. Why does this patient need urgent surgical debridement?

    Intravenous antibiotics alone will not cure the majority of patients with osteomyelitis. As devitalized bone becomes necrotic, it serves as a nidus for continual infection and is known as a sequestrum. This area must be debrided and any orthopedic hardware removed. Involucrum refers to the formation of new bone around the necrotic area. Wound cultures should be taken in the operating room to help tailor antibiotic therapy (Fig. 2.9).

61. Blood cultures from the patient have continued to be negative. Wound cultures have grown back methicillin resistant *Staphylococcus aureus*. What is your treatment plan?

    Blood cultures are negative in about half of all cases of osteomyelitis. Therefore, we must rely on surgical cultures to help dictate appropriate antibiotic therapy. Animal models have shown a 4-week revascularization period of bone, so patients are often given at least 4 weeks of antibiotics postoperatively. Specific antibiotic coverage will be discussed in the pharmacology section, but intravenous vancomycin is the antibiotic of choice for MRSA. Prognosis depends on the patient's medical comorbidities and nutritional status, location of the lesion (metaphyseal infections do better than diaphyseal lesions), and the severity of bone loss.

62. What other organisms are common causes of osteomyelitis? (Table 2.3)

ORTHOPEDIC PHARMACOLOGY

CASE 2-5

A 68-year-old female presents to your office with left lateral thigh pain for 1 month. She has a long history of osteoporosis and has been taking alendronate for over 7 years. The patient also takes lisinopril for hypertension, metformin for diabetes, and ibuprofen for pain. Radiographs reveal lateral cortical thickening in her left subtrochanteric femur region.

63. Which of her medications is the likely causal agent?

    Long-term bisphosphonate use is known to cause subtrochanteric stress reaction and fractures. Members of this drug class, such as alendronate, help to maintain bone mass by

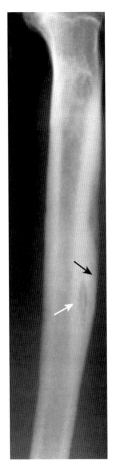

Figure 2.9. Sequestrum in osteomyelitis of the tibia (white arrow pointing to sequestrum and black arrow pointing to involucrum). (*Adapted from Canale ST, Beaty JH [eds]. Campbell's Operative Orthopaedics, 11th edn. Philadelphia, PA, Mosby Elsevier, 2007, p. 702.*)

Table 2.3. Organisms Causing Osteomyelitis

PATIENT GROUP	ORGANISM
Newborns	S. *aureus*, Group A and B *Streptococcus*, *Enterobacter*
Children and adolescents	S. *aureus*, Sc. *pneumoniae*, *Haemophilus influenzae*
Adults	S. *aureus*, occasionally Group A *Streptococcus*
HIV	*Bartonella henselae*
Sickle cell	S. *aureus*, *Salmonella*
Human or animal bites	*Pasturella multocida*, *Eikenella corrodens*
Nosocomial infections	*Pseudomonas aeruginosa*

inhibiting osteoclast resorption. Bisphosphonates are incorporated into the bony matrix and bind to the ruffled border on osteoclasts, stimulating apoptosis. Unfortunately, these drugs also prevent physiologic bone healing and remodeling, as their long-term use can lead to stress fractures of the femur. Osteonecrosis of the jaw is another rare, but concerning side effect from bisphosphonate use.

64. **What are some indications for bisphosphonates?**
Bisphosphonates are some of the best selling drugs on the market and have several indications in addition to osteoporosis. Patients with multiple myeloma or metastatic bone cancer benefit from treatment by a decreased risk of pathologic fractures. Osteoporotic patients with fragility fractures or vertebral compression fractures have fewer skeletal complications with bisphosphonate therapy. Bisphosphonates are also beneficial in patients with Paget's disease and early stage avascular necrosis.

65. **Describe the mechanism of action for ibuprofen?**
Non-steroidal antiinflammatory drugs (NSAIDs) such as ibuprofen *competitively inhibit the enzyme cyclooxygenase (COX)*, which is responsible for converting arachidonic acid into prostaglandins, and thromboxane. There are two isoforms of the enzyme: (1) COX-1 responsible for synthesizing prostaglandins that maintain and protect the gastrointestinal mucosa and (2) COX-2 synthesizes prostaglandins responsible for inflammation and pain. NSAIDs such as ibuprofen and naproxen inhibit *both* isoforms of cyclooxygenase causing decreased inflammation and pain, but with peptic ulcers as an unfortunate side effect. Prostaglandins have also been implicated in altering neurons in the hypothalamus causing an increase in body temperature, thus NSAIDs are an effective antipyretic. Since NSAIDs also block the synthesis of thromboxane, an important platelet aggregator, patients taking these drugs are at higher risk of bleeding. Some studies also suggest that NSAIDs inhibit bone healing and some orthopedists are reluctant to use these drugs in fracture patients.

66. **How does the mechanism of aspirin differ from other NSAIDs?**
Aspirin is a *noncompetitive inhibitor of cyclooxygenase*, and *binds irreversibly* to the enzyme's active site. It has the same effects on blocking prostaglandin synthesis as other NSAIDs. Some orthopedic surgeons take advantage of aspirin's antiplatelet activity and use the drug as prophylaxis against deep venous thrombosis. The half-life is 1 week, so patients should discontinue aspirin 7 days before surgery to prevent increased intraoperative bleeding.

67. **Since the inhibition of COX-1 results in an unfavorable side-effect profile, are there any selective COX-2 inhibitors?**
Celecoxib is the only FDA approved selective COX-2 inhibitor available in the United States. It does not affect platelet function or cause gastric ulcers and only inhibits prostaglandin synthesis responsible for inflammation and pain. Though the mechanism is not well understood, COX-2 inhibitors have a higher incidence of cardiac events. These side effects caused the popular drug rofecoxib to be pulled from the market in 2004.

CASE 2-5   continued

You admit the patient to the hospital for prophylactic fixation of her impending subtrochanteric femur fracture. Her immobility puts her at risk for developing a DVT.

68. **Which drug should this patient receive for DVT prophylaxis?**
Venous thromboembolic events are a major problem in orthopedics, especially with trauma and joint replacement patients. Aspirin is an option in patients at low risk for DVT and pulmonary embolism (PE). While strong data supporting the use of aspirin as an anticoagulant are lacking, the drug has been shown to decrease the frequency of symptomatic DVTs after total hip arthroplasty. Warfarin has long been used for DVT prophylaxis. This drug is a *competitive inhibitor of vitamin K dependent clotting factors (II, VII, IX, X, protein C, protein S)* and is quite effective at reducing the incidence of VTE. Coumadin is often used to treat deep venous thrombosis and pulmonary embolism, but requires frequent coagulation monitoring and has multiple drug interactions. Low-molecular-weight heparin (LMWH) has been shown to be as effective as warfarin and more effective than heparin at reducing DVT in hip replacement patients. LMWH works by

binding and increasing the activity of antithrombin III, which leads to inhibition of factors Xa and IIa. While it shares a similar mechanism of action to unfractionated heparin, LMWH preferentially inhibits factor Xa rather than IIa (Figs 2.10A and B). Inhibition of Factor Xa inhibits conversion of prothrombin to thrombin and prevents fibrin clot formation. LMWH also has a lower incidence of heparin-induced thrombocytopenia (HIT) compared to unfractionated heparin. LMWH is contraindicated in renal failure (Fig. 2.10).

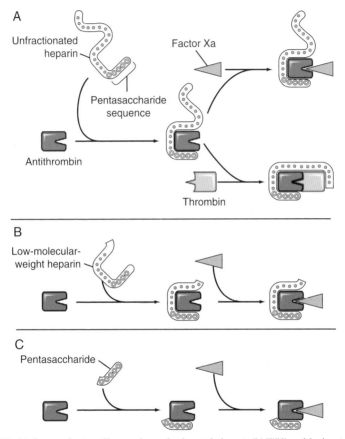

Figure 2.10. Mechanism of action of heparin, low-molecular-weight heparin (LMWH), and fondaparinux, a synthetic pentasaccharide. (A) Heparin binds to antithrombin via its pentasaccharide sequence. This induces a conformational change in the reactive center loop of antithrombin that accelerates its interaction with factor Xa. To potentiate thrombin inhibition, heparin must simultaneously bind to antithrombin and thrombin. Only heparin chains composed of at least 18 saccharide units, which correspond to a molecular weight of 5400 Daltons, are of sufficient length to perform this bridging function. With a mean molecular weight of 15 000 Daltons, all of the heparin chains are long enough to do this. (B) LMWH has greater capacity to potentiate factor Xa inhibition by antithrombin than thrombin because, with a mean molecular weight of 4500 to 5000 Daltons, at least half of the LMWH chains are too short to bridge antithrombin to thrombin. (C) The pentasaccharide only accelerates factor Xa inhibition by antithrombin because the pentasaccharide is too short to bridge antithrombin to thrombin. (*Adapted from Hoffman R [ed.]. Hematology: Basic Principles and Practice. Hematology, 5th edn. Philadelphia, PA, Churchill Livingstone, Elsevier, 2009.*)

69. Just prior to surgery, the patient receives a dose of antibiotics. Which antibiotics are most commonly used in preventing and treating orthopedic infections? (Table 2.4)

Table 2.4. Common Antibiotic Classes Used in Orthopedics

ANTIBIOTIC CLASS	MECHANISM OF ACTION	CLINICAL USES	ADVERSE EFFECTS	DRUGS
Penicillins	Inhibition of cell wall synthesis	Gram-positive bacteria, *Clostridium*. Ampicillin *drug of choice for Escherichia coli*	Hypersensitivity, hemolytic anemia	Penicillin V, penicillin K, amoxicillin, ampicillin
Penicillinase resistant	Inhibition of cell wall synthesis	Broad-spectrum gram-positive and gram-negative coverage	Same as penicillins	Oxacillin, nafcillin
Beta-lactamase inhibitors	Inhibition of beta-lactamase	Broad-spectrum gram-positive and gram-negative coverage, resistant bacteria	Same as penicillins	Amoxicillin–clavulanic acid, piperacillin–tazobactam
Cephalosporins	Inhibition of cell wall synthesis	Broad-spectrum coverage, surgical prophylaxis, UTIs	Small cross-reactivity with penicillin, hemolytic anemia	Cephalexin, cefuroxime, ceftriaxone, cefepime
Glycopeptides	Inhibition of cell wall synthesis and cross linking	Drug of choice for MRSA, resistant gram-positive bacteria, penicillin allergic patients	"Red man" syndrome, nephrotoxic, ototoxic	Vancomycin
Aminoglycosides	Binds to 30S ribosomal subunit, inhibits protein synthesis	Effective against gram-negative bacteria, pseudomonas, prophylaxis with grade III open fractures	Nephrotoxicity, ototoxicity	Gentamycin, tobramycin
Lincosamides	Binds to 50S ribosomal subunit, inhibits protein synthesis	Effective against anaerobes, gram-positive bacteria, some MRSA coverage	*C. difficile* colitis, hypersensitivity	Clindamycin
Fluoroquinolones	Inhibit DNA gyrase	Gram-negative bacteria, newer generations have some anaerobic and gram-positive coverage	Gastrointestinal (GI) symptoms, photosensitivity, tendonopathy, inhibits early fracture healing	Ciprofloxacin, levofloxacin
Sulfonamides	Inhibit folic acid synthesis	Broad aerobic gram-negative coverage, some gram positive and MRSA coverage, UTIs	Hypersensitivity, GI symptoms, myelosuppression, rash	Trimethoprim/ sulfamethoxazole

BASIC BIOMECHANICS AND BIOMATERIALS

70. **What is stress? What is strain?**
    Stress is the applied force (newtons) per unit area (square millimeters) and is measured in
    N/mm², or pascals (1 pascal = 1 N/m²). *Strain* is the increase in length (millimeters) as a
    fraction of the original length (millimeters). By definition, strain is not associated with a
    unit of measurement.

CASE 2-6

See a representative stress–strain curve below (Fig. 2.11).

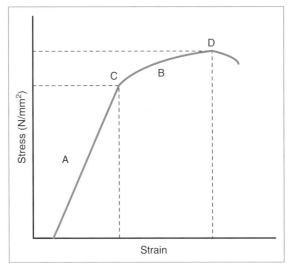

Figure 2.11. (A) Stress–strain curve. Line A is the elastic region, whose slope indicates Young's modulus of
the material. Point C is the yield point between elastic and plastic deformation (line B). Point D is the
ultimate strength of the material. (*Adapted from Golish SR, et al. Principles of Biomechanics and Biomaterials in
Orthopaedic Surgery. JBJS 2011.*)

71. **What does the slope of the stress–strain curve represent? Where is the linear**
    elastic region and the plastic region of the curve? What is the difference
    between yield strength and ultimate strength?
    The slope of a stress–strain curve is the *modulus of elasticity*, also known as *Young's modulus*.
    The greater the slope, the stiffer the material. Increases in stress lead to a proportional
    increase in strain in the *linear elastic region* of the curve, represented by the region A.
    In the linear elastic region, changes in shape of the material are reversible. Once the
    yield strength (C) is reached, the stress and strain increases are not proportional due to
    plastic deformation in the *plastic region* (B). In the plastic region, the material will not return
    to its original shape after the stress is removed. Failure then occurs when the *ultimate strength*
    (D) is reached.

72. **What is the difference between toughness and hardness? Can these be**
    represented in the stress–strain curves?
    Toughness is the amount of energy expended in deforming a material before it reaches its
    failure strength and breaks. This can be represented by the area under the elastic and
    plastic portions of the stress–strain curve. *Hardness* is the amount of energy it takes to
    deform a material. It has no association with the stress–strain curve.

73. **What is the difference between elastic and viscoelastic materials? What do the terms creep, stress relaxation, and hysteresis mean?**

An elastic behavior refers to an instantaneous change in strain when a stress is applied to a material. A viscoelastic behavior has characteristics of both an elastic material and a viscous material (one that resists strain when a stress is applied). It, therefore, has *time-dependent* characteristics, including creep, stress relaxation, and hysteresis. *Creep* refers to an increase in strain when the stress is held constant (the material progressively deforms as a constant force is applied), while *stress relaxation* refers to a decrease in stress when the strain is held constant. *Hysteresis* refers to the loss of energy (represented by the area under the stress–strain curve) with cyclic loading. While all materials exhibit some form of viscoelasticity, certain materials such as metals exhibit less viscoelasticity than biologic materials such as tendon, ligament, and cartilage.

CASE 2-7

A 40-year-old male is involved in a motor vehicle accident and presents to the trauma bay. He is found to have an isolated Schatzker VI tibial plateau fracture. You decide to take him to the operating room the next day for open reduction internal fixation of the tibial plateau fracture. You have the choice between using a titanium plate and a stainless steel plate.

74. **Titanium and stainless steel plates are typically composed of what elements?**

Orthopedic implants are typically made of alloys that are steel (iron-based), titanium-based, or cobalt-based. *316L stainless steel* is an iron-based alloy that also contains chromium, nickel, molybdenum, and carbon, as well as a small amount of manganese, phosphorous, selenium, and silicone. *Ti-6Al-4V* is a titanium-based alloy that also contains aluminum, vanadium, and small amounts of iron, niobium, and zinc. *Cobalt alloy* is another commonly used metal alloy that is primarily cobalt and chromium with smaller amounts of molybdenum, nickel, iron, carbon, manganese, and silicone.

75. **Is the modulus of elasticity of cortical bone closer to titanium or stainless steel? Which metal would lead to less stress shielding of bone?**

The modulus of elasticity of bone is less than titanium, which is less than stainless steel. Graphically, this means the slope of the stress–strain curve of bone is shallow compared to the two metals, and the slope would be lower in titanium than stainless steel. Relative values of modulus of elasticity of various orthopedic implant materials and biologic structures are as follows (from highest modulus of elasticity to lowest):

1. Ceramic
2. Cobalt-chrome
3. Stainless steel
4. Titanium
5. Cortical bone
6. PMMA
7. Polyethylene
8. Cancellous bone
9. Tendon and ligament
10. Cartilage

When the stiffness of the bone and a plate are different, a load, which is applied to the bone, is transferred to the implant. The strain in the bone adjacent to the implant will be reduced, which is termed *stress shielding*. Stress shielding manifests as reduction of bone density (osteopenia) via Wolf's law (previously discussed). Because titanium has a modulus of elasticity that is more similar to bone, less stress shielding of bone will occur with titanium than stainless steel.

76. **You are deciding between plates that are 3.5 mm and 4.5 mm in thickness. How does the bending stiffness relate to the thickness of the plate? How does bending stiffness relate to the diameter of an intramedullary nail?**

The bending stiffness of a plate is proportional to the *thickness of the plate to the third power*. Therefore, the bending stiffness of the 4.5 mm plate will be more than twice the bending stiffness of a 3.5 mm plate ($3.5^3 = 42.875$, $4.5^3 = 91.125$). For a solid intramedullary nail, the bending stiffness is proportional to the *diameter to the fourth power*.

77. **What is fatigue failure, and is fatigue failure greater in the titanium plate or the stainless steel plate?**

Fatigue failure is the resistance of the implant to repeated load. In general, *fatigue strength* is defined by the maximum stress at which the plate can withstand ten million cyclic loading cycles without failing. Titanium generally has slightly greater cycle fatigue resistance compared to stainless steel.

78. **What is corrosion and what are the different types that can occur with plates?**

Corrosion is the degradation of implants that is dictated by the environment in which the material is placed. While there are many forms of corrosion, the primary types related to orthopedic implants include galvanic, crevice, pitting, stress, and fretting corrosion. *Galvanic corrosion* occurs when two different types of metal are used. This leads to an electrochemical potential that leads to weakening of the materials. In particular, cobalt chromium and stainless steel should not be mixed together. *Crevice corrosion* refers to a confined space (crevice) of altered chemical environment between two parts of an implant. This occurs more commonly in passive metals, particularly stainless steel. *Pitting corrosion* is a very similar process that is even more localized to small holes (or pits) in the metal, but can potentially lead to insidious, yet destructive, propagation and catastrophic failure. *Stress corrosion* is weakening of the implant at the area of greatest stress concentration. Cracking of the metal occurs from tensile stresses. *Fretting corrosion* refers to damage that occurs at the contact surfaces of two metals during repetitive surface micromotion, such as a screw–plate interface.

CASE 2-8

A 60-year-old female presents to your office with 10 years of increasing left hip pain. Radiographs reveal severe degenerative changes at the hip joint. She no longer can tolerate the pain and has exhausted conservative measures. You suggest she undergo total hip arthroplasty for pain relief and function.

79. **Preoperatively, you discuss the various bearing surfaces that are available to this patient. What bearing surfaces are commonly used, and what are the advantages and disadvantages of each?**

The most common bearing surfaces include metal on conventional polyethylene and newer alternative bearing surfaces, including highly cross-linked polyethylene, metal-on-metal, and ceramic-on-ceramic. *Metal on polyethylene* has a long track record of success. However, over time, the polyethylene wears and produces particulate debris that can lead to osteolysis. Because of osteolysis (bone resorption by osteoclasts in response to polyethylene wear) the acetabular and femoral components can become loose. This problem has increased interest in the development of alternative bearing surfaces.

Highly cross-linked polyethylene can be produced by using higher doses of radiation during the sterilization process. The process leads to a highly cross-linked polymer that is more resistant to wear and oxidative degradation than conventional polyethylene. The disadvantage of highly cross-linked polyethylene is that other material properties are diminished, including fracture toughness. This can lead to delamination and fracture when a thin polyethylene component is used with large head sizes.

Metal-on-metal is a hard-on-hard bearing surface and, therefore, has excellent wear resistance. This bearing surface gives surgeons the option of larger head sizes to reduce the incidence of dislocation without the risk of mechanical failure. However, there are many disadvantages to this bearing surface. Patients have elevated levels of metal ions in their blood, and some patients will develop reactions to the metal debris, including metallosis, delayed-type hypersensitivity, and pseudotumor formation.

Ceramic-on-ceramic, like metal-on-metal, is a hard-on-hard alternative bearing surface that has excellent wear resistance. Ceramic is harder than metal, and so there is little concern of wear with this bearing surface. The initial ceramic-on-ceramic implants were susceptible to catastrophic failure (fracture of the components), but recent improvements in manufacturing have led to a very low fracture rate. Unlike the metal ion release in metal-on-metal bearing surfaces, ceramic is inert and does not cause systemic reactions. However, *stripe wear* from edge loading of the ceramic ball within the ceramic acetabulum can occur in this bearing surface. Also, ceramic on ceramic has been reported to cause squeaking in some patients, which can be bothersome.

80. **Describe how the forces around the hip change after the operation as described by the Charnley concept of total hip arthroplasty.**

The biomechanical concept of Charnley's original total hip arthroplasty was to medialize the acetabulum and center of the femoral head. This gives a mechanical advantage to the abductor musculature by increasing its moment arm (Fig. 2.12).

The *moment* about a point is the cross product between a *force* and the *moment arm*:

$$M = r \times F$$

where M is the moment and the cross product between *r*, the moment arm, and *F*, the force. As shown in the figure above, the force produced by the abductors is perpendicular to the moment arm, which is the distance between A and B. When the acetabulum is medialized, the moment arm is increased (distance between A1 and B1). With an increase in moment arm (*r*), less abductor force is required to produce the same moment.

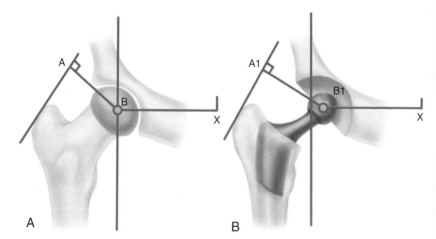

Figure 2.12. A diagram depicting joint reactive forces across the hip joint in a native hip (A) and prosthesis (B). Point B is the center of rotation, point X is the center of gravity, A represents the vector of the pull of the abductors. (*From Canale ST, Beaty JH [eds]. Campbell's Operative Orthopaedics, 12th edn, pp. 158–310.e10. Copyright © Mosby, 2013.*)

81. **During the early postoperative period, the patient uses a cane to assist in her ambulation. Which hand should the cane be held in and why?**

A cane is used to counteract weak hip abductors. The patient should hold the cane in the contralateral hand from the affected leg in order to decrease the joint reactive forces. The moment arm from the affected hip to the contralateral hand is much greater than the moment arm from the affected hip to the ipsilateral hand. Therefore, a greater moment can be generated by using the cane in the contralateral hand.

BIOSTATISTICS

CASE 2-9

You are planning to do a study on patients with tiba fractures to see if time to union was affected by three different types of implants. You hypothesize that there is no difference between the implants in terms of time to union. A chart review is done for 15 patients in each group, and plain films taken at set intervals are reviewed for bony union.

82. **What is the difference between independent and dependent variables? Which would be the independent variable and which would be the dependent variable in this case?**

Independent variables (i.e., the variable that you have control over) are variables that are thought to determine the value of dependent variables. *Dependent variables* are variables that are thought to be affected by independent variables. In this case, the type of implant would be the independent variable (the factor that you control), and the dependent variable would be the time to union.

83. **What are confounders? Give examples of potential confounders in this case.**
Confounders are variables that are related to and affect the relationship between the independent and dependent variables. Potential confounders in this proposed study include age, smoking, diabetes, and fracture severity.

84. **Is time to union a continuous, ordinal, or categorical type of data? What about type of implant?**
Time to union is categorized under continuous data, while type of implant is classified as categorical data. *Continuous data*, also referred to as nominal data, contain values that are ordered sequentially, and the differences between values are meaningful. Other examples include age, range of motion, or temperature. *Ordinal data* can be grouped together and put in order, but the interval between groups may be uneven. Examples are pain scales or the severity of a disease (mild, moderate, severe). *Categorical data* can be grouped, but not ordered sequentially or differentiated by mathematical methods. Examples include gender, hand-dominance, or ethnicity.

85. **What is the difference between parametric and non-parametric data? Would time to union in this case be parametric or non-parametric?**
Parametric data assume that the sample in question has a standard, or normal, distribution, meaning that the majority of data points center around the mean, or average, of the population, with few points at one extreme or the other (Fig. 2.13). *Non-parametric data* do not follow a normal distribution. With the small number of patients in each group, the time to union data are likely non-parametric. However, deciding whether data are parametric and non-parametric can be complex and may require further formal statistics (Kolmogorov–Smirnov test) in order to determine whether those data follow a normal distribution.

Gaussian distribution ("bell-shaped" curve)

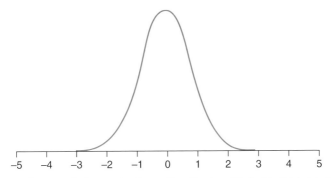
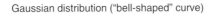

Figure 2.13. An illustration of a Gaussian distribution. (*From Rosenbaum SH. Statistical Methods in Anesthesia. In: Miller RD et al. [eds] Miller's Anesthesia, 7th edn. Philadelphia, Copyright © Churchill Livingstone/Elsevier, 2010.*)

86. **With a normal distribution, how much of the population is within one standard deviation of the mean? What about two or three standard deviations?**
Approximately 69% of the sample falls within one standard deviation of the mean, while 95% falls within two standard deviations and 99% within three standard deviations.

87. **What statistical test would you use to determine if the time to union (three groups with continuous data) was different between the three different implants? What about if the data were ordinal or categorical?**
In this case, *a Kruskal–Wallis test* would be most appropriate for non-parametric data with three or more groups. The type of statistical test is dependent on the number of groups and

type of data. If the data are continuous, it must be decided whether the data are parametric or not (Table 2.5). In this case, if the data were parametric, an ANOVA (*analysis of variance*) test would be used; if the data were categorical, a *Pearson chi-square test* would be most appropriate. For comparing only two groups; a *Student t test* would be used to compare parametric continuous data, while a *Mann–Whitney U test* would be used for ordinal data or non-parametric continuous data. Two groups of categorical data could be tested using a *Fisher exact test*. For paired samples, the most appropriate tests are different.

Table 2.5. Statistical Tests for Comparing Groups

		INDEPENDENT GROUPS	PAIRED SAMPLES
Continuous			
Normal	Two	Student t test	Paired t test
Non-normal	Two	Mann–Whitney U test	Wilcoxon signed-rank test
Normal	Three or more	Analysis of variance	Repeated-measures analysis of variance
Non-normal	Three or more	Kruskal–Wallis test	Friedman test
Ordinal	Two	Mann–Whitney U test	Wilcoxon signed-rank test
	Three or more	Kruskal–Wallis test	Friedman test
Categorical	Two	Fisher exact test	McNemar test
	Three or more	Pearson chi-square test	Cochran Q test

Adapted from Kocher and Zurakowski, JBJS 2004.

88. **After statistical testing, you find a *P*-value of 0.16 between implant type and time to union. What does a *P*-value of 0.16 mean?**
Our null hypothesis (the hypothesis that we can prove to be false) is that there is no difference in time to union with different implants. A *P*-value of 0.16 means that there is a 16% probability that a difference equal to or larger than the one found in our group will be observed. Typically, a *P*-value (or alpha) of 0.05 is accepted as statistically significant. With a *P*-value of 0.16, we cannot reject our null hypothesis. This means we cannot prove that there is a difference in time to union with different implants.

89. **What are type I and type II errors? What are alpha and beta? What is power?**
Alpha is the probability of a *type I error*, which is the error that occurs when the study shows a difference when there is no true difference. *Beta* is the probability of a *type II error*, which is the error that occurs when the study shows no difference when there is a true difference. *Power* is 1–beta and represents the probability of the study showing no association when there truly is no association.

90. **What is the level of evidence of this study?**
This is a retrospective comparative study and therefore it is a Level III study. The levels of evidence are shown in Table 2.6. A stronger study would be a prospective study following a specific population with a specific exposure or treatment over time (Level II). The gold standard study would be a randomized double-blind, placebo-controlled trial.

91. **In this study, what types of bias may possibly result in incorrect study conclusions?**
A non-random systematic error of design or execution results in bias. In this study, since the data collector was not blinded to the groups, *measurement bias* during the reading of plain films may result in favorable outcomes for a group using one implant over another. *Selection bias* describes situations in which two groups are different in ways other than the variable of interest. Any conclusion from a retrospective study such as this one should be evaluated for potential confounding variables, and results should be statistically adjusted for these confounders.

Table 2.6. Levels of Evidence for Primary Research Question

	TYPES OF STUDIES			
	Therapeutic Studies – Investigating the Results of Treatment	Prognostic Studies – Investigating the Effect of a Patient Characteristic on the Outcome of Disease	Diagnostic Studies – Investigating a Diagnostic Test	Economic and Decision Analyses – Developing an Economic or Decision Model
Level I	• High-quality randomized controlled trial with statistically significant difference but narrow confidence intervals • Systematic review of Level-I randomized controlled trials (and study results were homogenous)	• High-quality prospective study (all patients were enrolled at the same point in their disease with ≥80% follow-up of enrolled patients) • Systematic review of Level-I studies	• Testing of previously developed diagnostic criteria in series of consecutive patients (with universally applied reference "gold" standard) • Systematic review of Level-I studies	• Sensible costs and alternatives; values obtained from many studies; multiway sensitivity analyses • Systematic review of Level-I studies
Level II	• Lesser-quality randomized controlled trial (e.g., <80% follow-up, no blinding, or improper randomization) • Prospective comparative study • Systematic review of Level-II studies or Level-I studies with inconsistent results	• Retrospective study • Untreated controls from a randomized controlled trial • Lesser-quality prospective study (e.g., patients enrolled at different points in their disease of <80% follow-up) • Systematic review of Level-II studies	• Development of diagnostic criteria on basis of consecutive patients (with universally applied reference "gold" standard) • Systematic review of Level-III studies	• Sensible costs and alternatives; values obtained from limited studies; multiway sensitivity analyses • Systematic review of Level-II studies
Level III	• Case-control study • Retrospective comparative study • Systematic review of Level-III studies	• Case-control study	• Study of nonconsecutive patients (without consistently applied reference "gold" standard) • Systematic review of Level-III studies	• Analyses based on limited alternatives and costs; poor estimates • Systematic review of Level-III studies
Level IV	Case series	Case series	• Case-control study • Poor reference standard	• No sensitivity analyses
Level V	Expert opinion	Expert opinion	Expert opinion	Expert opinion

Adapted from Wright JG, Swiontkowski MF, Heckman JD. Introducing levels of evidence to the journal. J Bone Joint Surg Am. 2003 Jan;85-A(1):1–3.

CASE 2-10

For your next study, you decide to look specifically at tibia fracture nonunions. In your chart review, you find that over the past 10 years, 100 patients had a tibia fracture surgically treated and subsequently developed a nonunion. In the work-up for nonunion, a CRP was drawn for every patient to rule out infection as a cause. Infection was deemed to be the reason for the nonunion in 20 patients. In these 20 patients, the CRP was elevated in 19 patients and was not elevated in 1 patient. In the remaining 80 patients without nonunion, the CRP was elevated in 20 patients and was not elevated in 60 patients.

92. Construct a 2x2 table and label the true positives, false positives, true negatives, and false negatives (see Table 2.7).

Table 2.7. Two by Two Table

	(+) NON-UNION	(−) NON-UNION
CRP positive	19	20
CRP negative	1	60

93. What are sensitivity and specificity? What is the sensitivity and specificity of CRP as a marker for infectious nonunion in this case?
    By definition, *sensitivity* is the number of true positives divided by the true positives and false negatives. Sensitivity, in this case, is the ability of the CRP test to detect an infectious nonunion when there is one. In this case, the sensitivity would be 19/20 or 95%.
    Specificity is the number of true negatives divided by the true negatives and false positives. Specificity, in this case, is the ability of the CRP test to not falsely label a nonunion as infectious when it is really not due to an infection. In this case, the specificity would be 60/80 or 75%.

94. What are the positive predictive value and the negative predictive value?
    The *positive predictive value* (PPV) is the probability of a patient having a nonunion when the patient has a positive CRP. The PPV in this case is 19/(19+20), which is 48.7%.
    The *negative predictive value* (NPV) is the probability of a patient not having a nonunion when the patient has a negative CRP. The NPV in this case is 60/(60+1), which is 98.4%.

95. In this case, the sensitivity of the CRP was 95% and the specificity was 75%. Would a diagnostic test with this sensitivity and specificity be better for ruling in or ruling out a disease?
    A test with a high sensitivity will be useful in ruling out a disease. When a sensitive test is negative, it is very likely that the patient does not have the disease. On the other hand, if a highly specific test is positive, it is very likely the patient does have the disease. An easy way to remember this is SNOUT (SeNsitivity rule OUT) and SPIN (Specificity rule IN).

BIBLIOGRAPHY

1. Bauer TW, Muschler GF. Bone graft materials: An overview of the basic science. Clin Orthop Relat Res 2000;371:10–27.
2. Canale ST, Beaty JH, editors. Campbell's Operative Orthopaedics. 11th ed. Philadelphia, PA: Mosby Elsevier; 2007.
3. Einhorn TA, O'Keefe RJ, Buckwalter JA, editors. Orthopaedic Basic Science: Foundations of Clinical Practice. 3rd ed. Rosemont, IL: American Academy of Orthopaedic Surgeons; 2007.
4. Fischgrund JS, editor. Orthopaedic Knowledge Update 9. Rosemont, IL: American Academy of Orthopaedic Surgeons; 2008.
5. Kocher MS, Zurakowski D. Clinical epidemiology and biostatistics: A primer for orthopaedic surgeons. JBJS 2004;86:607–20.
6. Koh JS, Goh SK, Png MA, et al. Femoral cortical stress lesions in long-term bisphosphonate therapy: a herald of impending fracture? J Orthop Trauma 2010;24(2):75–81.
7. Lee SK, Wolfe SW. Peripheral nerve injury and repair. J Am Acad Orthop Surg 2000;8:243–52.
8. Lieberman JR, editor. AAOS Comprehensive Orthopaedic Review. Rosemont, IL: American Academy of Orthopaedic Surgeons; 2009.
9. Miller MD, editor. Review of Orthopaedics. 5th ed. Philadelphia, PA: Saunders; 2008.
10. Ulrich-Vinther M, Maloney MD, Schwarz EM, et al. Articular cartilage biology. J Am Acad Orthop Surg 2003;11:421–30.

GREAT TOE DISORDERS

CASE 3-1

A 52-year-old woman presents complaining a painful "big toe" that makes it unbearable to wear high-heeled shoes. She has noticed that her big toe seems to be pointed more outward in the past few years and she has a noticeable bump on the inside part of her toe. She also states that she remembers her mother suffering from similar problems.

1. **What is hallux valgus?**
   Hallux valgus is lateral deviation of the first proximal phalanx on the first metatarsal. Often, this deformity is associated with a medial deviation of the first metatarsal. The common name for this deformity is "bunion" (Fig. 3.1).

2. **What causes hallux valgus?**
   The most common cause of hallux valgus is narrow-toed, high-heeled footwear (one reason that the condition is much more common in females). Hereditary factors are also implicated in the deformity, as up to 70% of patients have a positive family history of the condition. Other causes include pes planus (flat feet), metatarsus primus (rotation and angulation of the first metatarsal away from the second metatarsal), and conditions such as rheumatoid arthritis, cerebral palsy, and ligamentous laxity.

3. **What are the anatomical deformities that occur with hallux valgus?**
   There are multiple changes in the bony and soft tissue anatomy as hallux valgus progresses: (1) the proximal phalanx deviates laterally; (2) the first metatarsal deviates medially; (3) the sesamoid complex moves laterally in relation to the metatarsal head; and (4) the medial capsule becomes attenuated while the lateral capsule contracts.

4. **How do the vector forces of tendons acting on the hallux change in regards to the deformity seen with hallux valgus?**
   Multiple changes in vector forces occur with the hallux valgus deformity. The abductor hallucis becomes slightly more plantar along the medial aspect of the first metatarsophalangeal (MTP) joint. This leaves the adductor tendon unopposed as an increasing deforming force laterally with its attachment to the proximal phalanx and the lateral sesamoid. Lastly, the flexor hallucis brevis, flexor hallucis longus, and extensor hallucis longus all increase their valgus moment on the MTP joint and further deviate the first ray.

5. **What are the radiographic measurements used to measure the severity of hallux valgus?** (See Table 3.1.)

6. **What are the non-surgical options available for the treatment of hallux valgus?**
   Many patients can be treated successfully with non-surgical treatment. The most successful option is footwear modification with a wide toed shoe with a low heel to take pressure and stress off the first MTP joint. Padding and orthoses are also options to relieve any discomfort, such as wearing a spacer in the first web space.

7. **What are the surgical options?** (See Fig. 3.2.)

CASE 3-2

A 53-year-old laborer comes in complaining of joint pain and swelling in his great toe. He has noted that when he squats or crawls in tight spaces at work, the pain in his great toe is excruciating. He denies having any rheumatologic disorders or recent injuries to the toe.

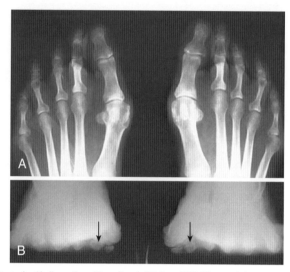

Figure 3.1. Radiograph of hallux valgus. *(From Canale ST, Beaty JH [eds], Campbell's Operative Orthopaedics, 12th edn, pp. 3805–6.e5. Copyright © Mosby, 2013.)*

Table 3.1. Hallux Valgus Angles and Normal Values		
ANGLE	**LOCATION**	**NORMAL**
HVA	Between long axes of 1st proximal phalanx and 1st metatarsal	<15°
IMA	Between long axes of 1st and 2nd metatarsal	<9°
DMAA	Between line bisecting MT shaft and through base of cartilage cap	<15°
PPAA	Articular angle at base of proximal phalanx in relation to longitudinal axis	<10°

HVA: Hallux valgus angle; IMA: intermetatarsal angle; DMAA: distal metatarsal articular angle; PPAA: proximal phalangeal articular angle.

8. **What is hallux rigidus?**
   Hallux rigidus is a degenerative arthritic disease of the first MTP joint. It leads to significant limitation in the range of motion of the first MTP joint. Like other degenerative arthritic processes, the formation of osteophytes is quite common. These osteophytes can lead to a mechanical hindering of MTP dorsiflexion (Fig. 3.3).

9. **What is the common etiology of hallux rigidus?**
   No primary etiology of hallux rigidus has been defined. However, it is believed that repetitive microtrauma or an acute traumatic event can be the cause. This is similar to the etiology of degenerative disease seen in other joints.

10. **What are the most common symptoms of hallux rigidus?**
    Patients typically present with joint pain, swelling, and limited dorsiflexion of the first MTP joint. Some patients can even note shoe wear irritation on the dorsum of the MTP joint from the formation of dorsal osteophytes.

11. **What surgical options are available for hallux rigidus?**
    There are various surgical options available for the treatment of hallux rigidus (Table 3.2).

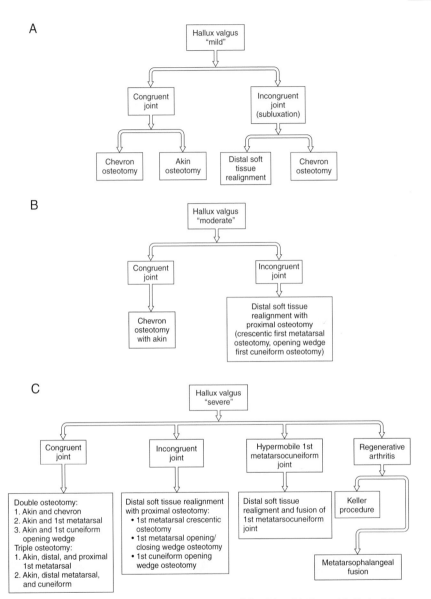

Figure 3.2. Algorithm for treatment of hallux valgus. (*From Haskell A, Mann RA. Foot and Ankle. In: DeLee JC et al., [eds], DeLee and Drez's Orthopaedic Sports Medicine, 3rd edn. Copyright © Saunders, Elsevier Inc., 2010.*)

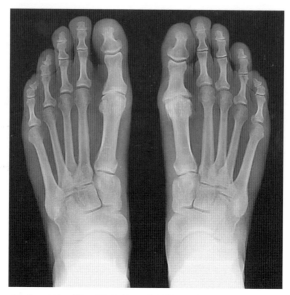

Figure 3.3. Bilateral hallux rigidus. (*From Wexler D, et al. Hallux Rigidus. In: Frontera WR, et al. [eds]. Essentials of Physical Medicine and Rehabilitation, 2nd edn. Copyright © 2008, Saunders, Elsevier Inc.*)

Table 3.2. Treatment of Hallux Rigidus Based on Disease Severity	
DISEASE SEVERITY	**INTERVENTION**
i. Mild	Joint debridement and synovectomy
ii. Moderate	Chielectomy
iii. Moderate	Dorsal closing wedge osteotomy
iv. Moderate	Resection arthroplasty
v. Severe	Arthrodesis

CASE 3-3

A 19-year-old college running back is tackled during a practice scrimmage. At the time of being tackled, one of the defensive linemen falls on the posterior aspect of the player's left leg while his foot is plantarflexed. He notes immediate pain on the plantar aspect of his left foot while attempting to run.

12. **What is turf toe?**
   Turf toe is a term used to describe injury to the capsule surrounding the first MTP joint. Most commonly the injury is caused by a hyperextended MTP joint with an axial load applied to the plantar flexed foot.

13. **What radiographic findings are possible in a turf toe injury?**
   Often, there are no radiographic findings for turf toe injuries. However, in a severe injury in which there is complete rupture of the plantar plate of the joint capsule, proximal migration of the sesamoids can be appreciated on the AP radiographic view.

14. **What are the treatment options for turf toe?**
   Most turf toe injuries are treated with rest and analgesia. A hard-soled shoe may be needed to prevent constant extension of the MTP joint during push-off with walking. Surgical treatment is rarely indicated. When radiographic findings as described above are

noted, surgery is deemed necessary. Surgery involves restoration of the plantar plate and flexor tendons.

LESSER TOE DISORDERS

CASE 3-4

A 42-year-old executive comes into your clinic with complaints of a "bump" on her small toe that has become quite painful when she is wearing high-heeled shoes. She always noted that her small toe "angled in", but lately she has noted a painful callous form over the bump. She had been treated in the past by a podiatrist who recommended wider shoes and pads.

15. What is a bunionette?

    A bunionette (or "tailor's bunion") is a prominence of the lateral aspect of the fifth metatarsal head. It is often associated with a varus MTP joint and with pes planus.

16. How are bunionettes classified? What type of imaging is necessary for classification?

    Bunionettes are classified on weight-bearing AP plain radiographs of the foot. There are three categories in the radiographic classification:
    1. Enlarged 5th MT head
    2. Congenital lateral bowing of the 5th MT
    3. Increased intermetatarsal angle between 4th and 5th MT (>8°) (Fig. 3.4).

CASE 3-4   continued

The patient is found on x-ray to have a Type I bunionette.

17. Why does radiographic classification of a bunionette matter?

    The radiographic classification of a bunionette can help determine the surgical option necessary to correct the deformity.

18. What is the best surgical option for this patient?

    The best surgical option for a Type I bunionette is a lateral condylectomy, which involves excision of the lateral bony prominence and reefing of the lateral MTP joint capsule (Fig. 3.5).

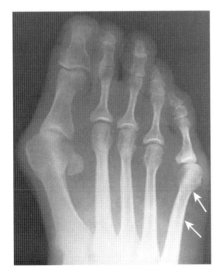

Figure 3.4. Bunionette deformity. (*From Canale ST, Beaty JH [eds]. Campbell's Operative Orthopaedics, 12th edn, pp. 3979–4026. Copyright © Mosby, 2013.*)

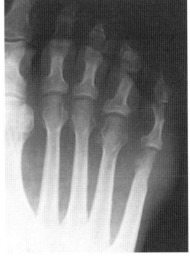

Figure 3.5. Bunionette after surgery. (*From Haskell A, Mann RA. Foot and Ankle. In: DeLee JC et al., [eds], DeLee and Drez's Orthopaedic Sports Medicine, 3rd edn. Copyright © Saunders, Elsevier Inc., 2010.*)

19. **What are the surgical options available for Type II and Type III bunionettes?**
    Type II: Distal chevron osteotomy with resection of the lateral prominence
    Type III: Oblique mid-diaphyseal metatarsal rotational osteotomy.

CASE 3-5

A worried mother brings in her 6-year-old son because she has noticed that his little toes seem to come over top of the adjacent toe. She is concerned because she remembers a cousin who had an issue with her toes that caused her to develop callouses on the top of her toes and to have pain with wearing certain shoes. The son denies any problems with wearing shoes.

20. **What is congenital overlapping fifth toe? When is it operative and what options are there?**
    Congenital overlapping fifth toe is a common familial trait in which the small toe is dorsiflexed and rests on top of the fourth toe. In severe cases, the capsule and extensor tendon on the dorsal aspect of the fifth MCP joint are shortened and prevent passive correction of the deformity. Stretching of mild deformities is often enough to correct the problem. Only symptomatic cases require surgery in the form of realignment or even amputation.

CASE 3-5 continued

You assure the mother that there is nothing to be concerned of at this time. Unless her son begins to develop painful shoe-wear that is unable to be treated with conservative treatment, surgery is not indicated. The patient goes on to ask what toe disorder her cousin likely suffered from.

21. **What is the most common deformity seen in the lesser toes?**
    Hammer toe deformity.

22. **What is a hammer toe deformity?**
    A hammer toe occurs when there is a flexion deformity at the PIP and an extension deformity at the MTP and distal interphalangeal (DIP) joints.

23. **What is the difference between a hammer toe, mallet toe, and claw toe?**
    The difference between the lesser toe deformities depends on the flexion or extension seen at the MTP, proximal interphalangeal (PIP), and DIP joints. (See Table 3.3.)

Table 3.3. Individual Joint Position with Toe Deformity

JOINT DEFORMITY	MTP JOINT	PIP JOINT	DIP JOINT
Mallet Toe	Neutral	Neutral	Hyperflexion
Hammer Toe	Extension	Flexion	Extension
Claw Toe	Extension	Hyperflexion	Hyperflexion

24. **What is the preferred treatment for the lesser toe deformities?**
    In all cases of lesser toe deformities, the preferred initial treatment is aimed at modifying patient shoe-wear. High-toed shoes with adequate space and plantar pads or toe sleeves are also implemented.

HEEL PAIN

CASE 3-6

A 50-year-old woman comes into the clinic complaining of worsening heel pain. She is a poor historian and states that she does not recall when the symptoms started. When asked where the heel hurts, she repeatedly just grabs the entire heel.

25. What are the etiologies of heel pain?
    There are many causes of heel pain:

Plantar fasciitis	Calcaneal stress fracture	Gout
Plantar fascia rupture	Fat pad atrophy	Sever's disease
Infection	Contusion	Neuropathy
Tarsal tunnel syndrome	1st branch lateral plantar nerve entrapment	

26. What is the first step in diagnosing the cause of heel pain?
    Physical examination is the first and often the most useful step in diagnosing the cause of heel pain.

CASE 3-6   continued

After examining the patient and finding her maximal point of tenderness at the anteromedial aspect of the heel pad, she confesses that her pain seems worse in the very beginning of the morning when she first gets out of bed (Fig. 3.6).

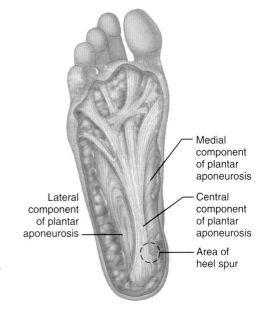

Medial component of plantar aponeurosis

Lateral component of plantar aponeurosis

Central component of plantar aponeurosis

Area of heel spur

Figure 3.6. Painful heel. (*From Canale ST, Beaty JH [eds]. Campbell's Operative Orthopaedics, 12th edn, pp. 3907–78.e7. Copyright © Mosby, 2013.*)

27. What causes plantar fasciitis?
    Plantar fasciitis is a degenerative process that involves microtears in the plantar fascia from repetitive trauma. Half of patients suffering from plantar fasciitis have a plantar heel spur that is not considered to be the generator of the pain.

28. How does pain in plantar fasciitis present?
    Patients with planta fasciitis will typically complain of pain in the morning when they first get out of bed and start walking. As they continue to ambulate throughout their day, patients will note a "relaxation" of the pain. However, vigorous physical activity (especially on hard surfaces) can lead to pain exacerbation. The point of maximum tenderness is located at the proximal medial origin of the plantar fascia at the anterior aspect of the heel pad.

CASE 3-6   continued

The patient asks about receiving an "injection" to make the pain go away. She has had injections in the past for knee pain.

29. What is the risk when giving the patient a corticosteroid injection?
The risk of corticosteroid injections include plantar fascia rupture and fat pad atrophy. Both can lead to more pain and further complications.

30. What is the best treatment for plantar fasciitis?
Plantar fasciitis is best treated in a step-wise fashion starting with a conservative approach. First, patients can be treated with night splinting, stretching exercises, and shoe inserts. Most patients will have their symptoms resolve with these modalities. Second, patients are given ultrasound shockwave treatment. This can be painful and takes months of treatment until results are noted. Lastly, if all other treatments fail, a surgical release of the plantar fascia can be performed.

31. What nerve can often be entrapped and associated with plantar fasciitis?
The first branch of the lateral plantar nerve (mixed sensory and motor) can often be entrapped in patients with plantar fasciitis. The nerve passes deep to the deep fascia of the abductor hallucis (they will complain of pain at this muscle's origin). This nerve is responsible for innervation of the flexor digitorum brevis and abductor digiti minimi.

CASE 3-7

Last week, you saw a patient with a similar complaint of heel pain. That patient was a 72-year-old female who had been treated with corticosteroid injections for her plantar fasciitis years ago. She did not have the complaint of "start up" pain.

32. What is central heel pain?
Central heel pain is caused by a mild-to-moderate amount of traumatic periostitis associated with an atrophied heel pad. The condition is often seen in older patients. Causes of fat pad atrophy can be age, inflammatory disease, or prior corticosteroid injection (i.e., reason to avoid injections of plantar fasciitis).

33. What difference in presentation is there from a patient suffering from plantar fasciitis?
Patients with central heel pain will note that their symptoms do not improve with initial ambulation. Additionally, dorsiflexion of the toes will not aggravate the symptoms like it does in stretching an inflamed plantar fascia. Lastly, the localization of the pain will be more central and diffuse than seen in the patient with plantar fasciitis.

ANKLE ARTHROSCOPY

CASE 3-8

A 33-year-old professional ballet dancer comes to your clinic with complaints of right anterior ankle pain, swelling, and decreased range of motion. She notes the pain is exacerbated when she is in positions that require dorsiflexion of the ankle. She states that she has noted the symptoms over the past year, but they are getting progressively worse to the point that she cannot perform. She is concerned about an ankle sprain.

34. What is tibiotalar impingement?
Tibiotalar or anterior bony impingement is a degenerative process that involves the anterior distal tibia where it articulates with the superior aspect of the talus. Patients typically present with complaints of pain in the anterior aspect of the ankle that is exacerbated when the foot is maximally dorsiflexed (Fig. 3.7).

35. How is tibiotalar impingement classified radiographically?
Tibiotalar impingement is classified according to the radiographic findings of anterior ankle osteophytes in regards to their size and presence of arthritis. It is best appreciated on a weight-bearing lateral radiograph:
Grade I: Synovial impingement, up to 3 mm tibial spur
Grade II: Tibial spur >3 mm
Grade III: Significant tibial exostosis, with or without fragmentation; secondary spur formation on talus
Grade IV: Talocrural arthritic changes (Fig. 3.8).
A Grade IV change is not considered suitable for arthroscopic repair.

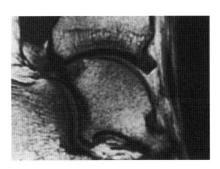

Figure 3.7. Anterior impingement syndrome of the talus. (*From Richardson DR. Ankle injuries. In: Canale ST, Beaty JH [eds], Campbell's Operative Orthopaedics, 11th edn. Philadelphia, Elsevier, 2008.*)

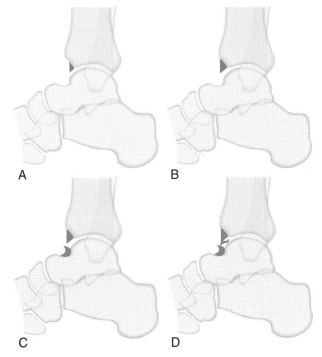

Figure 3.8. Classification of anterior impingement syndrome. (*Redrawn from Ferkel RD, Scranton PE. Current concepts review: Arthroscopy of the ankle and foot. J Bone Joint Surg Am 1993;75:1233–42.*)

A   B

C   D

CASE 3-8 continued

You get a lateral weight-bearing x-ray of the patient's right ankle and note a Grade II anterior ankle osteophyte. You explain to the patient that an arthroscopic surgical procedure could rid her of her pain.

36. What are the surgical indications for ankle arthroscopy?
    Ankle arthroscopy is a surgical option for the treatment of anterior tibiotalar impingement, osteochondral lesions of the talus, post-traumatic synovitis debridement, and cartilage debridement in the setting of arthrodesis.

37. Where are the portal placements for ankle arthroscopy? What structures are at risk when placing these portals? (See Fig. 3.9.)
    There are three essential portals used in ankle arthroscopy:
    1. Anteromedial portal: This portal is placed medial to the tibialis anterior tendon and slightly proximal to the medial malleolus tip. The structures at greatest risk with this

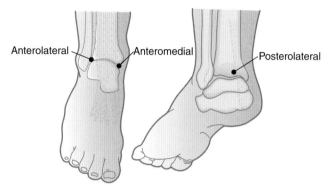

Figure 3.9. Ankle arthroscopy portals. *(From Miller MD, Osborne JR, Warner JJP, Fu FH [eds]. MRI-Arthroscopy Correlative Atlas. Philadelphia, WB Saunders, 1997, p. 134.)*

portal are the greatest saphenous nerve and saphenous vein, which are located medial to the portal site.

2. Anterolateral portal: This portal is placed just lateral to the peroneus tertius tendon and medial to the lateral malleolus at the level of the ankle joint. The structure at greatest risk with this portal placement is the superficial peroneal nerve, which lies lateral to the portal site. The most common mistake with this portal placement is placing the portal too distally which interrupts visualization of the ankle joint. This portal is usually 0.5 to 1 cm proximal to the level of the anteromedial portal.

3. Posterolateral portal: This portal is placed between the Achilles tendon and the peroneal tendons at a level 2 cm proximal to the tip of the lateral malleolus. The structures at greatest risk with this portal are the sural nerve and the lesser saphenous vein, which lie lateral to the portal.

38. **What techniques are used to treat anterior tibiotalar impingement arthroscopically?**
Under the guidance of an arthroscope, the anterior distal tibia is visualized and osteophytes are taken down with the use of an arthroscopic burr or shaver. If bone spurs are larger in size, an osteotome can be introduced into the portals and used to detach them. Any soft-tissue scarring or changes can be excised with the use of electrothermal probes and shavers. Similar techniques can be used for the treatment of synovitis, anterolateral soft-tissue impingement, and syndesmotic impingement.

CASE 3-8 continued

During the diagnostic part of the arthroscopy, you note a defect in the patient's talar dome cartilage.

39. **What is the etiology and treatment of osteochondral lesions of the talus?**
Osteochondral lesions of the talus typically occur from trauma or idiopathic osteonecrosis. Many terms have been used to describe these lesions, including osteochondritis dissecans, osteochondral fracture, and talar dome fracture. Treatment includes cast immobilization, microfracture, internal fixation, osteochondral mosaicplasty, and osteochondral allograft or other bone grafting techniques. Smaller lesions that are not involving the shoulders of the talus are more amenable to arthroscopic treatment.

40. **What is the Berndt and Hardy classification of osteochondral lesions of the talus? What imaging modality is it based on?**
Berndt and Hardy classification of osetochondral lesions of the talus is based on plain film radiography:
    Type I: Compression fracture
    Type II: Partially detached osteochondral fragment
    Type III: Completely detached fragment but non-displaced
    Type IV: Completely detached fragment, displaced.

41. What is the Ferkel and Sgaglione CT staging system for osteochondral lesions of the talus?

The Ferkel and Sgaglione staging system is based on CT scan:

Stage I: Cystic lesion within the talar dome with intact roof

Stage IIa: Cystic lesion within talar dome with communication to surface

Stage IIb: Open articular surface lesion with non-displaced fragment

Stage III: Non-displaced lesion

Stage IV: Displaced fragment.

TENDON DISORDERS

CASE 3-9

A 42-year-old lawyer is referred to your office after playing basketball over the weekend when he heard a loud "pop" in the back of his leg as he went for a rebound. He was seen in a nearby Emergency Room and was told he had an Achilles tendon rupture.

42. What is the typical presentation of a patient with an Achilles tendon rupture?

Achilles tendon ruptures tend to happen in males between 30 and 40 years of age. They tend to happen in the "weekend warrior" athlete who is not properly conditioned. Three-quarters of ruptures are reported to occur during sporting activity. Patients often describe the sensation of a "pop" and the feeling like they were kicked in the back of the leg. Immediate weakness with ambulation is noted as patients have difficulty plantarflexing the foot during the pushoff phase of gait.

43. Where does the tendon usually rupture?

Most Achilles tendon ruptures occur about 4 cm proximal to its calcaneal insertion. This region is a watershed area for tendon blood supply and is often found to have degenerative changes, which can lead to eventual rupture.

44. What is the evaluation of a patient with a suspected Achilles tendon rupture?

Physical examination is typically all that is needed in a patient with a complete Achilles tendon rupture. The patient is noted to have weakness with ankle plantarflexion. A palpable defect can often be felt where the cord-like attachment of the Achilles once was. Lastly, the Thompson test can prove disruption of the musculotendinous mechanism when the calf is squeezed and there is no plantar flexion noted in the foot. This test is best performed with the patient in the prone position with the knee flexed at 90° (Fig. 3.10).

45. What are the benefits of surgical repair? What are the risks with surgical repair?

Surgical repair of the Achilles tendon restores the appropriate tension on the musculotendinous mechanism. There is also decreased risk of re-rupture with surgical repair (1% with surgery vs. 8–40% without surgery).

The risk of surgery includes wound complications, such as skin necrosis, infection, skin adhesions, and dehiscence.

46. How should patients have their foot and ankle splinted or casted after surgical repair?

It is important to cast the patient in a few degrees of plantar flexion following surgical repair of an Achilles rupture to ensure that tension is kept off the repair site during healing.

47. If this patient had complained of chronic posterior heel pain and swelling, without a "pop", what would be the more likely diagnosis?

Patients who present with pain, warmth, and swelling at the Achilles' insertion site with a recent change in activity level may have Achilles tendonitis or paratenonitis. This is an overuse injury caused by repetitive microtrauma that can lead to inflammation in the tendon, paratenon, or retro-calcaneal bursa. Patients are noted to have pain and swelling overlying the region of inflammation with tenderness to palpation most notable at the

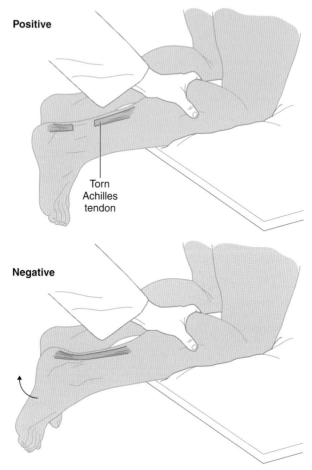

Positive

Torn
Achilles
tendon

Negative

Figure 3.10. Thompson test for Achilles tear. (*From Stretanski MF. Achilles Tendinitis. In: Frontera WR, et al., Essentials of Physical Medicine and Rehabilitation, 2nd edn. Copyright © 2008, Saunders, Elsevier Inc.*)

Achilles insertion site (such inflammation can occur in other regions of the Achilles tendon as well). MRI imaging typically demonstrates increased fluid signal and tendon breakdown at the insertional site.

Conservative treatment is favored for this disorder with focus on eccentric strengthening, stretching of the gastrocnemius–soleus complex, rest, NSAIDs, icing, and even immobilization with a removable boot.

Cases that do not respond well to conservative therapy are considered for surgical debridement of the diseased tendon or paratenon and possible excision of bony spurring. If greater than 50% of the tendon is found to be involved, a tendon transfer should be performed to maintain ankle plantarflexion function. The most commonly used tendon for transfer is the flexor hallucis longus.

CASE 3-10

An obese 53-year-old female with known "flat feet" arrives to your clinic with complaints of gradual onset of pain on the inside of her ankle and foot and the sensation of her foot "turning out."

48. **What is the function of the posterior tibial tendon?**
The posterior tibial tendon serves as an invertor of the hindfoot while adducting and supinating the forefoot during the stance phase of gait. It is also secondary to the Achilles as a plantar flexor of the ankle. During the toe-off phase of gait, the posterior tibial tendon is responsible for locking the transverse tarsal joints to provide a rigid lever arm. The posterior tibial tendon is able to provide such functions due to its various insertions:
    1. Anterior limb: 1st cuneiform, navicular tuberosity
    2. Middle limb: 2nd/3rd cuneiform, cuboid, 2nd to 5th metatarsals
    3. Posterior limb: anterior sustentaculum tali.

49. **What happens to a patient's foot with posterior tibial tendon insufficiency (PTTI)?**
Patients who suffer from PTTI develop a flatfoot deformity. The four classic findings of a patient suffering from PTTI are: collapsed medial arch, hindfoot valgus, forefoot abduction, and varus (Fig. 3.11).

    A good test for assessing these features is the "too many toes" sign in which the patient stands, facing away from the examiner, with his/her feet facing straight ahead.

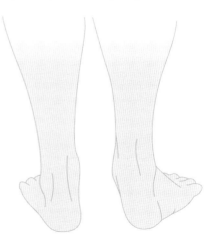

Figure 3.11. Too many toes sign. (*From Haskell A, Mann RA. Foot and Ankle. In: DeLee JC et al., [eds], DeLee and Drez's Orthopaedic Sports Medicine, 3rd edn. Copyright © Saunders, Elsevier Inc., 2010.*)

50. **What is the classification for staging of PTTI? (Table 3.4)**
Treatment for PTTI is based on the stage of the disease:
    Non-surgical treatment: Stage I and II disease is best treated with a period of immobilization in a walking cast and NSAIDs. Patients can then be advanced to a custom molded in-shoe orthosis. Stage III and IV disease is only treated non-surgically in patients who cannot tolerate surgery. For these patients, a brace that crosses the ankle joint (AFO) is required.

Table 3.4. Characteristics Associated with each Stage of PTTI

STAGE	DEFORMITY	FLEXIBILITY	ABILITY TO HEEL RISE	SUBTALAR ARTHRITIS	ANKLE VALGUS
I	Absent	Normal	Yes	No	No
II	Pes planovalgus	Normal	Difficult/unable	No	No
III	Pes planovalgus	Decreased/fixed	Unable	Possible	No
IV	Pes planovalgus	Decreased/fixed	Unable	Possible	Yes

Surgical treatment: Surgery is indicated in patients with Stage I/II disease who fail conservative measures or in patients with Stage III/IV disease. Achilles lengthening is almost always considered regardless of surgical option chosen. Surgical options are as follows:

Stage I: Tenosynovectomy

Stage II: FDL tendon transfer with medial calcaneal displacement osteotomy; lateral column lengthening

Stage III: Hindfoot arthrodesis (triple arthrodesis: subtalar joint, calcaneocuboid joint, talonavicular joint)

Stage IV: Pantalar arthrodesis.

51. **What is the function of the peroneal tendons?**
The primary function of the peroneal tendons is to evert the hindfoot. They also serve as secondary plantar flexors of the foot with the peroneus longus having specific function on the first ray.

52. **What is the injury mechanism that places the peroneal tendons at risk of rupture?**
Inversion injuries or sudden dorsiflexion injuries of the inverted foot are capable of causing peroneal tendon rupture. Tears usually occur in the peroneal brevis tendon at the level of the fibular groove as it travels adjacent to the bone. These tears are longitudinal in nature. Patients with a history of peroneal subluxation/dislocation are at increased risk of rupture.

53. **What is peroneal subluxation/dislocation?**
Peroneal subluxation occurs as a result of a disruption in the fibro-osseus tendon sheath that occurs during an inversion injury to the dorsiflexed ankle. Patients can often have a shallow peroneal groove that leads to the peroneal tendons "popping" out of the groove. The subluxation can often be elicited on examination with forceful positioning from inversion and plantar flexion to eversion and dorsiflexion (Fig. 3.12).

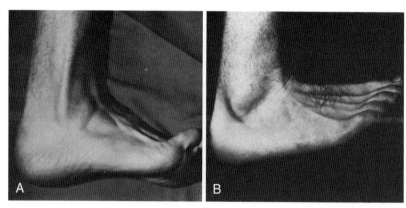

Figure 3.12. Subluxation of peroneal tendons. (*From Haskell A, Mann RA. Foot and Ankle. In: DeLee JC et al., [eds], DeLee and Drez's Orthopaedic Sports Medicine, 3rd edn. Copyright © Saunders, Elsevier Inc., 2010.*)

54. **What is the treatment option for peroneal subluxation, dislocation, and rupture?**
Patients with acutely subluxing or dislocation peroneal tendons can often be treated in a cast for ankle immobilization. This allows time for the tendon sheath to heal. In patients who are high-level athletes or have chronic subluxation, a surgical deepening of the peroneal groove can be performed on the fibula.

Patients who have low ambulatory status, are bed bound, or are poor surgical candidates can have rupture of the peroneal tendons treated non-surgically with rest, NSAIDs, icing, and immobilization similar to treatment for tendonitis. The success rate for such treatment is poor so surgical repair is favored in healthy, active patients. Surgical repair consists of debridement and suture repair. If more than 50% of the tendon is found to be damaged at the time of surgery, then a peroneal brevis to longus tenodesis can be done.

CASE 3-11

A 16-year-old male arrives in the emergency room after kicking his foot through a glass door. He has a deep laceration of the anterior aspect of the distal tibia with a moderate amount of non-pulsatile bleeding. You identify tendon exposed in the wound. When you ask the patient to dorsiflex his foot on the injured side, he is notably weaker than the contralateral side.

55. **What are the common etiologies of anterior tibial tendon ruptures?**
   Anterior tibial tendon ruptures tend to occur from laceration or from a closed injury. In younger patients, the closed injury is often the result of a strong eccentric contraction of the muscle. In older patients, closed ruptures tend to occur in the setting of diabetes, inflammatory arthritis, or history of local steroid injection.

56. **How do patients with anterior tibial tendon ruptures present?**
   Patients with an anterior tibial tendon rupture often complain of difficulty walking. Since the tibialis anterior is responsible for ankle dorsiflexion, patients with a rupture will note difficulty in clearing the foot while walking. Similarly, the loss of eccentric strength may cause a slap-foot gait pattern. Lastly, anterior ankle swelling, a palpable defect at the anterior ankle, and weak dorsiflexion can all be appreciated.

CASE 3-11   continued

Upon further inspection of the wound, you note that the exposed tendon is completely lacerated. The patient is an avid student-athlete and is concerned about his ability to play sports again.

57. **What is the treatment for anterior tibial tendon ruptures?**
   Partial ruptures can often be treated with immobilization via casting for about 6 weeks. If symptoms persist after this time period, an AFO brace can be used for 4–6 months until resolved. Complete ruptures are treated with end-to-end repair in the acute setting. If the tendon has avulsed from its insertion site, suture anchors can be used to repair the tendon to bone. If the tendon quality is poor, a free tendon graft repair or extensor hallucis longus (EHL) tenodesis can be performed to restore ankle dorsiflexion.

CASE 3-12

A 17-year-old baseball player limps into the Emergency Department still in his baseball uniform. He claims that he was sliding into second base when he "rolled" his ankle. He is complaining of pain on the lateral aspect of his foot and difficulty bearing weight. You palpate the base of the fifth metatarsal and the patient screams out in pain. You immediately get x-rays of his injured foot and see a fracture at the base of the 5th metatarsal.

58. **How many fracture zones are there at the base of the 5th metatarsal?**
   (See Fig. 3.13.)
   The base of the 5th metatarsal is divided into 3 zones, and the mechanism of injury has a large influence on the fracture pattern:
   Zone I: Hindfoot inversion
   Zone II: Forefoot adduction
   Zone III: Repetitive microtrauma.

59. **Which of the above zones has the most difficult time to union? Why?**
   Injuries seen in Zone II are referred to as Jones fractures. These fractures can fail to unite because there is a vascular watershed area between the metaphysis and diaphysis.

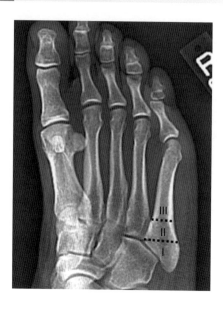

Figure 3.13. Zones of injury for 5th metatarsal base. (*From Banerjee R et al. Foot Injuries. In: Browner BD et al., Skeletal Trauma, 4th edn. Philadelphia: Basic Science, Management, and Reconstruction. Saunders, Elsevier, 2009.*)

60. **Which of the above zones has the best chance of union?**
    Zone I injuries have very high union rates. They represent bony avulsion injuries from the pull of the peroneus brevis tendon or lateral aspect of the plantar fascia.

61. **What is the preferred treatment for fracture of the base of the 5th metatarsal?**
    Non-operative treatment is the preferred treatment for these fractures. Zone I injuries are often treated with a walking cast or fracture boot while Zone II and III injuries are treated with non-weight-bearing for 6–8 weeks until radiographic evidence of healing has occurred.

62. **What if the patient was a competitive athlete? Would that change your proposed treatment plan?**
    Percutaneous intramedullary screw fixation can be offered for a Jones fracture in an athlete. This may increase the likelihood of union.

DIABETIC FOOT
CASE 3-13

A 74-year-old male presents to the Emergency Room with an ulcerated lesion on the plantar aspect his forefoot. He has a 30-year history of non-insulin-dependent diabetes. He states that he does not recall an injury to his foot and only noticed the injury after he noted some bloody drainage on his sock. Despite the significant size and depth of the ulcer, the patient denies any significant pain (Fig. 3.14).

63. **What associated underlying condition increases the risk of developing an ulcer in a patient with diabetes mellitus?**
    Peripheral neuropathy is the greatest cause of foot pathology in diabetic patients. It is present in 50–80% of all diabetic patients. Diabetic neuropathy causes nerve dysfunction in three different ways: sensory, motor, and autonomic function:
    1. Sensory neuropathy: This neuropathy is the most prevalent nerve dysfunction seen in diabetic patients (approximately 70% of patients). The typical pattern of sensation disturbance is in the "glove and stocking" distribution, meaning the loss affects the entire distal extent of the limb rather than following a specific nerve dermatome. This distribution of decreased sensation starts distally and progresses

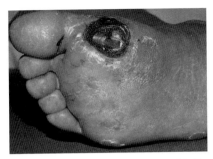

Figure 3.14. Diabetic foot ulcer. *(From James WD, et al. Andrews' Diseases of the Skin: Clinical Dermatology, 11th edn, pp. 45–61. Copyright © Elsevier Inc., 2011.)*

proximally as axons "die off." This places the patient at increased risk of injury with lack of protective sensation.

2. Motor neuropathy: This neuropathy is one of the most obvious in clinical presentation as it leads to the development of contracture and deformity. Weakness of the intrinsic muscles leads to the development of claw toes. Additionally, contracture of the Achilles tendon places the foot in the equinus position. These deforming forces lead to areas of increased pressure on the foot that accelerate skin breakdown and ulcer development.

3. Autonomic neuropathy: This neuropathy is often forgotten, but is an integral part of diabetic foot pathology. The autonomic nervous system is responsible for control of blood vessel tone and sweat gland function. A decrease in this neurologic control leads to increased drying of the skin and decreased oxygenation of the tissues. Combined, these two changes in autonomic function place the foot at increased risk of gangrene and infected wounds.

64. **What physical exam tests are best suited to assess a patient's sensory exam?**
Skin sensation in the diabetic foot can be assessed both qualitatively and quantitatively. Qualitative studies of light touch and pin-prick are quick and easy to get a general understanding of sensory neuropathy severity. More quantitative measures include the use of Semmes–Weinstein monofilaments that gradually increase in diameter and force needed to bend against a patient's skin. The size of the smallest filament felt against the skin is considered the patient's threshold of sensation. Typically, protective sensation is considered intact if the patient can feel a 5.07 monofilament.

CASE 3-13   continued

You decide to probe the ulcer in order to get a better examination of the patient's wound. There is visible tendon and foul-smelling fluid oozing from the site. The tissue edges show good vascularity. You take a swab to culture the depths of the ulcer and order some basic labs while he is in the Emergency Department.

65. **How do you classify the ulcer?**
This patient's ulcer would be classified as a Brodsky 2A (deep ulceration with exposed tendon and/or bone; adequate vascularity). The Brodsky classification of diabetic foot ulcers is based on two factors: Depth and Ischemia (Table 3.5). Alternatively, the wound could be classified under the Wagner classification system as a Grade 2 ulcer (Table 3.6).

The most appropriate treatment for this wound would be surgical debridement. Any deep ulceration is best treated with surgical care in the operating room. Superficial ulcers can be treated with a total contact cast used to relieve regions of increased pressure. For patients with at-risk feet (history of ulceration or neuropathy), treatment is preventative with footwear adjustments, regular scheduled examinations of the feet, and patient education on foot care.

Table 3.5. Brodsky Depth/Ischemia Classification

DEPTH CLASSIFICATION

Grade	Definition
0	At-risk foot; previous ulcer or neuropathy that may cause ulceration
1	Superficial ulceration, no infection
2	Deep ulceration exposing tendon/joint (infection may exist superficially)
3	Extensive ulceration with exposed bone and/or deep infection

ISCHEMIC CLASSIFICATION

Grade	Definition
A	No ischemia
B	Ischemia without gangrene
C	Partial gangrene (forefoot)
D	Complete gangrene of foot

Table 3.6. Wagner Classification

GRADE	SKIN DESCRIPTION
0	Skin intact
1	Superficial
2	Deeper, full-thickness extension
3	Deep abscess formation or osteomyelitis
4	Partial gangrene of the forefoot
5	Extensive gangrene

66. **What would you expect the cultures to show?**
Infections of diabetic feet tend to be polymicrobial with aerobic gram-positive skin flora (*Staphylococcus aureus*) being the most common bacteria (46% incidence). The second most common organism is *Streptococcus* species (35% incidence). However, patients with chronic wounds and prior treatments of antibiotics aimed at gram-positive flora can also present with gram-negative infections (*Enterococcus, Proteus*). Patients with advanced disease (ischemic feet, gangrene) are also at risk for anaerobic infections.

67. **What antibiotic choice would best suit the treatment of this patient's infection?**
Typically, coverage for *Staphylococcus* is included in the initial broad-spectrum coverage of a diabetic ulcer. First-generation cephalosporins are great for coverage of MSSA. However, with the growing incidence of MRSA, vancomycin or a similar agent is often chosen as the initial antibiotic. Coverage of gram-negative organisms can often be achieved with a fluoroquinolone (e.g., ciprofloxacin).

68. **What other studies could help determine the cause, prognosis, and pathology of the patient's disease?**
Obtaining a detailed history, including medical co-morbidities, prior treatments, and smoking history, is essential. The physical examination should include lower extremity vascular status, such as peripheral pulses and capillary refill, and skin integrity.

Further vascular testing includes the studies of ABI (ankle–brachial index). ABIs are a percentage calculated by dividing the systolic pressure of the lower extremity by that of the brachial artery. An ABI of 0.45 is the minimum considered necessary for adequate healing of diabetic wounds. Additionally, absolute toe pressures and flow waveforms can be more specifically analyzed. The minimum absolute toe pressure needed for healing an ulcer is 60 mmHg. Meanwhile, a pressure of 45 mmHg is considered necessary for healing of an amputation. Waveforms are depicted on pulse–volume recordings and are documented as triphasic (normal), biphasic, or monophasic. The waveform characteristics reflect the compliance of the arterial wall being examined and allow a critical interpretation of the pressures.

69. In what scenario can a poorly vascularized limb have elevated absolute pressures?
    Calcified vessels have decreased elasticity and can give falsely elevated absolute pressure readings. In this instance, it is important to evaluate the waveforms as calcified vessel walls will not produce the normal triphasic wave.

CASE 3-13   continued

The patient's foot has good vascularity. However, given the extent of his ulcer wound, surgical debridement and antibiotics are indicated to treat the wound. Prior to taking the patient to the OR, you request imaging of the foot.

70. What imaging studies are most helpful in evaluating the diabetic foot?
    As with any orthopedic condition, plain radiography is the first imaging study ordered. Plain films are useful in evaluating for foreign bodies, fractures, and progression of bony deformity. In rare cases, bony changes consistent with osteomyelitis can be appreciated on plain film radiography.
    Often, the use of MRI can be helpful to reveal soft-tissue infection and abscesses. It is more sensitive for detecting oteomyelitis than plain films. However, it can be difficult to differentiate Charcot arthropathy from infection on MRI.

CASE 3-13   continued

Imaging of the patient's foot shows the plantar ulceration and the soft-tissue swelling around the wound site. There does not appear to be any osteomyelitis and no abscess collection appreciated on MRI. In addition, there does not appear to be any Charcot arthropathy changes in the foot. You proceed to the OR with the patient the following day.

71. What are the goals in the operating room?
    The goals of surgical debridement of diabetic foot ulcers are to remove any area of infected or devitalized tissue and lavage areas in need of drainage. Wounds may be packed open with wet-to-dry dressings or a vacuum-assisted dressing can be applied. The wound care that follows surgical debridement should accomplish the following goals: provide a moist environment, absorb any drainage or exudates, serve as a sterile barrier to the outside environment, and relieve any pressure points.

CASE 3-13   continued

After successful debridement and a few days of daily wet-to-dry dressing changes, you decide to place the patient in a total contact cast to provide relief of the plantar ulcer.

72. What is the purpose of a total contact cast (TCC)?
    TCC is considered the gold standard for off-loading pressure ulcers on the plantar aspect of the foot. The goal of TCC is to evenly distribute the pressure and sheer forces over the foot so that relief of the ulcer allows it to heal. Although it seems contradictory, the casts have little padding inside to allow for proper formation of the plaster around the contours of the foot in order to distribute forces equally.
    TCC should be changed every 2–4 weeks with constant reassessment of the wounds until the erythema, drainage, and edema have resolved. At the time of cast change, the ulcer wounds can be debrided as needed for further healing.

TCC can be used as treatment anywhere from 6 weeks up to 6 months. A study by Myerson found 90% of Wagner Grade 1 and 2 lesions healed in an average of about 6 weeks. Thirty-one percent of the ulcers recurred during the 1.5 year follow-up period, but 81% of those recurrences were healed successfully with a repeat TCC of 2 weeks.

CASE 3-13   continued

You tell the patient to follow-up in the office in 2 weeks for removal of the cast and assessment of his wounds. His cultures came back positive for MSSA and after receiving IV antibiotics in the hospital, you plan to send him out on an oral cephalosporin. Before leaving, the patient becomes worried about an eventual amputation. You explain that if he is compliant with his care and continues to control his blood glucose levels, he should be able to avoid any chance of amputation.

73. **What are the amputation options available to patients who have not had success with more conservative treatments?**
   Amputation for diabetes-related extremity disease accounts for about 80 000 amputations a year in the United States. With advancements in prosthetics and limb salvage, amputation of various levels can offer patients a very functional lifestyle. There are various levels of amputation of the lower extremity (Fig. 3.15):
   1. Toe amputation:
      a. Hallux amputation: These amputations are indicated for ulceration of the great toe. The concern for hallux amputation is the increased pressure and stresses transmitted to the lesser toes and metatarsal heads. This could lead to further ulceration and subsequent amputations.

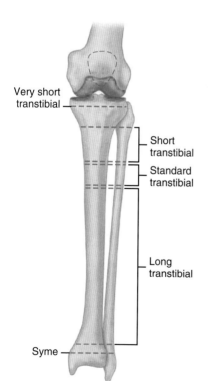

Very short transtibial

Short transtibial

Standard transtibial

Long transtibial

Syme

Figure 3.15. Levels of transtibial amputation. (*From Canale ST, Beaty JH [eds]. Campbell's Operative Orthopaedics, 12th edn, pp. 637–50. Copyright © Mosby, 2013.*)

b. Lesser toe amputation: These amputations are indicated for ulceration of lesser toes without proximal extension. The greatest risk with this amputation is in reference to the second toe in which the absence of the digit can lead to the development of hallux vaglus.

2. Ray amputation: These amputations allow for preservation of the metatarsal base, which preserves Lisfranc joint stability. Patients tend to tolerate this type of amputation better on the lateral aspect of the foot more than on the medial aspect. Amputation of the 5th ray is the most common ray amputation performed. Amputation of the 1st ray increases the weight-bearing load on the other rays and can lead to decreased dorsiflexion secondary to loss of the tibialis anterior insertion.

3. Transmetatarsal amputation: The benefit of a transmetatarsal amputation is that it allows the patient to maintain a distal weight-bearing limb and requires less energy expenditure for ambulation than a higher level of amputation. The risk with this amputation is imbalance of muscles responsible for plantar and dorsiflexion. Disruption of extensor digitorum longus and tibialis anterior insertions leads to unopposed pull of the Achilles tendon, which can place the residual foot in equinus.

4. Syme amputation: The main benefit of a Syme amputation is preservation of a long weight-bearing residual limb, as compared to transtibial amputation. Patients considered for a Syme amputation require a viable heel pad with no infection, good vascularity, and the ability to ambulate with a prosthesis.

5. Transtibial ("below-the-knee") amputation: This amputation is the best choice for a patient with complete foot and ankle involvement. The benefit of a transtibial amputation over a transfemoral amputation is preservation of the knee joint, better prosthetic options, and lower energy expenditure with gait.

74. What is the end-stage bony change often seen in patients with diabetes and neuropathy?

Charcot arthropathy is the progressive destruction of bone and soft tissue that leads to fracture, dislocation, and deformity. It is typically seen in the weight-bearing areas of the body, such as the foot and ankle. Up to 7.5% of patients with diabetes and neuropathy develop Charcot arthropathy.

75. What are the classifications of Charcot arthropathy?

The most common classification systems for Charcot arthropathy are the Eichenholtz classification (Table 3.7) and Brodsky anatomic classification (Table 3.8).

Table 3.7. Eichenholtz Classification of Charcot Arthropathy

STAGE	CHARACTERISTICS
0	Acute inflammation: swollen foot
1	Developmental/fragmentation phase: periarticular fracture; joint subluxation with risk of deformity
2	Coalescence stage: Resorption of bone debris; soft tissue normalizes
3	Consolidation stage: Foot restabilizes with bony and/or fibrotic arthrodesis

Table 3.8. Brodsky Anatomic Classification

STAGE	LOCATION
Type 1	Tarsometatarsal and naviculocuneiform joints
Type 2	Subtalar, talonavicular, calcaneocuboid joints
Type 3	Tibiotalar joint

76. **What is the goal for surgical correction of a Charcot arthropathy?**

The goal of surgical correction of a late Charcot deformity is to create a plantigrade foot that will not result in recurrent ulceration. Surgery is indicated in Charcot arthropathy when the foot suffers from recurrent ulcers or instability that is not controlled with an orthosis. Surgical options include exostectomy, osteotomy, and arthrodesis.

ANKLE ARTHRITIS

CASE 3-14

A 57-year-old man comes into clinic in noticeable pain. He states that he has been dealing with pain in his right ankle ever since a motor vehicle accident when he was in his early 20s. He did not go to the Emergency Room when the injury occurred. He states that the pain makes it difficult to bear weight.

77. **What is the most common etiology of ankle arthritis?**

Arthritis of the tibiotalar (ankle) joint is usually post-traumatic (66% of cases). Patients often have a history of severe injury to the ankle that results in cartilage defects or non-anatomic articular surface healing. Primary osteoarthritis accounts for less than 10% of tibiotalar arthritis. Inflammatory arthritides such as rheumatoid arthritis, psoriartic arthritis, gout, and infection account for the remainder of cases. Overall, the incidence of ankle arthritis is much less than that of the hip and knee joints.

78. **How do patients with ankle arthritis often present?**

Patients with ankle arthritis will often report pain in the anterior ankle with weight-bearing and during the push-off stage of the gait cycle. They will also often have a reduced and painful range of motion.

CASE 3-14   continued

The patient hands you some x-ray films of his right ankle that his primary care physician had ordered about a year ago. You quickly look at the films and realize that they are non-weight-bearing.

79. **What type of radiograph is most important in evaluation of ankle arthritis?**

Weight-bearing ankle x-rays are most important. Typically, weight-bearing AP, lateral, and oblique views of the ankle are obtained for assessment of the ankle joint.

80. **What are the treatment options for a patient with ankle arthritis?**

Non-surgical treatment is the first-line treatment. NSAIDs, bracing, and activity modification can often successfully treat painful and debilitating ankle arthritis.

If conservative therapy fails, surgical treatment is available. Ankle debridement and anterior tibial/dorsal talar exostectomy can help relieve impingement and improve symptoms in mild cases. Arthrodesis (fusion) is the gold standard treatment for end-stage ankle arthritis. It is preferable for older and less active patient populations. There is a 10% nonunion rate, which can be negatively influenced by such factors as smoking, diabetes, avascular necrosis, and prior arthrodesis. Ankle arthroplasty is also an option in low-demand indivdiuals.

CASE 3-14   continued

The patient is admittedly a two-pack-per-day smoker. He is also notably overweight.

81. **What is the increased risk of nonunion seen in smokers versus non-smokers?**

Tobacco use increases the risk of arthrodesis nonunion by almost 300%.

82. **What are the indications and contraindications to total ankle arthroplasty?**

Patient selection is the most crucial aspect to successful ankle arthroplasty. Indications for joint replacement include elderly patients with post-traumatic or inflammatory arthritis. Contraindications to joint replacement include severe osteoporosis, obesity, young patients, laborers, Charcot joint, ankle instability, osteonecrosis, and uncorrectable deformity.

ANKLE SPRAINS AND INSTABILITY

CASE 3-15

A 23-year-old woman limps into the Emergency Room smelling of alcohol and complaining of left ankle pain. She states that she was walking home from the bar when her high-heeled shoe became caught in a steel-grate on the sidewalk and she twisted her ankle.

83. **How are ankle sprains classified?**
   Acute lateral ankle instability (sprain) is classified into three grades based on ligament injury, swelling, tenderness, and pain with weight bearing (Table 3.9).

Table 3.9. Characteristics Associated with Grade of Ankle Sprain

GRADE	LIGAMENT INJURY	SWELLING, TENDERNESS, ECCHYMOSIS	PAINFUL WEIGHT BEARING
I	None	Minimal	None
II	Stretch	Moderate	Mild
III	Rupture	Severe	Severe

84. **Where do most patients have pain on examination of an ankle sprain?**
   Most patients suffer an inversion injury placing stress on the lateral ankle ligaments. The anterior talofibular ligament (ATFL) and calcaneofibular ligament (CFL) are the most commonly injured ligaments, more so than the posterior talofibuar ligament (PTFL). Patients will have palpation tenderness at the insertion sites of these ligaments. Some patients will display a positive anterior drawer sign and/or talar tilt sign.

85. **How is the anterior drawer test administered, and what constitutes a positive anterior drawer test?**
   The anterior drawer test is performed by stabilizing the distal tibia with one hand and grasping the posterior heel with the other. An anterior force is applied to the posterior heel in an effort to displace the talus anteriorly. A large shift anteriorly, or even a palpable clunk in severe cases, indicates a positive anterior drawer test. The uninjured ankle should always be examined for comparison.

86. **What is the talar tilt test?**
   The talar tilt test examines the integrity of the calcaneofibular ligament and the anterior talofibular ligament. It is performed by grasping the foot and heel while attempting to invert the talus on the tibia. Normal individuals rarely have a talar tilt test >5°.

87. **Which lateral ligament is most commonly injured?**
   The lateral ligament most commonly injured is the ATFL, which is the primary lateral stabilizer of the ankle in plantar flexion. The CFL is a secondary stabilizer and resists inversion of the talus and calcaneus; thus it plays a major role in stability of the subtalar joint. The CFL is usually disrupted in association with a tear of the ATFL. The PTFL resists dorsiflexion–external rotation forces in the ankle and is rarely sprained. Of the lateral ankle ligaments, the CFL is by far the strongest, followed by the PTFL, and lastly the ATFL.

CASE 3-15   continued

Although she is very tearful and upset, the patient does not complain of any significant tenderness to palpation. She was also witnessed walking (albeit limping) to her assigned room in the Emergency Department.

88. **Is it appropriate to get x-rays of this patient?**
   The Ottawa rules were developed in the early 1990s by a group of physicians to determine when it is appropriate to get foot or ankle x-rays after an injury.

Per the Ottawa rules, x-rays should be obtained if any of the following conditions are present:
1. Bone tenderness along the distal 6 cm of the posterior edge of the medial malleolus
2. Bone tenderness along the distal 6 cm of the posterior edge of the lateral malleolus
3. An inability to bear weight immediately or upon presentation for 4 steps
4. Bone tenderness at the base of the 5th metatarsal
5. Bone tenderness at the navicular.
   In most cases, this patient's presentation does not warrant x-rays. However, given her intoxicated state, her exam cannot be trusted and she should get x-rays.

CASE 3-15   continued

The patient gets x-rays of her left ankle. They are negative for any bony injury.

89. **What is the treatment for an acute ankle sprain? How effective is this treatment?**
    Treatment of an acute ankle sprain is strictly non-operative. It involves rest, ice, compression, and elevation (RICE). Ninety percent of ankle sprain injuries resolve with this treatment and functional rehabilitation.

CASE 3-15   continued

Your patient follows all of the directions for her conservative care, but returns to the office about 2.5 months later with continued symptoms.

90. **What is the next study indicated in this patient?**
    A patient who suffers an acute ankle sprain and still complains of symptoms after 8 weeks or more should undergo an MRI of the foot and ankle. This imaging study is suitable for detecting osteochondral lesions, occult fractures, bone edema, or peroneal tendon injury.

CASE 3-15   continued

After discussing further with your patient, she recalls that her last episode of an ankle sprain was not the first. She recalls multiple episodes of inverting her ankle since an old gymnastics injury in high school. She states that she feels the ankle is often "giving way."

91. **What are the symptoms of chronic lateral ankle instability?**
    Patients with chronic ankle instability will often complain of frequent giving way, pain, and instability.

92. **What is the first line of treatment in chronic lateral ankle instability?**
    The first line of treatment in chronic lateral ankle instability is bracing and physical therapy. If this treatment fails, patients can undergo surgical repair in the form of anatomic repair (direct repair of attenuated ligaments) or tendon rerouting techniques to recreate the stability provided by the injured ligaments.

CASE 3-15   continued

Your patient admits she does not remember much from the night she was evaluated in the Emergency Room. She is curious if she suffered a "high ankle sprain" or "low ankle sprain."

93. **What is a "high ankle sprain"?**
    A high ankle sprain is one in which the injury pattern is a combination of dorsiflexion and external rotation. The force of the injury travels up the leg and results in injury to the syndesmosis. It represents fewer than 10% of all ankle sprain injuries.

94. What structures make up the syndesmotic ligaments? What is the function of the syndesmosis?

Four ligaments form the syndesmotic ligament complex: (1) the anterior inferior tibiofibular ligament, (2) the posterior inferior tibiofibular ligament, (3) the transverse tibiofibular ligament, and (4) the interosseous ligament. The four ligaments maintain the integrity between the distal tibia and the fibula and resist the axial, rotational, and translational forces that would otherwise separate the two bones.

95. In a patient with a suspected eversion ankle sprain, how is a syndesmosis sprain diagnosed? How is it treated?

Patients often have extreme tenderness over the syndesmosis, a positive squeeze test, pain with abduction or external rotation of the ankle, pain with weight bearing, and a positive stress external rotation or gravity stress radiograph. Treatment should be supervised, consisting of RICE, toe-touch weight bearing until pain free, gradual mobilization and range-of-motion exercises, progressive strengthening exercises, and proprioceptive training.

96. What is the squeeze test?

The squeeze test is performed by squeezing the distal fibula and tibia together. A positive test is demonstrated by tenderness over the syndesmosis that is consistent with an injury to this area (Fig. 3.16).

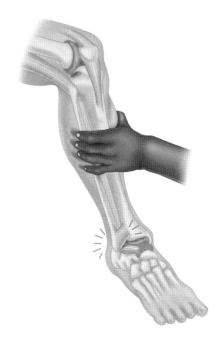

Figure 3.16. Squeeze test. *(From Canale ST, Beaty JH [eds]. Campbell's Operative Orthopaedics, 12th edn, pp. 4213–53.e4. Copyright © Mosby, 2013.)*

97. How is a complete syndesmosis injury (tibiofibular diastasis) diagnosed? How is it treated?

In this injury, the ligaments holding the tibia and fibula have ruptured completely; thus the ankle mortise is unstable. Patients have similar exam findings to those with a syndesmosis sprain. Radiographs typically show widening of the medial clear space (between the medial malleolus and medial talar dome) relative to the lateral clear space (between the lateral malleolus and lateral talar dome). The mortise needs to be reduced and held together with syndesmosis screws. The distance between the tibia and fibula is fixed and stable after reduction and screw fixation. Careful reduction is paramount, as the most common complication of surgical intervention is malreduction.

NEUROLOGIC DISORDERS OF THE FOOT AND ANKLE

CASE 3-16

A 56-year-old female comes to your office complaining of a recurring burning sensation that occurs between her 3rd and 4th toe of her left foot. She states that she has no history of fungal foot infections or injury. She notices that wearing high heels makes the pain seem worse. She also claims to feel a small nodule between those toes.

98. What is Morton's neuroma (interdigital neuritis)?

Morton's neuroma is a perineural thickening of the common digital nerve at the webspace of the foot. It is most commonly seen in women (4:1, female-to-male ratio). The etiology is uncertain; possibilities include anatomic factors, direct trauma, and extrinsic pressure. It is most commonly found between the third and fourth toes (third webspace) (Fig. 3.17).

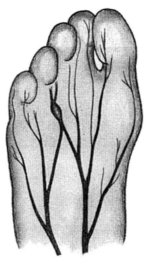

Figure 3.17. Morton's neuroma. (*From Mercier L, Practical Orthopedics, 6th edn, pp. 243–75. Copyright © Mosby, 2008.*)

99. What are the symptoms of a Morton's neuroma?

Morton's neuroma usually presents as pain on the plantar aspect of the foot between the metatarsal heads, which is often associated with burning or tingling of the involved toes. Pain increases with activity and when wearing shoes with a narrow toe box. Typically the pain is resolved with removal of the shoe and massage of the foot.

100. What is Mulder's sign?

The Mulder sign is elicited by squeezing the foot while palpating the webspace. A tangible "click" can be felt that indicates the presence of a Morton's neuroma.

101. What diagnostic and/or radiographic tests are helpful in diagnosing Morton's neuroma?

The diagnosis of a Morton's neuroma is based on history and physical examination. In one-third of patients the nerve and its neuroma can be palpated. It is important to differentiate metatarsal phalangeal joint tenderness from interdigital tenderness.

102. What diagnostic approach can help differentiate MTP joint synovitis from interdigital neuroma?

Differential injections can help in this difficult diagnosis. An injection of local anesthetic into the web space between the metatarsal heads causing resolution of the patient's symptoms favors a diagnosis of Morton's neuroma. If no relief is obtained, a second injection can be administered to the MTP joint, with a repeat exam noting any improvement in the patient's symptoms.

103. What is the non-surgical management of Morton's neuroma?

Always try non-surgical treatment first, because approximately 80% of patients will have complete resolution of symptoms. The goals are to alleviate pressure on the nerve by decreasing tension on the intermetatarsal ligament and to reduce compression of the forefoot, which may be accomplished through the use of shoes with a wide toe box, firm sole, and a more rigid arch support. Metatarsal pads also may help to relieve pressure on the nerve. Anti-inflammatory medication rarely offers any benefit. Local corticosteroid injection may be helpful in relieving symptoms, but repeated injections are contraindicated.

104. Do all patients improve after excision of a Morton's neuroma?

Surgery should only be reserved for patients who fail non-surgical treatment. Very few patients consider the operation to be either a failure or only marginally beneficial. It is important to inform the patient that surgical excision does not always provide relief and recurrence is possible.

CASE 3-17

A 36-year-old man comes to your office with vague complaints of foot numbness on the plantar aspect of his foot. He says that the symptoms are worse with working and while running, but resolve when he is resting. He has no history of vascular problems. He can't seem to localize the origin of the pain/numbness.

105. Define tarsal tunnel syndrome.

Tarsal tunnel syndrome is analogous to carpal tunnel syndrome and involves compression of the posterior tibial nerve or its branches (the calcaneal branch, lateral plantar nerve, and medial plantar nerve). The cause of the syndrome can be identified in only 50% of cases. Etiologies include fracture callus, ganglion of the tendon sheath, lipoma, exostosis, engorged venous plexus, and excessive pronation of the hind foot.

106. What is the tarsal tunnel and what structures lie within it?

The tarsal tunnel is a fibro-osseous tunnel formed by the flexor retinaculum, the medial wall of the calcaneus and talus, and the medial malleolus. The tunnel contains (from anterior to posterior) the tibialis posterior tendon, flexor digitorum longus tendon, posterior tibial artery and vein, tibial nerve, and flexor hallucis longus tendon. The mnemonic "Tom, Dick, And Very Nervous Harry" may be helpful in remembering the order of the structures:

T = tibialis posterior
D = flexor digitorum longus
A = posterior tibial artery
V = posterior tibial vein
N = tibial nerve
H = flexor hallucis longus (Fig. 3.18).

107. What are the most common symptoms of tarsal tunnel syndrome?

Patients with tarsal tunnel syndrome complain of plantar numbness, diffuse plantar burning, and tingling pain that increases with activity and decreases with rest. Occasionally, the pain radiates along a branch of the posterior tibial nerve or proximally along the posterior tibial nerve.

108. How is tarsal tunnel syndrome diagnosed?

The best diagnostic physical exam finding for tarsal tunnel syndrome is a positive Tinel's sign over the tarsal tunnel. Patients will note that tapping this region elicits symptoms. Confirmation of the diagnosis can be made with a positive electromyelogram documenting entrapment of the posterior tibial nerve or one of its branches.

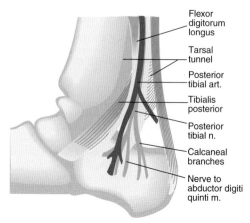

Flexor digitorum longus
Tarsal tunnel
Posterior tibial art.
Tibialis posterior
Posterior tibial n.
Calcaneal branches
Nerve to abductor digiti quinti m.

Figure 3.18. Tarsal tunnel. (*From Haskell A, Mann RA. Foot and Ankle. In: DeLee JC et al., [eds], DeLee and Drez's Orthopaedic Sports Medicine, 3rd edn. Copyright © Saunders, Elsevier Inc., 2010.*)

CASE 3-17 continued

The patient has a positive Tinel's test and you decide to send him for an EMG study. The EMG comes back confirming the diagnosis of tarsal tunnel syndrome. The patient wants to know what the next step to fix his problem is.

109. **How is tarsal tunnel syndrome treated?**
Initial treatment for tarsal tunnel syndrome consists of NSAIDs and local corticosteroid injection. Orthotics may help to reduce tension on the nerves by limiting pronation in the patient with a hindfoot deformity. When conservative modalities fail, surgical treatment consisting of a tarsal tunnel release is indicated.

CASE 3-18

A 32-year-old male comes into your office with complaints of a progressive deformity of his foot. He has noted some weakness in his feet over the past few years and has seen his foot slowly progress in a deformity that "flexes his toes" and "increases his arch." He states that he has an uncle who suffers from Charcot–Marie–Tooth disease and ended up truly debilitated from the condition. He is concerned about his disease progression.

110. **What is Charcot–Marie–Tooth disease?**
Charcot–Marie–Tooth (CMT) disease is the most common inherited neuropathy. It is a degenerative neuropathy of the peripheral nerves and most commonly affects the leg, ankle, and foot. It is characterized by loss of intrinsic muscle mass and touch sensation. The eventual positioning of the foot affected by CMT is a cavovarus foot in equinus.

111. **What are the characteristic deformities of a Charcot–Marie–Tooth disease foot?**
The symptoms of CMT usually begin in late childhood or early adulthood. A footdrop is often first noticed. The hindfoot develops a varus position to compensate for the forefoot valgus and because of the unopposed pull of the tibialis posterior that inverts the hindfoot. The imbalance continues to the intrinsics and extrinsics of the foot, which results in an elevation of the foot arch (pes cavus). The loss of intrinsics also results in claw toes. Lastly, the weakened tibialis anterior is unable to oppose the gastrocnemius–soleus and the foot ends up in equines (Fig. 3.19).

112. **What is the Coleman block test?**
The Coleman block test is used to determine the progression of CMT. It specifically is used to see if the hindfoot is flexible and to determine if the deformity of the foot is a result of first ray plantarflexion or if the hindfoot is also involved (Fig. 3.20).

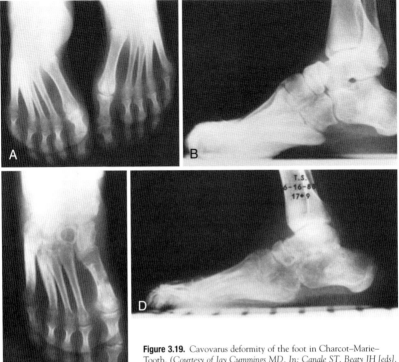

Figure 3.19. Cavovarus deformity of the foot in Charcot–Marie–Tooth. *(Courtesy of Jay Cummings MD, In: Canale ST, Beaty JH [eds], Campbell's Operative Orthopaedics, 12th edn, pp. 1335–61.e5. Copyright © Mosby, 2013.)*

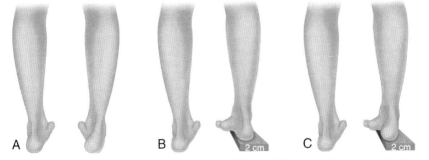

Figure 3.20. Coleman block test. *(From Canale ST, Beaty JH [eds]. Campbell's Operative Orthopaedics, 12th edn, pp. 1335–61.e5. Copyright © Mosby, 2013.)*

The test is performed with a patient weight-bearing on his/her hindfoot and lateral forefoot on a block. If the hindfoot corrects itself to neutral or everts, then the deformity is caused by the first ray plantar flexion. If the foot does not correct, then the hindfoot is also involved in the deformity.

113. **What is the treatment of a CMT-afflicted foot?**

Treatment of CMT can be either surgical or non-surgical. Non-surgical treatment focuses on non-impact exercise, strengthening and stretching of affected muscles, and orthotics that correct the deformity. Surgical treatment is reserved for when patients fail conservative treatment, have symptoms from their deformity, or develop contractures from the muscle weakness. Surgical correction typically involves bony and soft-tissue procedures in the form of osteotomies and tendon transfers.

CHAPTER 4

HAND

Joshua A. Gordon and Adam Griska

ANATOMY OF THE HAND

GENERAL CONSIDERATIONS

1. What are the general functions of the hand and what anatomical considerations exist?
   1. *Sensation* in the hand is crucial. Many social and functional interactions occur through hand sensation. Additionally, a hand without sensation is soon destroyed from ulceration and trauma (as seen in leprosy). The most important areas for fine sensation are supplied by the median nerve, which innervates the thumb, index finger, long finger, and radial aspect of the ring finger. The ulnar nerve is also vital in that it inervates the ulnar aspect of the ring finger and the entire volar aspect of the small finger.
   2. *Motor function for gripping.* Through various forms of grip, we perform daily activities of life. Gripping objects is accomplished by a combination of many muscles, including the forearm wrist extensors and the forearm finger flexors. The thumb secures gripped objects by grasping over the fingers. Manipulation of small objects using two-point pinch or three-point chuck involves the intrinsic hand muscles.

2. How do you describe which surface of the hand you are referring to?
   In the anatomic position, the dorsal surface faces posterior, while the palmar or volar surface faces anterior.

ANATOMY OF THE HAND AND WRIST

Bones and Joints

3. What osseous structures make up the anatomy of the hand?
   Twenty-seven bones contribute to the skeleton of the hand. These bones include carpal, metacarpal, and phalangeal bones. Each finger and the thumb have a metacarpal bone, which articulates at its distal most extent with the proximal phalanx. The thumb's proximal phalanx articulates directly with the distal phalanx, while each finger has the addition of a middle phalanx between the two. Each finger, with its phalanges, is combined with the metacarpal of that finger to form a "ray". This means that there are 5 rays, one for each finger. There are also multiple, small sesamoid bones of the hand with some anatomic variation (Fig. 4.1).

4. What is the volar plate?
   The volar plate, also sometimes called the palmar plate, is a fibrous structure that re-enforces the palmar side of the joint capsule of the MP and IP joints. It acts to limit hyperextension, and if injured during hyperextension, can scar and lead to flexion contractures.

5. What is Dupuytren's contracture and what structure is involved?
   Dupuytren's contracture is a painless, but progressive flexion contracture of the fingers caused by diseased palmar fascia. It commonly starts with the ring finger and small finger, but it may involve the entire hand. The disease has a hereditary component and is seen more commonly in men of Northern European descent. Its gene has been mapped.

CASE 4-1

A 22-year-old male presents to the Emergency Department after a fight. He has a small laceration over the dorsal aspect of his hand at the ring finger metacarpophalangeal (MP) joint. He is unable to recall how he got the laceration. The patient complains of minimal pain at the site of the laceration, and there is no drainage from the laceration site.

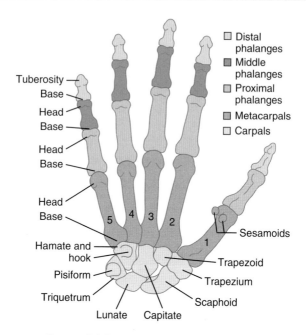

Bones of right wrist and hand (palmar view)

Figure 4.1. Osseous anatomy of the hand. *(From Pratt NE, Anatomy and Kinesiology of the Hand: Skirven TM, et al. [eds], Rehabilitation of the Hand and Upper Extremity, 6th edn. Mosby, 2011.)*

6. **What is the most likely diagnosis and what are the important considerations?**
   Any small laceration on the *dorsum of the hand* especially around the MP joint should be considered a *"fight bite"* until proven otherwise. Damage of deep structures is frequent. Some case series suggest that 70% of "fight bites" result in damage to deep structures such as the extensor tendon, joint capsule, bone, and/or cartilage. It is difficult to assess the deep structures from inspection at the site of the laceration because most injuries are sustained in a flexed position (with the fingers in a fist). However, when the examination is done, the fingers are typically extended so the position of the deeper structures is altered relative to the skin. Due to the high bacterial content of the human mouth, these injuries are always assumed to be contaminated. Irrigation and debridement in the operating room with antibiotic coverage for *Eikenella corrodens* (and other gram-negative organisms) as well as *Staphylococcus* and *Streptococcus* species is imperative.

7. **What are the carpometacarpal joints of the hand?**
   Carpometacarpal (CMC) joints: There are five CMC joints with each metacarpal articulating with different carpal bones:
   1st metacarpal: trapezium
   2nd metacarpal: primarily with the trapezoid, but also trapezium and capitate
   3rd metacarpal: capitate
   4th metacarpal: capitate and hamate
   5th metacarpal: hamate.

8. **Name the bones of the proximal and distal carpal rows.**
   From radial to ulnar, the bones of the proximal carpal row are the scaphoid, lunate, triquetrum, and pisiform. In a similar radial to ulnar direction, the bones of the distal row are the trapezium, trapezoid, capitate, and hamate.

To remember the organization of these bones, one can use the pneumonic: *Some Lovers Try Positions That They Can't Handle.* Proximal row: Scaphoid, Lunate, Triquetrum, and Pisiform (also a sesamoid bone). Distal row: *Trapezium* (*um* for under the thumb), Trapezoid, Capitate, and Hamate.

Although there is great individual variability, the carpal bones start to ossify with the capitate in a counterclockwise fashion (when considering the volar surface of the right hand) from several months to 10 years of age. The pisiform is the exception to the counterclockwise rule as it is the last to ossify.

9. Besides being the last to ossify, what is special about the pisiform?
It is a sesamoid bone in the tendon of the flexor carpi ulnaris (FCU).

10. How is the wrist stabilized?
Ligaments stabilize the wrist during its many mechanical functions. These ligaments are generally named for their attachments and can be divided into two groups. Intrinsic ligaments connect carpal bones. Extrinsic ligaments connect the non-carpal bones (i.e., the radius and ulna) to the carpal bones and are considered capsular expansions (Fig. 4.2).

11. What is the space of Poirier?
The space of Poirier is a weak area of the volar capsule that is devoid of stout ligaments. Perilunate dislocations are associated with a capsular rent in this space and potential displacement of the lunate through the defect.

12. Where do most wrist ganglia originate?
The most common ganglion is the dorsal wrist ganglion, which originates from the scapholunate ligament and accounts for approximately 60–70% of all hand ganglia. The second most common ganglion is the volar ganglion, which accounts for 20% of ganglia and typically originates from the radioscaphoid or scapho-trapezial-trapezoid (STT) joint. Ganglia of the flexor tendon sheath at the A-1 pulley are the third most common and are called volar retinacular cysts.

CASE 4-2

A 25-year-old male presents 2 days after a fall on an outstretched hand with forced hyperextension of the wrist. He complains of tenderness just proximal to the base of his thumb and in his wrist. His wrist appears mildly swollen, and on examination, there is tenderness in the anatomic snuffbox with pain on motion of the wrist.

13. Which carpal bone has likely been fractured?
The scaphoid is the most commonly fractured carpal bone, representing as high as 70% of all carpal fractures.

14. What is important to remember about the anatomy of the scaphoid in terms of: (a) the blood supply to the scaphoid and (b) the anatomic borders of the "snuff box"?
The blood supply to the scaphoid is predominantly retrograde and enters at the distal pole. This is important in determining the prognosis for various scaphoid fractures. Fractures that are more proximal have a higher likelihood of nonunion and avascular necrosis.

The snuffbox lies just distal to the radial styloid. The radial border is composed of the abductor pollicis longus and extensor pollicis brevis. The ulnar border is the extensor pollicis longus. The floor of the snuffbox is the scaphoid and, therefore, palpation of the snuffbox is a physical exam maneuver used to evaluate for possible scaphoid fractures.

Muscles and Tendons

CASE 4-3

A 34-year-old male presents to the Emergency Room after his car fell on his right hand while changing a tire. The emergency room staff have obtained plain films and evaluated the hand. They have not identified any fractures or dislocations and have documented normal radial and ulnar pulses. The hand "looks good", but the physician would like the hand surgery service to evaluate the patient prior to discharge. On evaluation, the patient is found to have significant pain, extensive swelling on the dorsal aspect of the hand, and is holding his hand in an intrinsic minus position.

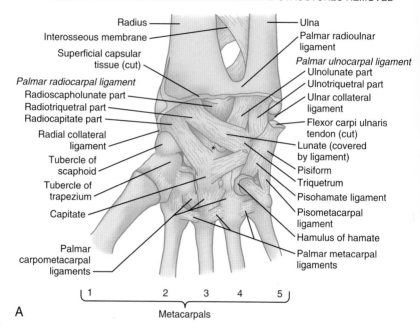

PALMAR VIEW WITH FLEXOR RETINACULUM AND STRUCTURES REMOVED

Radius
Interosseous membrane
Superficial capsular tissue (cut)
Palmar radiocarpal ligament
Radioscapholunate part
Radiotriquetral part
Radiocapitate part
Radial collateral ligament
Tubercle of scaphoid
Tubercle of trapezium
Capitate
Palmar carpometacarpal ligaments

Ulna
Palmar radioulnar ligament
Palmar ulnocarpal ligament
Ulnolunate part
Ulnotriquetral part
Ulnar collateral ligament
Flexor carpi ulnaris tendon (cut)
Lunate (covered by ligament)
Pisiform
Triquetrum
Pisohamate ligament
Pisometacarpal ligament
Hamulus of hamate
Palmar metacarpal ligaments

1 2 3 4 5
Metacarpals

A

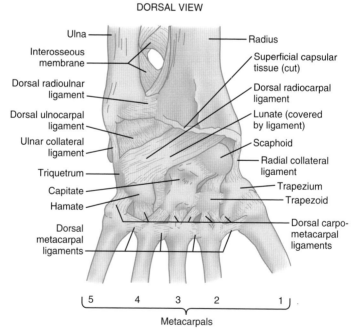

DORSAL VIEW

Ulna
Interosseous membrane
Dorsal radioulnar ligament
Dorsal ulnocarpal ligament
Ulnar collateral ligament
Triquetrum
Capitate
Hamate
Dorsal metacarpal ligaments

Radius
Superficial capsular tissue (cut)
Dorsal radiocarpal ligament
Lunate (covered by ligament)
Scaphoid
Radial collateral ligament
Trapezium
Trapezoid
Dorsal carpo-metacarpal ligaments

5 4 3 2 1
Metacarpals

B

Figure 4.2. Ligaments of the wrist. (A) The volar extrinsic ligaments are the most important ligaments in providing stability to the wrist and include the radial collateral ligament, radiocapitate ligament, radioscaphoid ligament, radiotriquetral ligament, ulnotriquetral ligament, capitotriquetral ligament, and ulnar collateral ligament. The space of Poirier (*) is a gap in the volar ligaments and the site of potential weakness. (B) The intrinsic (intercarpal) ligaments interconnect the individual carpal bones. The most important of these are the scapholunate ligament and the lunotriquetral ligament. (*Redrawn from Netter FH: Atlas of Human Anatomy, 3rd edn. Teterboro, NJ, Icon, 2003.*)

15. What is the most likely diagnosis, and what is the treatment?
   This patient most likely has *compartment syndrome* of the hand due to a crush injury (compartment syndrome may also result from reperfusion after an ischemic event). The compartments of the hand should be released by an emergent *fasciotomy* to avoid muscle necrosis and permanent contracture.

16. How many fascial compartments are there in the hand and what are their contents?
   There are 10 compartments of the hand: 3 volar interosseous muscles, 4 dorsal interosseous muscles, the thenar compartment, the hypothenar compartment, and the adductor compartment. If there is concern for compartment syndrome of the hand, each of these compartments should be surgically released.

17. List the contents of the six dorsal wrist compartments (extrinsic extensors.)
   The dorsal wrist compartments are numbered from radial to ulnar and contain the extensor tendons.

Dorsal Wrist Compartments

Compartment	Contents
1 (2)	Abductor pollicis longus (APL)
	Extensor pollicis brevis (EPB)
2 (2)	Extensor carpi radialis longus (ECRL)
	Extensor carpi radialis brevis (ECRB)
3 (1)	Extensor pollicis longus (EPL)
4 (2)	Extensor digitorum communis (EDC)
	Extensor indicis proprius (EIP)
5 (1)	Extensor digiti minimi (EDM)
6 (1)	Extensor carpi ulnaris (ECU)

18. Are these compartments treated with fasciotomy in the case of compartment syndrome of the hand?
   No, these compartments only contain the extensor tendons as they pass across the wrist. They do not contain muscle, and as a result, they do not become ischemic in the setting of compartment syndrome of the hand.

19. What is the common used name for 1st dorsal compartment tenosynovitis?
   1st dorsal compartment tenoysnovitis is also called De Quervain's tenosynovitis. It presents as radial-sided wrist pain which worsens with ulnar deviation. It is diagnosed by a positive Finkelstein's test, which involves ulnar deviation of a flexed thumb held in a clenched fist. Typically, it is treated with thumb spica splinting and a corticosteroid injection. Recalcitrant symptoms are treated with surgical release of the first dorsal compartment.

20. What are the intrinsic muscles of the hand?
   The intrinsic muscles are those that both attach and insert in the hand. They consist of four groups (Fig. 4.3):
   1. Adductor muscle (Table 4.1)
   2. Thenar muscle group (Table 4.2)
   3. Hypothenar muscle group (Table 4.3)
   4. Central muscle group (Table 4.4).

Table 4.1. Adductor Muscle

MUSCLE	ORIGIN	INSERTION	INNERVATION	ACTION
Adductor pollicis: a. Oblique head b. Transverse head	a. Capitate and base of 2nd and 3rd metacarpal b. Palmar surface of 3rd metacarpal	Ulnar side of the base of the proximal phalanx of the thumb	Deep branch of the ulnar nerve (C8–T1)	Adduction of the thumb

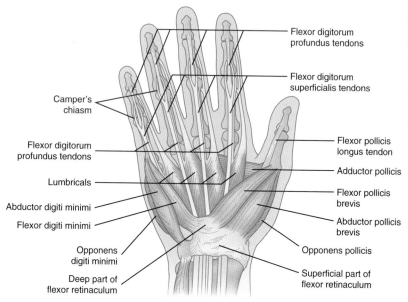

Figure 4.3. Palmer anatomy of the hand showing the thenar and hypothenar compartments as well as the superficial muscles of the central compartment. (*From Shin EK, Hand Fractures and Joint Injuries: Skirven TM, et al. [eds], Rehabilitation of the Hand and Upper Extremity, 6th edn. Mosby, 2011.*)

Table 4.2. Thenar Muscle Group

MUSCLE	ORIGIN	INSERTION	INNERVATION	ACTION
Abductor pollicis brevis (APB)	Scaphoid, trapezium, and transverse carpal ligament (TCL)	Palmar radial base of the proximal phalanx of the thumb	Median nerve, motor recurrent branch (C8–T1)	Abduction/ palmer pronation
Opponens pollicis (OP)	Trapezium and TCL	Radial border of metacarpal of the thumb	Median nerve, motor recurrent branch (C8–T1) with possible contribution of deep ulnar branch (C8–T1)	Opposition against other digits
Flexor pollicis brevis (FPB): a. Superficial head b. Deep head	a. TCL and trapezium b. Trapezoid and capitate	Radial aspect of the proximal phalanx of the thumb	a. Median nerve, motor recurrent branch (C8–T1) b. Deep ulnar branch (C8–T1)	Flexes thumb MP joint

Table 4.3. Hypothenar Muscle Group

MUSCLE	ORIGIN	INSERTION	INNERVATION	ACTION
Palmaris brevis (PB)	Palmer aponeurosis	Dermis of the ulnar aspect of hand	Ulnar nerve, superficial branch (C8–T1)	Tension of skin over ulnar palmar hand
Abductor digiti minimi (ADM)	Pisiform and flexor carpi ulnaris	Ulnar base of proximal phalanx and dorsal aponeurosis of the small finger	Ulnar nerve, deep branch (C8–T1)	Abduction of small finger
Opponens digiti minimi (ODM)	Hamulus of hamate and transverse carpal ligament (TCL)	Ulnar aspect of small finger metacarpal	Ulnar nerve, deep branch (C8–T1)	Opposition of small finger
Flexor digiti minimi (FDM)	Hamulus of hamate and TCL	Ulnar base of proximal phalanx of small finger	Ulnar nerve, deep branch (C8–T1)	MP joint flexion of small finger

Table 4.4. Central Muscle Group

MUSCLE	ORIGIN	INSERTION	INNERVATION	ACTION
Lumbrical muscles (radial 2) 1 and 2 (a.)	a. Flexor digitorum profundus (FDP) tendons, arise from the radial aspect of radial two tendons (unipennate)	Radial aspect of the dorsal digital expansion	Median nerve	Flex metacarpophalangeal (MP) joints and extend interphalangeal (IP) joints
Lumbricals (ulnar 2) 3 and 4 (b.)	b. FDP tendons: three ulnar tendons each attaching to the ulnar and radial aspect of the adjacent tendons (bipennate)	Radial aspect of the dorsal digital expansion	Ulnar nerve, deep branch (C8–T1)	Flex MP joints and extend IP joints

Continued on following page

Table 4.4. Central Muscle Group *(Continued)*

MUSCLE	ORIGIN	INSERTION	INNERVATION	ACTION
Dorsal interossei (4) (bipennate)	Each arises from two heads (bipennate), one on each adjacent metacarpal	Base of the proximal phalanx and dorsal extensor expansions	Ulnar nerve, deep branch (C8–T1)	**Ab**duction and assist the lumbricals in MP joint flexion and IP joint extension
Palmer interossei (3) (unipennate)	The 1st arises from the ulnar aspect of the second metacarpal, while the 2nd and 3rd arise from the radial aspect of the 4th and 5th metacarpals	Insert into the proximal phalanx distally on the same side as their origin	Ulnar nerve, deep branch (C8–T1)	**Ad**duction and assist the lumbricals in MP joint flexion and IP joint extension

21. What mnemonic can help you differentiate the function of the dorsal and palmar interossei?

    DAB and *PAD*: Dorsal *Ab*duct; Palmer *Ad*duct.

    In addition, both dorsal and palmar interossei act to flex the MP joints and assist in extension of the IP joints (Fig. 4.4).

22. What extrinsic flexor tendons enter the hand?

    Extrinsic muscles have origins outside of the hand and traverse the wrist to insert within the hand:

    Superficial flexors: flexor carpi radialis (FCR), palmaris longus (PL), flexor digitorum superficialis (FDS), and flexor carpi ulnaris (FCU).

    Deep flexors: FDP and flexor pollicis longus (FPL).

23. What percentage of people lack a palmaris longus tendon?

    It is estimated that 10–20% of people lack a PL.

24. What is intrinsic plus and intrinsic minus (also termed lumbrical plus or minus)?

    Intrinsic plus is the position of the hand in which the lumbrical muscles are in action: MP joints flexed and IP joints extended. Intrinsic minus describes the opposite position with the intrinsic or lumbrical muscles not in action: MP joints extended and the IP joints flexed.

25. Why are patients' hands placed in the intrinsic plus position when splinted?

    The metacarpal head is ovoid in shape. As a result, the collateral ligaments are at variable length depending on the position of the proximal phalanx. This mechanical property is referred to as the "cam" effect. In the intrinsic plus position, the collateral ligaments are taut.

    If a patient is placed in intrinsic plus position (Fig. 4.5) while splinted, the ligaments will be taut, which will make it easier for the ligaments to move into the loose position (intrinsic minus) when therapy is initiated. Alternatively, if splinted in intrinsic minus, the collateral ligaments may contract while in the "loose" position, causing the inability to achieve the intrinsic plus position (contracture and stiffness).

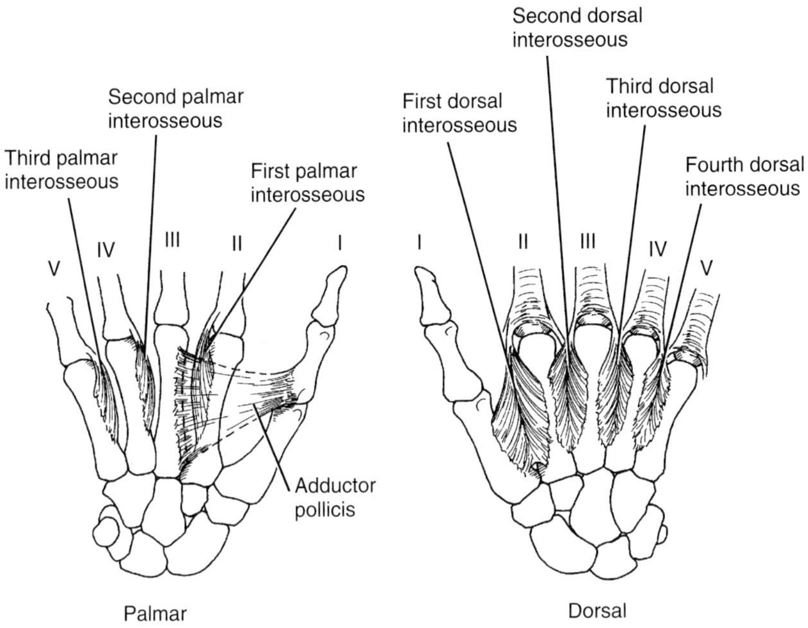

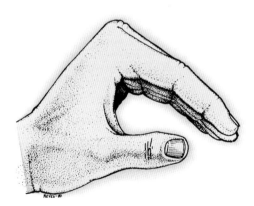

Figure 4.4. Dorsal and volar (palmer) interossei, with adductor pollicis. Recall DAB: Dorsal Abduct. PAD: Palmer Adduct. *(From Trumble TE, [ed]: Principles of Hand Surgery and Therapy. Philadelphia, WB Saunders Company, 2000.)*

Figure 4.5. Intrinsic plus position, also called the "safe" position of the hand. *(From Day CS, Fractures of the Metacarpals and Phalanges: Wolfe SW, et al. [eds], Green's Operative Hand Surgery, 6th edn. Churchill Livingstone, 2011.)*

26. **What is unique about the lumbrical muscles?**

The lumbrical muscles are unique in that they originate from a tendon. Arising from the FDP tendons in the palm, these muscles join the dorsal aponeurosis and act primarily as extensors of the IP joints. As a result of their tendinous origin, the lumbricals are the only muscles that relax an antagonist (FDP) with contraction. The lumbricals also flex the MP joints.

Nerves and Vessels

CASE 4-4

A 22-year-old female presents to the Emergency Department after incurring a laceration to her wrist from a broken champagne glass. On examination, the patient has a 6 cm laceration on the volar and ulnar aspect of the wrist. Although there is only a small amount of active bleeding, the patient reports having had pulsatile bleeding at the time of the injury. The patient is unable to voluntarily flex the ring and small fingers. The patient has decreased sensation on the palmar surface of the ring and small fingers and she cannot abduct or adduct the fingers. She has a 2+ radial pulse, and brisk capillary refill of all fingers.

27. **What structures are likely injured and what is the next step?**
    In this clinical scenario, there are probably injuries to the flexor tendons of the ring and small fingers, the ulnar artery, and the ulnar nerve. The next step is surgical exploration with irrigation, debridement, and repair of critical structures. The timing of this intervention is controversial in the setting of a hand that is well-perfused by collateral circulation.

28. **What is the blood supply to the hand?**
    The radial and ulnar arteries supply the hand; both arise from the brachial artery (Fig. 4.6):
    The deep palmer arch is primarily supplied by the deep branch of the radial artery: The radial artery enters the wrist dorsally in the anatomic "snuff box" and gives rise to the *dorsal carpal branch*, which provides the primary vascular supply to the dorsum of the hand. The radial artery then perforates the two heads of the first dorsal interosseous muscle and then branches into the *princeps policis* and the *deep branch of the radial artery*, which becomes the deep palmar arch. The ulnar artery also contributes a deep branch to the deep palmar arch. The deep palmar arch lies proximal to the superficial arch at the level of the base of the metacarpals.
    Princeps policis (a branch of the radial artery that supplies the thumb): This artery provides vascular supply to the radial aspect of the index finger, as well as the two digital arteries of the thumb. However, the vascular supply to the thumb is highly variable.
    The superficial palmer arch is primarily supplied by the ulnar artery: The ulnar artery enters the wrist through Guyon's canal, on the radial side of the ulnar nerve. It gives off the deep branch which wraps around the hook of the hamate and continues into the palm as a contributor to the deep palmer arch, joining the deep branch from the radial artery. The ulnar artery is the primary contributor to the superficial palmar arch. This superficial arch gives rise to 3–4 common digital arteries, which bifurcate into the proper digital arteries, and traverse the radial and ulnar sides of the fingers deep to the digital nerves.

29. **What is Guyon's canal?**
    Guyon's canal is defined by the transverse carpal ligament (TCL) and hypothenar muscles as the floor, the hook of the hamate radially, the pisiform and abductor digiti minimi (ADM) ulnarly, and the volar carpal ligament as the roof. The ulnar nerve and ulnar artery traverse the canal, with the nerve on the ulnar side of the artery. The ulnar nerve may be compressed within Guyon's canal, leading to ulnar tunnel syndrome.

30. **What are the symptoms of ulnar tunnel syndrome?**
    Patients with ulnar tunnel syndrome have numbness in the volar aspect of the small finger and ulnar half of the ring finger. Because the dorsal sensory branch of the ulnar nerve splits prior to Guyon's canal, these patients do not have numbness on the dorsal ulnar aspect of the hand. This can help to distinguish ulnar tunnel syndrome from cubital tunnel syndrome. Furthermore, if the compression is severe enough, patients can have weakness and atrophy of the intrinsic muscles of the hand.

31. **What is the Allen's test?**
    The Allen's test evaluates the vascular contribution of the radial and ulnar arteries to the hand (Fig. 4.7). With pressure on the radial and ulnar arteries at the wrist, the patient is asked to open and close their fist several times, which removes all of the blood from the

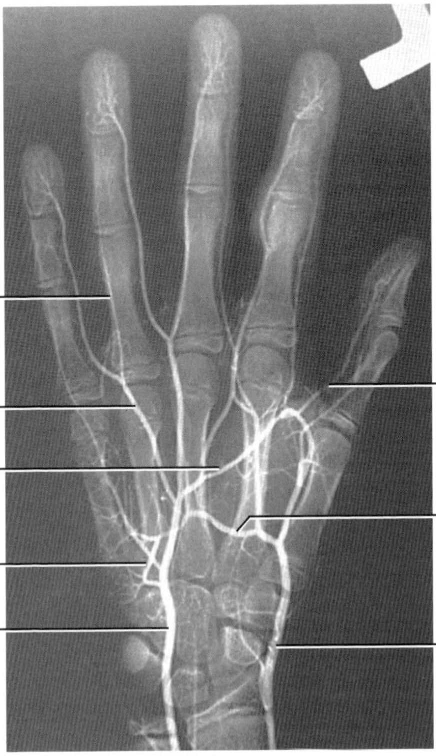

Figure 4.6. Arteriogram of the hand which demonstrates the ulnar artery contribution to the superficial palmar arch. (*Courtesy of Dr D. Armstrong, Associate Professor of Radiology, University of Toronto, Ontario, Canada. In: Mailhot T, Lyn ET, Rosen's Emergency Medicine: Concepts and Clinical Practice, 8th edn.*)

hand. Next, the patient opens their fist. The examiner releases the radial or ulnar artery, and the hand is observed for return of circulation to the fingers. The hand should flush immediately after release of either of the arteries. The procedure is repeated with release of the other artery. Failure to flush, or a slow return, suggests occlusion of one of the arteries or an incomplete arch. This test should be performed prior to any surgery around the wrist. If there is an iatrogenic injury to the dominant vessel to the hand (radial or ulnar artery), this would necessitate immediate repair.

32. **What are the sensory nerve distributions of the hand?**
    Radial nerve: This superficial radial nerve supplies the dorsal aspect of the thumb, index finger, long finger, and radial aspect of ring finger proximal to about the proximal interphalangeal joint (PIPJ). Furthermore, it supplies the dorsal-radial side of the hand. It is best evaluated at the dorsal surface of the first web space.
    Ulnar nerve: The ulnar nerve supplies the small finger and the ulnar half of the ring finger on both the dorsal and volar aspects. The dorsal aspects are supplied by the dorsal sensory branch of the ulnar nerve, which branches proximal to the wrist. Overall, the ulnar nerve is best evaluated at the tip of the small finger.
    Median nerve: This nerve supplies the thumb, index finger, long finger, and radial side of the ring finger on the palmar aspect. Furthermore, it supplies the dorsal aspect distal to about the PIPJ of these same fingers. It is best evaluated at the tip of the index finger.

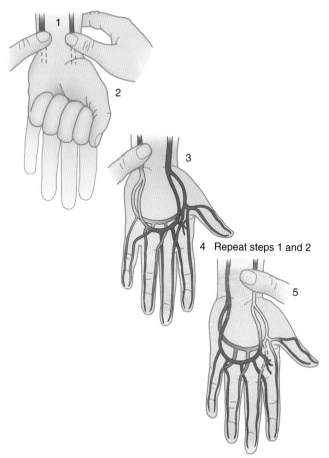

Figure 4.7. An illustrated step-by-step guide to Allen's test. (*From American Society for Surgery of the Hand: The Hand: Examination and Diagnosis, 3rd edn. New York, Churchill Livingstone, 1990, p. 46.*)

33. **What examination can be used to test specific motor nerve function of the hand?**
   Radial nerve: Wrist extension
   Posterior interosseous nerve (PIN): Finger/thumb extension
   Median nerve (motor recurrent branch): Thumb opposition
   Anterior interosseous nerve (AIN): Index finger distal interphalangeal joint (DIPJ) flexion and thumb IP flexion
   Ulnar nerve (proximal to wrist): Small finger DIPJ flexion
   Ulnar nerve (deep branch): Index finger/small finger abduction and adduction (crossing fingers).

34. **What muscles are innervated by the median nerve distal to the carpal tunnel?**
   The mnemonic *LOAF* can be helpful. The median nerve supplies motor branches to the index finger and long finger *L*umbricals, *O*pponens pollicis, *A*bductor pollicis brevis, and the superficial head of the *F*lexor pollicis brevis. Opposition of the thumb is tested by having the patient touch the tips of the thumb and small finger.

35. **What are the borders of the carpal tunnel?**
   The carpal canal is defined by the TCL as the roof, the scaphoid tubercle and trapezium radially, the hook of the hamate and pisiform radially, and the carpus as the floor.

36. **What are potential causes of carpal tunnel syndrome (CTS)?**
    CTS or compression of the median nerve can be caused by any factor that increases carpal tunnel pressures. This includes anatomic abnormalities (proximal lumbrical muscles), trauma (distal radius fractures), fluid imbalances (pregnancy), inflammatory conditions (rheumatoid arthritis), associated medical conditions (diabetes), and positional factors. Psychosocial factors are also known to contribute to the diseased state.

37. **How is CTS diagnosed and treated?**
    CTS is a clinical diagnosis. Most patients complain of numbness in the median nerve distribution (radial 3½ fingers), which typically is worse at night and with activity. As CTS progresses, the numbness can become more constant, and patients often complain of clumsiness or thenar weakness. A nerve conduction velocity (NCV) study and electromyography (EMG) is useful for confirming the diagnosis and documenting severity.
    CTS is initially treated with night-time wrist splints, which prevent hyperflexion of the wrists. If symptoms continue to persist, a corticosteroid injection or carpal tunnel release is considered.

Flexor Tendons

38. **List the contents of the carpal tunnel.**
    The carpal tunnel contains the median nerve and nine flexor tendons. Specifically, these tendons are the four FDS, the four FDP, and the FPL (Fig. 4.8).

39. **What are the vinculae tendinum?**
    The vincula are thin synovial folds that transmit blood vessels to the dorsal side of the flexor tendons. Each FDS and FDP tendon has a vinculum brevis and a vinculum longus.

40. **What pulleys make up the fibro-osseous flexor pulley system for the fingers?**
    There are five annular (A) and three cruciate (C) pulleys, which are numbered from proximal to distal. The A1, 3 and 5 pulleys are located at the MP, PIP and distal interphalangeal (DIP) joints, respectively. The A2 and A4 pulleys are located at the mid portion of the proximal phalanx and the middle phalanx, respectively. The three cruciate pulleys are less well-developed than the annular pulleys and are located between A2 and A3, between A3 and A4, and between A4 and A5. They act as accordions, taking up slack in the sheath with flexion of the finger.

41. **Which of the pulleys of the flexor tendon sheath are most important in preventing bowstringing?**
    Although biomechanical studies have shown the A1 pulley to be the strongest, the A2 and A4 pulleys are the most important in preventing the tendons from bowstringing. Often, patients with bowstringing of the flexor tendons have ruptured multiple pulleys, including A-3.

42. **What is the clinical significance of the A1 pulley?**
    The A1 pulley is involved in trigger finger or stenosing tenosynovitis, which is a discrepancy between the flexor tendons and the sheath. Clinically, this presents as triggering or locking of the finger and is frequently seen in patients with diabetes and/or hypothyroidism.

43. **What is the treatment for trigger fingers?**
    Typically, trigger fingers are initially treated with a corticosteroid injection, which is successful approximately 50–60% of the time. If patients fail one or more corticosteroid injections, they are candidates for surgery, which involves release of the A1 pulley.

CASE 4-5

A 24-year-old student cut the palmar surface of his ring finger on a can just proximal to the PIP joint crease. The finger lies in the extended position and does not follow the normal "cascade" of the fingers. Additionally, the patient complains that he is unable to flex his ring finger at either the PIP or DIP joints. The patient is in moderate pain but his sensation in the finger is intact, and the distal digit remains well-perfused.

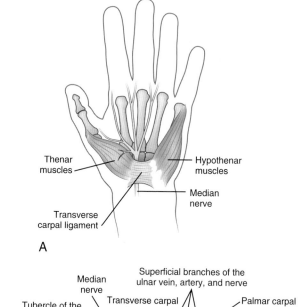

A

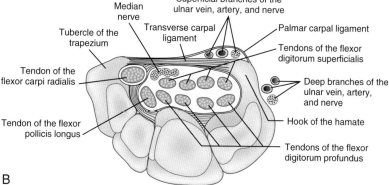

B

Figure 4.8. The carpal tunnel (A) seen from a palmer view, illustrating the relationship of the median nerve to the TCL and (B) a cross-sectional view at the level of the distal carpal row, demonstrating the relationships between the contents of the carpal tunnel: nine tendons and one nerve. If the median nerve is compressed or irritated, this results in the symptoms of CTS. (*Redrawing based on an illustration by Li-Guo Liang. In: Yu HL, Chase RA, Strauch B: Atlas of Hand Anatomy and Clinical Implications, Philadelphia, Mosby, 2004, p. 513.*)

44. **What structures are likely injured?**
    Based on his lack of finger flexion and complete loss of the resting cascade, it is likely that both the FDS and FDP have been completely transected. If only the FDS had been lacerated, the cascade could appear normal.

45. **How do you test the function of the FDS and FDP?**
    To test FDP function, the PIP joint is stabilized in extension, and the patient is asked to flex the DIP joint. Given that both the FDP and the FDS flex the PIP joint, testing of the FDS is more difficult. In order to do so, the FDP must be limited from functioning within the finger. This is accomplished by holding all the other fingers in extension. By doing this, all the FDP tendons are incapacitated because they are connected at the wrist, and flexion of the finger at the PIP must result from FDS function. Because the FDP of the

index finger is usually not connected to the other FDP tendons at the wrist, it is often not possible to test the FDS of the index by this method.

46. **What is the tenodesis effect and how may this be applied to testing patients with possible tendon lacerations?**
This is the effect of flexion and extension of the wrist on flexion and extension of the fingers. With intact tendons, extension of the wrist will produce flexion of the fingers, and flexion of the wrist will cause extension of the fingers. This maneuver is quite useful in the unconscious or uncooperative patient.

47. **What other methods can be used to diagnose a flexor tendon injury?**
In the normal hand, the tone of the forearm muscles and the intact tendons hold the fingers in a position of slight flexion, with the index being the least flexed and the small finger being the most flexed. This formation is referred to as the normal finger "resting cascade." Following a tendon laceration, the injured finger lies extended, and this cascade is disrupted. In a child or in an uncooperative patient, gentle pressure on the musculature in the forearm will generally cause some slight finger flexion confirming the continuity of the flexor tendon (Fig. 4.9).

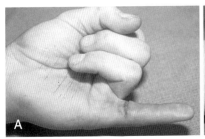 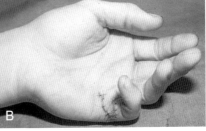

Figure 4.9. (A) Laceration of the flexor digitorum superficialis and flexor digitorum profundus tendons with inability for the patient to flex the finger. (B) After surgical repair, flexion and the normal resting cascade is restored.

48. **What zones are used to describe the location of flexor tendon injuries and where is "No Man's Land"?**
There are five zones of flexor tendon laceration (Fig. 4.10). "No man's" land is the area in which *both* flexor tendons of the fingers pass through the tight fibro-osseous tunnel. Designated as Zone II, it is the area between the distal palmar crease and the insertion of the FDS at the mid-portion of the middle phalanx. Repair of tendon lacerations in this region requires meticulous technique, and complications are more frequent:
Zone I: From the insertion of the FDP at the distal phalanx to just distal to the insertion of the FDS on the middle phalanx
Zone II: From the insertion of the FDS on the middle phalanx to the distal palmar crease
Zone III: From the distal palmar crease to the distal edge of the carpal tunnel
Zone IV: Carpal tunnel
Zone V: From the proximal edge of the carpal tunnel to the musculotendinous junction.

49. **What are the main factors that determine the strength of flexor tendon repair at the time of surgery?**
Several factors are considered important for a strong tendon repair. The size, ultimate tensile strength and elongation of the suture material are important. The number of suture strands crossing the repair site has been shown to be roughly proportional to the strength of the repair. Four strands of suture in the core of the tendon are generally needed to be able to withstand the stress of an early active motion therapy program. Also, the method of attaching the suture to the tendon is important and locking stitches are considered to provide a stronger attachment than grasping stitches.

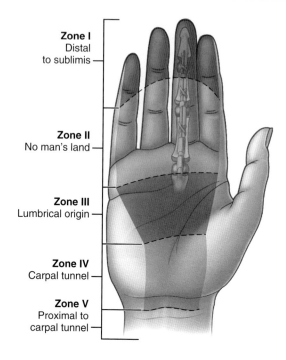

Figure 4.10. Zones of injury for flexor tendons. (*Reprinted from Cannon DL, Campbell's Operative Orthopaedics, pp. 3247–3304.e5. © 2013 Copyright by Mosby, an imprint of Elsevier Inc.*)

Zone I
Distal to sublimis

Zone II
No man's land

Zone III
Lumbrical origin

Zone IV
Carpal tunnel

Zone V
Proximal to carpal tunnel

50. **What are the most frequent complications after repair of flexor tendons?**
Flexor tendon repairs, especially in Zone II, are at risk for complications because of the tight pulley system and the need for smooth gliding, or excursion, of the tendon through the pulleys to flex the finger. Tendon re-rupture can occur if motion is too vigorous before healing has occurred. If motion is initiated too late, adhesions form around the tendon, leading to stiffness and decreased motion. Both of these complications typically require re-operation and can result in significant loss of function.

CASE 4-6

A 20-year-old football player attempted to stop an opposing player from breaking loose by grabbing his jersey. At that moment, the opposing player broke away. The patient states that he felt immediate pain in his ring finger and was unable to flex it fully. He continued to play but noticed increasing swelling of the finger.

51. **What is the most likely diagnosis in this patient?**
A jersey finger is an avulsion of the FDP tendon from its insertion into the distal phalanx. It is commonly a sports injury that occurs when a player tries to grab another player's jersey. The resisted, forceful extension causes the tendon to avulse from the distal phalanx (Fig. 4.11). The diagnosis is made by the inability of the patient to flex the distal phalanx. On radiographic evaluation, a fleck of bone may be found on the palmar surface of the finger. This injury should be treated by early surgical repair, especially if the tendon has retracted proximally.

CASE 4-7

A 21-year-old male presents to the Emergency Department with the inability to completely extend his middle finger after sustaining a puncture wound from a shard of glass. On exam the patient maintains some ability to extend at the IP joints, but is unable to extend at the MP joint.

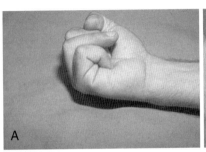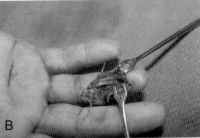

Figure 4.11. A jersey finger with inability of the patient to flex the distal interphalangeal joint. The flexor digitorum profundus insertion can be seen avulsed from the attachment to the distal phalanx.

52. **What is the diagnosis? Why is some extension of the fingers spared?**
    The extensor tendon alone is responsible for the extension of the MP joint, while the intrinsics aid in IP joint extension (Fig. 4.12).

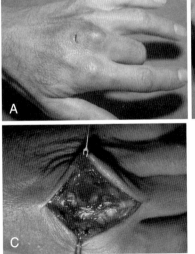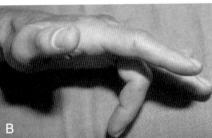

Figure 4.12. Patient's puncture wound (A), physical exam findings (B), and intraoperative visualization of an extensor tendon laceration (C).

53. **What are the zones of extensor tendon injury?**
    Described by Kleinert, and Verdan and later modified by Doyle, there are nine zones of extensor tendon injury (Fig. 4.13).

54. **How are extensor tendon lacerations repaired?**
    The primary suture repair configuration, as well as the size and type of suture used, is often dependent on the zone of the tendon injury. After primary repair, patients are typically placed in a palmar splint holding the MP joint in 20–30° of flexion and the PIP and DIP joints in extension. Recently, early active protocols have been gaining popularity.

55. **Can you describe the extensor mechanism?** (Fig. 4.14)
    The EDC to each finger, along with the EIP to the index finger and the EDM to the small finger, form the common extensor tendon. Without attaching to the proximal phalanx,

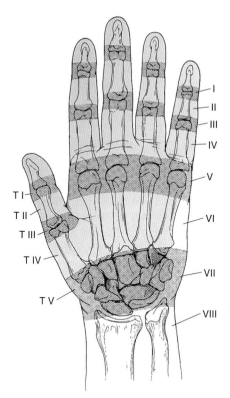

I
II
III
IV
V
VI
VII
VIII

T I
T II
T III
T IV
T V

Figure 4.13. Zones of extensor tendon injury, with the zones for the finger labeled on the small finger, and the distinct thumb (T) zones labeled along the thumb. Diagram excludes Zone IX, which involves the proximal forearm. *(From Trumble TE, et al. [eds]: Core Knowledge in Orthopaedics: Hand, Elbow, and Shoulder. Philadelphia, Mosby, 2006, p. 203.)*

this tendon extends the MP joint via the sagittal bands, which travel in a volar direction from the extensor tendon around the MP joint to join the volar plate. The sagittal bands serve to centralize the common extensor tendon, but also functionally pull the proximal phalanx into extension.

At the level of the proximal phalanx, the extensor tendon is joined by the lateral bands, which are the terminal tendinous extensions of the intrinsic muscles of the hand (the lumbricals and the interossei). These lateral bands join the extensor tendon to extend the PIP joint via the central slip. The tendons of the intrinsic muscles lie palmar to the axis of motion at the MP joint and, therefore, flex the MP joint; however, they lie dorsal to the axis of the PIP joint and, therefore, are the primary extensors of the PIP joint. At the PIP joint, the lateral bands divide and travel distally to form the terminal tendon that extends the DIP joint. This is the sole extensor of the DIP joint.

CASE 4-8

An 18-year-old male presents to the Emergency Department after a basketball injury and is unable to extend at the DIP joint of the long finger. While attempting to rebound the ball, he "jammed" his finger. On exam, the patient's finger is held in a flexed position. Although the finger can be extended passively, the patient is unable to actively extend the DIP joint. An image of the patient's finger can be seen below (Fig. 4.15).

Posterior (dorsal) view

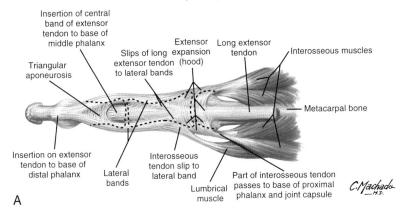

- Insertion of central band of extensor tendon to base of middle phalanx
- Triangular aponeurosis
- Slips of long extensor tendon to lateral bands
- Extensor expansion (hood)
- Long extensor tendon
- Interosseous muscles
- Metacarpal bone
- Insertion on extensor tendon to base of distal phalanx
- Lateral bands
- Interosseous tendon slip to lateral band
- Part of interosseous tendon passes to base of proximal phalanx and joint capsule
- Lumbrical muscle

C.Machado —M.D.

A

Finger in extension: lateral view

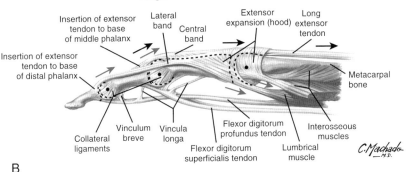

- Insertion of extensor tendon to base of middle phalanx
- Lateral band
- Central band
- Extensor expansion (hood)
- Long extensor tendon
- Insertion of extensor tendon to base of distal phalanx
- Metacarpal bone
- Collateral ligaments
- Vinculum breve
- Vincula longa
- Flexor digitorum profundus tendon
- Flexor digitorum superficialis tendon
- Interosseous muscles
- Lumbrical muscle

C.Machado —M.D.

B

Finger in flexion: lateral view

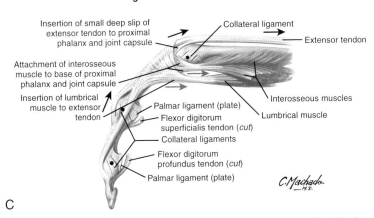

- Insertion of small deep slip of extensor tendon to proximal phalanx and joint capsule
- Collateral ligament
- Extensor tendon
- Attachment of interosseous muscle to base of proximal phalanx and joint capsule
- Insertion of lumbrical muscle to extensor tendon
- Palmar ligament (plate)
- Flexor digitorum superficialis tendon (*cut*)
- Collateral ligaments
- Flexor digitorum profundus tendon (*cut*)
- Palmar ligament (plate)
- Interosseous muscles
- Lumbrical muscle

C.Machado —M.D.

C

Figure 4.14. Extensor tendon anatomy. (A–C: Netter illustrations adapted with permission from Netter's Orthopaedics, Chapter 16, pp. 335–362. Copyright © 2006 by Elsevier Inc. All rights reserved.)

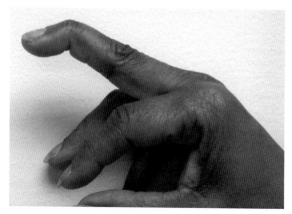

Figure 4.15. Patient presenting to Emergency Room with inability to extend the right long finger distal interphalangeal joint. *(From Roberts JR, et al. [eds], Roberts and Hedges' Clinical Procedures in Emergency Medicine. 6th edn, pp. 954–998.e2. Copyright © Saunders, Elsevier Inc., 2014.)*

56. What is a mallet finger?

Mallet finger describes a flexion deformity of the DIP joint due to loss of continuity of the extensor tendon (Fig. 4.16). It may be due to a tearing of the extensor tendon or an avulsion fracture of the tendon at the tendon insertion. It is considered a Zone I extensor tendon injury.

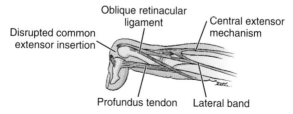

Figure 4.16. Diagram of mallet finger injury with disruption of the extensor tendon. *(From Roberts JR, et al. [eds], Roberts and Hedges' Clinical Procedures in Emergency Medicine, 6th edn, pp. 954–998.e2. Copyright © Saunders, Elsevier Inc., 2014.)*

57. What are the types of mallet finger injuries?

Type 1: Closed injury with loss of tendon continuity with or without a small avulsion fracture

Type 2: Open injury with loss of tendon continuity

Type 3: Open injury with loss of skin and tendon substance

Type 4: Large fractures of the articular surface.

58. How do you treat a mallet finger?

Type 1: The preferred treatment method is DIP joint extension splinting. Classically, this involves 6 weeks of full-time splinting and 6 weeks of night-time splinting. However, the period of splinting is dependent on healing and physician preference.

Types 2 and 3: Because they are open injuries, these are usually treated with open repair +/− DIP joint pinning, followed by splinting.

Type 4: These injuries can be treated open or closed. Many surgeons advocate surgical treatment if the fracture involves greater than 30% of the articular surface or if the joint is subluxated in a volar direction. The procedure often involves DIP joint pinning to maintain reduction.

59. **What are some key points to remember with regard to mallet finger?**
    1. Radiographic evaluation is necessary to determine if there is a fracture.
    2. Only the DIP needs to be splinted.
    3. A closed injury with no fracture can be treated with continuous splinting.
    4. If a fracture involves greater than 30–50% of the joint surface and/or the joint is subluxated, surgery is typically recommended.

CASE 4-9

A 22-year-old woman sustained a minimally displaced fracture of her distal radius. She was treated in a cast. At her 6-week clinic visit, you remove the cast and you notice that she is unable to extend the thumb.

60. **What is the most likely diagnosis?**
    Rupture of the EPL tendon can be seen following fractures of the distal radius. It is usually secondary to hematoma compression and subsequent attrition of the tendon within the third dorsal compartment. It is more common with minimally displaced fractures in which the third dorsal compartment is still intact.

CASE 4-10 (Fig. 4.17)

A 30-year-old man had a window fall on the dorsal aspect of the PIP joint of his small finger. Initially, he appeared to have extension of the PIP joint, and he was given a finger splint to hold the joint in extension. He was non-compliant with this treatment and did not wear the splint. As he continued to use the finger, he became unable to extend the PIP joint, and the DIP joint developed a hyperextended position.

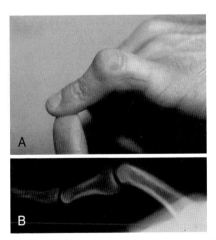

Figure 4.17. Photo (A) and radiograph (B) of the above patient's disease process.

61. **What is the diagnosis and why does this often develop weeks or months after the injury?**
    This finger has a flexed PIP joint and a hyperextended DIP joint, also called a boutonnière deformity. Initially, even though the central slip is injured, the two lateral bands lie on the dorsal aspect of the PIP joint and allow for extension. However, over time, the lateral bands slowly migrate in a palmar direction with the PIP joint button-holing between

them. As the lateral bands reach a critical point palmar to the axis of the joint, they pull the PIP joint into flexion rather than extension.

ARTHRITIS AND ARTHROPLASTY OF THE HAND AND WRIST

CASE 4-11

A 61-year-old female is referred for pain at the base of her right thumb, which has been steadily increasing over the past 5 years. She describes the pain as a dull and constant ache that becomes sharp while writing or playing video games with her grandchildren. The patient denies trauma. On physical examination, the patient has normal range of motion of the thumb but has pain with axial loading with thumb-index finger pinch. There is a prominent swelling at the base of the thumb, and Finkelstein test is negative. There is marked laxity in the radioulnar plane and crepitus is elicited with motion. Lastly, on testing of strength, the patient is found to be significantly weaker compared to the contralateral side.

62. **What is the differential diagnosis for this patient?**
    In a patient with pain at the base of the thumb there are several considerations, including De Quervain's tenosynovitis, thumb stenosing tenosynovitis, thumb CMC joint arthritis, and FCR tendonitis. With a negative Finkelstein test (pathognomonic of De Quervain's), smooth flexion and extension of the joint with no triggering, thumb CMC joint arthritis is the most likely diagnosis.

63. **What are the radiographic findings and anatomic considerations associated with thumb basal joint arthritis?**
    The thumb CMC joint is a saddle joint, which allows for circumduction as well as flexion–extension and radial-ulnar motion. This joint is very mobile but has a high incidence of degenerative arthritis. The severity of thumb basal joint arthritis is characterized by radiographic findings and is staged from I to IV:
    Stage I: Normal radiographs or joint space widening secondary to synovitis
    Stage II: Mild joint space narrowing and osteophyte formation less than 2 mm
    Stage III: Significant joint space narrowing osteophyte formation greater than 2 mm
    Stage IV: Similar to stage III, but with associated STT joint involvement.

64. **Who is at greatest risk for CMC arthritis? (Figs 4.18, 4.19)**
    Osteoarthritis of the thumb CMC joint, also known as basal joint arthritis, has a predilection for postmenopausal women, affecting as many as 50% of women after menopause.

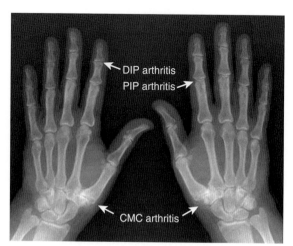

Figure 4.18. Plain radiographs of thumb carpometacarpal arthritis, with some degree of distal interphalangeal and proximal interphalangeal joint arthritis. (*From Sears ED, Chung KC, Arthroplasty Procedures in the Hand: Chung KC, Evans GRD, [eds], Hand and Upper Extremity Reconstruction, 1st edn. Saunders, 2009.*)

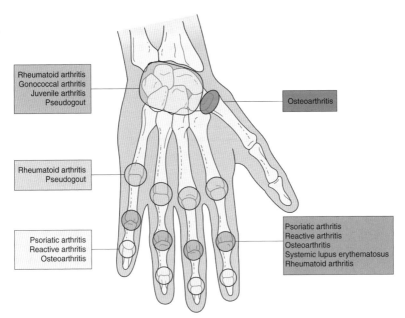

Figure 4.19. Common sites of arthritis; it is notable that rheumatoid arthritis is distal interphalangeal (DIP) sparing while psoriatic arthritis most frequently involves the DIP joint. Although osteoarthritis is common in many joints (actually more common in the DIP joint) it is very frequently found in the carpometacarpal joint of the thumb. (*Adapted from Longo DL, Fauci AS, Kasper D, et al. Harrison's Principles of Internal Medicine, 18th edn. New York, McGraw Hill, 2011.*)

65. Describe the treatment options for CMC arthritis of the thumb.
    Conservative treatment includes activity modification, thumb spica splinting, oral non-steroidal antiinflammatories (NSAIDs), and corticosteroid injection. The indications for operative intervention include pain that is unresponsive to conservative measures, loss of function, and/or joint instability. Surgical options include trapeziectomy with or without ligament reconstruction and/or tendon interposition. The combination of a tendon interposition and ligament stabilization is known as the LRTI (Ligament Reconstruction Tendon Interposition) procedure.

66. What are the key aspects of the LRTI procedure?
    1. Resection of the trapezium
    2. Anterior oblique ligament reconstruction to improve joint stability
    3. Tendon interposition to preserve the joint space.

67. What other treatment options are available for CMC arthritis of the thumb?
    CMC arthrodesis or fusion is a suitable option in a young patient with an occupation demanding forceful use of the hand. Various prosthetic implants including silastic (silicone based), metal, and other substances have been used, but none has demonstrated superiority to the LRTI procedure.

CASE 4-12

A 55-year-old right handed man has been referred by his primary care provider with pain in his right long finger DIP joint and to a lesser extent also the ring finger PIP joint. There is minimal deformity noted, but his pain is severe. The patient works as a carpenter and describes the pain as dull but progressively worsening as the day progresses. The patient has tried NSAIDs, which have helped in the past, without success. The patient is otherwise healthy.

68. **What is the most likely diagnosis, and how is this treated?**
    This patient likely has osteoarthritis of the DIP joint. Non-operative management with antiinflammatory medication, activity modification, and possibly bracing, is the first line of treatment. DIP arthrodesis is the typical surgical intervention of choice.

69. **What are Heberden's nodes?**
    Heberden's nodes are bone spurs or exostoses that form from osteoarthritis on the dorsal aspect of the DIP joints. Although typically small, these exostoses around the DIP joint may give the joint a "knobby" appearance.

70. **What are Bouchard's nodes.**
    Bouchard's nodes are osteophytes that develop on the dorsal aspect of the PIP joints, a less frequent site of osteoarthritis. These are commonly associated with rheumatoid arthritis.

71. **What is the most common indication for surgical intervention in cases of DIP arthritis?**
    Pain is the most common indication for the surgical treatment of DIP joint arthritis.

72. **What are the available arthroplasty options for MCP and PIP joints?**
    For both metacarpophalangeal (MCP) and PIP joints, there are silicone implants, pyrolytic carbon implants, and surface replacement arthroplasty options available. There is no clearly superior implant, based on the current literature, and all implants are prone to subsequent infection, instability, wear, and/or fracture.

73. **What is the most commonly used arthroplasty for the digits?**
    Silicone elastomer based resection arthroplasty is the most commonly used arthroplasty technique for MP and PIP joints.

74. **What are the primary indications for surgical intervention in MCP, PIP and DIP arthritis?**
    1. Pain
    2. Deformity.

75. **Which patients are at risk of developing degenerative arthritis after a fracture of the distal radius?**
    Patients with intra-articular extension of the fracture into the radiocarpal joint or the distal radioulnar joint (DRUJ) are at greatest risk for developing degenerative arthritis. Specifically, fractures extending into the radiocarpal joint that subsequently heal with greater than 2 mm of intra-articular incongruity have been shown to be at increased risk for developing degenerative arthritis.

RHEUMATOID ARTHRITIS

CASE 4-13 (Fig. 4.20)

A 50-year-old women presents to clinic after referral from her rheumatologist for surgical evaluation. The patient complains of ongoing finger and wrist pain, which is worse in the mornings and improves through the course of the day. The pain is predominantly in her hands; however, the patient also has had a significant amount of jaw and neck pain recently. On examination there is marked ulnar deviation of her fingers bilaterally and moderate deformity including boutonnière deformities with varied severity in all the fingers. The deformity is passively correctable at the time of examination.

76. **What is the pathophysiology of rheumatoid arthritis?**
    Rhematoid arthritis (RA) is a systemic autoimmune disorder that involves the synovial tissue. It is typically bilateral and involving multiple joints (**polyarthritis**). Synovial inflammation and hyperplasia lead to the formation of synovial tissue referred to as pannus. This inflammatory process can lead to joint deformity, then joint destruction, and eventually joint ankylosis.

77. **What is a Brewerton view?**
    A Brewerton view is a variation of the antero-posterior (AP) radiograph of the hand. It can be useful in evaluating patient's with rheumatoid arthritis. The fingers are placed

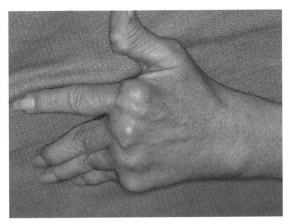

Figure 4.20. Rheumatoid arthritis patient seen with marked finger deformity.

flat on the radiographic plate, and the metacarpals are inclined at an angle of 65°. The x-ray tube is then inclined 15° toward the ulnar side of the hand. The Brewerton view may show bony erosive changes beneath the collateral ligaments of the MP joints early in the course of RA, when standard AP radiographs of the hand demonstrate little change.

78. **In advanced rheumatoid arthritis, what MP joint deformity is typically seen? What are the underlying causes?**
    The classic deformity seen in rheumatoid arthritis is ulnar drift of the digits and volar subluxation of the proximal phalanges. Various factors are responsible for the pathophysiology, including MP joint synovitis, articular cartilage erosion with bony destruction, extensor tendon ulnar subluxation or dislocation (due to selective stretching of the radial support structures), ligamentous disruption, intrinsic tightness, and forces of gravity. The ulnar drift of the fingers is often accompanied by radial deviation of the wrist, creating the characteristic Z-deformity seen in RA patients.

79. **What is one contraindication to synovectomy?**
    Synovectomy is not a useful procedure in patients with rapidly progressive joint disease. In these patients, reconstructive surgery is the preferred method and is optimally preformed prior to significant deformity.

80. **What non-surgical perioperative considerations are of particular importance for RA patients?**
    Prior to undergoing a procedure to correct RA deformity or other sequelae of disease, one should consider cervical spine instability (for anesthesia), temporo-mandibular joint involvement (for anesthesia), pulmonary involvement, immunologic compromise (from either Felty's syndrome or disease modifying pharmacotherapy), and thrombocytopenia (as a result of disease modifying agents). Regardless of the apparent stage of disease, these patients should be evaluated in consultation with a rheumatologist.

81. **What is caput ulnae syndrome?**
    Caput ulnae syndrome refers to the destructive process initiated by synovitis of the DRUJ. Characteristic findings include loss of wrist rotation (pronation and supination), dorsal prominence of the distal ulna, instability of the distal ulna, and soft-tissue swelling over the ulnar head (Fig. 4.21). There is a loss of the normal action of the ECU tendon. The extensor tendons to the ring and small fingers may rupture due to ongoing synovitis resulting in loss of the ability to extend the ring and small finger.

82. **What are the indications for total wrist arthroplasty?**
    The ideal indication for total wrist arthroplasty is wrist pain due to advanced rheumatoid RA in a patient with a contralateral wrist arthrodesis. While the procedure can be

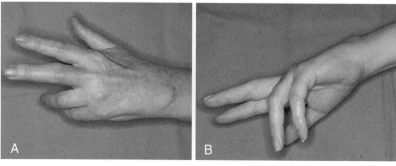

Figure 4.21. Caput ulnae syndrome with characteristic findings (A and B) dorsal prominence of the ulnar head.

beneficial for post-traumatic or degenerative arthritis, it is less frequently the treatment of choice in those circumstances. The operation is best suited for patients who have involvement of other joints in the upper extremities, with limited finger, forearm, elbow, and/or shoulder motion. Total wrist arthroplasty is desirable in such patients because some upper extremity motion is conserved. Wrist arthrodesis, however, is still the preferred procedure for most patients with advanced wrist arthritis because it provides pain relief with few complications (Fig. 4.22).

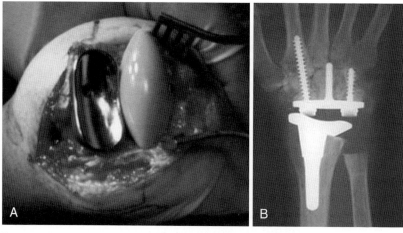

Figure 4.22. (A) Intraoperative photograph of a total wrist prosthesis during implantation. (B) and (C) Postoperative radiographs after total wrist arthroplasty. *(A and B: Stanley J, Arthroplasty and Arthrodesis of the Wrist: Wolfe SW, et al. [eds], Green's Operative Hand Surgery, 6th edn. Churchill Livingstone, 2011. C: From Sestero AM, et al., Rheumatoid Arthritis – Hand and Wrist: Trumble TE, et al. [eds], Skeletal Reconstruction: Core Knowledge in Orthopaedics – Hand, Elbow, and Shoulder, 1st edn. Mosby, 2006.)*

83. **What are the contraindications for total wrist arthroplasty?**
The only true contraindication for total wrist arthroplasty is active infection. However, soft tissue concerns, including tendon quality, can also exclude this as a treatment option. Furthermore, young and/or active patients are not recommended to have a total wrist arthroplasty due to the high rate of failure.

84. **What are the most common complications of total wrist arthroplasty?**
The most common complication of total wrist arthroplasty is loosening of the distal component, which has been found in approximately 20% of wrists over a 5-year period.

A second potential complication is dislocation of the prosthesis. Both of these complications may cause swelling and secondary carpal tunnel syndrome. Failure of total wrist arthroplasty typically requires conversion to a wrist fusion, although this can be challenging in the setting of bone loss.

Additional complications include:

Other implant component loosening and failure

Peri-prosthetic fracture

Infection.

85. **What is one concern particular to implants that use silicone?**

Silicone synovitis is a complication unique to these implants. Silicone debris can cause an inflammatory reaction, resulting in proliferative synovitis and subsequent bone erosion. This complication is most often seen in wrist and MP arthroplasty and can lead to revision surgery.

86. **Which flexor tendon most commonly ruptures in rheumatoid arthritis?**

The FPL is the tendon that most commonly ruptures in RA (Mannerfelt syndrome). The rupture is usually due to attrition as the tendon passes over a bone spur or erosion on the scaphoid. Treatment usually consists of surgical reconstruction with a tendon graft or a tendon transfer using an FDS tendon. The responsible bone spur must be resected to avoid future, recurrent rupture.

87. **Why does boutonnière deformity occur in rheumatoid arthritis?**

The deformity has three components:

1. Flexion of the PIP joint
2. Hyperextension of the DIP joint
3. Hyperextension of the MP joint.

The primary inciting event is synovial proliferation within the PIP joint, which stretches the extensor mechanism. With damage to the central slip, the joint "button holes" through the lateral bands, which move palmar to the axis of the PIP joint. Ultimately, the lateral bands become fixed in this palmar position. Shortening of the oblique retinacular ligaments results in hyperextension and limited active flexion of the DIP joint. Patients compensate for the flexion deformity of the PIP joint by hyperextending the MP joint. The deformity tends to progress from a supple and passively correctable condition to a fixed condition that may be functionally disabling (Fig. 4.23).

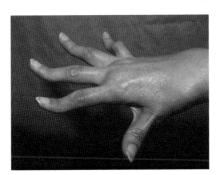

Figure 4.23. Notable boutonnière deformities.

88. **What is swan neck deformity?**

Like boutonnière deformity, swan neck deformity can occur in patients with RA, but is not limited to this condition. Swan neck deformity is characterized by:

1. Hyperextension of the PIP joint
2. Flexion of the DIP joint.

The primary cause of swan neck deformities can be located at the MP joint (intrinsic tightness), PIP joint (volar plate laxity), or the DIP joint (mallet finger).

UNUSUAL ARTHRITIC DISORDERS

CASE 4-14

A 37-year-old African-American female is referred from her rheumatologist with a known case of systemic lupus erythematosus and hand involvement. The patient complains of bilateral hand and wrist swelling and pain. On examination, the patient has mild ulnar deviation of her digits and swan neck deformities, which are passively correctable. Although she has had significant pain in her thumb, there is no deformity noted. The patient's plain films show no erosive changes to her phalanges.

89. **What characteristic manifestations are found in the hands of patients with systemic lupus erythematosus (SLE)?**
    SLE is a connective tissue disorder that occurs primarily in young adult women (more commonly in African-American women). A common clinical feature of SLE is polyarthritis, usually involving the small bones of the hands and feet. Ligamentous laxity with subsequent instability of the DRUJ, intercarpal joints, MP joints, and thumb joints is a distinctive feature of the disease. Raynaud's phenomena may also exist in up to 50% of patients.

90. **What is Jaccoud's arthropathy (or the lupus hand)?**
    Jaccoud's arthropathy, also known as lupus hand, is a classic finding in patients with lupus. The typical constellation of findings includes flexion deformities and ulnar deviation of the MP joints, swan neck deformities of the digits, and Z-deformity of the thumb (CMC joint flexion and MP joint extension). Although these deformities may resemble those found in RA, this condition is not associated with synovitis or with bone erosion.

91. **What is the primary surgical concern in patients with lupus involving the hand?**
    Reconstruction of soft-tissue deformity is often avoided due to a high recurrence rate. Many surgeons favor early arthrodesis and/or arthroplasty, prior to the occurrence of a fixed deformity.

92. **What is the pathophysiology of psoriatic arthritis?**
    Although the mechanisms are not fully elucidated, psoriatic arthritis manifests differently in the various regions of the body. The disease is a seronegative spondyloarthropathy and is most closely associated with the HLA-B27 genotype.

93. **What are some of the typical manifestations of psoriatic arthritis?**
    Arthritic changes in psoriatic arthritis are less frequently symmetric when compared to RA. They also differ from RA in that they less frequently involve the tendons, lack rheumatoid nodules, and are often accompanied by psoriatic skin changes. Common findings include:
    1. DIP joint arthritis
    2. Psoriasis of the skin
    3. Onycholysis (destruction and pitting of the nails)
    4. Ankylosis of the spine (ankylosing spondylitis)
    5. Dactylitis (commonly referred to as sausage digits).

94. **What are the common x-ray findings associated psoriatic arthritis of the hand?**
    Classically, erosive articular destruction can lead to the commonly associated "pencil in cup deformity" seen on radiographic evaluation (Fig. 4.24). Other common findings include distal phalangeal osteolysis and fusion of the DIP joints.

95. **What is arthritis mutilans?**
    This term describes the condition of severe destruction and foreshortening of the fingers or toes that can result from RA or psoriatic arthritis. As the fingers become foreshortened and collapse, the telescoping nature of the collapse leads to an "opera glass hand," which is a classically described deformity found in arthritis mutilans (Fig. 4.25).

CASE 4-15 (Fig. 4.26)

A 45-year-old women presents to clinic after recent evaluation by her rheumatologist for her longstanding scleroderma. Her hands demonstrate the characteristic flexion contractures and skin fibrosis associated with scleroderma. She is referred to you for evaluation of a chronically non-healing ulcer on the distal tip of her left index finger and newly observed white chalky material that has "built up" underneath her skin in different locations on the hands.

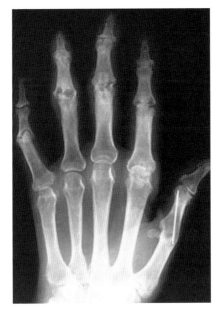

Figure 4.24. Common radiographic appearance of psoriatic arthritis. *(Reprinted from Mettler FA, Jr., Essentials of Radiology, 8, pp. 185–268. Copyright © 2014, 2005, 1996 by Saunders, an imprint of Elsevier Inc.).*

96. What is scleroderma?
    Scleroderma is a systemic connective tissue disorder characterized by changes in the skin, GI tract, lungs, kidneys, and heart. There are several characteristic hand findings including Raynaud's phenomenon (vasospasm affecting circulation to the digits), calcinosis (Fig. 4.27), and characteristic skin changes with resultant flexion contracture.

97. What is CREST syndrome?
    Crest syndrome describes a variant of systemic sclerosis. The name is an acronym and stands for Calcinosis, Raynaud's, Esophageal dysmotility, Sclerodactyly and Telangiectasia.

98. When is surgery indicated for patients with various forms of systemic sclerosis?
    This is patient dependent, but surgery can often be indicated for chronic non-healing ulcers created by vascular and mechanical compromise of fibrotic skin. Additionally, calcinosis and deformities can be corrected with surgical intervention and are indicated depending on the patient's symptoms (calcinosis can cause significant painful discomfort) and functional status.

FRACTURES AND DISLOCATIONS OF THE HAND AND CARPUS

INTRODUCTION

99. What bones are most frequently fractured in the hand?
    Fractures of the metacarpals and phalanges represent up to 10% of all fractures. Of these fractures, the distal phalanx is the most frequently fractured bone representing approximately 45% of such injuries.

FRACTURES AND DISLOCATIONS OF THE DISTAL PHALANX

100. Which distal phalanx is most commonly fractured?
    The thumb and long finger distal phalanx are most commonly fractured.

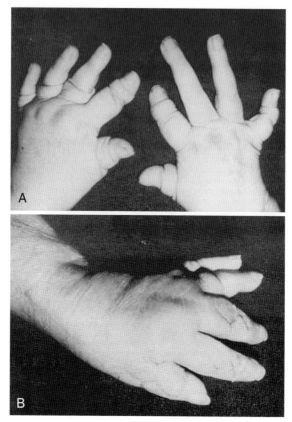

Figure 4.25. (A) Arthritis mutilans with telescoping "opera glass" hand deformity. (B) After fusion of the interphalangeal and metacarpophalangeal joints of the thumb, index finger and long finger. (*From Feldon P, et al., Rheumatoid Arthritis and Other Connective Tissue Diseases: Wolfe SW, et al. [eds], Green's Operative Hand Surgery, 6th edn. Churchill Livingstone, 2011.*)

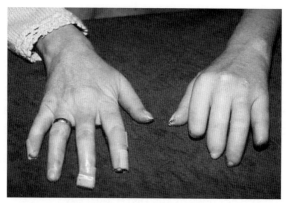

Figure 4.26. Patient with scleroderma with characteristic flexion contractures of the hands. (*From Lubahn JD, et al., Joint Replacement in the Hand and Wrist: Surgery and Therapy: Skirven TM, et al. [eds], Rehabilitation of the Hand and Upper Extremity, 6th edn. Mosby, 2011*)

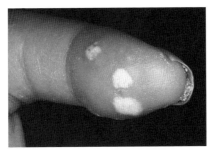

Figure 4.27. Calcinosis on the pulp of the finger seen in a patient with scleroderma. *(From Connolly MK, Systemic Sclerosis (Scleroderma) and Related Disorders: Bolognia JL, et al., Dermatology, 3rd edn. Saunders, 2012.)*

101. **What categories of distal phalangeal fractures are described?**
Distal phalanx fractures can be classified into three groups:
1. Tuft fractures
2. Shaft fractures
3. Articular fractures.

102. **What categories of distal phalanx tuft fractures are often described?**
Simple vs. Comminuted.

103. **What categories of distal phalanx intra-articular fracture are often described?**
1. Volar (with flexor digitorum profundus avulsion)
2. Dorsal (with extensor tendon avulsion, "mallet finger").

104. **What is the treatment for distal phalangeal fractures?**
In general, most distal phalanx fractures are treated with splint immobilization. However, displaced fractures, unstable fractures, and open fractures often require surgery. After fracture reduction, K-wires are often used to maintain fracture alignment.

105. **What structure is frequently injured in crush injuries of the distal phalanx?**
The nail bed is frequently involved in crush injuries, and nail bed injuries are often accompanied by subungual hematoma. Following this type of injury, the nail should be removed so that the nail bed can be repaired. This should be done with a fine, absorbable suture. Fractures of the distal phalanx rarely require more than simple splinting for protection. If there is wide displacement, open or closed reduction and fixation may be required.

106. **What is the normal rate of growth of a nail?**
Although this may vary for adults and children, the average adult's nail grows approximately 3 mm each month. As a result, it takes about 4 months to grow back entirely.

FRACTURES AND DISLOCATIONS OF THE PROXIMAL AND MIDDLE PHALANGES

107. **Do proximal and middle phalangeal fractures generally require surgery?**
The majority of these fractures are closed, non-displaced, and/or stable after reduction and, therefore, do not require surgery.

108. **What are the operative indications for proximal and middle phalangeal fractures?**
Indications for surgery include:
1. Displaced or unstable fractures that cannot be adequately reduced or maintained in a cast or splint
2. Intra-articular fractures with articular incongruity

3. Fractures with angular or rotational deformity
4. Multiple fractures are more likely to need surgery as the splinting function of the adjacent digits is lost
5. Open fractures with associated soft-tissue injury.

109. What methods of fixation are used for phalangeal fractures?

The most common fixation method is K-wires. Intramedullary fixation has been described, but is rarely used. External fixation is usually reserved for situations with problematic soft-tissue coverage or articular comminution. Screw fixation is useful across oblique and spiral fractures. Plates are considered for very unstable or transverse fractures.

110. What are the most common complications of phalangeal fractures?

The two most common complications of phalangeal fractures are stiffness and malunion.

111. How long does a phalangeal fracture take to heal?

It takes approximately 4–6 weeks to achieve "clinical healing." Gentle mobilization is usually initiated around 2–4 weeks. Solid radiographic union may take up to 6 months. The benefit of secure fixation is the ability to start mobilization earlier thereby preventing stiffness.

CASE 4-16 (Fig. 4.28)

A 30-year-old worker sustains a fracture of the proximal phalanx of the small finger when his finger is crushed under a heavy piece of wood. There is a deep laceration, but the tendons and neurovascular structures appear to be intact.

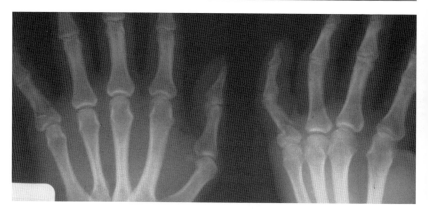

Figure 4.28. Anterior–posterior and oblique plain films obtained after the patient sustained a crush injury to the hand.

112. What is the diagnosis?

Based on the physical examination and the radiographs, this can be described as an open, comminuted, proximal phalanx fracture of the small finger with articular involvement. It is angulated ulnarly and the apex of the fracture is volar.

113. How would you treat this injury?

This is an open fracture and needs thorough irrigation and debridement, especially considering the possibility of retained wood fragments. As with all open fractures, the patient requires a course of antibiotics. Given the displacement, the fracture must be reduced, and then, stability should be assessed. If unstable, the reduction can be maintained using K-wires or a low profile plate.

CASE 4-17 (Fig. 4.29)

A 23-year-old male sustains a twisting, supination injury to his small finger while attempting to fix his bicycle. The patient complains of swelling and pain. On examination, there is slight malrotation in supination. The following radiographs are obtained.

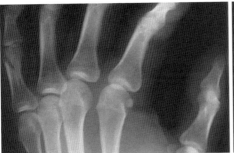 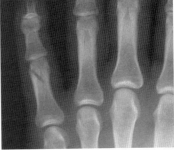

Figure 4.29. Radiographic evaluation of a supination injury of the 5th digit.

114. **What is the diagnosis?**
Closed proximal phalangeal spiral fracture.

115. **In such an injury, which way would the finger flex?**
As a result of the supination deformity of the finger, it will flex towards the ring finger and cross over it.

116. **What is the treatment?**
Reduction is needed and may be possible in a closed manner, followed by percutaneous wire or screw fixation under fluoroscopic guidance. If reduction is unable to be accomplished in a closed manner, open reduction and fixation is required.

CASE 4-18 (Fig. 4.30)

A 17-year-old boy dislocated his finger while playing football. The patient described an injury resulting from hyperextension with axial compression while attempting to intercept a pass. The team trainer was able to reduce the dislocation after an initial x-ray was obtained. Plain films are seen below.

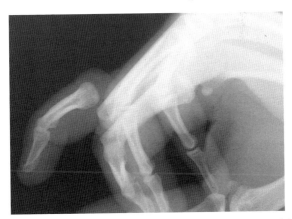

Figure 4.30. A 17-year-old boy after sustaining a football injury when his finger was hyperextended and compressed.

117. **What is the most common direction of PIP joint dislocations?**
The most frequent dislocations of the PIP joint are dorsal.

118. **What structure is ruptured in dorsal dislocations of the PIP joint?**
The volar plate is always ruptured in dorsal PIP dislocations.

119. **After reduction what is the next treatment step?**
    These injuries can typically be treated with early range of motion. Initially, a dorsal blocking splint is used to avoid hyperextension and recurrent instability. Subsequently, the patient can be transitioned from a splint to buddy taping. However, early motion is required to avoid volar plate scarring and a flexion contracture.

CASE 4-19 (Fig. 4.31)

A 30-year-old man sustained this injury when a basketball hit on the end of his finger in an axial direction. Radiographs were obtained after presentation to the Emergency Department.

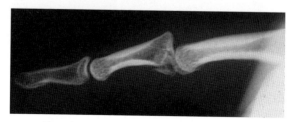

Figure 4.31. 30-year-old patient with a basketball injury.

120. **What is the diagnosis?**
    PIP dorsal fracture dislocation.

121. **What are the indications for surgery? What are the possible surgical treatment options?**
    The indication for surgery is a non-concentric PIP joint. Reduction can usually be obtained by flexing the joint. If a concentric reduction can be achieved, a dorsal block splint in flexion for several weeks with gradual initiation of extension motion is the treatment of choice. Otherwise, several external fixation devices are available to maintain reduction, while allowing early motion. If over 40% of the joint surface is involved, open surgery will likely be needed to restore the joint congruity. Depending on the size of the fragment and functional status of the patient, options include ORIF, volar plate arthroplasty, and hemi-hamate arthroplasty.

FRACTURES AND DISLOCATIONS OF THE METACARPALS AND MP JOINTS

122. **How do you classify metacarpal fractures?**
    Generally metacarpal fractures are subdivided into four main categories:
    1. Metacarpal head fractures:
       a. Subcapital
       b. Intra-articular
    2. Metacarpal neck fractures
    3. Metacarpal shaft fractures:
       a. Transverse
       b. Oblique or spiral
    4. Metacarpal base fractures.

CASE 4-20 (Fig. 4.32)

A 25-year-old man presents with 3 days of right hand pain just proximal to the 5th MP joint. The patient states that his hand started hurting after he punched a wall during a night of drinking 2 days previously. The pain was significantly more severe when he awoke the next morning and has continued since that time. He also noticed that his knuckle seemed to have "changed" after the fight. On exam, the patient has tenderness and swelling over the ulnar aspect of the hand and a prominent bump on the dorsum of the hand. Radiographs of the injured hand are seen below.

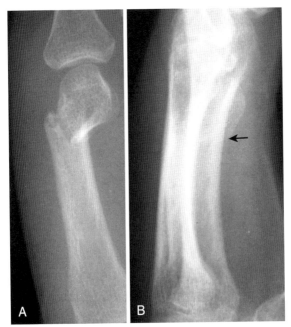

Figure 4.32. Angulation of fracture fragments. AP (A) and lateral (B) views of a "boxer's fracture" of the distal 5th metacarpal demonstrates typical radial and volar angulation of the distal fragment (arrow). (*Reprinted from Rogers LF, Grainger & Allison's Diagnostic Radiology: A Textbook of Medical Imaging, Elsevier Ltd., pp. 977–1027, 2007.*)

123. **What is the most likely diagnosis?**
  The diagnosis is a fracture of the 5th metacarpal neck, also commonly termed a "boxer's fracture." The fracture is typically angulated with the apex of the fracture in the dorsal direction. These fractures are usually treated non-operatively with or without a closed reduction. Given that most of these fractures are stable, patients are usually given an ulnar gutter splint but are quickly transitioned to early range of motion. Indications for surgery are significant angulation of the fracture (often between 40° and 70°), rotatory malalignment, or the presence of pseudoclawing consisting of hyperextension of MCP joint and flexion of the proximal interphalangeal (PIP) joint. An open fracture must be treated with open irrigation and debridement. When indicated, surgery may consist of open or closed reduction combined with percutaneous pinning or open fixation.

124. **Why are most metacarpal fractures dorsally angulated?**
  The major deforming force is supplied by the interosseous muscles, which function to flex the MP joint, leading to dorsal angulation of the fracture.

125. **What cosmetic finding do patients often complain of after sustaining a metacarpal neck fracture?**
  Patients often complain of loss of prominence of the metacarpal head, or "knuckle," and sometimes of a reciprocal prominence on the palmar aspect of the hand. This is due to the dorsal angulation of the fracture placing the head in a volar position.

126. **What problems may occur if there is greater than 40° of flexion at the fracture site?**
The problems that may occur with healing in >40° of flexion are a slight extensor lag and a metacarpal head prominence in the distal palm.

127. **What degree of angulation is tolerated for each of the metacarpal necks?**
There is no clear-cut consensus; however, the following may be used as general parameters:
Small finger: 40–70°
Ring finger: 30–40°
Middle finger: <15°
Index finger: <15°.

128. **Why does the accepted degree of angulation increase as you move from radial to ulnar?**
As you move ulnarly, the accepted angulation that can be tolerated increases because there is increased mobility of the CMC joints of the ulnar fingers.

129. **How can rotational malalignment be evaluated?**
Very small rotational discrepancies at the base of the finger can cause overlap or divergence of the digits with flexion. To evaluate rotational alignment, the patient is asked to make a fist, and the alignment of the fingers is observed. The fingers should all point toward the scaphoid. Furthermore, the plane of the nail can be compared to adjacent fingers and to fingers of the contralateral hand (Fig. 4.33).

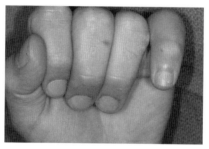

Figure 4.33. Malrotation of the small finger results in divergence of the finger and a nail that is slightly rotated compared with the ring finger.

130. **What is a complex dislocation of the MP joint?**
Dorsal dislocations of the MP are divided into simple or complex dislocations. Both are caused by hyperextension injuries. Simple dislocations can be treated with closed reduction and splinting or buddy taping. Complex dislocations require open reduction secondary to the interposition of the volar plate between the metacarpal head and the proximal phalanx. Improper reduction of simple dislocations may convert them to complex dislocations.

131. **How can you determine if a dislocation is simple or complex?**
Simple dislocations present with the proximal phalanx hyperextended (60–90°) on the dorsum of the metacarpal head. The joint surfaces are still partially in contact on a lateral radiograph. Complex dislocations present with the digit in a less dramatic position. The MCP is slightly hyperextended, and the PIP is slightly flexed. A hollow defect can be felt proximal to the dorsal base of the proximal phalanx, and the metacarpal head is prominent in the palm. Furthermore, the skin is often puckered in the palm. On radiographs, the joint surfaces demonstrate bayonet positioning. A pathognomonic finding is the presence of a sesamoid within the joint space on a radiograph. The sesamoid is within the volar plate, which is interposed between the phalanx and the metacarpal head (Fig. 4.34).

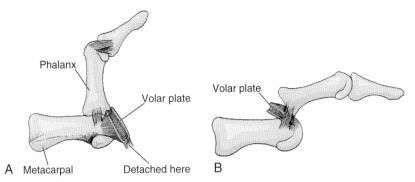

Figure 4.34. Depiction of simple and complex MP joint dislocations. *(From De Palma AF, Management of Fractures and Dislocations: An Atlas. Philadelphia: Saunders, 1970, pp. 1177. Reproduced by permission.)*

THUMB FRACTURES AND DISLOCATIONS

CASE 4-21

An 18-year-old female sustained a Bennett's fracture after falling off her bike. The fracture involved 30% of the articular surface. Initially, she was placed in a thumb spica cast, but radiographs now show a 2 mm step off at the articular surface and "slight" proximal displacement of the metacarpal.

132. What is a Bennett fracture?

A Bennett fracture is a fracture-dislocation of the thumb CMC joint. The volar ulnar aspect of the metacarpal base remains attached to the anterior, or volar, oblique ligament which holds this fragment steady while causing destabilizing the thumb. The adductor pollicis and APL are the primary deforming forces and combine to supinate, adduct, and flex the metacarpal shaft.

133. What treatment is needed?

The articular portion of the fracture must be fully reduced. Without stabilization, the metacarpal will tend to further displace. To avoid this, a K-wire can be inserted to hold the metacarpal in anatomic alignment. Reduction can be accomplished with axial traction, palmar abduction, and slight pronation. If an anatomic reduction cannot be obtained, then the joint should be open reduced and stabilized with a K-wire or screw fixation (Fig. 4.35).

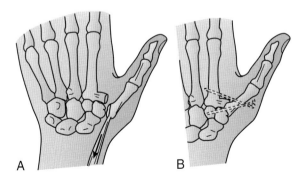

Figure 4.35. Bennett's fracture before (A) and after (B) closed reduction percutaneous fixation with a K-wire. *(From Townsend CM, et al. [eds]: Sabiston Textbook of Surgery, 19th edn. pp. 1952–2002. Copyright © Saunders, Elsevier Inc., 2012)*

134. **What other named fractures exist at the base of the thumb?**

Rolando fractures can be viewed as a comminuted Bennett's fracture with a second, large dorsal fragment that creates a T- or Y-shaped pattern (Fig. 4.36). Treatment should be directed at restoration of the articular surface.

CASE 4-22

A 24-year-old woman falls while skiing and sustains a forced abduction injury of her thumb as it contacts her ski pole. She has swelling, pain, and tenderness on the ulnar side of the MP joint of her thumb.

135. **What is the most likely diagnosis?**

The patient has most likely sustained a "gamekeeper's thumb," also known as "skier's thumb."

136. **What is gamekeeper's thumb?**

The term *gamekeeper's thumb* refers to an injury of the ulnar collateral ligament (UCL) of the thumb MP joint. Historically, it describes an occupational injury of the hands that occurred in British gamekeepers due to their methods of killing rabbits with forced abduction of the MP joint of the thumb. This caused a slow stretch of the UCL over time. *Skier's thumb* is a more appropriate name for an acute injury, which occurs from a fall onto the thumb, causing a forced abduction and an acute rupture of the UCL.

137. **What treatment is indicated for a thumb UCL injury?**

The key is to determine the stability of the thumb MP joint. First, the MP joint is examined for tenderness on its ulnar aspect. Then, in extension and 30° of flexion, a gentle abduction stress is placed on the joint to assess for the competency of the UCL. If the ligament is intact, there will be a discernable end-point. This exam should be compared to the contralateral side. Often, laxity can be difficult to assess secondary to patient guarding. If there is any question of stability, an MRI can be obtained or the patient should be re-evaluated in approximately 1 week.

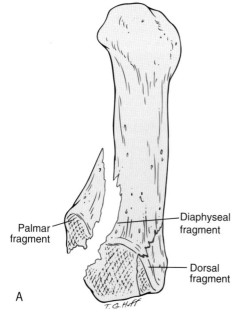

Palmar fragment

Diaphyseal fragment

Dorsal fragment

A

T. G. Huff

Figure 4.36. Diagram (A) and radiographs (B) of a Rolando fracture. (A: *Reprinted from Jupiter JB, Skeletal Trauma: Basic Science, Management, and Reconstruction, pp. 1221–1341. Copyright © 2009 by Saunders, Elsevier Inc. B: Reprinted from Calandruccio JH, Campbell's Operative Orthopaedics, pp. 3305–3365.e2. Copyright © 2013 by Mosby, Elsevier Inc.*)

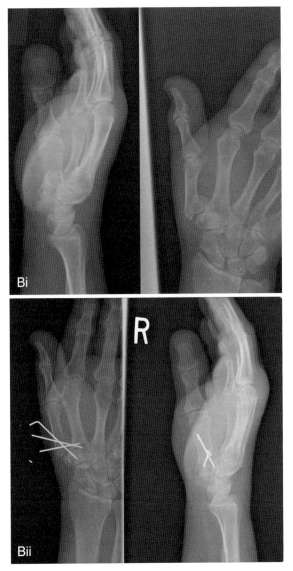

Figure 4.36, continued

If a complete tear of the ligament is diagnosed, the treatment options are thumb spica cast immobilization vs. open UCL repair. Recently, surgery has been favored to avoid problems secondary to a Stener lesion (Fig. 4.37).

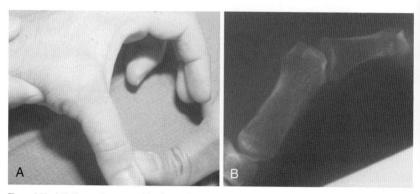

Figure 4.37. (A) Testing for an unstable ulnar collateral ligament showing opening on the ulnar side. (B) Radiographic confirmation.

138. **What is a Stener lesion?**
Stener reported a series of cases in which the adductor pollicis aponeurosis remains intact, and the UCL, with a small piece of the bone avulsed off the proximal phalanx, is positioned superficial to the adductor. The bone and ligament are blocked from healing to the phalanx by the aponeurosis. In these instances, open UCL repair is necessary (Fig. 4.38).

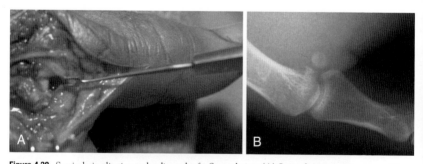

Figure 4.38. Surgical visualization and radiograph of a Stener lesion. (A) Stener lesion seen at surgery with the adductor aponeurosis interposed between the joint and a small avulsion fracture which lies superficial. (B) Radiograph showing a small "chip" of bone indicating a possible complete tear of the ligament and an avulsion fracture from the ligamentous attachment.

FRACTURES AND LIGAMENT INJURIES OF THE CARPAL BONES

139. **Which carpal bone is fractured most often?**
The scaphoid is the most commonly fractured carpal bone. It functions as a link between the proximal and distal carpal rows, which makes it vulnerable to injury. Approximately 80% of fractures occur in the middle third of the scaphoid.

140. **What other carpal bones are frequently fractured?**
By far, the most common carpal bone fractured is the scaphoid:
Scaphoid: >50% of all carpal fractures   Capitate: ~2%
Triquetrum: ~20%   Hamate: ~2%
Trapezium: ~5%   Pisiform ~1%
Lunate: ~4%   Trapezoid <1%.

141. **Fractures at which location in the scaphoid have the lowest rate of healing? Why?**
The major blood supply to the scaphoid is a branch of the radial artery that enters the dorsal ridge of the scaphoid. Because the vessels travel from distal to proximal, a fracture across the bone compromises the proximal blood supply and can lead to delayed or nonunion and subsequent avascular necrosis of the proximal segment. For this reason, proximal pole fractures have the lowest healing rates while tuberosity distal fractures have the highest healing rates.

142. **What should be done if no fracture is seen on the radiograph but the "snuff box" is tender?**
When the snuff box is tender to palpation, it is best to assume that there is a scaphoid fracture even if it is not apparent on plain radiographs in the acute setting. An occult scaphoid fracture should be treated with thumb spica cast/splint immobilization. Furthermore, radiographs should be repeated in 2–3 weeks, or, a CT scan versus an MRI should be obtained.

143. **How are scaphoid fractures described?**
Scaphoid fractures are often described according to the location of the fracture (i.e., proximal pole, waist, or distal pole). They may also be described as transverse or oblique.

144. **Which type of scaphoid fracture is at greatest risk for future complications?**
Due to the vascular anatomy, proximal pole fractures are at greater risk for nonunion and avascular necrosis.

145. **How are scaphoid fractures treated?**
Scaphoid fracture treatment is determined by fracture displacement and location. Displaced fractures are almost uniformly treated with ORIF using a headless compression screw fixation. Treatment of non-displaced fractures is more complicated. Typically, non-displaced distal pole fractures are treated non-operatively with a thumb spica cast, while non-displaced proximal pole fractures are treated operatively with ORIF. Non-displaced scaphoid waist fractures can be treated either non-operatively or operatively, and this decision is usually dependent on patient and surgeon preference.

146. **What is the "Terry Thomas" sign?**
Named after the British comedian Terry Thomas, who was famous for a noticeable gap between his two front teeth, the "Terry Thomas" sign refers to the radiographic finding of a widened scapholunate interval. It suggests that the scapolunate ligament has been damaged allowing the two bones to separate like Mr. Thomas's two front teeth.

147. **What is a SLAC or SNAC wrist?**
Tears of the SL ligament lead to separation of the scaphoid and lunate. A wide SL interval (Terry Thomas sign) is seen on radiographic evaluation. This lesion should be considered in all radius fractures and suspected scaphoid fractures. SLAC wrist refers to ScaphoLunate Advanced Collapse, which is the most common form of arthritis in the wrist. The degenerative change follows a specific sequence and is initiated by SL ligament disruption. This causes the scaphoid and lunate to separate and the capitate to migrate proximally with a "collapse" of the normal architecture of the wrist. The degenerative arthritis initially involves the radioscaphoid joint and ultimately advances to complete collapse as the capitate moves towards the radius. Scaphoid nonunion advanced collapse (SNAC) progresses through a similar set of stages toward arthritis of the wrist. This is the direct result of nonunion of a previous fracture of the scaphoid (Fig. 4.39).

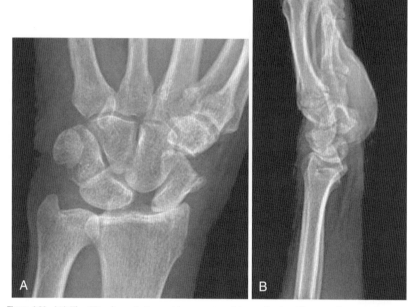

Figure 4.39. (A) The AP radiograph shows wide separation of the scaphoid and lunate with proximal capitate migration. (B) On the lateral radiograph, the lunate is extended and the scaphoid is flexed, which is called a dorsal intercalary segment instability pattern. (*Reprinted from Nolla JM, Essentials of Physical Medicine and Rehabilitation: Musculoskeletal Disorders, Pain, and Rehabilitation, pp. 193–201. Copyright © 2008, 2002 by Saunders, Elsevier Inc.*)

BIBLIOGRAPHY

1. American Society for Surgery of the Hand. The Hand: Examination and Diagnosis. 3rd ed. New York: Churchill Livingstone; 1990.
2. Ashkenaze DM, Ruby LK. Metacarpal fractures and dislocations. Orthop Clin North Am 1992;23:19.
3. Azar FM. Arthrodesis of shoulder, elbow, and wrist. In: Canale ST, editor. Campbell's Operative Orthopaedics. 9th ed. St. Louis: Mosby; 1998. p. 203–6.
4. Beer TA, Turner RH. Wrist arthrodesis for failed wrist implant arthroplasty. J Hand Surg 1997;22A:685–93.
5. Bodin ND, Spangler R, Thoder JJ. Interposition arthroplasty options for carpometacarpal arthritis of the thumb. Hand Clin 2010;26:339–50, v–vi.
6. Branam BR, Tuttle HG, Stern PJ, et al. Resurfacing arthroplasty versus silicone arthroplasty for proximal interphalangeal joint osteoarthritis. J Hand Surg [Am] 2007;32:75–88.
7. Bucholz RW, Heckman JD, editors. Rockwood and Green's Fractures in Adults. 7th ed. Philadelphia: JB Lippincott; 2010.
8. Carmine D. Clemente: Anatomy: A Regional Atlas of the Human Body. 5th ed. Baltimore: Lipincott Williams & Wilkins; 2007.
9. Cooney WP III, Dobyns JH, Linscheid RL. Non-union of the scaphoid: Analysis of the results from bone grafting. J Hand Surg 1980;5:343.
10. Dalbeth N, Pui K, Lobo M, et al. Nail disease in psoriatic arthritis: distal phalangeal bone edema detected by magnetic resonance imaging predicts development of onchyolysis and hyperkeratosis. J Rheumatol 2012;39:841–3.
11. Davis DI, Catalano L. Treatment of advanced carpometacarpal joint disease: carpometacarpal arthroplasty with ligament interposition. Hand Clin 2008;24:263–9, vi.
12. Doyle JR. Extensor tendons: Acute injuries. In: Green DP, editor. Operative Hand Surgery. 4th ed. New York: Churchill Livingstone; 1999. p. 1950–87.
13. Drake ML, Segalman KA. Complications of small joint arthroplasty. Hand Clin 2010;26:205–12.

14. Egol KA, Koval KJ, Zuckerman JD. The Handbook of Fractures. 4th ed. Philadelphia: Lippincott Williams and Wilkins; 2010.
15. Ford DJ, Ali MS, Steel WM. Fractures of the fifth metacarpal neck: Is reduction or immobilization necessary? J Hand Surg 1989;14B:165.
16. Gelberman RH. The wrist: total wrist arthroplasty. New York: Raven Press; 1994. p. 253–78.
17. Geyman JP, Fink K, Sullivan SD. Conservative versus surgical treatment of mallet finger: A pooled quantitative literature evaluation. J Am Board Fam Pract 1998;11:382–90.
18. Goldstein EJ, Citron DM. Susceptability of Eikenella corrodens to penicillin, ampacillin and twelve new cephalosporins. Antimicrob Agents Chemother 1984;26:947–8.
19. Goldstein EJ, Caffee HH, Price JE, et al. Human bite infections. Lancet 1977;17;2(8051):1290.
20. Gordon JA, Stone L, Gordon L. Surface markers for locating the pulleys and flexor tendon anatomy in the palm and fingers with reference to minimally invasive incisions. J Hand Surg 2012;37:913–18.
21. Hardy MA. Principles of metacarpal and phalangeal fracture management: a review of rehabilitation concepts. J Orthop Sports Phys Ther 2004;34:781–99.
22. Hornbach EE, Cohen MS. Closed reduction and percutaneous pinning of fractures of the proximal phalanx. J Hand Surg [Br] 2001;26:45–9.
23. Hubbard LF. Metacarpal phalangeal dislocations. Hand Clin 1988;4:39.
24. Kaur JM. The distal radioulnar joint: Anatomic and functional considerations. Clin Orthop 1992;275:37.
25. Knirk JL, Jupiter JB. Intra-articular fractures of the distal end of the radius in young adults. J Bone Joint Surg 1986;68A:647–58.
26. Landsmeer JMF. Atlas of Anatomy of the Hand. Edinburgh: Churchill Livingstone; 1976.
27. Lanzetta M, Herbert TJ, Conolly WB. Silicone synovitis. A perspective. J Hand Surg [Br] 1994;19:479–84.
28. Leddy JP, Packer JW. Avulsion of the profundus tendon insertion in athletes. J Hand Surg 1977;2A:66–9.
29. Lichtman DM, Alexander AH, editors. The Wrist and Its Disorders. Philadelphia: WB Saunders; 1997.
30. Lins RE, Gelberman RH, McKeown L, et al. Basal joint arthritis: Trapeziectomy with ligament reconstruction and tendon interposition arthroplasty. J Hand Surg 1996;21A:202–9.
31. Livesley PJ. Conservative management of Bennett's fracture-dislocation: A 26 year follow-up. J Hand Surg 1990;15B:291.
32. Lubahn JD. Mallet finger fractures: A comparison of open and closed technique. J Hand Surg 1990;14A:394.
33. Mannerfelt L, Norman O. Attrition ruptures of flexor tendons in rheumatoid arthritis caused by bony spurs in the carpal tunnel. J Bone Joint Surg 1969;51B:270–7.
34. Matloub HS, Yousef NJ. Peripheral nerve anatomy and innervation patterns. Hand Clin 1992;8:201.
35. Melone CP Jr. Rigid fixation of phalangeal and metacarpal fractures. Orthop Clin North Am 1986;17:421–35.
36. Netter FH. Atlas of Human Anatomy. Summit, NJ: Ciba-Geigy; 1989.
37. Ono S, Shauver MJ, Chang KW, et al. Outcomes of pyrolytic carbon arthroplasty for the proximal interphalangeal joint at 44 months' mean follow-up. Plast Reconstr Surg 2012;129(5):1139–50.
38. Palmer AK, Werner FW, Murphy D, et al. Functional wrist anatomy: A biomechanical study. J Hand Surg 1985;10A:39.
39. Pugliese D, Bush D, Harrington T. Silicone synovitis: longer term outcome data and review of the literature. J Clin Rheumatol 2009;15:8–11.
40. Rizzo M, Cooney WP. Current concepts and treatment for the rheumatoid wrist. Hand Clin 2011;27:57–72.
41. Romanes GJ. Cunningham's Manual of Practical Anatomy, vol. 1. 15th ed. Upper and Lower Limbs. Oxford: Oxford University Press; 1986.
42. Royle SG. Rotational deformity following metacarpal fracture. J Hand Surg 1990;15B:124.
43. Sahu A, Gujral SS, Batra S, et al. The current practice of the management of little finger metacarpal fractures—a review of the literature and results of a survey conducted among upper limb surgeons in the United Kingdom. Hand Surg 2012;17:55–63.
44. Seiler JG III, Fraser JLL. Digital flexor sheath: Repair and reconstruction of the annular pulleys and membranous sheath. J South Orthop Assoc 2000;9(2):8190.
45. Siegel D, Gebhardt M, Jupiter JB. Spontaneous rupture of the extensor pollicis longus tendon. J Hand Surg 1987;12A:1106–9.
46. Smith RJ. Intrinsic muscles of the fingers: Function, dysfunction, and surgical reconstruction. Instructional Course Lectures, vol. 24. St. Louis: Mosby; 1975.
47. Squitieri L, Chung KC. A systematic review of outcomes and complications of vascularized toe joint transfer, silicone arthroplasty, and pyrocarbon arthroplasty for posttraumatic joint reconstruction of the finger. Plast Reconstr Surg 2008;121:1697–707.
48. Staiano J, Graham K. A tooth in the hand is worth a washout in the operating theater. J Trauma 2007;62(6):1531–2.
49. Strickland JW. Flexor tendons: Acute injuries. In: Green DP, editor. Operative hand surgery. 4th ed. New York: Churchill Livingstone; 1999. p. 1851–97.
50. Strickland JW. Flexor tendon injuries: Part I and part II. J Am Acad Orthop Surg 1995;3:44–62.

51. Swanson AB, de Groot Swanson G, Ishikawa H. Flexible implant resection arthroplasty. In: Strickland JW, editor. Master Techniques in Orthopaedic Surgery: The Hand. Philadelphia: Lippincott-Raven; 1998. p. 421–38.
52. Thompson JC. Netter's Concise Orthopaedic Anatomy. 2nd ed. Philadelphia: WB Saunders; 2010.
53. Tubiana R, editor. The Hand, vol. 5. Philadelphia: WB Saunders; 1999.
54. Vaccaro AR, Kupcha PC, Salvo JP. Accurate reduction and splint of the common boxer's fracture. Orthop Rev 1990;19:994.
55. Ward CM, Kuhl T, Adams BD. Five to ten-year outcomes of the universal total wrist arthroplasty in patients with rheumatoid arthritis. J Bone Joint Surg Am 2011;93:914–19.
56. Wolfe SW, Hotchkiss RN, Pederson WC, et al. Green's Operative Hand Surgery. 6th ed. New York: Elsevier, Churchill Livingstone; 2011.
57. Yoong P, Goodwin RW, Chojnowski A. Phalangeal fractures of the hand. Clin Radiol 2010;65:773–80.

ORTHOPEDIC ONCOLOGY

J. Gabriel Horneff III and Stephan G. Pill

CHAPTER 5

GENERAL ORTHOPEDIC ONCOLOGY

CASE 5-1

A 40-year-old woman comes to your office with a pile of radiographs and MRIs stating that she has recently been diagnosed with a lesion in her right femur. She states that she has no history of cancer and scans of her entire body show no other concerning lesions. She has been doing some "research" on the internet and is concerned she has a sarcoma.

1. What is a sarcoma? How is it different from a carcinoma?

   A sarcoma is a malignancy arising in mesenchymal tissue (fibrous tissue, muscle, bone, adipose). A carcinoma arises from epithelial cells. Sarcomas tend to rapidly grow in a centripetal fashion and typically metastasize hematogenously, whereas carcinomas typically metastasize through the lymphatic system.

2. What is the most common site for metastases of soft-tissue sarcomas?

   The most common site for hematogenous spread of a sarcoma is to the lungs.

3. How are primary orthopedic tumors staged?

   The Enneking system is the most commonly used staging system for primary orthopedic tumors. This system is based on three characteristics of the tumor: histologic grade (G), anatomic site (T), and metastases (M).

   Grade (G), is an assessment of histologic grade, radiographic classification, and clinical course. Tumors are classified as benign (G0), low-grade malignant (G1), or high-grade malignant (G2). Anatomic site (T) places tumors into intracompartmental (T1) or extracompartmental (T2) groups. Intracompartmental tumors are contained within an anatomic compartment that serves as a natural barrier to tumor extension. These natural barriers include cortical bone, articular cartilage, joint capsule, and fascia. Extracompartmental tumors span at least one of these natural barriers. Tumors that have either regional or distant metastases are labeled M1, and those with no metastases are designated M0.

   Benign lesions (G0) are staged into one of three groups. Benign stage 1 lesions are latent, static lesions. Benign stage 2 lesions are progressive, and may expand a fascial or cortical margin but do not broach it. Benign stage 3 lesions are aggressive and have breached compartments or have metastasized.

   Malignant lesions without metastases are grouped into Stage I (G1) or Stage II (G2). Malignant lesions of either grade with local or distant metastases are grouped into Stage III. Each of these malignant stages is further stratified based on anatomic site. Intracompartmental lesions are labeled "A," and extracompartmental lesions are labeled "B." (See Table 5.1.)

4. What are the most common orthopedic tumors seen in patients under the age of 30 years?

   The most common orthopedic tumors in patients under 30 years old are **A**neurysmal bone cyst, **E**wing's sarcoma, **I**nfection (abscess), **O**steosarcoma, **U**nicameral bone cyst, and giant cell tumor.

   Remember the pneumonic: AEIOU.

CASE 5-1 continued

As stated before, your patient is a 40-year-old female. You begin to create a differential diagnosis in your head as you start to go through her films.

Table 5.1. Enneking System for Staging Primary Orthopedic Tumors

Stage	IA	IB	IIA	IIB	IIIA	IIIB
Grade	G1	G1	G2	G2	G1/G2	G1/G2
Site	T1	T2	T1	T2	T1	T2
Metastases	M0	M0	M0	M0	M1	M1

5. What are the most common orthopedic tumors seen in patients over the age of 30 years?

The most common orthopedic tumors in patients over 30 years old are **M**etastatic tumors, **A**dult **R**ound cell tumors (myeloma, lymphoma), **C**hondrosarcoma, **O**steosarcoma, and giant cell tumor.

Remember the pneumonic: MARCO.

6. What are the most common orthopedic tumors found in the:
   a. Spine:

   The most common orthopedic tumors found in the spine are plasmacytoma (multiple myeloma), metastatic tumors, chordoma, giant cell tumor, and chondrosarcoma.
   b. Phalanges:

   The most common orthopedic tumors found in the phalanges are enchondroma, abscess, metastatic tumor (especially lung), pigmented villonodular synovitis, and giant cell tumor.
   c. Intra-articular:

   The most common intra-articular orthopedic tumors are synovial cell carcinomatosis and pigmented villonodular synovitis.
   d. Epiphysis:

   Giant cell tumor (Fig. 5.1).
   e. Metaphysis:

   Osteosarcoma (Fig. 5.2).
   f. Diaphysis:

   Ewing's sarcoma (Fig. 5.3).
   g. Anterior tibial diaphysis:

   Cortical fibrous dysplasia (males in first 2 decades) and adamantinoma.
   h. Proximal tibial metaphysis:

   Chondromyxoid fibroma.

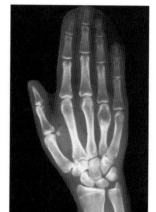

Figure 5.1. Radiograph of giant cell tumor. *(From Bullough P [ed.]: Orthopaedic Pathology, 5th edn, pp. 449–476. Copyright © Mosby, Elsevier Inc., 2010.)*

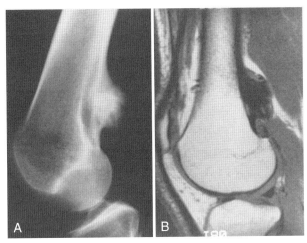

Figure 5.2. Radiograph (A) and MRI (B) of osteosarcoma. *(From Resnick D, Kransdorf M [eds]: Bone and Joint Imaging, 3rd edn. Copyright © Elsevier Inc., 2005.)*

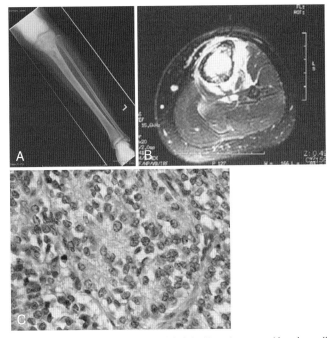

Figure 5.3. Radiograph (A), MRI (B), and histologic slide (C) of Ewing's sarcoma. Note the small round cells found on histology. *(From Niederhuber JE, et al. [eds], Abeloff's Clinical Oncology, 5th edn, pp. 1693–1752.e9. Copyright © Churchill Livingstone, Elsevier Inc., 2014.)*

7. What are the common bone forming tumors?

When the plain films show bone formation within or surrounding the tumor, think osteoid osteoma, osteoblastoma, osteochondroma, osteosarcoma, blastic metastasis, and Paget's disease lesion.

8. What are the common cartilage forming tumors?

When cartilage is seen within the tumor, (such as on histology) think osteochondroma, chondromyxoid fibroma, chondroblastoma, chondrosarcoma, and endochondroma.

PRINCIPLES OF DIAGNOSIS AND TREATMENT OF MUSCULOSKELETAL TUMORS

CASE 5-2

A 29-year-old male began noting pain in his left forearm after a rigorous workout at the gym about 5 months ago. He initially thought that he had just strained a muscle, but began to notice a firmness presenting as swelling in his arm that would not go away. His primary care physician got x-rays, which were negative. He has been referred to you for further work up of his symptoms. He denies any recent weight loss, but has noted continued pain in the arm.

9. What questions are important to add to a standard orthopedic history to consider the possibility of an orthopedic tumor?

Have you experienced any weight loss?

Do you have any history of night pain?

Do you have any history of malignancy?

Do you smoke?

Do you have any history of masses or lesions?

Keep in mind these are non-specific questions.

10. If a patient with a known chronic lesion develops pain, what two things should be considered?

The onset of pain could signify a pathologic fracture or malignant transformation, and a work-up is indicated.

CASE 5-2 continued

You decide that the patient needs further imaging studies to better qualify what the lesion is.

11. What are the benefits of:
    a. CT scan:
       CT scan is good for showing bone detail and soft-tissue calcification.
    b. MRI:
       MRI is useful for showing the extent of a lesion within bone itself or into the soft tissue. It is also useful in determining whether a lesion is a solid tumor (enhancing) or cystic (non-enhancing/rim enhancing) if gadolium is administered.
    c. Technitium bone scan:
       Technitium bone scans are important for skeletal surveys in disease that is widespread throughout the skeleton. It displays active bone-forming lesions as "hot" and lytic lesions without bony reaction as "cold" or normal as seen in multiple myeloma.

CASE 5-2 continued

The patient asks why nothing showed up on his x-ray.

12. How much bone is typically destroyed before a lesion is noticeable on plain radiography?

In general, 30% to 40% of bone must be destroyed before a lesion is evident on x-ray.

CASE 5-2 continued

You explain to the patient that depending on the results of the imaging, you may have to perform a biopsy on the left forearm if there is a concerning lesion.

13. **What is the principle goal of a biopsy?**
The goal is to establish a histologic diagnosis without affecting subsequent treatment. Primary bone tumors are very heterogeneous and sampling error can lead to misdiagnosis. Therefore, it is often best to get a frozen biopsy to ensure adequate specimen is available for diagnosis. In general, the biopsy is best obtained by a surgeon who can provide final management of the tumor. In many cases, this necessitates referral to an orthopedic oncologist.

14. **What are three different types of biopsy?**
The biopsy can be obtained three ways: needle biopsy, excisional biopsy, or incisional biopsy. Needle biopsy has the advantage of less morbidity, but may not provide sufficient tissue for a diagnosis and is subject to sampling error. They are often helpful for anatomically inaccessible areas such as the spine or pelvis. Excisional biopsy consists of removing the entire lesion and is most often used with small, benign appearing lesions. Open incisional biopsy remains the gold standard when the underlying diagnosis is uncertain.

15. **What are some important rules to follow when obtaining an incisional biopsy?**
Incisional biopsies must be performed meticulously, with the definitive surgical procedure in mind. Frozen sections should be obtained whenever possible as the tumor is often necrotic and more tissue is better for diagnosis. The surgeon should accompany the specimen to the pathology lab. If the fresh frozen specimen suggests malignancy, the biopsy tract will be considered contaminated and must be removed at the time of tumor resection. No Esmarch should be used for possible risk of disseminating the tumor into the surrounding tissue. The biopsy incision should be longitudinal, to allow for an extensile approach, and as small as possible. Rather than following internervous planes as routinely done in orthopedic surgery, a more direct ("one compartment") approach should be used to minimize the contamination of surrounding areas. Neurovascular structures should be particularly avoided when possible. Minimal retraction should be used to reduce the risk of soft-tissue contamination. A multilayered water-tight closure should be done once sufficient tissue has been obtained, as determined by the pathologist. Drains should exit in line with the incision so that the tract can be excised if needed.

16. **When surgically removing a tumor, name the types of excision used from most to least conservative?**
Curettage can be used for benign bony lesions. This involves scooping the tumor out then scraping the surrounding walls to induce healing. Marginal excision involves removing a small amount of "reactive zone", which is host tissue attempting to "wall off" the tumor. This is typically used for benign soft-tissue lesions. Wide excision involves excising a small amount of normal tissue to ensure "clean" margins. This is used for malignant lesions that invade surrounding tissue. Lastly, radical excision involves removing the entire compartment containing the lesion. This is reserved for highly malignant tumors, but is often not necessary with the advent of limb salvage technique with adjuvant chemotherapeutic and radiation therapies.

17. **What are the advantages of preoperative radiation therapy?**
Preoperative radiation therapy can (1) decrease the size of the tumor, (2) decrease the vascularity of the tumor, and (3) increase the firmness of the lesion making it easier to resect.

18. **What are the disadvantages of preoperative radiation?**
Radiation therapy can (1) damage normal tissue surrounding the lesion and (2) inhibit wound healing following resection.

19. **Name some orthopedic tumors that are particularly sensitive to chemotherapy?**
Rhabdomyosarcoma, **E**wing's sarcoma, **M**yeloma, and **O**steosarcoma are all chemosensitive.
Remember pneumonic: REMO rhymes with CHEMO.

20. Name the tumors associated with each of the following stains.
   a. Keratin:
      Metastatic carcinoma, synovial cell sarcoma, adamantinoma, epithelioid sarcoma.
   b. Vimentin:
      Sarcomas (negative in carcinomas).
   c. Desmin and actin:
      Rhabdomyoma/rhabdomyosarcomas, leimyoma/leimyosarcoma, and occasionally seen in desmoid tumors and primitive neuroectodermal tumors (PNET).
   d. S-100:
      Tumors from neural, chondroid, and melanocytic differentiation.
   e. Factor VIII related antigen (vWF):
      Benign and low-grade vascular lesions (not typically seen in high-grade angiosarcomas).

BENIGN BONE LESIONS
CASE 5-3

A 25-year-old female comes to your office after being referred by her primary care physician for constant knee pain that started about a month ago without any prior injury. She states that the pain is worse at night. She has tried non-steroidal antiinflammatory drugs (NSAIDs) for the pain and has had some relief, but feels that the duration of her symptoms and lack of an injury are concerning. She brings an x-ray which doesn't show any abnormality.

21. Name two benign bone forming tumors?
   Osteoid osteoma and osteoblastoma are primary benign bone forming tumors.

22. What is an osteoid osteoma?
   An osteoid osteoma is a benign osteoblastic lesion characterized by a well-demarcated central nidus of ≤1.5 cm surrounded by dense reactive bone. It typically occurs in the metaphyseal regions of long bones (femur or tibia) or in the posterior elements of the spine in the first 2 decades of life. Patients present with night pain, which increases over time and is relieved by NSAIDs. Lesions in the posterior elements of the spine can produce a painful scoliosis. CT scans are occasionally helpful to locate the nidus if not apparent on x-ray.
   Remember the pneumonic: three N's of osteoid osteoma: **N**idus, **N**ight pain, **N**SAIDs. (See Fig. 5.4.)

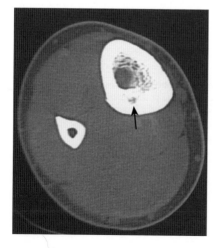

Figure 5.4. CT scan of osteoid osteoma. (*From Adam A, et al. [eds], Grainger & Allison's Diagnostic Radiology, 5th edn, pp. 1029–1057. Copyright © Churchill Livingstone, Elsevier Inc., 2008.*)

CASE 5-3 continued

You order a CT scan of the patient's knee and note that there is a small lytic nidus that looks like a "target" with significant sclerosis surrounding it. It is located on the lateral aspect of the proximal tibia. You diagnose the patient with an osteoid osteoma.

23. **How do you treat an osteoid osteoma?**

    Medical treatment with NSAIDs is acceptable as most lesions regress over 4 years. Surgical treatment by en bloc excision of the nidus or intralesional curettage can be done if symptoms are poorly controlled. Percutaneous radiofrequency ablation is also an option for osteoid osteomas in the extremities.

CASE 5-3 continued

The patient states that she had done some searching on the internet and was concerned that she may have an osteoblastoma.

24. **How does an osteoblastoma compare to an osteoid osteoma?**

    An osteoblastoma is larger than an osteoid osteoma and often does not have a rim of reactive bone around it. Also, it can often behave quite aggressively so treatment is wide resection. Similar to osteoid osteoma, it is commonly located in the posterior element of the spine. It can also be found as a blastic or lytic lesion in the metaphyseal region of long bones.

25. **Name three benign cartilage forming tumors.**

    Enchondroma, chondroblastoma, and chondromyxoid fibroma are primary benign cartilage forming tumors.

26. **What is a common radiographic appearance seen with cartilage forming lesions?**

    Scalloping is a common radiographic characteristic of cartilage forming tumors (Fig. 5.5).

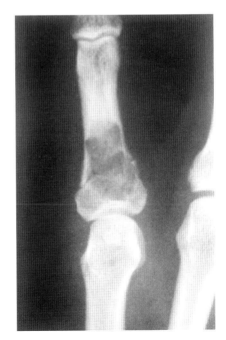

Figure 5.5. Radiograph demonstrating scalloping. *(From Kumar V, et al. [eds], Robbins and Cotran Pathologic Basis of Disease, Professional Edition, 8th edn. Copyright © Saunders, Elsevier Inc., 2010.)*

CASE 5-4

A 50-year old woman presented to the orthopedic office with left shoulder pain. A routine AP radiograph was obtained, which showed a lesion in the proximal humerus (Fig. 5.6). She is very nervous about what the lesion could be.

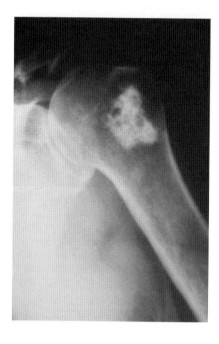

Figure 5.6. Radiograph of enchondroma. (*From Weidner N, et al. [eds], Modern Surgical Pathology, 2nd edn, pp. 1784–1840. Copyright © Saunders, Elsevier Inc., 2009.*)

27. **What is an enchondroma?**
An enchondroma is a benign nest of mature cartilage within a bone, located typically in the center of the metaphysis. They calcify slowly over many years. They are the most common primary bone tumor in the hand, but enchondromas can be found in any bone. They are usually asymptomatic.

28. **What is the typical radiographic appearance of an enchondroma?**
A "popcorn" pattern of stippled calcification is seen on x-ray. They appear "hot" on technetium bone scans. They may cause cortical expansion in small or flat bones.

29. **What eponyms are associated with multiple enchondromas?**
Ollier disease is the presence of multiple enchondromas. Maffucci disease is associated with multiple enchondromas and soft-tissue angiomas.

30. **What is the risk of malignant transformation of an enchondroma?**
There is a 1% risk of malignant transformation of an enchondroma to chondrosarcoma, so annual surveillance MRIs may be helpful.

31. **If you see chondroid calcification on x-ray, what lesions should you consider?**
Enchondroma and chondrosarcoma both have chondroid calcification. Enchondromas are non-painful, while chondrosarcomas are typically painful and expansile.

32. **What is a chondroblastoma?**
A chondroblastoma is a painful benign tumor characteristically located in the epiphysis of a male adolescent. The pain they cause may limit joint motion. On MRI, there

is often significant edema. Histologically, the stromal cells of chondroblastomas are polyhedral with clear halos around the nuclei resulting in the characteristic "chicken wire" appearance. About 2% of chondroblastomas are metastatic to the lungs.

33. **What is on the differential diagnosis for a chondroblastoma?**
Osteochondritis dissecans lesions and infection are possible pathologies that should be on the differential for a suspected chondroblastoma.

34. **What is a chondromyxoid fibroma?**
A chondromyxoid fibroma is a rare benign cartilage tumor that contains spindle cells in a collagenous matrix and varying amounts of immature chondroid. The tumor is more commonly found in males and occurs usually in the first 3 decades of life. It is classically found in the proximal tibia but may also be seen in the femur and pelvis. The lesion is lytic and sharply demarcated from the surrounding normal bone. It looks like a large non-ossifying fibroma. It causes cortical thinning but does not affect the periosteum. It is treated with marginal resection.

CASE 5-5

A 30-year-old female had x-rays of her left knee performed in a local Emergency Room after being involved in a car accident. She had no fracture, but there was a mass noted on the distal femur described on the radiographic report as a "pedunculated osseous mass confluent with the cortex." The patient is concerned about malignancy of the lesion.

35. **What is an osteochondroma?**
Osteochondromas are the most common benign bone tumor. They are both bone and cartilage forming. They appear as metaphyseal or epiphyseal cartilage-capped cortical out-growths (do not sit on an intact cortex). The most common sites are the distal femur, proximal tibia, proximal humerus, distal radius, and distal tibia. They are thought to arise as the result of aberrant growth plate cartilage and grow through enchondral ossification, until the growth plate from which they arose stops growing. They exist in sessile and pedunculated forms, and in each case, the cortical margins of the osteochondroma are continuous with the cortical margin of the rest of the bone. They are typically painless, but can cause irritation of surrounding soft tissues (Fig. 5.7).

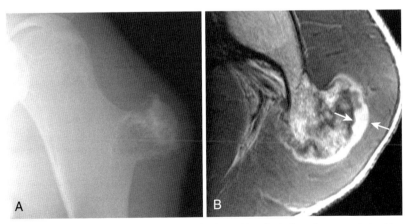

Figure 5.7. Radiograph (A) and MRI (B) of an osteochondroma. Note the thick cartilage cap as depicted by the arrows on the MRI. (*From Resnick D, Kransdorf M [eds]: Bone and Joint Imaging, 3rd edn. Copyright © Elsevier Inc., 2005.*)

36. **What is the risk of malignant transformation of osteochondromas? What are the warning signs?**

    Malignant transformation, typically to a low-grade chondrosarcoma, occurs in <1% of osteochondromas. An osteochondroma that becomes painful may signify a fracture, soft-tissue irritation, or malignant transformation. Osteochondromas that continue to grow after puberty or that have >3 cm cartilage caps are concerning due to possible malignant transformation.

37. **Are there any hereditary forms of osteochondromas?**

    Yes, multiple hereditary exostoses is an autosomal dominant hereditary form and represents about 10% of patients with osteochondromas. It is associated with short stature in 40% of patients, ulnar shortening, ankle valgus deformity, and leg-length discrepancy.

38. **What is a non-ossifying fibroma?**

    A non-ossifying fibroma (NOF) is the most common benign bone tumor in children and is often found incidentally on radiographs. They are eccentric metaphyseal bone lesions and are often well-marginated with a distinct multilocular appearance. The lesions tend to have an irregular pattern and are surrounded by a reactive rim of bone. As the lesion grows, it moves towards the diaphysis and becomes intracortical (Fig. 5.8).

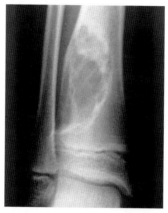

Figure 5.8. Radiograph of non-ossifying fibroma. *(From Kumar V, et al. [eds], Robbins and Cotran Pathologic Basis of Disease, Professional Edition, 8th edn. Copyright © Saunders, Elsevier Inc., 2010.)*

39. **How do you treat an NOF?**

    Unlike what the name would suggest, NOFs often heal in with bone after adolescence. Therefore, the treatment is usually observation. For large lesions that are symptomatic or at risk of an impending pathologic fracture, open biopsy with bone grafting can be done.

CASE 5-6

A 63-year-old female presents to your office with increasing right wrist pain over the past 3 months. You get an x-ray which shows a large expansile lesion in the distal radius with some cortical thinning of the bone. There does not appear to be any periosteal reaction in the bone. You schedule the patient for an open biopsy of the lesion.

40. **What is a giant cell tumor?**

    Giant cell tumors (GCTs) are aggressive benign lesions often found juxta-articularly in long bones. They are often found around the knee joint (distal femur of proximal tibia), but they also have a predilection for the distal radius. They are most commonly seen in patients after skeletal maturity and up to age 50 years. The tumor causes cortical thinning and is expansile in nature with a moth-eaten margin on x-ray. A periosteal reaction does not typically occur since the tumor remains contained within a thin cortical shell. In time, the surrounding bone may appear as if it has dissolved. On histology, the tumor has multinucleated giant cells interspersed between mononuclear stromal cells with mitotic figures (Fig. 5.9).

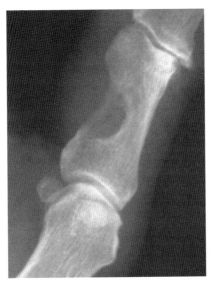

Figure 5.9. Radiograph of giant cell tumor. (*From Firestein GS, et al. Kelley's Textbook of Rheumatology, 8th edn, pp. 1883–1902. Copyright © Saunders, Elsevier Inc., 2009.*)

41. Can GCTs metastasize?
    GCTs metastasize to the lungs in 2% of patients.

42. How are GCTs treated?
    GCTs are treated with wide resection.

43. What is an adamantinoma?
    Adamantinoma is a rare tumor of unknown origin often found in long bones, specifically the anterior cortex of the midshaft of the tibia (90% of cases). It commonly affects both sexes between the ages of 20 and 50 years old. It has a "soap-bubble" appearance on radiographs. The overlying skin may be thin and shiny. On histological examination, the lesion appears as a low-grade spindle cell sarcoma with islands of epithelial cells or neoplastic cells surrounded by columnar cells in a palisading fashion. Treatment involves wide-margin resection. The differential diagnosis for adamantinoma should include cortical fibrous dysplasia.

44. What is the appearance of Paget's disease?
    Paget's disease presents as a lytic bone lesion early in its course and blastic late. The lesion has coarse trabeculae with thickened cortices.

MALIGNANT BONE TUMORS

45. Name a malignant primary bone-forming tumor.
    Osteosarcoma is a malignant primary bone-forming tumor.

46. How many types of osteosarcomas are there and which is the most common?
    There are four types of osteosarcomas: classic, periosteal, parosteal, and telangiectatic. Classic osteosarcoma is the most common type.

CASE 5-7

A 16-year-old hockey player had a fall while playing in a game about 3 weeks ago that resulted in continued left thigh pain. He had x-rays performed by his primary care physician who found the results to be concerning on the radiology report. A distal metaphyseal femoral lesion was seen on x-ray and is described as having a "sunburst" appearance.

47. **What is a classic osteosarcoma?**

An osteosarcoma is a malignant tumor that produces osteoid and often presents with soft-tissue extension. They are typically metaphyseal. The knee is the most common location. Patients present with pain, a mass, or occasionally a pathologic fracture. They tend to affect males more than females. A bimodal age distribution exists, with patients in their 2nd or 3rd decade and then again after their 6th decade being most frequently affected. Patients with Paget's disease are prone to developing osteosarcoma.

48. **What is the radiographic appearance of an osteosarcoma?**

Osteosarcomas show a "sunburst" or "hair on end" lesion on x-ray (Fig. 5.10).

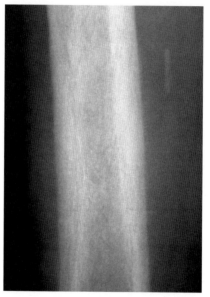

Figure 5.10. Radiograph demonstrating sunburst pattern. (*From Adam A, et al. [eds], Grainger & Allison's Diagnostic Radiology, 5th edn, pp. 1059–1081. Copyright © Churchill Livingstone, Elsevier Inc., 2008.*)

49. **What is the laboratory marker for osteosarcoma?**

An increased alkaline phosphatase may be found in patients with osteosarcoma.

CASE 5-7   continued

You explain to the patient your concern for a tumor and the need for biopsy. Biopsy results confirm your concern for osteosarcoma. The patient wants to know what the treatment is for his diagnosis.

50. **How are osteosarcomas treated?**

Osteosarcomas are treated with surgical excision and chemotherapy.

51. **What is telangiectatic osteosarcoma?**

Telangiectatic osteosarcoma is an aggressive and high-grade form that accounts for 5% of all osteosarcomas. It produces lytic lesions in the diaphysis or metaphysis. Periosteal reactions and Codman triangles are seen on x-ray. Grossly, it appears as a multi-cystic "bag of blood" lesion.

52. **What is parosteal osteosarcoma?**
Parosteal osteosarcoma accounts for another 5% of all osteosarcomas. It is a less malignant (Grade I) tumor that is slow to grow and metastasize. It is commonly found on the posterior aspect of the distal femur.

53. **What is periosteal osteosarcoma?**
Periosteal osteosarcoma accounts for only 1–2% of all osteosarcomas. It is often found on the anterior diaphyses of the tibia, femur, and humerus. It typically displays the "sunburst" pattern of periosteal reaction common to osteosarcoma. It can range from low to high grade.

54. **What are the primary malignant cartilage-forming bone lesions?**
Chondrosarcoma is the only primary malignant cartilage-forming bone lesion.

55. **What histological changes occur as cartilage shifts from benign to malignant?**
Increased cellularity, plump dark nuclei, and binucleate cells are signs of malignant transformation. More than one cell is seen in each lacunae or even outside of the lacunae. The matrix often becomes more myxoid and more mitotic figures are seen.

56. **What is a chondrosarcoma?**
A chondrosarcoma is a malignant, cartilage-forming tumor most commonly occurring in patients 40–60 years of age. Common sites include the pelvis (30%), proximal and distal femur, ribs, proximal humerus, and proximal tibia. Pelvic lesions are often misdiagnosed or diagnosed late.

57. **What is the radiographic appearance of chondrosarcoma?**
Chondrosarcoma displays endosteal scalloping, cortical thinning and expansion, and "speckled" calcification on x-ray. It destroys host bone as it grows.

58. **What is the most malignant form of chondrosarcoma?**
Dedifferentiated chondrosarcoma is the most malignant cartilage-forming tumor. This tumor most often occurs in the distal and proximal femur and the proximal humerus. The prognosis is poor, with less than 10% long-term survival.

59. **What is a chordoma?**
Chordomas are low-grade sarcomas from notochord remnant. They are most commonly found in the sacrum or the base of the brain. Patients usually present between the ages of 40 and 70 years old. Low back pain, pelvic pain, or perineal pain and numbness are common complaints. These tumors are often difficult to see on plain radiographs, but CT will show bony destruction and soft-tissue mass. Histologically, these tumors are characterized by "foam" cells, which are vacuolated and surrounded by a myxoid mucinous matrix and strands of syncytial cells. Grossly, these masses appear to have a mucinous and runny texture. Treatment involves surgery with pre- and postoperative radiation.

60. **What is Ewing's sarcoma?**
Ewing's sarcoma is a small round blue cell tumor possibly related to primitive neuroectodermal cells. Patients are usually males in their first 2 decades of life. Twenty percent of the patients have constitutional symptoms including fever, anemia, leukocytosis, and an increased sedimentation rate. The tumor is characteristically diaphyseal and affects the femur most commonly, but can be seen in other long bones and in the pelvis in about 20% of cases. It is often associated with a soft-tissue mass. Radiographs reveal the typical "onion skin" periosteal reaction. Treatment typically involves surgery with neoadjuvant and adjuvant chemotherapy.

61. **What should be on the differential diagnosis for Ewing's sarcoma?**
Osteomyelitis has a similar histologic appearance (numerous dense blue PMNs) as opposed to small round blue cells seen in Ewing's sarcoma.

62. **How does the histologic appearance of Ewing's sarcoma compare to neuroblastoma?**
Neuroblastoma has pseudo-rosettes, which are circles or round cells surrounding a pink ground substance.

63. **What are two hematopoietic tumors that affect bone?**
Lymphoma and myeloma are hematopoietic tumors that can be found in bone.

64. **What is the effect of lymphoma on bone?**
Although very permeative, lymphoma is minimally destructive to bone. It typically fills the medullary canal first and then spreads to the soft tissue in almost ghost-like fashion. Because of its minimal destruction of bone, lymphoma may present with normal radiographs. An MRI is often needed to show marrow replacement and the soft-tissue mass.

65. **What other condition can cause intramedullary edema similar to that seen with lymphoma?**
Stress fractures can cause intramedullary edema similar to that seen with lymphoma.

66. **What is plasmacytoma?**
Plasmacytoma is a solitary monoclonal plasma cell-derived malignancy.

67. **What is a multiple myeloma?**
Multiple myeloma is a neoplastic condition whereby malignant monoclonal plasma cells form medullary lytic lesions. The lesions often have sharp margins with little reaction of the surrounding tissue. It typically affects patients over the age of 40 years. The lesions are found in many locations including the skull, spine, ribs, pelvis, and proximal long bones. Patients often present with malaise, bone pain, or a pathologic fracture. Diagnostic blood tests include anemia (90%), elevated ESR, and elevated monoclonal immunoglobulin "g" protein levels. Diagnosis is confirmed with a bone marrow biopsy in which >20% plasma cells are seen. On histology, these plasma cells are seen to have prominent chromatin in a "clock face" pattern with eccentric cytoplasm (Fig. 5.11). Treatment for multiple myeloma involves radiation.

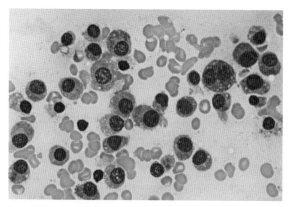

Figure 5.11. Histological appearance of plasma cell. (*From Jaffe ES, et al. [eds], Hematopathology, 1st edn, pp. 410–435.e5. Copyright © Saunders, Elsevier Inc., 2011.*)

68. **What imaging study should be performed in a patient with multiple myeloma?**
A skeletal survey can be useful to determine the location of other lesions.

69. **What other tumors cause multiple lesions in the bone?**
Other tumors that appear with multiple lesions are metastases, enchondroma, histiocytosis, fibrous dysplasia, and non-ossifying fibroma.

70. **What are the most common pediatric and adult round cell tumors?**
(See Table 5.2.)

Table 5.2. Most Common Pediatric and Adult Round Cell Tumors	
PEDIATRIC	**ADULT**
Ewing's sarcoma	Lymphoma
Neuroblastoma	Myeloma

BENIGN SOFT-TISSUE TUMORS AND REACTIVE LESIONS
CASE 5-8

A 30-year-old male presents to your office with a recently developed soft-tissue mass on the lateral aspect of his forearm. It is non-painful and feels mobile under the skin. It is not very large, but the patient is concerned for the mass. You order an MRI, which shows the mass to be very bright on T1 imaging (Fig. 5.12).

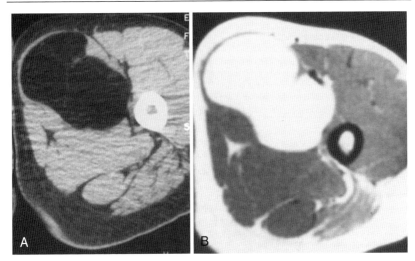

Figure 5.12. Fat-suppressed (A) and T1 (B) MRI demonstrating a lipoma. Note the similar appearance of the lipoma and the subcutaenous fat. (*From Resnick D, Kransdorf M [eds]: Bone and Joint Imaging, 3rd edn. Copyright © Elsevier Inc., 2005.*)

71. What is the most common benign soft-tissue tumor found in adults?
    Lipoma.

72. What is a lipoma?
    Lipomas are benign soft-tissues masses comprised of mature adipocytes. Their appearance is consistent with normal subcutaneous fat on MRI (bright on T1 and T2 images; dark on fat-suppressed and STIR images). They are homogeneous without any interstitial markings. They can be treated with observation.

CASE 5-8 continued

The patient wants to know the chances of this mass becoming malignant and whether he should have it removed.

73. What is an atypical lipoma? Is it malignant or benign?
    Atypical lipomas are also known as well-differentiated liposarcomas. They have a surrounding layer of fibrous tissue that causes them to have a low signal on T1 images. They have a 10% chance of malignant transformation.

74. What characteristic of angiolipoma separates it from other lipomas?
    Angiolipomas are tender when palpated. They are usually located in the upper extremity and are often found in children. They are typically located deep within muscle tissue as opposed to the superficial location of other lipomas.

75. **What is a desmoid tumor?**
Desmoid tumors are benign soft-tissue tumors that are locally invasive. They are typically found as firm masses in adolescents and young adults.

76. **What is the preferred treatment of a desmoid tumor?**
Wide resection is the preferred treatment of a desmoid tumor to prevent local tissue invasion.

77. **What is fibrous dysplasia?**
Fibrous dysplasia is a developmental abnormality of bone that is often seen as a long lesion in a long bone (i.e., femur). Radiographs of bone often show a "ground-glass" appearance representing medullary calcification. In addition, there is often cortical thinning with no periosteal reaction. Histologically, the major finding is numerous fibroblasts responsible for creating a dense collagenous matrix.

78. **What should be in the differential diagnosis of every benign bone lesion?**
Fibrous dysplasia has a variable appearance, so should be on the differential diagnosis for all benign bone lesions.

79. **What is a hemangioma?**
A hemangioma is a tumor comprised of a conglomeration of blood vessels. It is the most common benign soft-tissue tumor found in children. They appear as a heterogeneous lesion with serpiginous borders, characterized by a honey-comb pattern. These are most commonly found in the vertebral bodies. When present in the extremities, the lower extremities are more commonly affected than the upper extremities. They are occasionally symptomatic and can be treated by radiation therapy or embolization.

80. **What marker is positive in hemangiomas?**
Factor VIII related antigen (vWF) is a marker for vascular differentiation and is positive in hemangiomas. This marker is not typically seen in high-grade vascular tumors (angiosarcoma).

81. **What is myositis ossificans?**
Myositis ossificans is a reactive process of heterotopic bone formation that occurs after an episode of blunt trauma. Patients often do not recall the specific trauma. Radiographs show the formation of peripheral maturation and calcification with a lucent center. The lucent center has aggressive-looking immature cells when examined histologically.

82. **What should be on the differential for myositis ossificans and why?**
Sarcoma should be included on the differential for myositis ossificans as both have an inactive center with an active periphery.

83. **What is a schwannoma?**
A schwannoma, also called a neurofibroma, is a benign peripheral nerve sheath tumor. It tends to occur in middle-aged adults and can occasionally cause pain.

84. **When should there be concern for neurofibrosarcoma?**
A diameter greater than 5 cm is concerning for malignancy.

85. **What are Antoni A and Antoni B?**
These are histological classifications of areas found within schwannomas. Antoni A areas are hypercellular areas of compact spindle cells; whereas, Antoni B areas are hypocellular areas that are less organized. When lesions show a predominance of Antoni A area, there is greater concern for malignancy.

86. **What marker is positive in a patient with a schwannoma?**
Schwannomas are S-100 positive, which is a marker found in tissues including neural, chondroid, and melanocytic-derived tissue.

87. **What is a myxoma?**
Myxoma is the most common benign muscle tumor in adults. It typically occurs in middle-aged females in the hip region.

88. What is on the differential for a myxoma?
    A myxoid fibrosarcoma is on the differential diagnosis, so a biopsy of the lesion must be performed.

MALIGNANT SOFT TISSUE TUMORS

89. What age group tends to get soft-tissue sarcomas? How do they present?
    Soft-tissue sarcoma is predominately a disease of older persons.

90. How do soft-tissue sarcomas typically present?
    Soft-tissue sarcomas typically present as a painless mass. The thigh and buttock are the most common location.

91. How should a patient with a suspected soft-tissue sarcoma be worked up?
    Plain radiographs are used to determine bony involvement and to see if there is calcification within the lesion. An MRI is used to determine the extent of the local disease. A CT scan of the chest is obtained to rule out metastatic disease. Positron emission tomography (PET) scans are being investigated as another option for discovering metastatic lesions. A biopsy is necessary for tissue diagnosis, but should be done after imaging is obtained.

92. What are the most common soft-tissue sarcomas?
    Malignant fibrous histiocytoma is the most common soft-tissue sarcoma. Liposarcoma and synovial sarcoma are other common sarcomas.

93. What is malignant fibrous histiocytoma?
    Malignant fibrous histiocytoma is a poorly defined and highly destructive tumor of spindle and histiocytic cells. The cells are arranged in a cartwheel pattern histologically. It commonly presents as a painless mass that becomes symptomatic when it becomes large.

94. What is a liposarcoma?
    Liposarcomas are malignant tumors comprised of lipoblasts. They tend to occur in the thigh, retroperitoneum, and popliteal fossa. Paradoxically, they typically do not contain fat. They are treated with wide excision and combinations of pre- and postoperative radiation and chemotherapies. Radiation can be given postoperatively if margins are positive, and chemotherapy is given if the mass is large.

95. What are the types of liposarcoma?
    Liposarcomas can be classified into four types: myxoid (low grade), well-differentiated (low grade), round cell (high grade), and pleomorphic (high grade). High-grade liposarcomas tend to be more vascular and appear denser on MRI.

CASE 5-9

A 29-year-old male with 2 months of ankle pain with no injury presents to your office with recent x-rays showing calcification around the ankle joint. You decide to take the patient to the OR for biopsy of the ankle.

96. What is a synovial sarcoma?
    Synovial sarcomas are cystic high-grade malignant tumors derived from an unknown cell of origin. They present as painful masses adjacent to joints (the knee is most common, followed by hands and feet). It is the most common sarcoma found in the foot. They tend to occur in patients less than 40 years of age. They have a strong predilection for metastases to the lymph nodes and lungs. X-rays may demonstrate calcification. Histologically, the tumor is typically biphasic with epithelial and spindle cell components.

97. How are synovial sarcomas treated?
    Biopsy is necessary followed by wide surgical excision and adjuvant radiation therapy.

98. Besides synovial sarcoma, what other soft-tissue malignancies have a strong predilection for metastasizing to the lymph nodes and lungs?
    Epithelioid sarcomas and rhabdomyosarcomas also tend to metastasize to the lymph nodes and lungs.

99. **What is the most common soft-tissue malignant tumor in children?**
Rhabdomyosarcoma.

100. **What is rhabdomyosarcoma?**
Rhabdomyosarcoma is a highly malignant tumor of muscle tissue. It is composed of spindle cells, multinucleated giant cells, and tennis racquet-shaped cells. The lesion is typically found in the head, neck, genitourinary tract, and pelvis of children. It is rapidly growing with a high rate of metastasizing to lymph nodes. They tend to be chemo sensitive.

METASTATIC BONE DISEASE

101. **Which metastases are osteoblastic?**
The "blastic" metastatic diseases are prostate and breast cancers.
Remember the pneumonic: **P**rostate and **B**reast...**P**roduce **B**one.

102. **What cancers commonly metastasize to bone?**
The cancers that most commonly metastasize to bone are **B**reast, **L**ung, **T**hyroid, **K**idney, and **P**rostate.
Remember the pneumonic: **BLT** on a **K**aiser roll with a **P**ickle.

103. **Which cancers frequently metastasize in children?**
Neuroblastoma, Ewing's sarcoma, lymphoma, and leukemia frequently metastasize.

104. **Which metastases are highly vascular?**
Renal cell and thyroid cancers are usually highly vascular, often requiring preoperative embolization if surgical biopsy or excision is planned.

MISCELLANEOUS LESIONS

105. **What should be in the differential diagnosis of every intramedullary lesion in a young person?**
Langerhans cell histiocytosis.

106. **What is a unicameral bone cyst? (Fig. 5.13)**
A unicameral bone cyst, also called simple bone cyst, is a cystic, symmetric expansion within bone. It is central and full width. The involved cortices may be thinned, but there is no periosteal reaction and the lesion is no wider than the widest portion of adjacent metaphysis. They are most commonly found in the proximal humerus and calcaneus. On histology, a thin layer of fibrous tissue is seen lining an empty space, and there are benign giant cells, few chronic inflammatory cells, and hemosiderin pigment. It can be treated with observation or intralesional steroid injection. Curettage and bone grafting may be performed for recalcitrant lesions.

107. **What is an aneurysmal bone cyst? (Fig. 5.14)**
An aneurysmal bone cyst is an expansile, eccentric metaphyseal lesion. The lesion is typically surrounded by a thin and fragile rim of expanded cortical bone. On histology, the lesion displays sponge-like spaces filled with unclotted blood. The lesion is typically seen in patients under the age of 20 years old. Secondary ABCs can be seen in osteosarcoma and Ewing's sarcoma. Treatment involves wide resection, as simple curettage has a recurrence rate of approximately 30%. Other methods to reduce recurrence include burring, phenol, and cauterization. Bone grafting is often done to reduce postoperative pathologic fracture (Figs 5.13, 5.14).

108. **What is Langerhan's cell histiocytosis?**
Langerhan's cell histiocytosis is an inflammatory condition characterized by intramedullary lytic lesions occurring most commonly in patients in their first three decades of life. The inflammation can cause an aggressive periosteal reaction. It should be included in the differential diagnosis of an intramedullary lesion in a young patient. Its histology displays many small round cells with histiocytes (large cells with ill-defined borders and indented nuclei), lymphocytes, neutrophils, and eosinophils (Fig. 5.15). It can be treated with simple curettage or observation, as most lesions will resolve spontaneously.

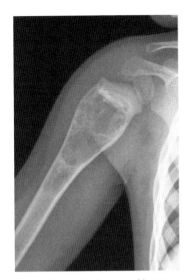

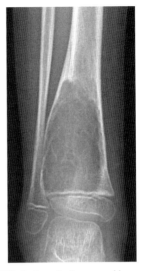

Figure 5.13. Radiograph of unicameral bone cyst. *(From Gilbert-Barness E, et al. [eds]. Potter's Pathology of the Fetus, Infant, and Child, 2nd edn, pp. 1797–1897. Copyright © Mosby, Elsevier Inc., 2007.)*

Figure 5.14. Radiograph of aneurysmal bone cyst. *(From Gilbert-Barness E, et al. [eds], Potter's Pathology of the Fetus, Infant, and Child, 2nd edn, pp. 1797–1897. Copyright © Mosby, Elsevier Inc., 2007.)*

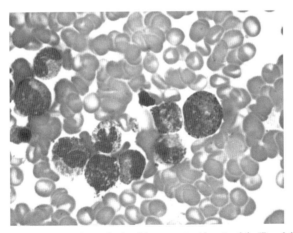

Figure 5.15. Histologic appearance of Langerhan's cell histiocytosis with eosinophils. *(From Jaffe ES, et al. [eds], Hematopathology, 1st edn, pp. 777–787.e1. Copyright © Saunders, Elsevier Inc., 2011.)*

BIBLIOGRAPHY

1. Aboulafia AJ, Kennon RE, Jelinek JS. Benign bone tumors of childhood. J Am Acad Orthop Surg 1999;7:377–88.
2. Bridge JA, Schwartz HS, Neff JR. Bone sarcomas. In: Abeloff MD, Armitage JO, Lichter AS, et al., editors. Clinical Oncology. 2nd ed. Orlando, FL: Harcourt Brace; 2000. p. 2160–72.
3. Capanna R, Campanacci DA. The treatment of metastases in the appendicular skeleton. J Bone Joint Surg Br 2001;83:471–81.
4. Enneking WE, Spanier SS, Goodman MA. A system for the surgical staging of musculoskeletal sarcoma. Clin Orthop Rel Res 1980;153:106–20.
5. Gilbert NF, Cannon CP, Lin PP, et al. Soft-tissue sarcoma. J Am Acad Orthop Surg 2009;17:40–7.
6. Gitelis S, Schajowicz F. Osteoid osteoma and osteoblastoma. Orthop Clin North Am 1989;20:313–25.
7. Kneisl JS, Simon MA. Medical management compared with operative treatment for osteoid osteoma. J Bone Joint Surg 1992;74A:179–85.
8. Lackman RD. Musculoskeletal oncology. In: Vaccaro AR, editor. Orthopaedic Knowledge Update, vol. 8. Rosemont, IL: American Academy of Orthopaedic Surgeons; 2005. p. 197–215.
9. Mankin HJ, Hornicek FJ. Diagnosis, classification, and management of soft tissue sarcomas. Cancer Control 2005;12:5–21.
10. Miller M. Review of Orthopaedics. 4th ed. Philadelphia, PA: Saunders; 2004. p. 440–500.
11. Weber K, Damron TA, Frassica FJ, et al. Malignant bone tumors. Instr Course Lect 2008;57: 673–88.
12. Yasko AW. Giant cell tumor of bone. Curr Oncol Rep 2002;4:520–6.

CHAPTER 6

PEDIATRIC ORTHOPEDICS

Eileen A. Crawford, Corinna C.D. Franklin, David A. Spiegel and Keith D. Baldwin

THE LIMPING CHILD

TODDLER'S FRACTURE

CASE 6-1

A 2-year-old boy is brought to the Emergency Room (ER) by his mother. She reports that he started limping earlier in the day, and now he is asking to be carried everywhere rather than walking himself. She did not see him fall or hurt himself, though he was playing with his older brother in the other room for a while as she was putting away laundry. He has been very fussy while they waited in the ER. Upon examination, you notice that he withdraws his right leg with any attempts to examine it. There is no deformity or significant swelling, but he has definite tenderness over the anterior mid-tibia. X-ray is shown in Figure 6.1.

1. What is a toddler's fracture?
   A "toddler's fracture" is a spiral fracture of the tibia in an approximately 24–36-month-old child. Most toddler's fractures occur in children less than 30 months old, and the mean age of incidence is 27 months. They occur more frequently in boys than in girls. The right leg is more commonly involved than the left.

2. What is the mechanism of injury?
   The mechanism of injury involves external rotation of the foot with the knee in a fixed position, creating a torsional force on the tibia. These fractures can also occur from a low-energy fall.

3. What is the clinical presentation?
   Children with a toddler's fracture typically present with a history of irritability and a limp, with or without a known injury. They may outright refuse to walk or bear weight on the involved leg. Point tenderness over the fracture site and pain with ankle dorsiflexion are other potential findings, though not always elicited with this fracture or age group. It is important in this age group to do a thorough examination of the entire lower extremity in an attempt to localize the site of involvement since any pathology from the hip to the foot may present similarly. Occult metatarsal fractures are also a common cause for limp in this age group, especially with a history of jumping off a couch.

4. What imaging studies should be performed to evaluate a suspected toddler's fracture?
   Antero-posterior (AP) and lateral views of the entire tibia should be obtained, but are often normal as toddler's fractures are frequently non-displaced. Non-displaced fractures should be apparent on x-ray by the presence of periosteal new bone 10–14 days following the injury.

5. How are toddler's fractures treated?
   Placement of a long-leg cast without manipulation is the recommended treatment for all fractures in acceptable alignment. After 3 weeks, the long-leg cast can be converted to a short-leg cast for another 2–3 weeks if still symptomatic or until the fracture is healed. Note the child will often limp for an additional week after the cast is removed.

6. What should be done for toddlers who have a history and exam consistent with fracture but negative x-rays?
   The first step is to rule out other potential causes of leg pain that may have unremarkable x-rays, such as infection. A toddler's fracture may be presumed when no other cause is found, and treated with a long leg cast. This will result in unnecessary casting of about half of patients, but avoids the mistreatment of an occult fracture. The downsides of casting in the absence of fracture include a temporary limp when the cast is removed and skin breakdown.

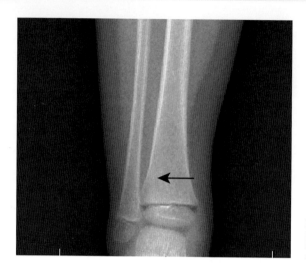

Figure 6.1. Antero-posterior projection of the distal tibia showing a subtle crack in the distal tibial metaphysis.

7. **What complications are seen with this fracture?**
Complications are very rare with toddler's fractures because of the remarkable healing and remodeling potential of children in this age group. There may be a slight rotational malalignment if the fragments slide inside the cast, but this is clinically insignificant and not noticeable unless the limbs are directly compared.

8. **Are there concerns for growth plate involvement?**
Yes. Be suspicious for toddler's fractures that spiral down to the distal tibial physis, resulting in a Salter–Harris II fracture. Physeal involvement may be difficult to appreciate on x-ray because the distal epiphysis does not typically appear radiographically until 2 years of age.

SEPTIC ARTHRITIS
CASE 6-2

A 6-year-old girl has been febrile for the past 24 hours. She refuses to bear weight on her left leg. You come to see her in the Emergency Room. She holds her left leg in a flexed and abducted position (frog-legged). She will not let you examine her. Her temperature is 38.5°C. She has a white count of 17 000 WBC/mm³. Her erythrocyte sedimentation rate (ESR) is 50 mm/h, her C-reactive protein (CRP) is 5.3 mg/dL.

9. **What are the different ways bacteria can enter the joint?**
Bacteria gain access to the joint via hematogenous dissemination, by local spread of disease (e.g., osteomyelitis), or via direct inoculation from trauma or surgery. The metaphysis is intra-articular in the proximal radius, proximal humerus, proximal femur, and distal fibula. As a result, direct spread from a metaphyseal osteomyelitis is a higher risk at the elbow, shoulder, hip, and ankle. In these joints, bacteria may directly invade the joint from the metaphysis in children up to 12–18 months of age after which the pattern of circulation changes and the physis forms a more effective barrier to spread.

10. **What factors increase a patient's risk for developing septic arthritis?**
Young age, prior trauma to the joint, systemic diseases affecting the joint (e.g., rheumatoid arthritis, hemophilia), and immunocompromised states all increase susceptibility to septic arthritis.

11. **What organism is most commonly implicated in septic arthritis in neonates? In children less than 2 years old? In children greater than 2 years old?**
Staphylococcus aureus is the most common pathogen of septic arthritis in all of these age groups. *Haemophilus influenza* has been a common cause of septic arthritis in children less than 2 years old, but the *H. influenza* type B vaccine has decreased the incidence of *H. influenza*-related septic arthritis.

12. **What organisms are found in septic arthritis associated with trauma?**
    Gram-negative bacilli, anaerobes, and *S. aureus* are the most common pathogens found in septic arthritis associated with trauma.

13. **What organisms are found in septic arthritis associated with hemophilia?**
    S. aureus, streptococci, and gram-negative bacilli are the most common pathogens found in septic arthritis associated with hemophilia.

14. **What organisms are found in septic arthritis in immunocompromised patients?**
    S. aureus, mycobacteria, and fungi are the most common pathogens found in septic arthritis in immunocompromised patients.

15. **What are the signs and symptoms of lower extremity septic arthritis in children?**
    Children often present with a history of limping, refusal to walk or bear weight, fussiness, fever, and/or recent trauma to the joint. On exam, the joint may be swollen, warm, and erythematous. A patient will hold a septic hip in flexion and external rotation, and a septic knee in flexion because these positions maximize volume within the capsule and tend to be more comfortable. Pain with short-arc passive range of motion ("micro-motion pain") is characteristic of septic arthritis. Absence of micro-motion pain decreases the likelihood of septic arthritis, although the entire clinical picture must be used in making a diagnosis. A high index of clinical suspicion is required, as no algorithm has been universally accepted thus far. "Kocher" criteria are also useful in judging septic hip arthritis in children. These criteria include inability to weight bear on the affected side, an ESR of 40 mm/h or more, fever, and a WBC count of >12000 cells/mm^3. When one-quarter of these is present there is a 3% chance of septic arthritis, ranging to 99% chance when all four are present. More recent studies suggest that CRP is a useful adjunct to this prediction model.

16. **What are the signs and symptoms of lower extremity septic arthritis in neonates?**
    Neonates have a less robust inflammatory response, and the characteristic signs of infection (fever, swelling, erythema, and pain with motion) may be absent. It is crucial to have a high suspicion with reports of irritable behavior, failure to thrive, asymmetric extremity movement, and coincident infections.

17. **Should x-rays be obtained to evaluate for septic arthritis?**
    Yes, x-rays of the symptomatic joint should be obtained in a patient being evaluated for septic arthritis. They can help narrow the differential diagnosis as it may reveal fractures or bone lesions that are sources of joint pain. Radiographs can also increase your suspicion for septic arthritis if a joint effusion, localized soft-tissue swelling, or evidence of osteomyelitis is present. However, a normal x-ray does not rule out septic arthritis (or an occult fracture).

18. **What other imaging studies are useful for evaluating septic arthritis?**
    Ultrasonography is particularly useful in septic arthritis of the hip since an effusion is not appreciable on clinical exam as with the knee or ankle. It can also be used to guide aspiration of a hip effusion to send for laboratory studies. MRI will demonstrate a joint effusion and often synovial inflammation or hypertrophy, but should not delay intervention when the characteristic signs and symptoms are present. Radionuclide bone scans will highlight regions of inflammation, but are not specific and, therefore, are rarely used in evaluating septic arthritis.

19. **How is septic arthritis diagnosed?**
    The definitive diagnosis of septic arthritis is based on culturing a pathogen from the synovial fluid of the affected joint. Because culture results can take days to identify an organism, the cell count and Gram stain are used as a preliminary indicator. A white blood cell count greater than 50000 cells/mm^3 and a differential of >90% polymorphonuclear cells is suggestive of septic arthritis, although occasionally other pathologies (JIA, Lyme) may have similar values. Immunocompromised patients may have a lower white blood cell count in the setting of septic arthritis. Culture-negative septic arthritis is not uncommon in children, so treatment should not be aborted early if the cultures fail to grow an organism.

20. **What landmarks are used to aspirate an ankle? A knee? A hip?**
For an ankle aspiration, insert the needle approximately 1 cm anterior to the lateral malleolus at the level of the joint line just lateral to the extensor digitorum longus. For a knee aspiration, insert the needle laterally at the level of the superior pole of the patella. Alternatively, with the knee flexed 30–40°, the needle can be inserted medial or lateral to the patellar tendon at the level of the joint line. A hip aspiration should be performed under ultrasound or fluoroscopic guidance. The needle can be inserted anteriorly (1 inch lateral and distal to the inguinal ligament), medially (inferior to the adductor longus tendon), or laterally (inferior and anterior to the greater trochanter).

21. **How quickly does joint destruction occur?**
Damage to articular cartilage begins within 18–24 hours from the start of the infection, and irreversible changes likely occur after several days. By 4 weeks, the articular surface may be destroyed. A delay in treatment can result in irreversible joint damage. Avascular necrosis of the hip may also occur due to tamponade of blood vessels from a tense effusion, mandating early diagnosis and prompt drainage of septic arthritis.

22. **How is septic arthritis treated?**
While repeated aspiration is an option in smaller joints, larger joints are typically managed with surgical drainage and irrigation and antibiotic therapy (typically 3–6 weeks). Septic arthritis of the hip is treated as a surgical emergency. Intravenous antibiotics are administered initially, and are often switched to an oral regimen within a few days based on the patients' clinical response. Empiric antibiotics should ideally be started after a sample of synovial fluid is obtained. The choice of antibiotic should then be tailored to the culture and sensitivity results when available. Patients are monitored for response to both interventions. Failure to improve should prompt adjustment of antibiotics, repeat surgical drainage, or a search for an alternate diagnosis.

TRANSIENT SYNOVITIS

CASE 6-3

You are called to the Emergency Room to see an 8-year-old girl with left hip pain and a limp that has been going on for 2 days. She has no history of trauma. According to her parents, she started complaining of pain in her left hip 2 mornings ago, but they thought she just bruised something while playing soccer. Last night she started limping and seemed more irritable. They took her temperature, and it was normal. In the ER she is also afebrile. She is resting on the stretcher with her right leg straight and her left hip flexed and externally rotated and her left knee flexed. She gets upset and grabs your hands when you gently rotate her hip. The ER physicians performed an ultrasound of the hip, which demonstrated a moderate effusion (Fig. 6.2). Her bloodwork has also just come back and is unremarkable other than a mildly elevated erythrocyte sedimentation rate (ESR) of 41 mm/h. You decide to aspirate her hip under ultrasound guidance. Results of the synovial fluid analysis reveals 186 white blood cells/mm³ with a normal differential. The Gram stain is negative for bacteria.

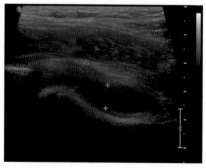

Figure 6.2. Ultrasound of the hip showing a moderate-sized effusion between the two white crosses.

23. **What is transient synovitis of the hip?**
Transient synovitis is a self-limiting, benign condition of the hip characterized by the acute onset of a limp, often associated with mild discomfort. There may be a history of a

recent viral-type illness, and occasionally a mild fever but no significant constitutional signs or symptoms that accompany the hip pain. The etiology of transient synovitis of the hip is unknown, though a viral etiology is suspected.

24. **Is transient synovitis of the hip a common condition?**
Yes. It is among the most common causes of limp in the young child. An individual has approximately a 3% risk of having at least one episode of transient synovitis in his or her childhood. Boys are affected twice as often as girls.

25. **What would you expect to find on physical examination of a child with transient synovitis of the hip?**
The child will walk with an antalgic gait or may refuse to walk altogether. The hip is most comfortable in a position of flexion and external rotation. Passive range of motion of the hip is mildly restricted, usually due to guarding, and there may be some discomfort at the end ranges of rotation (especially internal rotation). The physical findings may be similar to septic arthritis, although patients with septic arthritis usually have more pronounced discomfort (which is present at rest) and pain is elicited throughout the range of motion.

26. **Are imaging studies useful in the diagnosis of transient synovitis of the hip?**
In general, imaging studies are of limited value in the diagnosis of transient synovitis of the hip. Radiographs occasionally show an enlarged joint space from a hip effusion. Ultrasound is more sensitive than radiography for detecting an effusion, but still is not specific for the diagnosis. MRI may be useful to detect joint effusions or subperiosteal abscesses.

27. **What are the Kocher criteria?**
The Kocher criteria are four physical examination or laboratory findings used to differentiate transient synovitis from septic arthritis. Although these criteria are not validated by other studies, they are the most frequently utilized for clinical decision making. The four criteria are history of fever, inability to bear weight, ESR greater than 40 mm/h, and white blood cell count greater than 12 000 cells/mm^3. The presence of all four criteria predicted a 99% chance that the diagnosis was septic arthritis. Three positive criteria correlated with a 93% chance, two positive criteria with a 40% chance, and only one positive criterion with a 3% chance of the patient having septic arthritis. Recent evidence suggests that a CRP level greater than 2 mg/dL is a strong independent factor in differentiating septic arthritis from transient synovitis.

28. **How is septic arthritis excluded in cases that mimic transient synovitis of the hip?**
Hip joint aspiration with cell count, Gram stain, and culture should be performed in cases for which septic arthritis is suspected.

29. **How is transient synovitis of the hip treated?**
Conservative management is the rule for transient synovitis of the hip. Antiinflammatories tend to have a remarkable and quick effect on the pain and may shorten the duration of the condition. Weight-bearing of the affected hip may be restricted until the symptoms resolve. Most patients experience significant relief by 5–7 days, although complete resolution may take up to 4–6 weeks. Prolonged symptoms should prompt reevaluation to rule out other diagnoses.

OSTEOMYELITIS

30. **What physical exam findings should you look for in a case of suspected osteomyelitis?**
Fever, limp, refusal to bear weight, erythema, warmth, swelling, and point tenderness over the metaphysis are all common signs of osteomyelitis. It is important to look for open wounds in children who are non-ambulatory or have chronic diseases that limit their mobility or sensation. Recent puncture wounds can also be suggestive of osteomyelitis that developed after a trauma.

31. **What indicators of osteomyelitis may be detectable on x-ray? Ultrasound? MRI?**
Plain radiographs are an important first step in the evaluation of osteomyelitis because they can often rule out other diagnoses and may be sufficient to establish the diagnosis.

Soft-tissue swelling, periosteal reaction, and bone resorption are the most likely x-ray findings, though bony changes typically take 10–14 days to develop. Early-stage osteomyelitis may have normal x-rays, in which case further imaging with MRI may be warranted. MRI features of osteomyelitis include bony edema, intra-osseous or subperiosteal abscesses, soft-tissue inflammation, effusion, and myositis. Bone scans are used less frequently in the workup of osteomyelitis because severe infections can show low activity due to compromised osseous microcirculation, and they can be more difficult to interpret in small children.

32. **What laboratory studies should be obtained for suspected osteomyelitis?**
    A complete blood count (CBC) with differential, ESR, CRP, and blood cultures should be obtained. A normal white blood cell count does not exclude osteomyelitis. Aspiration of the metaphyseal region should be considered when there is point tenderness on examination, as a subperiostial abscess may be identified and the fluid sent for culture.

33. **Which marker, ESR or CRP, takes longer to return to normal following resolution of osteomyelitis?**
    ESR takes longer to return to normal levels following infection – typically about 3 weeks. CRP is an acute-phase reactant that rises and descends more quickly than ESR in the setting of infection. CRP level may normalize within a week of initiation of effective treatment; as such, CRP is a better marker to monitor the response to treatment.

34. **What is a sequestrum? What is an involucrum?**
    These are terms related to chronic osteomyelitis. A sequestrum is a fragment of necrotic bone that has been walled off by the infection. Sequestrae may be partially or completely resorbed by the host response. It must be removed to clear the osteomyelitis. An involucrum represents the host response, and involves periosteal new bone formation which serves to wall off sequestrae and restore mechanical stability to the involved segment of bone. Sequestrectomy should be delayed until sufficient involucrum has been formed, otherwise segmental bone loss may occur.

35. **What is the most common causative organism in cases of pediatric osteomyelitis?**
    As with septic arthritis, *S. aureus* is the most common causative organism for pediatric osteomyelitis. Neonatal osteomyelitis may be caused by *Escherichia coli*, Group B *Streptococci*, *Enterobacteriae*, or *Candida albicans*.

36. **How is osteomyelitis treated?**
    All cases of osteomyelitis are treated with intravenous antibiotics based on culture and sensitivity results. If a causative organism is not isolated, antibiotics are selected empirically. After response to intravenous antibiotics has been demonstrated, conversion to an oral antibiotic regimen can be considered. In fact, recent evidence supports earlier switch to oral antibiotics based on organism and clinical response. Antibiotic treatment typically lasts for 6 weeks.

37. **When is surgical intervention appropriate for osteomyelitis?**
    If diagnosed early, uncomplicated cases of osteomyelitis do not require surgical intervention. However, the presence of a drainable intra-osseous or subperiosteal abscess, or bony destruction on x-ray, is an appropriate indication for surgery. Patients who do not respond to intravenous antibiotics after 48 hours are also candidates for surgical intervention. All cases of chronic osteomyelitis warrant surgical débridement and removal of any devitalized tissues as the primary treatment strategy, and antibiotics serve as an adjunct in these cases.

38. **What is a concern of metaphyseal osteomyelitis in the growing child?**
    The physis can be damaged in metaphyseal osteomyelitis, leading to physeal arrest with limb-length discrepancies or angular deformities.

39. **What type of musculoskeletal infection is more common in children, osteomyelitis or septic arthritis?**
    Septic arthritis occurs approximately twice as frequently as osteomyelitis in children. They also tend to affect different age groups, with septic arthritis more common in patients less than 5 years old and osteomyelitis more common in patients 5–10 years old.

40. **Does osteomyelitis ever occur concomitantly with septic arthritis?**
Yes, septic arthritis and osteomyelitis affect the same joint simultaneously in about 20–30% of cases. In infants, this dual infection is thought to occur because the epiphyseal and metaphyseal circulation communicate. After approximately 12–18 months of age, the physis serves as a barrier to the spread of infection. Joints in which the metaphysis is intra-articular (proximal femur, distal fibula, proximal radius, proximal humerus) are more prone to direct spread from a metaphyseal focus of osteomyelitis.

LYME DISEASE

41. **What causes Lyme disease?**
Lyme disease is caused by the spirochete *Borrelia burgdorferi*.

42. **What other infection with orthopedic manifestations is caused by a spirochete?**
Syphilis is also caused by a spirochete named *Treponema pallidum*, which can be transmitted across the placenta from an infected mother to the fetus. Congenital syphilis manifests in the proximal tibia with cortical thickening ("saber shins"). Chronic arthralgias may occur throughout the body.

43. **How is the spirochete of Lyme disease transmitted?**
Ticks of the *Ixodes* family are the primary vectors of *Borrelia burgdorferi* that transmit Lyme disease. Ixodes dammini and Ixodes pacificus are the most common vectors in the US and are found in forests of the northeast and mid-Atlantic states. These ticks feed on a variety of animals, but are classically associated with deer ("deer-ticks") and rodents. Children presenting with Lyme disease may have a known tick-bite or have played recently in wooded areas. Transmission is more common in the spring and summer months. When ticks are discovered and removed within 24 hours of the bite, there is a low risk of developing the disease because transmission takes approximately 48–72 hours.

44. **Where did the name "Lyme disease" originate?**
An outbreak of 51 cases occurred in and around the town of Lyme, Connecticut in the 1970s.

45. **What is the pathognomonic sign of Lyme disease?**
The erythema migrans rash is the pathognomonic sign of Lyme disease. It begins as a small red macule or papule that develops a surrounding annular component, creating a "bulls-eye" or "target" lesion.

46. **What organ systems can be involved in Lyme disease?**
The cutaneous, cardiac, neurologic, and musculoskeletal systems may be involved. The cutaneous stage appears first within a month of infection with the classic erythema migrans rash. Cardiac and neurologic involvement (the early disseminated stage) is less common, usually manifesting as atrioventricular block, Bell's palsy, or meningoencephalitis. Untreated patients develop chronic arthralgias due to inflammatory arthritis in approximately 60% of cases.

47. **What are the orthopedic symptoms of Lyme disease?**
The arthralgias of Lyme disease can last for 2 weeks and may be monoarticular or polyarticular with migration to different joints. The knee is the most commonly involved joint. Arthritis can recur after the initial symptomatic period or even become chronic. Children are more likely than adults to present with joint pain as the initial symptom of Lyme disease. The most common presenting scenario is a child with a significant effusion but minimal discomfort, and often just a mild limp.

48. **How is Lyme disease diagnosed?**
The diagnosis is often initially suspected clinically based an erythema migrans rash, and emperic treatment is initiated. The diagnosis may be confirmed with serum testing for the presence of antibodies specific to *Borrelia burgdorferi*, using ELISA and Western blot techniques. ELISA has been criticized, however, as not having the minimum 95% sensitivity to be considered a good screening test. All borderline and positive ELISA should be confirmed with a Western blot test. If the ELISA is negative and symptoms are highly suggestive, the test may be repeated several weeks later. Synovial fluid analysis is non-specific, showing a leukocytosis with high percentage of polymononuclear cells.

49. **What other conditions have a similar clinical presentation to Lyme disease?**
    Inflammatory arthritis and bacterial septic arthritis have similar presentations and must be differentiated from Lyme disease.

50. **What is the treatment for Lyme disease?**
    The infection is treated with antibiotics, namely amoxicillin, a third-generation cephalosporin, or a tetracycline (e.g., doxycycline) if the patient is older than 8 years.

51. **What is the prognosis for Lyme disease?**
    The prognosis following a single course of antibiotics is excellent, with up to 95% of patients remaining asymptomatic. Even patients who are untreated have a low risk of developing chronic arthritis, though episodes of arthralgia may persist for some time.

LEGG–CALVE–PERTHES DISEASE

CASE 6-4

A 9-year-old boy presents to your clinic with his parents at the request of his pediatrician. He is a very healthy and active boy, so his parents grew concerned when they noticed that he seemed to be running strangely when playing outside a few weeks ago. They tell you that the problem has been worsening since then, and he now walks with an overt limp. When you ask him to walk, he takes shorter steps with his left leg and spends less of the stance phase on that limb. You ask him where he hurts, but he denies any pain. Examination of bilateral hips reveals significant limitations in both hips in internal and external rotation and abduction. His parents brought x-rays that were ordered by the pediatrician (Fig. 6.3).

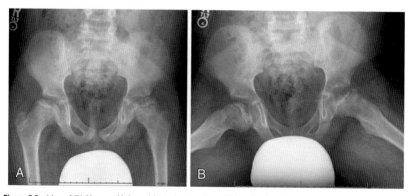

Figure 6.3. (A and B) X-rays of bilateral hips showing Legg–Calve–Perthes disease affecting both femoral heads, with the left femoral head more severely involved.

52. **What is Legg–Calve–Perthes disease?**
    Legg–Calve–Perthes disease (LCPD), frequently referred to simply as Perthes disease, is an idiopathic childhood disease involving loss of vascularity to the femoral head.

53. **What is the pathogenesis of LCPD?**
    For an as yet unidentified reason, the blood supply to the epiphysis of the femoral head (the capital femoral epiphysis) is temporarily disrupted. Theories for this disruption include infection, trauma, and blood hyperviscosity or hypercoagulability. The femoral head then goes through a series of stages in which there may be collapse, followed by revascularization and reconstitution. The avascular necrosis may also damage the proximal femoral physis, resulting in abnormalities of the femoral head and neck as well as leg-length discrepancy.

54. **What is the appearance of a femoral head affected by LCPD?**
    Early in the disease process there may be fragmentation within the capital femoral epiphysis, and there may be a subchondral fracture seen best on the frog lateral radiograph as a "crescent sign". There may be collapse of the femoral head. The ultimate shape of the

femoral head after reossification or healing varies in terms of sphericity, with the best outcomes associated with a spherical head rather than an aspherical head. There is commonly overgrowth of the femoral head (coxa magna), and damage to the proximal femoral physis may result in shortening (coxa breva) and widening of the femoral neck. There is some capacity for remodeling of the femoral head after healing, depending on the growth remaining. The capacity of the acetabulum to remodel also impacts the ultimate relationship between the femoral head and the acetabulum.

55. **What factors affect prognosis?**
    Once the process of new bone formation is underway, the femoral head will continue to remodel until skeletal maturity. Better prognosis is associated with age <8 years or involvement of <50% of the epiphysis. Ultimately, the final shape of the femoral head determines whether and at what age symptomatic osteoarthritis will ensue. If the head is incongruous with the acetabulum then arthritis may occur as early as the 3rd or the 4rth decade, whereas if the head is aspherical, but congruous, arthritis may be delayed until as late as the 6th decade. The shape of the head is particularly difficult to use for prognosis, because after the final shape of the head is known, there is little clinically that can be done. The Herring lateral pillar classification can predict ultimate shape of the femoral head, but can be difficult to interpret, because the classification is static, and the disease course may change the classification if the patient is followed longer.

56. **Who is more likely to present with LCPD: a 5-year-old boy or a 12-year-old girl?**
    A 5-year-old boy is more likely to have LCPD. The incidence is four to five times more common in boys than girls. The peak age of incidence is 4–8 years old.

57. **Is LCPD usually unilateral or bilateral?**
    Approximately 80% of cases are unilateral. When both hips are involved, they are typically at different stages along the course of the disease. Cases of bilateral involvement should be further evaluated to rule out other causes of hip deformity such as skeletal epiphyseal dysplasias, genetic syndromes, and endocrinopathies such as hypothyroidism.

58. **Where do you expect the patient with LCPD to complain of pain?**
    Groin pain is characteristic of intra-articular hip pathology in general, but the pain may be referred to the thigh or knee. All patients with complaints of knee pain should have a thorough hip evaluation as well. Despite all this, the most common presentation of LCPD is a *painless* limp.

59. **What are the early physical exam findings of LCPD? What findings indicate more advanced disease?**
    Gait abnormalities and limitations in range of motion due to synovitis typically present early in the course of the disease. Internal rotation and abduction are most affected. The pain and limp are worsened by activity and, over time, contractures (flexion and adduction) may occur. Muscle atrophy is common, and limb shortening may be apparent (from contractures and/or from femoral head collapse or damage to the physis).

60. **Should laboratory studies be performed to evaluate LCPD?**
    Laboratory studies are generally all within normal limits for patients with LCPD, though the ESR may be mildly elevated. Laboratory studies should be performed to rule out other causes of limping and hip pain, such as infection or inflammatory disease, if clinically indicated.

61. **What imaging should be obtained for the evaluation and management of LCPD?**
    Serial antero-posterior and frog-leg lateral x-rays are necessary and sufficient for diagnosis, staging, monitoring, and prognosis. In selected cases in which the early radiographic changes are not apparent, but the symptoms persist longer than might be expected for transient synovitis, an MRI may be useful in securing the diagnosis. The radiographic stages of LCPD are listed in the chart below. For surgical planning purposes, an arthrogram is another useful modality to show what interventions may optimize the ability to

Table 6.1. Waldenstrom Stages of Perthes Disease

STAGE	RADIOGRAPHIC FINDINGS
I	Small ossification center, lateralized femoral head, physeal irregularity, subchondral fracture
II	Epiphyseal fragmentation with varying radiolucent and radiodense regions
III	New bone formation that fills in radiolucencies
IV	Gradual remodeling of the reossified femoral head and remodeling of the acetabulum

maintain the femoral head/acetabulum relationship in the acetabulum. Arthrograms are dynamic studies which can evaluate for hinge abduction (the femoral head hinging on the edge of the acetabulum) and femoral head shape and congruence. Radiographic signs felt to indicate a poor prognosis include a horizontal physis, lateral subluxation of the epiphysis, calcification lateral to the epiphysis, and radiolucency in the lateral epiphysis and metaphysis (the Gage sign) (Table 6.1).

62. **How is LCPD classified?**
The most commonly used classification system is the Herring lateral pillar radiographic classification, which applies to the fragmentation stage. On antero-posterior x-ray, the femoral head epiphysis is divided into medial, lateral, and central segments or pillars. The central pillar is the largest, representing ~50% of the width of the epiphysis, with the medial and lateral pillars representing 20–30% each. The radiographic appearance of the lateral pillar is what determines the class. Group A refers to a normal lateral pillar. Most group A patients will have a spherical femoral head at skeletal maturity. In group B, there is lucency of the lateral pillar with >50% of pillar height remaining. Group B patients have a better prognosis if the onset of LCPD was prior to age 9. In group C, less than 50% of pillar height is maintained. Most group C patients have deformity of the femoral head at skeletal maturity. A B/C "border" group was recently added to increase reliability in which the lateral pillar is narrowed and poorly ossified with approximately 50% height (Fig. 6.4).

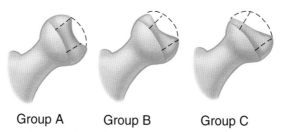

Group A   Group B   Group C

Figure 6.4. (A–C) Lateral pillar classification based on height of lateral pillar. (*From Canale ST, Osteochondrosis or Epiphysitis and Other Miscellaneous Affections: Canale ST, Beaty JH, (eds). Campbell's Operative Orthopaedics, 12th edn, pp. 1133–1199.e10. Copyright © 2013 by Mosby, Elsevier Inc.*)

63. **Is non-operative treatment ever appropriate for LCPD patients?**
The goals of treatment are to alleviate the symptoms, maintain range of motion and maintain containment of the femoral head in the acetabulum to facilitate healing of the femoral head in a spherical geometry. Mild cases may be amenable to simple activity restriction to control pain, with close monitoring of range of motion and periodic radiographs to evaluate the progression of healing and identify complications. Physical therapy may help restore or maintain range of motion. Other non-operative options for treating pain include antiinflammatory medications, crutches, bracing, casting, bedrest,

and traction. Selected patients with a poor prognosis, especially when subluxation is identified, may benefit from "containment" of the femoral head. Abduction braces and Petrie casting are non-operative methods for treatment of Perthes disease. Options for surgical containment include a femoral osteotomy, pelvic osteotomy, or combined osteotomies.

64. **What is an osteotomy?**
Osteotomy means cutting the bone, usually with a saw or an osteotome (a surgical instrument that resembles a chisel). After the bone is cut, it can be repositioned to achieve the goals of the procedure.

65. **How is the bone repositioned in a femoral osteotomy for LCPD?**
The proximal femur is repositioned in more varus (bending the distal fragment toward the midline). The goal is to place the anterior and lateral portions of the epiphysis (extruded segment) within the acetabulum to promote healing in a spherical position. Varus osteotomies are associated with shortening of the limb, as well as a decreased mechanical advantage of the abductor muscles resulting in abductor insufficiency and a limp.

66. **How is the bone repositioned in an acetabular osteotomy for LCPD?**
The bone is repositioned to provide more coverage of the femoral head laterally and anteriorly. Early in the disease process, as a containment strategy, this is most commonly achieved by a Salter innominate osteotomy, which redirects the acetabulum to provide greater anterior and lateral coverage with articular cartilage. Some authors have favored a shelf arthroplasty, which augments the acetabulum, and places extra bone anteriorly and laterally. The capsular tissue undergoes metaplasia, resulting in the formation of fibrocartilage, which is less durable when compared with hyaline cartilage. In patients in the healing phase of the disease, in whom symptomatic incongruence has developed between the femoral head and the acetabulum, a salvage option such as the Chiari osteotomy may provide symptomatic relief. In this surgery, the acetabulum is displaced medially, improving the coverage, and perhaps most importantly, reducing the joint reaction forces.

JUVENILE IDIOPATHIC ARTHITIS
CASE 6-5

A 12-year-old girl presents to the Emergency Room. She has had a fever of 38.0°C for 3 days. She complains of swelling and pain in her hands and feet for the past week. Her parents are distraught. They say she has not been herself all week. She has been lying in bed and sleeping 12–15 hours per day. She refuses to eat.

67. **What are the criteria for the diagnosis of juvenile idiopathic arthritis (JIA)?**
Patients must have onset of the disease by 16 years old, presence of symptoms for at least 6 weeks, and exclusion of other possible causes of the arthritis. JIA, formerly referred to as juvenile rheumatoid arthritis, is a diagnosis of exclusion.

68. **What are the three types of JIA?**
The three types of juvenile idiopathic arthritis are oligoarticular JIA (fewer than five joints involved), polyarticular JIA (five or more joints involved), and systemic onset JIA. Oligoarticular JIA is the most common form.

69. **How does oligoarticular JIA typically present?**
Oligoarticular JIA typically presents in Caucasian girls of 1–3 years of age. A single joint is involved in half of cases. The knee and ankle are the most frequently involved joints, so the patient often has a limp. A leg-length discrepancy may be present from reactive bony overgrowth due to stimulation of the physis of the affected joint(s).

70. **What other specialist should patients with oligoarticular JIA see routinely?**
Because anti-nuclear antibodies are present in a large proportion of patients with oligoarticular JIA, uveitis may occur and may be asymptomatic. These patients should see an ophthalmologist routinely for screening with a slit lamp.

71. **How is polyarticular JIA defined?**
Polyarticular JIA is defined as JIA with involvement of at least five joints. The small joints of the hands and feet are most commonly involved, with a symmetric distribution. Females are more commonly affected. Morning stiffness and decreased range of motion are common complaints.

72. **What laboratory finding is predictive of a more severe form of polyarticular JIA?**
A positive rheumatoid factor (RF) serology is predictive of a more severe form of polyarticular JIA. However, only 3% of patients with polyarticular JIA have a positive RF. The ESR, CBC, and antinuclear antibodies (ANA) are also useful studies to obtain for JIA, as is a synovial biopsy.

73. **What is the treatment for polyarticular JIA?**
Intra-articular corticosteroid injections, non-steroidal antiinflammatory medications, methotrexate, and tumor necrosis factor α inhibitors are used to treat polyarticular JIA. Systemic steroids can be avoided for most cases.

74. **What are the characteristic physical examination findings of systemic onset JIA?**
Systemic onset JIA typically presents with daily or twice-daily fever spikes accompanied by a salmon-colored truncal rash that waxes and wanes with the fever. Patients may also have lymphadenopathy and hepatosplenomegaly. The arthritis may be monoarticular or polyarticular and varies greatly in severity.

75. **What is macrophage activation syndrome (MAS)?**
Macrophage activation syndrome is a feature of systemic onset JIA that occurs during flares or following viral infections. In its most severe form, MAS can lead to disseminated intravascular coagulopathy. Signs of MAS include elevated D-dimer, and a relatively low ESR, white blood cell count, and platelet count, all of which are typically elevated in systemic onset JIA.

76. **How is systemic onset JIA treated?**
The combination of medications used to treat systemic onset JIA depends on the severity of the case. Systemic and intra-articular corticosteroids, non-steroidal antiinflammatory medications, methotrexate, tumor necrosis factor inhibitors, and cyclophosphamide are all potential treatment medications. Severe forms may require autologous stem cell transplantation.

PEDIATRIC TUMORS

CASE 6-6

You see a 14-year-old girl in clinic for a complaint of persistent left knee pain after getting hit in the leg with a field hockey stick over a month ago. The pain initially started to get better, but then she was left with a dull ache in the back of her knee. She has been favoring that leg when she walks. You notice that the circumference of her distal thigh is visibly larger on the left. She has a firm mass palpable in the back of her left knee. X-rays of her left knee are shown in Figure 6.5.

77. **What are the most common bone tumors in patients greater than 10 years old?**
The most common benign bone tumors in this age group are fibrous dysplasia, osteoid osteoma, non-ossifying fibroma, aneurysmal bone cyst, chondroblastoma, and osteofibrous dysplasia. The most common malignant bone tumors in this age group are osteosarcoma, Ewing sarcoma, and chondrosarcoma.

78. **What are the most common bone tumors in patients aged 5–10 years?**
The most common benign bone tumors in this age group are unicameral bone cyst, aneurysmal bone cyst, fibrous dysplasia, non-ossifying fibroma, osteoid osteoma, and Langerhans cell histiocytosis. The most common malignant bone tumor in this age group is osteosarcoma.

79. **What are the most common bone tumors in patients less than 5 years old?**
The most common benign bone tumor in this age group is Langerhans cell histiocytosis, or eosinophilic granuloma. The most common malignant bone tumors in this age group are Ewing sarcoma, leukemia, and metastatic tumors.

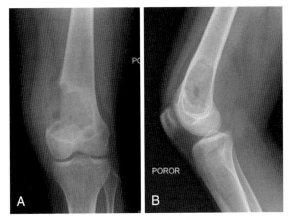

Figure 6.5. (A and B) Antero-posterior and lateral x-rays of the left knee showing an osteosarcoma of the distal femur with cortical destruction and extension into the soft tissue.

80. **What bone tumors are typically found in the epiphysis of a long bone? Diaphysis? Metaphysis?**
    Chondroblastoma, fibrous dysplasia, and giant cell tumors can all be found in the epiphysis of a long bone. A non-neoplastic lesion that can be found in the epiphysis is a Brodie's abscess. Tumors that have a predilection for the diaphysis include fibrous dysplasia, osteofibrous dysplasia, unicameral bone cyst, Ewing sarcoma, Langerhans cell histiocytosis, leukemia, and lymphoma. Virtually all tumors can affect the metaphysis of long bones but classic osteosarcoma often preferentially affects the metaphysis (Fig. 6.5).

81. **What are the important radiographic qualities that should be noted when classifying a bone tumor?**
    The lesion's margin – geographic, moth-eaten, or permeative – can be an important indicator of the aggressiveness of the lesion. Lesions with geographic margins tend to be benign, whereas permeative lesions are suspicious for aggressive or malignant tumors. Cortical destruction is another sign of an aggressive tumor. The periosteal reaction can also give clues to the diagnosis. Classic patterns include the sunburst reaction of osteosarcoma and the onion-skin appearance of Ewing sarcoma. A Codman triangle describes a triangular-shaped pattern of periosteal reaction that extends from the lesion where it breaks through the cortex to the adjacent normal cortex.

82. **What is the final step in diagnosis of a bone tumor?**
    Pathologic evaluation of tissue from the lesion is the final step in diagnosis. While some benign tumors have a classic appearance and a history that allows observation without surgery (such as a non-ossifying fibroma or fibrous cortical defect), any surgical procedures performed for a bone lesion must include biopsy regardless of the surgeon's level of confidence in the diagnosis.

83. **What other studies should be obtained prior to biopsy of a suspected malignant bone tumor?**
    Lesions suspected of being malignant should have an MRI of the primary lesion (whole bone to assure there are no "skip" lesions), CT scan of the chest, and whole body bone scan. These studies aid in diagnosis, staging, and monitoring response to treatment.

84. **Night-time pain relieved by non-steroidal antiinflammatory medications is characteristic of what type of bone tumor?**
    Osteoid osteomas typically cause an achy pain in the location of the lesion that is worse at night, but responds very well to non-steroidal antiinflammatory medications. They are intra-cortical lesions that have a self-limiting course, though it can take years for the pain to resolve. For this reason, many osteoid osteomas are treated by radiofrequency ablation or surgical excision.

85. **Why should some osteoblastomas be resected?**
    Although osteoblastomas are benign tumors, they are locally aggressive. They are most commonly observed in the posterior elements of the spine, and may impinge on the spinal cord or nerve roots (Fig. 6.6).

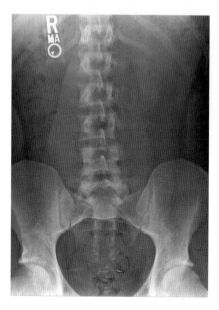

Figure 6.6. Antero-posterior radiograph of an 18-year-old boy with osteoblastoma of the left L2 transverse process. (*From Heck RK, Benign/Aggressive Tumors of Bone: Campbell's Operative Orthopaedics, 12th edn, pp. 887–908.e3. Copyright © 2013 by Mosby, Elsevier Inc.*)

86. **What is the radiographic appearance of an osteochondroma?**
    Osteochondromas are bony lesions that protrude from and are continuous with the normal cortex. They can be broad-based (sessile) or have a bony stalk (pedunculated). They are usually found in the metaphysis. As the lesions have a large cartilaginous cap, they are frequently much larger than they appear on plain radiographs (Fig. 6.7).

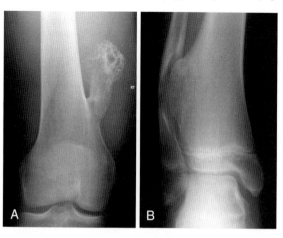

Figure 6.7. Osteochodroma. (A) Antero-posterior (AP) radiograph showing a typical pendunculated osteochondroma of the distal femur. (B) AP radiograph of the distal tibia showing a sessile osteochondroma with associated modeling deformity of the adjacent fibula. (*From Stoker DJ, Grainger & Allison's Diagnostic Radiology: A Textbook of Medical Imaging, 5th edn, pp. 1029–1057. Copyright © 2008, Elsevier Ltd, All rights reserved.*)

87. **Why should osteochondromas be monitored into adulthood?**
    Osteochondromas have a very small risk of transformation into chondrosarcoma (about 1%). Patients with a condition of multiple osteochondromas called

hereditary multiple exostosis have a risk of transformation that ranges from 0.5% to 8%.

88. **A geographic, lytic lesion in the epiphysis of a long bone is most likely to be what tumor?**

   This radiographic appearance is classic for a chondroblastoma. Surgical treatment is commonly recommended since these may invade the neighboring joint (Fig. 6.8).

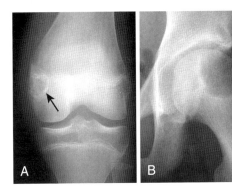

Figure 6.8. Chondroblastoma in the immature and mature skeleton. (A) Antero-posterior (AP) x-ray showing a lobulated, lytic lesion (arrow) adjacent to the open growth plate and limited to the epiphysis. (B) AP x-ray showing extension of the lesion across the fused growth plate. *(From Stoker DJ, Grainger & Allison's Diagnostic Radiology: A Textbook of Medical Imaging, pp. 1029–1057. Copyright © 2008, Elsevier Ltd.)*

89. **What is a non-ossifying fibroma?**

   A non-ossifying fibroma is a benign fibrous tissue lesion that occurs within normal bone, and may be viewed as a developmental variant. These may be identified in approximately 22% of pediatric patients, and most will involute over time. They are often detected as incidental findings when x-rays are performed for other reasons. They do not require treatment unless there is a pathologic fracture through the lesion, or when their size would be considered to be a risk for a pathologic fracture (Fig. 6.9).

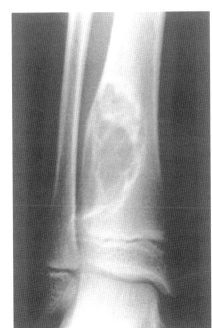

Figure 6.9. Non-ossifying fibroma of the distal tibial metaphysis producing an eccentric lobulated radiolucency surrounded by a sclerotic margin. *(From Rosenberg AE, Bones, Joints, and Soft-Tissue Tumors: Kumar V, et al. [eds], Robbins and Cotran Pathologic Basis of Disease, 8th edn. Copyright © 2010 by Saunders, Elsevier Inc.)*

90. **What is the classic radiographic appearance of fibrous dysplasia?**

    Fibrous dysplasia has a "ground glass" appearance on x-ray. It is usually located in the diaphysis and may cause local thinning of the cortex and expansion of the bone. Multiple lesions may be identified, and so a bone scan is typically recommended when the diagnosis is made or suspected (Fig. 6.10).

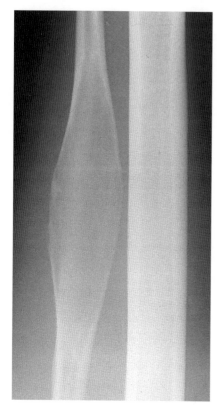

Figure 6.10. Fibrous dysplasia. A characteristic expansile lesion with a ground-glass appearance has caused thinning of the cortex in the mid-diaphysis of the fibula. (*From Whyte MP: Fibrous Dysplasia. In: Favus MJ [ed]: Primer on the Metabolic Bone Diseases and Disorders of Mineral Metabolism, 3rd edn. Philadelphia, Lippincott-Raven, 1996*)

91. **What is a "shepherd's crook" deformity?**

    A "shepherd's crook" deformity is a varus deformity of the proximal femur that occurs from repetitive microfractures occurring through a fibrous dysplasia lesion. The patient may develop a limp due to the deformity.

92. **What is McCune–Albright syndrome?**

    McCune–Albright syndrome is a syndrome that involves fibrous dysplasia affecting multiple locations (polyostotic), café-au-lait skin lesions, and precocious puberty.

93. **Half of all osteosarcomas are found in what two locations?**

    Half of all osteosarcomas are found in the distal femur and proximal tibia.

94. **What differences exist between a unicameral bone cyst and an aneurysmal bone cyst?**

    The term unicameral means that the cyst has only a single cavity, though unicameral bone cysts can contain septations. Aneurysmal bone cysts (ABCs) are multiloculated vascular lesions that contain chambers filled with blood. Unicameral bone cysts (UBCs) and ABCs are both benign lesions, but ABCs tend to exhibit more aggressive behavior with expansion and destruction of the surrounding bone. UBCs tend to be asymptomatic unless a fracture occurs through the lesion. ABCs may have dull, persistent pain in the absence of a fracture. Treatment for UBCs is aimed at preventing or treating pathologic fractures, usually with curettage and grafting (bone marrow, demineralized bone matrix, calcium sulfate pellets) of the lesion. Treatment for ABCs is more comprehensive because of its aggressive nature. In addition to curettage and bone grafting, adjuvants such as electrocautery, burring, and application of phenol to the cyst wall are utilized.

95. **What is the radiographic appearance of a UBC?**
A UBC typically appears as a geographic, lucent lesion in the metaphysis of a long bone, most commonly the proximal femur and proximal humerus. These lesions are less commonly identified in the calcaneus. Expansion of the surrounding bone is minimal, and a sclerotic rim may be seen surrounding the lesion.

96. **What is the radiographic appearance of an ABC?**
An ABC appears as a lytic lesion that expands and thins the nearby cortex, usually in the metaphysis of a long bone (Fig. 6.11). The lesion may have multiple septations and fluid-fluid levels on MRI representing the blood within the chambers. Of note, an ABC can exist within an osteosarcoma, so caution in treating these lesions is warranted.

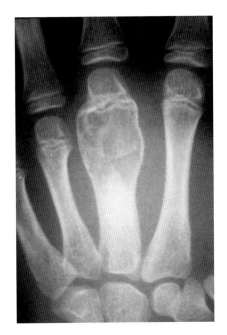

Figure 6.11. Aneurysmal bone cyst in middle finger metacarpal in skeletally immature patient. (*From Calandruccio JH, Jobe MT, Tumors and Tumorous Conditions of the Hand: Campbell's Operative Orthopaedics, pp. 3661–3692.e2. Copyright © 2013 by Mosby, Elsevier Inc.*)

97. **How are eosinophilic granuloma and Langerhans cell histiocytosis related?**
Eosinophilic granuloma (EG) is a solitary form of Langerhans cell histiocytosis, and is limited to the musculoskeletal system. Lytic lesions are identified on radiographs, and are filled with lipid-laden histiocytes (Langerhans cells). These are commonly encountered in the skull, long bones, pelvis, ribs, and spine, as isolated or multifocal lesions. Hand–Schuller–Christian disease is a form of Langerhans cell histiocytosis that involves skeletal lesions, exophthalmos, and diabetes insipidus. Letterer–Siwe disease is the most severe form of Langerhans cell histiocytosis, which presents in infants and can involve multiple organs and organ systems, including the liver, skin, and nervous system. Letterer–Siwe disease is rapidly fatal. Vertebra plana (or flattening of the vertebral body) is a radiographic finding in the spine that suggests EG.

98. **What is the treatment for eosinophic granuloma?**
EG is a benign condition that often spontaneously resolves over time. Once the diagnosis is confirmed by biopsy and the more severe forms of Langerhans cell histiocytosis are excluded, no further treatment is necessary.

99. **What is Ewing sarcoma?**
Ewing sarcoma is a malignant tumor characterized histologically by small, blue round cells. It is usually found in the diaphysis (or metaphysis) of long bones, presenting radiographically as an aggressive lesion with cortical destruction and a soft tissue component. Metastases are present at diagnosis in approximately 25% of cases. Treatment involves preoperative chemotherapy, wide resection of the primary tumor, and sometimes radiation therapy if wide resection is not possible.

100. **Skeletal involvement is most often associated with which type of leukemia?**
Skeletal lesions are seen most often in acute lymphoblastic leukemia.

101. **How are pathologic fractures acutely managed in children?**
As with all fractures, temporary stabilization of the fracture should be performed for pain control and correction of any deformity that may damage surrounding structures. Before a fracture is definitively stabilized, however, the diagnosis must be confirmed with biopsy. Standard methods for fracture fixation risk widening the necessary zone of resection in the event that the pathologic lesion turns out to be malignant. Generally fractures can be treated in several ways depending on the type of lesion. In benign lesions it is common to both treat the fracture and the lesion simultaneously. In some cases of benign lesions, treatment of the fracture alone may be enough, and the lesion may heal secondarily. When a malignant lesion is suspected, it is necessary to first establish the diagnosis, and fractures are temporarily stabilized by splinting or traction until a definitive surgical plan is developed, especially when limb salvage may be an option.

PEDIATRIC ORTHOPEDIC TRAUMA

GENERAL PRINCIPLES

102. **What are some differences in pediatric orthopedic trauma compared to adult orthopedic trauma?**
    a. *Thick, active periosteum*: Facilitates achieving and maintenance of reduction and makes closed treatment more successful in a child compared to an adult.
    b. *Open physes*: Allows for bony remodeling, particularly in younger children and when the injury is closer to the growth plate.
    c. *Possibility of non-accidental trauma*: Must be considered by the orthopedic physician, particularly in younger non-ambulatory children.
    d. *Large head*: creates unacceptable flexion of the c-spine if an adult spine board is used, use a pediatric spine board with a recessed head.
    e. *Large body surface area to mass ratio*: Increases the chances of hypothermia due to blood loss.

103. **What is the most important determinant of the outcome of pediatric polytrauma?**
Brain and central nervous system injury are the most important determining factors in outcome of pediatric polytrauma. Of note, care must be taken to prevent secondary injury due to hypoxia/hypovolemia. Brain injury is the most common cause of death in this population. Orthopedic surgeons should treat fractures as if the patient will achieve a full recovery.

104. **What are the recommendations for seating children in vehicles?**
    a. Infants/toddlers: Rear facing infant seat or rear-facing convertible seat until 2 years of age or until child reaches highest weight or height allowed by car seat's manufacturer.
    b. Toddlers/preschoolers: Forward-facing car seat with a harness up to highest weight or height allowed by seat manufacturer.
    c. School-aged children: Belt-positioning booster seat in the back seat until vehicle seat belt fits properly (typically 4 ft 9 inches in height and between 8 and 12 years of age).
    d. Older children: Lap and shoulder belts, in the rear seat until at least 13 years of age.

CASE 6-7

You are called to see a 15-month-old male in the Emergency Room with a femur fracture (Fig. 6.12). The mother is present. She reports that the child fell off the couch this afternoon. Upon chart review, you notice the EMT note specifies that the mother reported that the fracture occurred last night when the child fell off a bed. You noted some bruises around the child's chest as well.

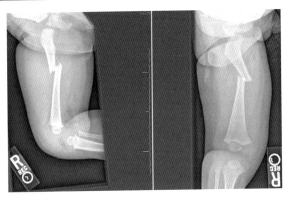

Figure 6.12. A femur fracture in an infant.

105. **What are some "red flags" that trauma in a child may be non-accidental?**
    a. Metaphyseal corner fractures
    b. Femur fractures in children who are not yet of walking age
    c. Inconsistent or implausible mechanism of injury as reported by caregivers
    d. Fractures in various stages of healing
    e. Posterior rib fractures
    f. Transphyseal separation of the distal humerus
    g. Other injuries such as bruises, burns or skin lesions.

106. **What are the most common injuries in non-accidental trauma?**
    Bruises and skin lesions are the number one injury; fractures are the second most common injury.

107. **What are some conditions that can be mistaken for non-accidental injury, and how can they be detected?**
    a. *Osteogenesis imperfecta*: blue sclera, poor dentition, family history of multiple fractures, biochemical testing
    b. *Rickets*: prematurity, vitamin D deficiency, metabolic and biochemical testing, wide physes, bow legs, "rachitic rosary"
    c. *Kidney disease*: history of dialysis, laboratory tests, urinalysis.

108. **What is the classification system used for growth plate fractures? Describe the classification system.**
    The classification used is the Salter–Harris classification described in 1963. The mnemonic "SALTR" can be used to remember the different types:
    Type I: "Slipped" – growth plate, the fracture propagates through the growth plate.
    Type II: "Above" – the growth plate, the fracture propagates through the growth plate and exits through the metaphysis. May have a large Thurston–Holland (metaphyseal) fragment that is useful for reduction and implant placement.
    Type III: "Lower" – the fracture crosses the physis and exits through the epiphysis (and usually into the joint)
    Type IV: "Through" – the metaphysis, the growth plate, and the epiphysis (through and through)
    Type V: "Rammed" – the growth plate is crushed, indistinguishable radiographically from a non-displaced type I fracture (Fig. 6.13).

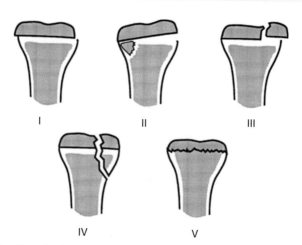

Figure 6.13. Salter–Harris classification of epiphyseal fractures in children. A type I fracture is straight across the epiphyseal plate and may have some lateral displacement of the epiphysis. This occurs 5% of the time. A type II fracture involves a portion of the epiphyseal plate and a corner fracture through the metaphysis. This occurs 75% of the time. A type III fracture involving part of the epiphysis occurs only about 10% of the time. A type IV fracture involving part of the epiphysis and part of the metaphysis occurs about 10% of the time. A type V fracture is direct impaction and has the most serious consequences for further growth. (*From Mettler FA, Skeletal System: Essentials of Radiology, 3rd edn, pp. 185–268. Copyright © 2014, 2005, 1996 by Saunders, Elsevier Inc.*)

109. Which growth plate injury is the most common? Which has the worst prognosis?

Type II is the most common, type V is the rarest and has the worst prognosis in terms of growth arrest.

HIP AND FEMUR TRAUMA

110. What is the mechanism of injury in a hip fracture in a child?

In general, hip fractures in children, adolescents, and young adults are the result of high-energy trauma such as motor vehicle accidents, fall from height, or auto vs. pedestrian. Femoral neck fractures are surgical emergencies as the blood flow to the femoral head is at risk, and avascular necrosis may result in premature degenerative changes requiring a total hip arthroplasty or other measures for salvage. THA is not a good option in active adolescents given the likelihood of multiple revisions during the patient's lifetime.

111. What is the major blood supply to the femoral head in different age groups?

At birth, the blood supply to the femoral head comes from metaphyseal vessels which arise from the medial and lateral femoral circumflex arteries. As the subcapital physis develops and the child matures, the metaphyseal vessels can no longer penetrate the head. By the time the child reaches the age of four, the majority of the blood supply of the head comes from the posterosuperior and posteroinferior retinacular complex of arteries. This system of arteries arises from the medial femoral circumflex artery.

112. What is the classification system used to describe hip fractures in children?

The *Delbet* classification was first reported in 1929, and divides fractures into four anatomic areas. A type I fracture is a separation of the capital femoral physis. A type II fracture is equivalent to a subcapital fracture in an adult. A type III fracture is equivalent to a basicervical fracture in an adult, and a type IV fracture is equivalent to an intertrochanteric fracture in an adult (Fig. 6.14).

113. What is the significance of the Delbet classification?

The Delbet classification has been found to be predictive of avascular necrosis of the femoral head. Type I fractures have an 80–100% rate of AVN, type II fractures have a 50%

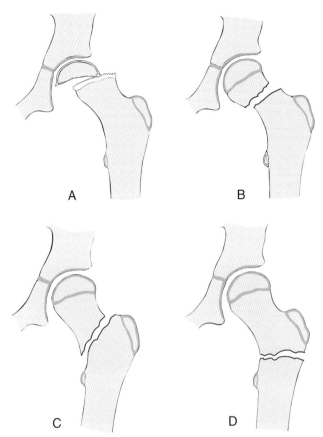

Figure 6.14. The Delbet classification of proximal femoral fractures in children. (A) Type I: Transepiphyseal fracture. (B) Type II: Transcervical fracture. (C) Type III: Cervicotrochanteric fracture. (D) Type IV: Intertrochanteric fracture. (*From Swiontkowski MF, Fractures and Dislocations About the Hip and Pelvis: Green NE, Swiontkowski MF, [eds], Skeletal Trauma in Children, 4th edn, pp. 355–396. Copyright © 2009 by Saunders, an imprint of Elsevier Inc.*)

rate of AVN, type III fractures have a 25% chance of AVN, and type IV fractures have a 10% chance of AVN.

114. **What is the treatment of choice for a pediatric hip fracture?**
Types II–IV fractures in children are generally treated with physeal sparing cannulated screw fixation. The screws may be placed across the physis in patients closer to skeletal maturity when required to obtain adequate fixation. In younger patients, smooth K-wire fixation with supplemental spica cast immobilization is required. Many surgeons feel that decompression of the intra-articular hematoma is beneficial in preventing avascular necrosis, though this has not been conclusively proven.

115. **What are the major complications of pediatric hip fractures?**
   a. *Osteonecrosis*: Ranges from 10% to 100% based on Delbet type.
   b. *Nonunion*: Less common than with adult fractures and is in the 5% range. Typically, nonunion is the result of non-anatomic reduction. Valgus osteotomy can be used to treat this problem.
   c. *Coxa vara*: Approximately 20% of cases are complicated by this problem which results in asymmetric premature physeal closure. This may be due to the injury or its treatment (malunion). Valgus subtrochanteric osteotomy may be required to correct the deformity.

116. **What is the mechanism of injury in a hip dislocation in a young child? In an adolescent?**

Young children can dislocate their hip with a low-energy mechanism such as a trip or fall. These dislocations are usually easily reduced with sedation. Stability of reduction should be evaluated with fluoroscopy. A CT or MRI is commonly obtained to evaluate the concentricity of reduction and rule out the presence of intra-articular fragments. Younger children are typically placed in a spica cast post reduction. Adolescents with hip dislocations are more typically the victims of high-energy trauma, such as dashboard injuries in an motor vehicle accident. The clinician should maintain a high index of suspicion for coexisting fractures of the femur and/or acetabular wall, or ipsilateral intra-articular knee injuries.

CASE 6-8

The trauma bay calls you to see a 16-year-old male with pain and deformity of his right thigh. He was hit by a car while skateboarding earlier that afternoon (Fig. 6.15). He has decreased lung sounds on his right size, and ecchymosis over his right chest. A chest x-ray reveals no pneumothorax, and a small amount of fluid at the right lung base. Base deficit and lactic acid levels are within normal limits. A head CT reveals no signs of intracranial injury. Of note, his lung injury was minor, and his lactic acid and base deficits were within levels acceptable for early total care (ETC) (Fig. 6.16).

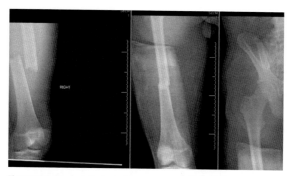

Figure 6.15. Femoral diaphysis fracture in a near skeletally mature patient.

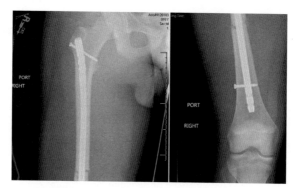

Figure 6.16. Femur fracture status post intramedullary fixation.

117. **What is the mechanism of injury in a diaphyseal femur fracture in a child? An adolescent?**

Younger children are more likely to fracture their femur in a playground or following a fall while running. Adolescent femur fractures are more often the result of higher-energy trauma such as motor vehicle accidents. These patients are at risk for ipsilateral femoral neck fracture and ipsilateral knee injuries. In very young children (<1 year of age) there is a high percentage (up to 40%) of non-accidental injuries.

118. **What are the treatment options for pediatric femoral shaft fractures (diaphyseal)?**
Recent AAOS guidelines detailed evidence based guidelines for treatment of pediatric femoral shaft fractures. A summary of their findings were:
Infants under 6 *months* may be treated in a spica cast or Pavlik harness
Children *6 months to 5 years* with a diaphyseal femur fracture with less than 2 cm of shortening may be treated with immediate spica casting or traction followed by spica casting
Children *5–11 years* of age may be treated with flexible intramedullary nailing techniques
Children *11 years of age to maturity* may be treated with flexible intramedullary nails (though results are less predictable in heavier children), rigid interlocked trochanteric or lateral entry intramedullary nailing or submuscular plating.
This patient in our case example was treated with reamed intramedullary nailing due to his skeletal maturity and large body habitus.
The panel recommends *against* piriformis entry nailing due to risk of avascular necrosis from disruption of the blood supply from the nail entry site. External fixation and bridge plating are other treatment options in selected cases, though the panel did not specifically address these options.

119. **What are some complications of spica casting for diaphyseal femur fractures?**
Skin breakdown or maceration is the most common. Additionally, malunion (typically varus) and excessive shortening can also occur. Typically a valgus mold is placed on the cast in order to try to reduce the risks. Some shortening (up to 1.5–2 cm) is acceptable, because younger children tend to overgrow a fractured limb by approximately 1 cm.

120. **What are some complications of external fixation of femur fractures?**
Pin site infection is the most common complication. Loss of reduction and nerve or vessel injury are also concerns during or after the placement of these devices, though these are uncommon. Knee stiffness commonly results from tethering of the distal pins on the iliotibial band, as well as patient apprehension often due to discomfort. Recurrence of the fracture is a concern, especially for transverse fractures. The risk of recurrent fracture may be reduced by placing fewer pins at greater distances from the fracture site, and allowing 50% translation of the fracture fragments to increase motion at the fracture site thereby stimulating callus formation.

121. **What are some complications of internal fixation of femur fractures?**
Flexible Nails: By far the most common complication of this treatment modality is symptomatic implants. The distal end of the nail is located in the soft tissue adjacent to the medial and lateral flare of the distal femur. This complication can be reduced by leaving the nails flush with the metaphysis, and having the tip of the nails at or above the level of the physis. The majority of these nails are removed in a second surgery. Additionally, flexible nails may be complicated by malunion (angular or rotational) and excessive limb shortening when utilized in length-unstable fractures. Rarely, fractures have occurred at the insertion site following removal.
Submuscular plating: Complications include hardware failure if the patient is non-compliant with weight bearing. Additionally, unless the plate is placed in a minimally invasive fashion with an aiming arm, there is a large scar with greater blood loss. Additionally, fractures through screw holes following removal have been reported.
Rigid intramedullary nailing: Complications include hip pain due to violation of the gluteal musculature, greater trochanteric growth arrest resulting in an abductor lurch (rarely in patients less than 9 years of age). Increase in lung injury secondary to fat embolism can be seen in polytrauma patients.

122. **What is the mechanism of a distal femoral physeal fracture?**
Distal femoral fractures are generally caused by hyperextension and valgus force. These injuries would normally result in a medial collateral injury in adults and adolescents, but in a younger child, the location of failure is the distal femoral physis.

123. **What is the treatment for a distal femoral physeal fracture, and what are the sequelae?**
Distal femoral physeal fractures are generally reduced in the operating room and then fixed with two large crossing pins. Cannulated screws may be utilized when there is a substantial metaphyseal component (Salter–Harris II or IV). The most commonly associated complication is growth arrest, which occurs in up to 40% of patients. Asymmetric arrest may result in limb shortening and an angular deformity, while complete arrest will result in only leg-length discrepancy. Distal femoral physeal fractures are the most likely fractures to experience growth arrest, due to the large surface area and undulations within the physis.

KNEE AND TIBIA FRACTURES

CASE 6-9

A 12-year-old male soccer player twists his knee while he is playing soccer. He has immediate pain and swelling in the knee. You see him the next day in the office. He is unable to extend his knee due to pain. There is a large effusion which you drain and find to contain blood. Tiny fat globules are visualized after the syringe is set down for a few minutes. X-rays are shown in Figure 6.17.

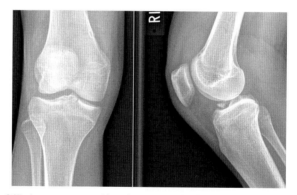

Figure 6.17. Antero-posterior and lateral projections of a tibial spine (eminence) fracture.

124. **What is a tibial eminence fracture?**
Tibial eminence fractures are the equivalent of anterior cruciate ligament (ACL) injuries in adults (Fig. 6.18). They typically result from a rapid deceleration or hyperextension of the knee. They can be associated with meniscal injuries. They present similarly to ACL injuries (pain and an immediate effusion).

125. **How are tibial eminence fractures classified?**
Tibial eminence fractures are classified by the *Meyers and McKeever* classification:
Type I: Non-displaced
Type II: Displaced with an intact posterior hinge
Type III: Completely displaced.

126. **What is the treatment of tibial eminence fractures?**
In general type I fractures will be placed in a long leg cast in 0–15° of flexion, following aspiration of hematoma. Type II fractures will be aspirated, close reduced then placed in

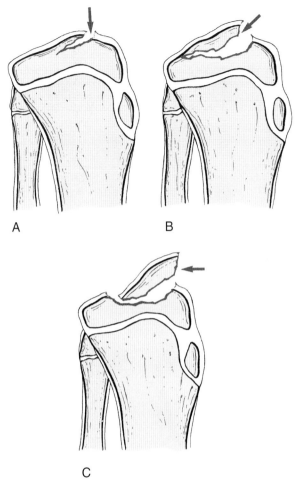

A

B

C

Figure 6.18. Meyers and McKeever classification of fractures of the anterior tibial spine. (A) Type I fracture with no displacement of the fracture. (B) Type II fracture with elevation of the anterior portion of the anterior tibial spine, but with the fracture posteriorly reduced. (C) Type III fracture that is totally displaced. (*From Zionts LE, Fractures and Dislocations About the Knee: Swiontkowski, MF [ed], Skeletal Trauma in Children, 4th edn. Copyright © 2009 by Saunders, an imprint of Elsevier Inc.*)

a cast in 0–15° of extension. Some type II fractures will be irreducible, owing to interposition of the *anterior horn of the medial meniscus* or intermeniscal ligament. In this case or in the case of type III fractures, surgery is indicated. Open or arthroscopic surgery is undertaken depending on surgeon preference and comfort. Fixation is obtained with either screws or a grasping stitch which is looped through the ACL and tied over a post in the tibia.

127. What is a tibial tubercle fracture?

This is a fracture through the secondary ossification center of the tibial tubercle, extending often into the anterior tibiofemoral joint. Effectively, it is an extensor mechanism injury. The typical patient is a male towards the end of their growth period. The mechanism of injury is forcible active knee extension, or eccentric loading of the quadriceps.

128. **What are the operative indications?**
All displaced fractures in which the extensor mechanism is disrupted should be treated by open reduction and internal fixation. Non-displaced fractures of the secondary growth center only can be treated in a cast in full extension.

129. **What are the complications associated with tibial tubercle fractures?**
Anterior compartment syndrome may result from disruption of the anterior tibial recurrent artery. Early closure of the secondary growth center may result in a recurvatum deformity as the posterior portion of the physis continues to grow longitudinally.

130. **What is a patellar sleeve fracture?**
Patellar sleeve fracture is a disruption of the extensor mechanism of the knee that typically occurs in children between 8 and 12 years of age. The fracture is the result of forcible active extension, or eccentric loading of the quadriceps. The disruption is between the cartilage of the inferior pole of the patella and the patella itself. The treatment is most often open reduction internal fixation unless the fracture is non-displaced (rare). Fixation can be accomplished with heavy suture fixation followed by immobilization. Alternatively, a tension band construct can be created with smooth wires and heavy suture.

131. **What is the danger of a proximal tibial physeal fracture in children?**
The physis is at the same level as the vascular trifurcation, and these vessels are tethered to the bone at this level. A careful neurovascular exam is mandatory. If the ankle-brachial index (ABI) is less than 0.90, more invasive testing is warranted. If there is a neurovascular compromise, the fracture should be stabilized with either smooth wire transphyseal fixation, or external fixation, and emergent vascular surgery consultation should be obtained. If the fracture is non-displaced and the vascular exam is normal, closed treatment can be considered. Vigilance must be maintained for compartment syndrome (Fig. 6.19).

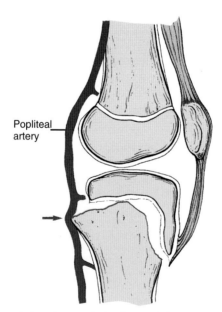

Popliteal artery

Figure 6.19. Lateral drawing of a knee showing a displaced proximal tibial physeal injury and demonstrating the risk of arterial injury because of the close proximity of the popliteal artery to the proximal end of the tibia. (*From Zionts LE, Fractures and Dislocations About the Knee: Swiontkowski MF [ed], Skeletal Trauma in Children, 4th edn. Copyright © 2009 by Saunders, an imprint of Elsevier Inc.*)

132. **What is the classic sign of compartment syndrome in a child?**
Pain and increasing narcotic requirement.

133. **What is the deformity commonly associated with proximal tibial metaphyseal (Cozen) fractures in children?**
Over time the limb may develop a valgus deformity. This deformity tends to be greatest at 18 months and then remodels with time. This deformity occurs in up to 50% of cases. It should be observed for at least 24 months. If the deformity does not remodel, reversible hemiepiphysiodesis (staple or plate) can be considered to correct the deformity.

134. **What are the classic deformities with pediatric tibial shaft fractures?**
Fractures of the tibia involve the fibula 30% of the time. When the fibula is involved, a valgus deformity may occur. If the fibula is intact, the tibia may drift into varus.

135. **What is the most common treatment of tibia fractures in children?**
Closed reduction and casting is the most common treatment. Acceptable reduction is 5° of varus or valgus, 50% cortical apposition, 1 cm of shortening, and 10° flexion or extension deformity. The cast is placed in 10° of knee flexion to prevent rotation and weight bearing. The cast may be wedged open to correct residual angulation.

136. **What are operative indications for tibia fractures in children?**
Open fractures, compartment syndrome, unacceptable alignment with closed treatment, neurovascular injury, and poly trauma. Treatment options include external fixation, flexible nailing, plating, or rigid intramedullary nailing. Rigid nails are reserved for skeletally mature patients. Flexible nails can be used in younger patients. External fixators are often the treatment of choice when there is a concomitant soft-tissue injury, especially when additional procedures for wound coverage are anticipated and when the fracture is length unstable or otherwise not amenable to flexible nailing.

FOOT AND ANKLE TRAUMA

137. **Describe treatment options for ankle fractures in children.**
Closed reduction and casting are generally sufficient for most ankle fractures in children. If there is an intra-articular component, anatomic reduction and fixation is indicated. For medial malleolar fractures, generally it is a Salter–Harris (SH) III or IV and an all epiphyseal screw is placed parallel to the physis. Many times there is an epiphyseal separation (SH II) that results from a plantar flexion force. If closed reduction fails, often it is due to interposition of periosteum, and open reduction and internal fixation is indicated. The lateral x-ray must be scrutinized to assure that sagittal alignment has been restored to avoid a loss of dorsiflexion and possible symptoms from impingement.

138. **What is a Tillaux fracture?**
A Tillaux fracture is a transitional injury which occurs in an older child due to forced external rotation of the foot. It is a SH III fracture of the distal tibial physis. The *anterior tibiofibular ligament* causes a fracture of the lateral physis which is the last to close. Operative indications are displacement and/or joint step-off of more than 2 mm after closed reduction. CT scanning is often employed to assess alignment following closed reduction (Fig. 6.20).

CASE 6-10

You are seeing a 15-year-old male in the Emergency Room who twisted his ankle earlier, falling off a skateboard. His ankle is moderately swollen. He has no open wounds and is neurovascularly intact. His CT scan is shown in Figure 6.21.

139. **What is a triplane fracture?**
A triplane fracture is a complex fracture of the distal tibial which occurs in all three planes. CT may be helpful to delineate the fracture pattern. This fracture results from the fact that the physis of the distal tibia closes first *centrally*, then *medially* then *laterally* (CML). These fractures occur only in older children whose growth is nearly completed.

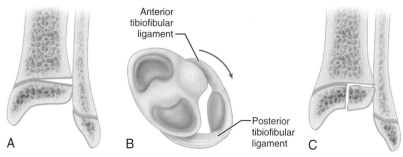

Figure 6.20. Mechanism of injury in Tillaux fracture. (A) Physis in older child closing medially but still open laterally. (B) External rotational force causes anterior tibiofibular ligament to avulse physis antero-laterally. (C) Avulsion produces Salter–Harris type III fracture because medial part of physis is closed. (*From Canale ST, Beaty JH, Fractures and Dislocations in Children: Canale ST, Beaty JH, [eds], Campbell's Operative Orthopaedics, 12th edn. Copyright © 2013 by Mosby, Elsevier Inc.*)

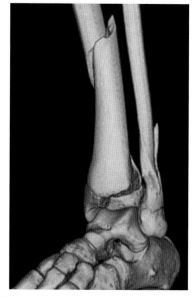

Figure 6.21. 15-year-old snowboarder status post fall.

140. **What is the most concerning complication of a crush injury to the foot in a child?**
Compartment syndrome is the biggest concern. Compartment syndrome can be difficult to diagnose in children, and the earliest warning sign is increasing pain and increasing narcotic requirements. Patients with crush injuries should be admitted and observed. If there is clinical concern for compartment syndrome, the child should be taken to the operating room for foot fasciotomies. Compartment pressures of the foot are unreliable, and the diagnosis is predominantly clinical.

SHOULDER FRACTURES AND DISLOCATIONS

141. **What is the pediatric equivalent of a sternoclavicular dislocation?**
In children (or adults under 25) a sternoclavicular dislocation can be a medial clavicular physeal fracture. They may be detected with a *serendipity* view (40° cephalic tilt), but the most appropriate diagnostic study is a CT scan with contrast, as displacement of these

fractures occurs in the axial plane. The CT scan will also help to delineate any compression of the trachea or vascular structures.

142. **What is the treatment of an anterior medial clavicle physeal separation? Posterior?**
Anterior medial clavicle separations and sternoclavicular dislocations are typically treated non-operatively with immobilization. Posterior dislocations are reduced in an urgent fashion if the patient is showing signs of vascular or airway compromise. While closed reduction (by manipulation or with a towel clip) is commonly practiced, the risk of recurrent displacement has led some to favor open reduction with suture fixation. These procedures are generally performed with a cardiothoracic surgeon available to assist in the rare case of a vascular injury. Metallic implants are avoided due to the risk of migration. Chronic dislocations are observed if asymptomatic.

CASE 6-11

A 16-year-old football player presents to the Emergency Room after having been tackled while playing football earlier in the day. He has pain and swelling in his left shoulder. You can feel a sharp piece of bone just deep to the skin over the area of the patient's collar bone. X-rays are shown in Figure 6.22.

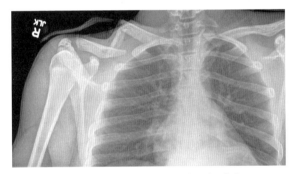

Figure 6.22. 16-year-old football player with a clavicle fracture.

143. **What is the treatment for clavicular fractures in children?**
Most clavicular fractures in children can be treated non-operatively. A sling or figure of 8 brace is effective, but a sling may be more comfortable and less restrictive.

144. **What exam should be performed in a newborn with a clavicle or humerus fracture?**
A clavicule fracture in a newborn can be an indication of birth trauma. A careful neurovascular exam should be performed to rule out brachial plexus palsy. The majority of brachial plexus palsies resolve on their own, but careful follow-up is necessary.

145. **What are the operative indications for clavicle shaft fractures in a child or adolescent?**
Common indications include open fractures, tenting of the skin, and/or neurovascular compromise. In some older children and adolescents, the adult indications of 100% displacement or 2 cm of fracture shortening should be considered, particularly when the patients dominant arm is involved or significant loading is anticipated (Fig. 6.23). Additionally, a throwing athlete with a dominant arm injury is more likely to be treated by open reduction and fixation.

146. **What are the operative indications for a proximal humeral fracture in a pediatric patient?**
Very few operative indications exist for proximal humerus fractures in children. Since 80% of the longitudinal growth of the humerus comes from the proximal physis, extensive

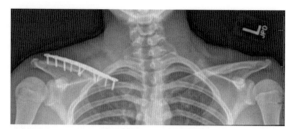

Figure 6.23. Clavicle fracture following open reduction internal fixation.

remodeling is expected in children. As such, non-operative treatment is the rule for these fractures. A closed reduction may be considered, depending on the degree of malalignment, followed by immobilization in a sling or shoulder immobilizer. The exception is an older adolescent that is close to skeletal maturity and who has little remodeling potential. Very displaced fractures may have interposition of the biceps tendon, though the consequences of this interposition are poorly understood.

147. **What is the standard treatment for a humeral shaft fracture in a child?**
Non-operative is the standard of care, typically in a shoulder immobilizer or Sarmiento cast brace. It is unclear whether a "hanging arm" (long arm) cast provides any true distraction to improve alignment or any added comfort versus a cast brace. In general, there is good remodeling potential for the humerus, and deformities can be well-tolerated. Additionally, children don't tend to be large enough for girth to cause the fracture to be pushed into varus. Operative indications include open fractures and vascular injury. Polytrauma is a relative indication to allow for early mobilization of patients with corresponding injuries. Consider pathologic processes, particularly when the mechanism of injury has low energy. Radial nerve palsies that present with the injury are occasionally encountered in distal third humeral shaft fractures, are considered to be traction injuries most commonly, and are typically treated non-operatively. If the palsy occurs following closed reduction, then nerve exploration should be considered.

ELBOW TRAUMA

148. **What are standard radiographic views in pediatric elbow trauma?**
Typically, antero-posterior, lateral, and oblique views are obtained. Internal oblique views are particularly useful in lateral condyle fractures to determine the degree of displacement.

149. **What does a fat pad sign typically indicate in a child?**
An anterior fat pad sign is often physiologic. When a posterior fat pad sign is present, it is generally indicative of an elbow effusion. This most commonly is due to a non-displaced supracondylar humerus fracture (SCH). Approximately 80% of positive posterior fat pad signs are the result of occult fractures.

CASE 6-12

A 6-year-old girl presents to the Emergency Room following a fall from the monkey bars earlier that day. She has a splint on her left arm that was placed by the EMT. She is tearful, but appears otherwise uninjured. X-rays and a clinical photo are shown in Figures 6.24 and 6.25.

150. **What neurovascular exam is particularly important in supracondylar humerus fractures?**
The anterior interosseous nerve is the most commonly injured structure in supracondylar humerus (SCH) fractures. This nerve injury generally occurs in extension type SCH fractures (>90% of fractures are extension type). This nerve is tested by flexion of the interphalangeal joint of the index finger and thumb. This nerve injury has been associated with vascular injury. The radial nerve is the second most commonly injured nerve. This nerve is tested by the distal most motor branch, the posterior interosseous nerve. This

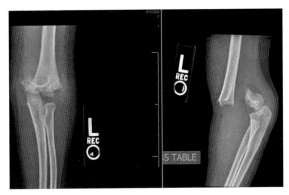

Figure 6.24. 6-year-old girl with an elbow injury after a fall.

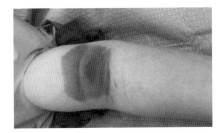

Figure 6.25. Clinical photograph of the patient's antecubital fossa.

nerve innervates muscles which extend the thumb and index finger interphalangeal joints. In a flexion type supracondylar humerus fracture, the ulnar nerve is most commonly injured and is tested by crossing of one finger over another. Most nerve palsies resolve with time.

151. **What other exam should be done in SCH fractures?**
A careful vascular exam is warranted. The brachial artery can be stretched over the proximal piece of the fracture resulting in vascular injury or spasm. The hand can either be "pink and pulseless", which suggests adequate perfusion from the collateral circulation, or "white and pulseless", which suggests inadequate perfusion from a vascular injury stretch/compression of the vessels. Fractures with vascular compromise are taken to the operating room in an urgent fashion for closed versus open reduction and stabilization. After reduction, the vascular status is reassessed. There is no indication for an arteriogram. If blood flow fails to return to the hand exploration, is indicated.

152. **What structure is in danger with a medial pin in a SCH fracture?**
Many orthopedists treat supracondylar humerus fractures with all lateral pinning. The ulnar nerve is in danger with a medial pin in SCH fractures. Generally, the lateral pins are placed percutaneously, and the medial pin is placed through a small incision with direct visualization to avoid placing this through the ulnar groove. The lateral pins are placed first, then the medial pin is placed with the elbow in more extension to allow the nerve to relax. If an ulnar neuropathy is identified following placement of a medial pin, especially when adequate visualization was achieved when placing the pin, one should suspect an unstable ulnar nerve which has subluxated anteriorly with the elbow in flexion, and is impinging on the wire. A careful postoperative exam must be documented.

153. **What deformity can occur with an untreated supracondylar humerus fracture?**
Cubitus varus is the most common deformity. It is generally cosmetically unappealing, but functionally of little consequence. It has been termed "gunstock deformity".

154. **What are the treatment options for lateral condyle fractures?**
Lateral condyle fractures historically have been classified as either through or medial to the capitellar ossification center (lateral to or through the trochlea). This classification system is less useful than newer classification systems, in which the stability of the fragment is a focus. A type I fracture is non-displaced and is generally stable and treated non-operatively in a cast. Close follow-up for displacement is warranted. Type II fractures are displaced, but not rotated, and are typically stable since there is preservation of an intact cartilaginous hinge. These fractures are sometimes treated in a cast, and often by closed reduction and percutaneous pinning. Type III fractures are displaced and rotated. These fractures require open reduction through a lateral (Kocher) approach and pinning.

155. **What are some complications of lateral condyle fractures?**
Delayed union and nonunion are risks. Additionally, osteonecrosis of the fracture fragment, resulting in nonunion, is possible if the dissection is carried too far posteriorly or if the injury results in posterior soft tissue stripping. A progressive drift into cubitus valgus may complicate a nonunion, often resulting in ulnar nerve palsy. Stiffness is also a potential complication of these injuries.

156. **How do medial epicondyle fractures occur?**
This injury typically results from a valgus stress or strong contraction that leads to an avulsion of the flexor-pronator wad of the elbow. Patients are usually between 9 and 14 years old. Up to half of injuries may be associated with elbow dislocation.

157. **What are the operative indications for a medial epicondyle fracture?**
Operative interventions for this fracture are a subject of debate. Absolute indications include the rare case of open fracture or when the fracture fragment becomes interposed within the joint. Displacement of the fracture cannot be gauged reliably on plain films. Displacement of greater than 5 mm is a relative indication for surgery, as is a concomitant elbow dislocation, particularly if the patient is an athlete, and it is a dominant arm injury. Bony union is far higher with operative compared to non-operative treatment. The long-term consequences of an non-united fracture are unknown.

158. **What are the treatment options for a radial head/neck fracture in a child?**
Radial head/neck fractures in children are generally closed reduced if the fracture is greater than 30° angulated in any plane, or translated more than 3–4 mm. The main risks of malunion are loss of motion, particularly forearm rotation. If a closed reduction fails, a percutaneous wire can be inserted to manipulate the fragment. The wire is kept anterior to avoid damage to the posterior interosseous nerve. If this maneuver is unsuccessful, an intramedullary implant (flexible nail) can be inserted in the radial styloid, advanced across the fracture site, and rotated to manipulate the fracture into acceptable alignment (Metizeau technique). If these maneuvers fail, an open procedure can be used, but this is avoided if possible due to the risk of nonunion and elbow stiffness.

159. **What should be considered if an olecranon sleeve fracture is encountered?**
If an olecranon sleeve fracture is encountered, the diagnosis of osteogenesis imperfecta should be ruled out.

160. **What is a Monteggia fracture dislocation, and how are they classified?**
Monteggia fractures are defined as a fracture of the ulnar shaft associated with a dislocation of the radial head. They are most commonly described by the Bado classification. Bado 1 is anterior dislocation of the radial head with apex volar angulation of the ulna and is the most common type. A Bado 2 is apex dorsal angulation with posterior dislocation of the radial head. Bado 3 is lateral dislocation of the radial head, and Bado 4 is both bone forearm fracture plus radial head dislocation. Many Monteggia fractures can be closed reduced and casted. If closed reduction fails and results in residual subluxation of the radial head, open reduction and internal fixation or closed reduction and intramedullary fixation of the ulna should be undertaken. Ulnar length is of utmost

importance in maintaining the reduction of the radial head. As a result, in the case of comminuted fractures or length unstable fractures, open reduction and plating should be considered. Plastic deformation may also result in radial head displacement and may require a large Steinmann pin in the ulna in order to correct (Fig. 6.26).

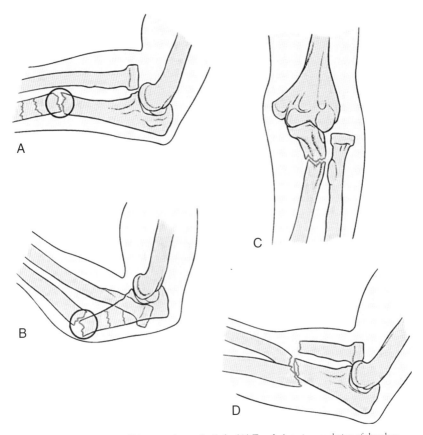

Figure 6.26. The classification of Monteggia lesions by Bado. (A) Type I: Anterior angulation of the ulnar fracture and anterior dislocation of the radial head. (B) Type II: Posterior angulation of the ulnar fracture and posterior dislocation of the radial head. (C) Type III: Fracture of the proximal ulna metaphysis and lateral dislocation of the radial head. (D) Type IV: Anterior dislocation of the radial head and fracture of the radial and ulnar shafts. (*From Jupiter JB, Kellam JF, Diaphyseal Fractures of the Forearm: Browner BD, et al. [eds], Skeletal Trauma: Basic Science, Management, and Reconstruction, 3rd edn. Copyright © 2009, Saunders, Elsevier Inc.*)

WRIST AND FOREARM

161. **What are the rotational forces acting on the segments of both bone forearm fractures?**

In proximal third forearm fractures, the supinator and biceps will tend to supinate the proximal segment, so the reduction maneuver involves supination of the distal segment. In distal third forearm fractures, the pronator quadratus pronates the distal third fragment; hence the forearm must be pronated. In middle third fractures, the proximal piece is supinated (biceps and supinator) and the distal piece is pronated (pronator teres and quadratus); hence the forearm is brought into neutral rotation to reduce the fracture.

162. **What is the epidemiology of pediatric distal radius fractures?**

They are the most common of all pediatric fractures and account for nearly 50% of all pediatric fractures. Peak incidence is 10–12 years of age.

163. **What is the treatment for distal radius fractures in children?**

The vast majority of distal radius fractures in children can be treated with closed reduction and casting. The majority will remodel without deformity. There is a low rate of growth arrest in distal radius fractures. In contrast, distal ulna fractures are at a high risk of growth arrest and subsequent angular deformity. As a result, these fractures require more careful monitoring.

PEDIATRIC SPINE

ADOLESCENT IDIOPATHIC SCOLIOSIS (AIS)

CASE 6-13

A 13-year-old girl accompanied by her mother presents to your clinic on referral from her pediatrician. She is healthy and active in sports but notes that she was told she needed to see a doctor after her entire gym class had their backs checked by the school nurse. Her mother recalls being told as a teenager that she had scoliosis, though she never received any treatment for it. When you ask your patient to bend forward and touch her toes, her right scapula is more prominent than the left. Her left iliac crest is also high with respect to the floor, but measurement of her leg lengths is equal. Her pediatrician ordered x-rays of her spine, which they brought with them (Fig. 6.27).

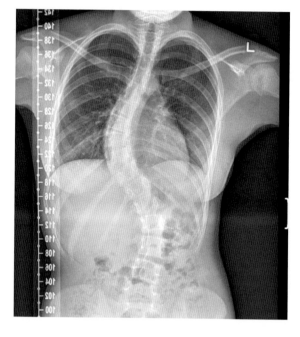

Figure 6.27. Patient with adolescent idiopathic scoliosis.

164. **What is idiopathic scoliosis?**

Idiopathic scoliosis is a curvature of the spine of unknown etiology. It is a complex three-dimensional deformity and is distinguished from scoliosis caused by congenital conditions, neuromuscular disease, and degenerative disease. Idiopathic scoliosis that occurs near the onset of puberty is known as adolescent idiopathic scoliosis (AIS). The other types of idiopathic scoliosis that affect the pediatric population are infantile (age 0–3) and juvenile idiopathic scoliosis (age 3–11).

165. **Is AIS heritable?**
Yes. Twin studies have shown a high concordance rate for both monozygous and dizygous twins. There is also about a 1 in 4 chance that a daughter of a woman with a curve greater than 15° will have scoliosis.

166. **Is AIS more common in boys or girls?**
While mild curves that do not need treatment (less than 10°) are equally common in boys and girls, progressive curves are more common in girls. The ratio of females to males is 10 to 1 for curves greater than 30°.

167. **How are children screened for AIS?**
School screenings have become the standard method for identifying children with scoliosis. Those noted to have spine asymmetry are referred to their pediatrician for diagnostic testing. Less than 1% of screened children will have a positive test, and of those, less than 10% will need treatment.

168. **What are the risk factors for curve progression?**
Risk factors for curve progression in skeletally immature patients include double thoracic and lumbar curves, a large curve at the time of presentation, amount of growth remaining (juveniles > adolescents), and female gender. Studies have shown that thoracic curves greater than 50° and lumbar curves greater than 30° can progress after skeletal maturity.

169. **What is the Risser classification?**
The Risser classification describes the progressive ossification of the iliac crest apophysis and is used as one index of skeletal maturity. Grade 1 is the presence of the lateral ossification center. Grade 2 is ossification of the lateral half of the apophysis. Grade 3 is ossification of the lateral three-quarters of the apophysis. Grade 4 is ossification to the medial side of the iliac crest, known as a "capped" apophysis. Grade 5 refers to complete fusion of the iliac crest apophysis. The Risser sign is accurate to +/− 9 months. The French version of the Risser classification is graded 0 to 4, instead of 0 to 5, as with the US version. (Fig. 6.28).

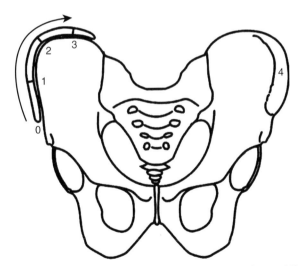

Figure 6.28. Scoliosis. Line diagram of the Risser grades (0 = iliac crest yet to ossify ▶ 4 = full closure of apophysis). (*From Offiah AC, Skeletal Radiology in Children: Non-traumatic and Non-malignant: Grainger & Allison's Diagnostic Radiology: A Textbook of Medical Imaging, pp. 1567–1609. Copyright © 2008, Elsevier Ltd.*)

170. **What are the symptoms of untreated AIS?**
The symptoms of untreated AIS may include back pain, decreased pulmonary function (only in thoracic curves greater than 90–100°), and psychosocial effects associated with the chest wall deformity. Mortality rates are not increased in patients with AIS compared to the general population.

171. **How is AIS diagnosed?**

    AIS is diagnosed based on physical exam findings and radiographs. Asymmetry of skin contour or rib prominence in standing and forward-bending positions is characteristic of scoliosis. Differences in shoulder height, iliac crest height, and apparent limb length may also be present. Abnormalities in gait, abnormal skin pigmentation or hair patterns, and foot deformities (particularly unilateral cavus) can all be indicative of non-idiopathic scoliosis and should prompt further investigation for congenital or neuromuscular causes.

    Posterior to anterior x-rays are used to confirm the diagnosis and characterize the severity of the curve. Lateral x-rays are often obtained to check for sagittal plane alignment. Bending x-rays, which are used to determine the flexibility of the curve, are only obtained when surgery is planned.

172. **How is the Cobb angle calculated?**

    To calculate the Cobb angle, you must first identify the superior and inferior end vertebrae of the curvature (last vertebra which tilts into the curve). These are the vertebrae that have maximally tilted endplates and delineate the length of the curve. Lines are drawn parallel to the superior end plate of the superior end vertebra and the inferior end plate of the inferior end vertebra. If the end plate is difficult to visualize, the lines can be drawn parallel to the pedicles. A perpendicular line is dropped from each of these lines, and the angle of their intersection is the Cobb angle.

173. **How is AIS classified?**

    There are multiple classification systems, the most recent of which have focused on surgical planning, and identifying which levels need to be instrumented and fused. The King classification focuses on thoracic curves and separates lumbar-predominant curves from the multiple types of thoracic-predominant curves. The Lenke classification is used most frequently and has good intraobserver and interobserver reliability. The curve is described based on which of the three regions (proximal thoracic, main thoracic, and thoracolumbar/lumbar) are structural and which are non-structural (compensatory). The structural criteria are based on Cobb angle and kyphosis. Modifiers are applied based on the lumbar spine alignment and thoracic sagittal alignment.

174. **What are the treatment options for AIS?**

    Treatment options are divided into observation, non-operative, and operative management. Observation is appropriate for patients with a curve of less than 20–25°. These patients should be followed every 6 months with serial x-rays to monitor curve progression. Curves that increase 5° or more between visits are considered to have progressed. Non-operative management involves bracing, which is recommended for progressive curves greater than 25 ° as long as sufficient growth is remaining. The goal is to prevent progression rather than to achieve correction. Studies suggest that about 75% of patients will be able to avoid progression using this strategy. Physical therapy and electrical stimulation have not been found to influence outcomes. Curves that are greater than 45–50° will not respond to bracing and operative management is offered to prevent progression.

175. **What type of brace is used in non-operative management?**

    The patient should be fitted for a thoracolumbosacral orthosis (TLSO). Schedules for brace wear vary between centers, from 16 to 23 hours per day. Patients are kept in the brace until they are at least Risser stage IV (females) or skeletally mature (males), and then they are gradually weaned from the brace. Compliance is a constant challenge due to the demanding bracing schedule in a patient population that is very sensitive to appearance and social normalcy. High thoracic curves may not be amenable to bracing with a TLSO. A cervicothoracolumbosacral orthosis (CTLSO) can be prescribed, but compliance with a brace that goes above the shoulders is typically poor.

176. **How is AIS corrected surgically?**

    The goal of surgical treatment is to arrest progression of the curvature, while achieving maximum correction of the curvature and maintaining or achieving a balanced spine (no trunk shift, shoulders level) in the coronal and sagittal planes. The typical spinal construct includes various points of fixation (hooks, wires, screws), which are attached to two rods. Correction is achieved by manipulation of the implants, which are secured when the correction has been completed. Correction is achieved in the coronal, sagittal, and axial (rotational deformity) planes. Most surgeons use cancellous allograft and locally obtained autograft to promote spinal fusion. While the major structural curve or curves are always included in the instrumentation and fusion, non-structural or compensatory curves may often be left out if they are flexible. A secondary goal is to preserve as many motion segments as possible.

177. **What is the surgical approach for spinal instrumentation and fusion?**
The surgical approach for most cases of AIS is a standard posterior approach to the thoracolumbar spine. An anterior spinal fusion with instrumentation may be useful in selected thoracolumbar and lumbar curvatures to reduce the number of segments fused. It typically allows for fusion of fewer levels but is more technically difficult and less familiar to most orthopedic surgeons. There are other indications for anterior spinal surgery in scoliosis. An anterior release involves removal of the discs and the anterior longitudinal ligament, and is indicated in rigid deformities to enhance the magnitude of correction achieved in the posterior procedure (anterior and posterior spinal fusion), as well as in very young patients in whom persistent anterior spinal growth might result in a progressive deformity despite a posterior fusion (crankshaft phenomenon). Combined anterior and posterior fusion has also been advocated in spina bifida to decrease the rate of pseudarthrosis.

178. **What can be used to minimize neurologic complications in surgical management of AIS?**
Spinal cord injury occurs in less than 1% of patients. Intraoperative spinal cord monitoring is perhaps most useful, and includes monitoring of both somatosensory and motor evoked potentials. Maintaining a stable blood pressure, and avoiding intraoperative hypotensive anesthesia, may enhance spinal cord blood flow and reduce the risks of microvascular ischemia. Intraoperative fluoroscopy or radiographs may help confirm positioning of the implants, and an intraoperative CT scan with navigation may potentially improve the ease of insertion and the positioning of pedicle screws. Avoiding overly aggressive attempts at correction will also minimize the risks of neurologic deterioration, especially with the latest generation implants which are capable of delivering substantial forces to the spine.

179. **What are the other most common complications following surgery for AIS?**
Wound infection, pseudarthrosis, and implant failure (loss of fixation, fracture, and disengagement) are other potential complications.

SCHEUERMANN DISEASE
CASE 6-14

A 16-year-old boy is brought to your clinic by his parents due to concern about his worsening posture. They state that they have been reprimanding him for slouching, but it only seems to be getting worse. He cannot fully straighten up, and he complains of activity related back pain which is dull in quality. On examination, you note that he has rounded shoulders with pronounced thoracic kyphosis and lumbar hyperlordosis. You are unable to passively extend the thoracic spine. Passive range of motion of his extremities reveals tightness in the hamstrings. When he lies down on the examination table, his shoulders rest off the table and his neck is hyperextended. The neurologic examination is normal. You order x-rays of the entire spine (Fig. 6.29).

180. **What is Scheuermann disease?**
Kyphosis refers to a sagittal plane curvature of the spine with the convexity of the curve pointing dorsally, and is a normal finding in the thoracic spine. The typical thoracic kyphosis measured from T3 to T12 is 20–50°, and values beyond this are termed hyperkyphosis. Postural hyperkyphosis is relatively common, and patients are able to voluntarily correct the deformity. There is no structural element in postural hyperkyphosis. In contrast, Scheuermann disease is a hyperkyphosis in which there is a structural component, and the deformity is not passively correctable. Characteristic findings

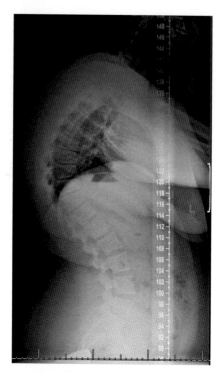

Figure 6.29. Patient with severe kyphosis.

include an apex that is lower than normal, wedging of more than 5° in three consecutive vertebrae, irregularities of the vertebral endplates, and Schmorl's nodes (protrusion of the intervertebral disk material into the vertebral body). Patients with Scheuermann kyphosis also develop compensatory cervical and lumbar hyperlordosis, and may have tight hamstrings.

181. **What is the etiology of Scheuermann disease?**
The etiology is unclear, but is likely genetic. Multiple theories have been proposed, including avascular necrosis, abnormalities of the anterior longitudinal ligament, osteoporosis, and cartilage defects.

182. **What symptoms are associated with Scheuermann disease?**
The most common symptom is back pain that is activity related and typically relieved by rest. The diagnosis is usually made in adolescence, and patients may experience more issues with the appearance of the deformity than with pain. Severe cases can cause cardiopulmonary compromise, typically when the curvature has surpassed 90°. Neurologic manifestations are uncommon, although associated spinal pathology such as a thoracic disc herniation or dural cysts can lead to neurologic symptoms at an earlier stage than they would in patients without the kyphotic deformity.

183. **What are the radiographic characteristics of Scheuermann disease?**
Anterior wedging of more than 5° of at least three adjacent vertebrae, narrow intervertebral disc spaces, endplate irregularities, and Schmorl's nodes are characteristic radiographic findings of Scheuermann disease. Schmorl's nodes are protrusions of intervertebral disc material into the endplates of adjacent vertebrae that are usually visible on x-ray, and better seen on an MRI. Lateral x-rays performed with hyperextension over a bolster will demonstrate the rigidity of the kyphosis.

184. **What is pseudo-Scheuermann disease?**

Pseudo-Scheuermann disease, also known as lumbar Scheuermann disease, is a painful condition of the thoracolumbar spine seen most frequently in adolescent males who do heavy lifting. It is characterized by a loss of lumbar lordosis, endplate irregularities, and Schmorl's nodes of the lumbar or lower thoracic vertebrae. Unlike Scheuermann kyphosis, it is a self-limiting condition that tends to improve with NSAIDs and activity modification, although bracing may be required to control the symptoms in a subset of cases. Juvenile discogenic disease should be considered in the differential diagnosis.

185. **What are the management options for Scheuermann disease?**

Non-operative management consists of bracing if the curve is more than 50° and the patient has significant growth remaining. As with AIS, bracing regimens are demanding, especially on the adolescent patient, so compliance may be an issue. This is particularly true since the brace must extend above the shoulders. Physical therapy focused on extension exercises can be a useful adjuvant to bracing. Patients with a progressive and symptomatic curve greater than 70° are candidates for surgical intervention.

186. **What are the surgical options for treating Scheuermann disease?**

An anterior release and posterior spinal fusion were commonly performed in the past. Anterior procedures involve lengthening of the spine, which may increase the risk of neurological complications. Currently, an instrumented posterior spinal fusion is combined with multiple osteotomies to shorten the posterior column. Correction of the deformity by shortening the spine presumably reduces the risks of neurological complications. The risk of neurologic injury is higher in kyphosis surgery when compared with surgery for idiopathic scoliosis.

SPONDYLOLISTHESIS AND SPONDYLOLYSIS

CASE 6-15

You are seeing a 12-year-old elite-level gymnast in your clinic for complaints of nagging back pain that is affecting her training. She reports a dull, aching pain in the lumbosacral region that bothers her throughout her practices. She took a couple of weeks off from gymnastics, thinking it was a muscle strain, but the pain returned as soon as she got back into her routine. The pain does not radiate, and she denies any numbness or tingling. Her lower extremity strength is normal and symmetric. She has tenderness at the lumbosacral junction and hyperextension of her spine reproduces the pain. She has a mild hamstring contracture. X-rays and a CT scan of her lumbar spine are shown in Figures 6.30 and 6.31.

187. **What does spondylolisthesis mean?**

Spondylolisthesis means the anterior translation of one vertebral body on the next.

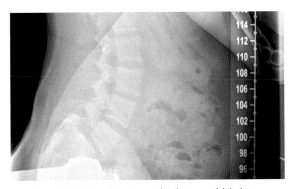

Figure 6.30. X-ray of a patient with isthmic spondylolisthesis.

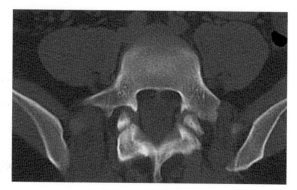

Figure 6.31. CT scan of isthmic spondylolisthesis.

188. **What does spondylolysis mean?**
Spondylolysis is a defect of the pars interarticularis, the region of the posterior elements between the pedicle and the superior articular process. Bilateral defects of the pars interarticularis allow spondylolisthesis to occur.

189. **What is the most common location for spondylolisthesis to occur in a child? What is the most common location for spondylolysis to occur in children?**
Spondylolisthesis typically affects children at the L5–S1 level. Spondylolysis is usually found at the L5 vertebra, but may be observed at one or more other levels in the lumbar spine.

190. **What are the two main types of spondylolisthesis that affect children?**
The two main types of spondylolisthesis that affect children are dysplastic and isthmic. Dysplastic spondylolisthesis (type I) refers to a congenital abnormality of the vertebral facets that allows one vertebra to slip on the next. Isthmic spondylolisthesis (type II) involves a defect of the pars interarticularis. The defect can be caused by a stress fracture (type IIA), an intact but elongated pars (type IIB), or an acute fracture (type IIC).

191. **What activities have been associated with fracture of the pars interarticularis and spondylolisthesis?**
Activities that accentuate the lumbar lordosis or involve repetitive extension of the lumbar spine (compressive loading of the posterior elements) increase the risk of spondylolysis and spondylolisthesis. Gymnastics, diving, rowing, weight lifting, and football are examples of such activities. Patients with Scheuermann disease are also at risk because they compensate for thoracic kyphosis with increased lumbar lordosis.

192. **What symptoms or findings occur with spondylolysis and spondylolisthesis?**
The classic presentation is an insidious onset of persistent low back pain that is worse with activity. An acute pars fracture (type IIB) is rare, and presents with an acute onset of pain following an injury. Focal neurologic signs and radicular symptoms are uncommon, although lumbar radiculopathy is often observed in patients with higher-grade spondylolisthesis. Symptomatic patients will often have a hamstring contracture or spasm, and some have suggested that the hamstrings are a "barometer" for the spine. Lumbar hyperextension often reproduces the patient's pain in a symptomatic spondylolysis or spondylolisthesis.

193. **What is the Phalen–Dickson sign?**
This is a physical finding in which the patient stands or walks with flexed hips and knees. It is thought to develop due to nerve irritation from spine instability and micromotion. This posture becomes more pronounced as the spondylolisthesis progresses. The patients commonly have hamstring tightness as well.

194. **What radiographic views are most useful for diagnosing spondylolisthesis and spondylolysis?**
The lateral x-ray is best to show spondylolisthesis. Oblique views show the pars interarticularis as a 'Scottie dog," with a pars fracture appearing as a lucency or "collar" on the dog (Fig. 6.30).

195. **What is the Meyerding classification?**
Meyerding classification describes the percentage of displacement or degree of slippage of the superior vertebral body on the inferior vertebral body as follows: Grade 0 (no displacement), Grade 1 (1–25%), Grade 2 (26–50%), Grade 3 (51–75%), Grade 4 (76–100%).

196. **What is the slip angle?**
The slip angle represents the degree of lumbosacral kyphosis, and is measured on the lateral radiograph as the angle between a line along the inferior body of the superior (slipped) vertebra, and a line perpendicular to the posterior cortex of the lower vertebra or sacrum. Normal angles are 0–10°. A slip angle greater than 55° is associated with a high risk of progression.

197. **What demographic factors increase the risk of progression? What characteristics of the spondylolisthesis increase the risk of progression?**
Younger age (i.e., more time left for skeletal growth) and female gender are risk factors for progression. Higher grade slips and dysplastic (type I) spondylolisthesis are also more prone to progression.

198. **What options are available for non-operative treatment of pediatric spondylolisthesis and spondylolysis?**
Activity modification, including rest from sports and other activities that aggravate the symptoms, physical therapy, and bracing are the best options for non-operative management. Braces counteract the lordotic posture of the lumbar spine, and are typically made with the lumbar spine in 15° of flexion to unload compressive stresses across the posterior elements, and should be worn for 3 to 6 months. Patients who have spondylolysis and spondylolisthesis related to an acute fracture tend to do best when bracing is initiated immediately after the injury. Non-operative management has a high success rate in patients with spondylolisthesis that is Grade 2 or less.

199. **What slip percentage is the usual threshold for operative treatment?**
A slip of 50% or greater at initial presentation is typically unresponsive to non-operative management and will likely progress over time, and surgery should be offered. This corresponds to a Grade 3 slip according to the Meyerding classification.

200. **What are the surgical options for treatment of spondylolysis and spondylolisthesis?**
A posterior instrumented "in situ" fusion of the involved vertebrae with autogenous bone graft is recommended for cases of spondylolysis and low-grade spondylolisthesis. When the spondylolysis is identified above the L5 level, consideration is given to achieving bony union across the defect by fixation and bone grafting without fusion. The treatment of higher-grade spondylolisthesis is more complex and prone to complications, and typically includes a wide decompression of the L5 and S1 nerve roots and an instrumented fusion from L4 to S1, with or without reduction of the slip. More recent thought has emphasized the importance of anterior column support (fibular graft placed through sacrum into L5, or a transforaminal metallic cage) to enhance stability and maximize the chance of a successful arthrodesis. While controversial, an instrumented reduction utilizes the implants to achieve gradual translation of the upper vertebra on the lower vertebra.

201. **What is the most common complication following surgical treatment of spondylolysis and spondylolisthesis?**
Neurologic injury is the most common complication following surgical treatment, most commonly an L5 radiculopathy resulting in foot drop, and less frequently a cauda equina

syndrome. Radiculopathy occurs more commonly when reduction of the slip is performed, but can also occur with in situ fusion.

CERVICAL SPINE

CASE 6-16

You are seeing a 6-week-old baby boy in clinic due to his parents' concern that his head is always positioned with a tilt toward his right shoulder, and mild rotation toward the left side. His delivery was prolonged due to breech positioning. Palpation of his neck reveals significant tightness of the right sternocleidomastoid muscle and a fullness within the muscle belly. While examining him, you also notice asymmetric thigh creases. Barlow and Ortolani tests are positive. X-rays demonstrate the described head positioning but show no bony abnormalities of the spine.

202. **What is congenital muscular torticollis?**
    Torticollis is a non-specific term used to describe tilting of the head and neck, and congenital muscular torticollis is caused by contracture of the sternocleidomastoid muscle. The contracture causes the head to tilt toward the affected side and the chin to rotate toward the opposite side (Fig. 6.32).

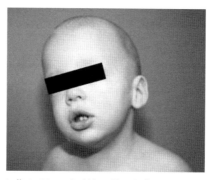

Figure 6.32. Congenital torticollis in 14-month-old boy. (*From Kelly DM, Campbell's Operative Orthopaedics, pp. 1119–1132.e2. Copyright © 2013 by Mosby, Elsevier Inc.*)

203. **What age group is most commonly affected by muscular torticollis?**
    Infants are affected by congenital muscular torticollis, and the right side is more frequently involved than the left side. There is greater concern when torticollis presents in an older infant or child who had no history or evidence of congenital muscular torticollis. The differential diagnosis is large in these cases, and a neurologic consultation is advised. Patients are often evaluated with an MRI of the brain.

204. **What is the etiology of congenital muscular torticollis?**
    MRI studies have suggested that a localized intramuscular compartment syndrome may result in fibrosis of the sternocleidomastoid muscle. Many patients will have a palpable mass of scar tissue within the substance of the muscle which gradually disappears over several weeks to months following delivery. The condition is often associated facial asymmetry and plagiocephally, presumably related to intrauterine deformation as well.

205. **What other congenital orthopedic conditions are frequently seen in association with congenital muscular torticollis?**
    Developmental dysplasia of the hip is associated with congenital muscular torticollis in approximately 8% of cases. Both conditions can be diagnosed with ultrasonography. Metatarsus adductus and other positional foot deformities are also observed in patients with congenital muscular torticollis.

206. **How is muscular torticollis treated?**
When the diagnosis is made before 1 year of age, 90–95% of patients will respond to stretching exercises alone. Patients older than 1 year of age typically require surgical intervention to correct the deformity. Surgical intervention involves release of the sternocleidomastoid muscle. This can be accomplished with a unipolar procedure, in which just sternal and clavicular heads are released, or a bipolar procedure in which release at the mastoid process is also accomplished. Postoperatively, patients are managed in a brace and stretching and strengthening exercises are performed after 6 weeks of immobilization.

207. **What are other causes of torticollis besides muscular torticollis?**
The differential diagnosis of torticollis is extensive, and includes congenital anomalies of the occipito-cervical spine (congenital scoliosis, Klippel–Feil syndrome, basilar invagination), posterior fossa tumors, ophthalmologic causes (extraocular muscle palsy or other), paroxysmal torticollis of infancy, fractures or dislocations of the cervical spine/occiput, inflammatory conditions (rheumatoid arthritis, retropharyngeal abscess), and esophageal reflux.

208. **What is atlantoaxial instability?**
Atlantoaxial instability refers to excessive translation at the joint between the first cervical vertebra (atlas) and the second cervical vertebra (axis) during flexion and extension. Instability at this joint can lead to stenosis of the spinal canal with neurologic complications.

209. **Why does cervical spine instability tend to occur at the atlantoaxial articulation?**
The C1–C2 articulation is surrounded by two joints that have relatively little motion, the atlanto-occipital joint (between the base of the skull and C1) and the C2–C3 joint. Abnormalities that may result in hypermobility at this joint include intrinsic weakness of the soft-tissue restraints, and/or loss of motion at the surrounding joints. For example, patients who have fusion of the atlanto-occipital joint also frequently have fusion of C2–C3, which leads to excessive stresses and compensatory hypermobility at C1–C2.

210. **What structural abnormalities lead to atlantoaxial instability?**
Deformities of the odontoid such as hypoplasia, fractures of the odontoid (os odontoideum), ligamentous hyperlaxity, and transverse atlantal ligament rupture can all lead to atlantoaxial instability.

211. **During which decade does atlantoaxial instability typically present?**
Symptoms of atlantoaxial instability usually occur during the third decade of life. Although it is a congenital problem, symptoms may be delayed because the pediatric spine and nervous system can accommodate minor instability. As the patient ages and degenerative changes begin to appear, the narrowing of the spinal cord can become worse and begin to cause impingement of the neural elements. Traumatic events are another reason for development of symptoms in a previously asymptomatic patient with atlantoaxial instability.

212. **What are the symptoms of atlantoaxial instability?**
The clinical presentation of atlantoaxial instability is quite variable and depends on where the spinal cord or brain stem is being compressed. Myelopathy manifests as episodic or progressive weakness and/or decreased physical endurance. Compression of the pyramidal tract causes muscle weakness and atrophy, spasticity, and hyperreflexia. Posterior cord compression from impingement against the posterior rim of the foramen magnum results in deficits in proprioception and vibratory responses. Impingement of cranial nerves can cause associated symptoms such as visual disturbances, dysphagia or tinnitus. Cerebellar involvement will lead to ataxia and deficits in coordination. Compression of the vertebral arteries can cause dizziness, syncope, vertigo, or seizures. Because the clinical picture can be so variable, it is important to have a high suspicion for atlantoaxial instability in patients at higher risk for the disorder.

213. **What congenital conditions are associated with atlantoaxial instability?**
Down syndrome, Morquio's syndrome, Marfan syndrome, Ehlers–Danlos syndrome, Klippel–Feil syndrome, Arnold–Chiari malformations, osteogenesis imperfecta, neurofibromatosis, spondyloepiphyseal dysplasia, and congenital scoliosis may all be associated with atlantoaxial instability. Patients with these conditions undergoing general anesthesia should have flexion–extension radiographs of the cervical spine before being anesthetized to identify the need for additional precautions with intubation.

214. **How is atlantoaxial instability recognized radiographically?**
The atlantodens interval (ADI) is the distance between the posterior border of the anterior ring of the atlas and the anterior border of the dens measured on lateral x-ray. A normal ADI in children should be ≤4 mm (≤5 mm in population with Down syndrome) and should be measured in both neutral and flexion (except in the setting of trauma when flexion could be dangerous). The ADI is most useful for acute cases of atlantoaxial instability in which excessive translation is due to incompetence or disruption of the transverse atlantal ligament. It can be normal in cases of congenital atlantoaxial instability, so the space available for the spinal cord (SAC) is also used. The SAC is the distance between the posterior border of the odontoid and the nearest posterior structure (foramen magnum or posterior ring of the atlas) as measured on lateral x-ray. Normal SAC increases with growth, so it should be compared against norms for the patient's age and the SAC for successive vertebral levels. Dynamic flexion–extension CT or MRI can also be used to diagnose neural impingement at the extremes of motion (Fig. 6.33).

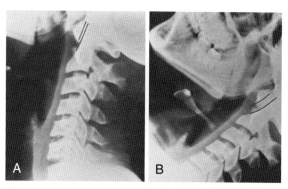

Figure 6.33. The atlantodens interval (ADI) is the distance on the lateral roentgenogram between the anterior aspect of the dens and the posterior aspect of the anterior ring of the atlas. In children, the ADI should not exceed 4.0 mm, whereas the upper limit in the normal adult is less than 3.0 mm. C1–C2 instability is vividly demonstrated in the extension (A) and flexion (B) views. *(From Torg JS, Glasgow SG: Criteria for return to contact activities following cervical spine injury. Clin J Sport Med 1:12–27, 1991.)*

215. **How is atlantoaxial instability treated?**
Patients with asymptomatic atlantoaxial hypermobility should avoid activities or sports that risk injury or hyperflexion/hyperextension to the cervical spine. They should also be followed clinically to monitor for radiographic progression or the development of any neurological signs or symptoms. Surgical treatment of atlantoaxial instability is reserved for cases of instability, with or without symptoms. Instability is treated by spinal stabilization (instrumented posterior spinal fusion). The location of the compression or impingement must first be identified to know in which position the fusion should occur to relieve the symptoms. Reduction should be performed prior to surgery with maintenance of reduction in traction or supported positioning prior to the procedure. Neurologic monitoring is also essential. Surgical stabilization of the atlantoaxial joint can be performed using sublaminar wires, screws across the C1–C2 joint, or by plate fixation.

216. **What is os odontoideum?**
Os odontoideum is an anomaly of the odontoid in which there is discontinuity between the upper or middle section of the odontoid and the base. It may be congenital or related

to prior fracture of the odontoid. Os odontoideum, as well as aplasia or hypoplasia of the odontoid, is commonly associated with atlantoaxial instability.

217. **What are the indications for surgical stabilization of an os odontoideum?**
The presence of neurologic symptoms, atlantoaxial instability of 10 mm or more from flexion to extension, and increasing instability over time are all indications for surgical intervention. Although patients without symptoms or instability are usually not treated with prophylactic stabilization, close observation and avoidance of activities that could stress or injure the cervical spine are important. A single minor trauma can be enough to cause devastating neurologic complications in these patients. If stabilization is not performed, patients should be followed clinically with routine flexion–extension radiographs to rule out progressive instability.

218. **What is Klippel–Feil syndrome?**
Klippel–Feil syndrome is a condition characterized by congenital failure of segmentation or fusion of two or more cervical vertebrae. It results from failure of the normal vertebral (cervical somite) segmentation that occurs in the fetus between 3 and 8 weeks of life.

219. **What is the classic triad of physical examination findings in patients with Klippel–Feil syndrome?**
A short neck, low posterior hairline, and limited neck range of motion make up the classic triad of Klippel–Feil syndrome. This triad is present in less than half of affected patients. While limited neck range of motion is the most common sign, patients with fusion of only two vertebrae or fusion of the mobile lower cervical vertebrae may not have a clinically detectable loss of neck range of motion. Unfused segments will see increased stresses, and may develop hypermobility or even instability.

220. **What plane of motion is best preserved in Klippel–Feil syndrome?**
Flexion–extension tends to be best preserved compared to lateral bending and rotation of the cervical spine.

221. **What is Sprengel's deformity?**
Sprengel's deformity is a congenital malformation involving the upper extremity in which there is hypoplasia and superior displacement of the scapula (unilateral or bilateral) due to failed descent of the bone during development. It is frequently seen in association with Klippel–Feil syndrome, and a fusion between the cervical spine and scapula (fibrous, cartilaginous, or bony) can be present (Fig. 6.34).

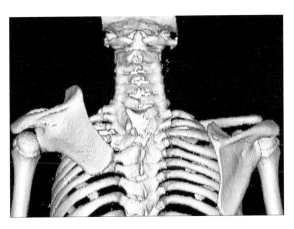

Figure 6.34. Sprengel's deformity: 3-D CT of thorax on bone windows. Elevated right scapula (Sprengel's deformity). Note also the spinal dysraphism (C5–T3) and failure of segmentation (T4/T5). (*From Offiah AC, Grainger & Allison's Diagnostic Radiology: A Textbook of Medical Imaging, pp. 1567–1609. Copyright © 2008, Elsevier Ltd, All rights reserved.*)

222. **Why does fusion cause neurologic symptoms in these patients?**
The uninvolved segments become hypermobile in order to compensate for the loss of motion at the involved segments. Hypermobility may progress to instability, and progressive joint degeneration may result in the gradual development of spinal stenosis, each of which may result in neurologic impairment.

223. **What is the most common musculoskeletal disorder that occurs with Klippel–Feil syndrome?**

Clinically significant scoliosis is present in up to 60% of patients with Klippel–Feil syndrome. Scoliosis may be congenital or compensatory in these patients.

224. **What other organ systems tend to be affected in patients with Klippel–Feil syndrome?**

Abnormalities of the genitourinary system (e.g., congenital absence of a kidney), nervous system (e.g., synkinesis or mirror motions), auditory system (e.g., deafness), and cardiopulmonary system (e.g., ventricular septal defect) can be observed. Upper-extremity abnormalities, such as syndactyly, supernumary digits, and hypoplasia of the thumb or upper extremity, are also associated with this condition.

225. **What radiologic studies should be performed to confirm the diagnosis of Klippel–Feil syndrome?**

Plain radiographs will confirm the diagnosis of Klippel–Feil syndrome. Hemivertebrae and wide, flattened vertebrae may be seen along with the fused vertebrae. MRI is useful to detect neurologic sequelae of Klippel–Feil syndrome, such as myelopathy and cord compression. Because of the high incidence of scoliosis, the thoracolumbar spine and sacrum should also be studied with radiographs.

226. **What are three radiographic patterns of Klippel–Feil syndrome?**

Pattern 1 involves fusion of C2 and C3 with occipitalization of C1. Pattern 2 is a long cervical fusion with an abnormal occipitocervical junction. Both patterns put abnormal stress at the C1–C2 articulation and can result in atlantoaxial instability. Pattern 3 involves 2 separate fused segments with a single uninvolved level between them (Fig. 6.35).

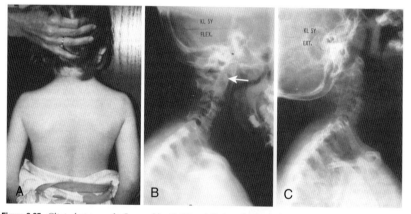

Figure 6.35. Clinical picture of a 5 year old with Klippel–Feil syndrome. (A) Note short neck and low hairline. Radiographs of the cervical spine (B, flexion; C, extension) demonstrate congenital fusion and evidence of spinal instability (arrow). (*From Drummond DS: Pediatric Cervical Instability. In: Weisel SE, Boden SD, Wisnecki RI, [eds], Seminars in Spine Surgery, pp. 292–309. Philadelphia, WB Saunders, 1996.*)

227. **How is Klippel–Feil syndrome treated?**

Asymptomatic patients with more than a single cervical fusion are instructed to avoid activities that risk trauma to the cervical spine. Symptomatic treatment includes analgesics and cervical immobilization. In patients with instability and/or stenosis, cervical decompression and/or fusion may be required. Brachial plexus injuries are a risk of traction and surgical stabilization because cervical nerve roots may have anomalous origins in these patients. Additionally, treatment of associated visceral problems or scoliosis may be required.

228. **What is basilar invagination?**

Basilar invagination is an abnormality of the upper cervical spine in which the base of the skull is indented by the impression of the cervical spine. It can interfere with flow of blood and/or cerebrospinal fluid (CSF) into and out of the skull. It can also result in impingement on the brain stem if the odontoid extends through the foramen magnum and into the skull.

229. **What are the two types of basilar invagination?**

Basilar invagination can be congenital (primary) or developmental (secondary). The congenital form is often associated with other congenital osseous abnormalities involving the skull and spine, such as atlanto-occipital fusion and odontoid deformities. The developmental form is thought to be related to a "softening" of the base of the skull due to metabolic bone disease or repetitive microtrauma.

230. **What bone disease is classically associated with developmental basilar invagination?**

Osteogenesis imperfecta (OI) has a relatively high incidence of basilar invagination, and other diseases in which basilar invagination may be associated include rickets, Paget's disease, osteomalacia, renal osteodystrophy, rheumatoid arthritis, neurofibromatosis, and ankylosing spondylitis.

231. **How is basilar invagination diagnosed?**

The diagnosis is based on clinical and radiographic findings. A wide range of neurologic symptoms may be present, depending on the degree of deformity and the existence of concurrent neurologic abnormalities. These may include parathesias, weakness, cerebellar dysfunction, nystagmus, and cranial nerve palsy. Headache and neck pain are also common. Traditionally, lateral or anteroposterior (AP) radiographs were used to evaluate for basilar invagination, and various measurement techniques have been utilized (e.g., Chamberlain's line, McGregor's line, McRae's line, Fischgold–Metzger line). These methods have largely been replaced by the use of CT and MRI.

232. **What other neurologic pathologies are often associated with basilar invagination?**

Arnold–Chiari malformation (herniation of the cerebellar tonsils through the foramen magnum), syringomyelia, and vertebral artery anomalies frequently coexist with basilar invagination. Therefore, MRI is frequently performed on patients with known or suspected basilar invagination.

233. **How is basilar invagination treated?**

Treatment must involve both decompression and stabilization. Decompression can be obtained with craniectomy and laminectomy for cases that respond to traction, or removal of the impinging bone for cases that do not respond to traction. Fusion must be performed for all cases.

PEDIATRIC HAND

CONGENITAL HAND ABNORMALITIES

234. **What are the seven categories in the classification system for congenital hand abnormalities?**

The seven categories of congenital hand abnormalities are: (1) failure of formation, (2) failure of differentiation, (3) overgrowth, (4) undergrowth, (5) duplication, (6) constriction band syndrome, and (7) generalized skeletal abnormalities.

235. **What is the difference between preaxial and postaxial?**

Preaxial refers to the lateral or radial (thumb) side of the hand whereas postaxial refers to the medial or ulnar (small finger) side of the hand.

236. **What embryologic structures influence the formation of the human upper limb bud?**

The apical ectodermal ridge influences the proximal–distal formation of the upper limb bud between 4 and 8 weeks' gestation of the human embryo. Apoptosis, or programmed cell death, results in separation of the distal limb bud into digits, so that a hand can be visualized as early as 7 weeks. Hypoplasia or hyperplasia of the apical ectodermal ridge in the upper limb bud leads to deformities such as cleft hand or polydactyly, respectively. The zone of polarizing activity is responsible for radioulnar differentiation via secretion of the Sonic Hedgehog protein.

237. **What non-syndromic hand deformities have an autosomal dominant inheritance pattern?**

Cleft hand deformity, symphalangism (ankylosis or fusion of phalanges), triphalangeal thumb, brachydactyly, camptodactyly (flexion deformity of the proximal interphalangeal (PIP)), and postaxial polydactyly all have an autosomal dominant inheritance pattern. Syndactyly can be autosomal dominant or a sporadic mutation.

238. **What is the most common level for a transverse deficiency (congenital amputation)?**

The proximal forearm is the most common level for a transverse deficiency. The mid-carpal region is the second most common level and may include "digital nubbins" that are rudimentary, non-functional digits. If a prosthesis is to be used, fitting should occur by the time the child is crawling.

239. **What are longitudinal deficiencies?**

Longitudinal deficiencies are failure of formation abnormalities other than transverse deficiencies. They are named for the bone that is absent or short. Examples include phocomelia, radial and ulnar clubhand, and cleft hand.

CASE 6-17

You are consulted for a newborn boy who is in the neonatal intensive care unit because of a cardiac birth defect. He has a deformity of the left upper extremity in which his thumb is missing and his entire hand is turned 90° from the wrist. His forearm also has a curve to it. There are no abnormalities of the right upper extremity or bilateral lower extremities. You order a forearm x-ray to characterize the extent of bony deformity (Fig. 6.36).

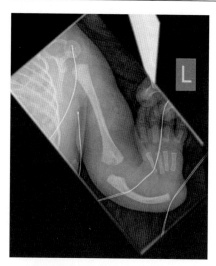

Figure 6.36. Child with radial club hand.

240. **What is radial clubhand?**

Radial clubhand, or radial longitudinal deficiency, refers to a failure of formation of the radial or preaxial aspect of the upper extremity, leaving a shortened or completely absent radius. Without the support of the distal radius, the hand deviates radially, giving an appearance similar to a clubfoot deformity of the lower extremity. The thumb is absent or hypoplastic in most cases of radial clubhand, even in the less severe types. The radial musculature does not develop normally, and neurovascular deficiencies or anomalies may be present. The ulna also develops a bowed morphology in more severe cases.

241. **What syndromes are commonly associated with radial clubhand?**
The most commonly associated syndromes include Fanconi anemia, Holt–Oram syndrome, thrombocytopenia-absent radius (TAR) syndrome, and VACTERL syndrome. Fanconi anemia is a severe pancytopenia that most often progresses to bone marrow failure requiring transplantation. Holt–Oram syndrome is a combination of cardiac and upper extremity congenital abnormalities. TAR syndrome may include cardiac deformities in addition to thrombocytopenia and absence of the radius. VACTERL syndrome includes Vertebral segmental defects, Anal atresia, Cardiac abnormalities, Tracheoesophageal fistula, Esophageal atresia, Renal abnormalities, and Limb agenesis. These syndromes can be life-threatening and their treatment should precede that of the limb deformity. All patients diagnosed with radial club hand must be tested with a complete blood count, renal ultrasound, and echocardiogram.

242. **How is radial clubhand treated?**
Stretching with bracing or casting may be enough to passively correct the radial clubhand if initiated early in infancy, though this does not address the thumb deficiency. Pollicization of another finger or toe may be performed at a later time. Surgical reconstruction for cases that do not respond to bracing or have a delayed presentation involves centralization or radialization of the hand on the ulna, sometimes with muscle transfers to replace the function of deficient muscle groups, and thumb reconstruction.

243. **How does ulnar clubhand differ from radial clubhand?**
In addition to the fact that the longitudinal deficiency exists on the ulnar, or postaxial, aspect of the extremity, ulnar clubhand has other important characteristics that contrast with radial clubhand. In ulnar deficiencies, the hand tends to be stable at the wrist (unlike radial clubhand), while the elbow is unstable. The associated anomalies of ulnar clubhand are almost purely musculoskeletal, whereas those of radial clubhand involve various other organ systems listed above. Ulnar deficiencies typically involve a partial absence of the ulna. Radial deficiencies more commonly have complete absence of the radius. Finally, hand abnormalities are more common in ulnar deficiencies, with up to 90% of patients having missing digits.

244. **What can be done to restore motion in a patient with ulnar clubhand and a dislocated radial head?**
When an ulnar clubhand is associated with radial head dislocation, extension of the elbow is blocked and function is further impeded. A potential solution is to perform osteotomies of the radius and ulna and fuse them into a single-bone forearm.

245. **What is cleft hand?**
Cleft hand is a congenital longitudinal deficiency characterized by absence of the central ray or rays (second, third, and/or fourth). It is also called a lobster claw deformity or ectrodactyly. The typical pattern has a deep V-shaped cleft in the center of the hand. The atypical pattern does not have the deep cleft and is more U-shaped with only a thumb and small finger present. Patients often have similar deformities involving the feet.

246. **How is cleft hand treated?**
Patients affected by cleft hand can often adapt to have a very functional hand. When function is lacking, surgical reconstruction is aimed at restoring pinch and grasp motions. This may involve closure of the cleft, contracture releases, tendon transfers, toe-to-hand transfers, or deepening of the palm for the atypical pattern.

247. **What is phocomelia? What drug has been implicated as a cause of phocomelia?**
Phocomelia describes a congenital abnormality in which there is an absence or hypoplasia of the humerus and/or forearm, leaving the hand in close proximity to the shoulder. The

term comes from the Greek word for "seal flipper." The hand itself is often deformed as well. Thalidomide, a drug used for treating pregnancy-related nausea in the 1950s, was implicated as a major cause of phocomelia in the early 1960s and was taken off the market in the US. While effective for other conditions unrelated to pregnancy, its use remains controversial today.

248. **What is syndactyly?**
Syndactyly is a congenital deformity of conjoined digits that results from a failure of differentiation. The degree of connection of the digits ranges from a simple skin bridge to fusion of one or more phalanges. It is the most common congenital hand abnormality (Fig. 6.37).

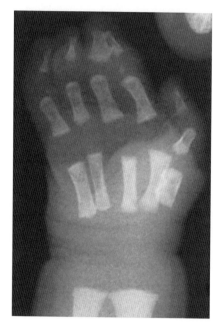

Figure 6.37. Complex syndactyly. Common bony elements are shared by involved fingers. (*From Jobe MT, Campbell's Operative Orthopaedics, pp. 3713–3794.e6. Copyright © 2013 by Mosby, Elsevier Inc.*)

249. **What fingers are most commonly involved in syndactyly?**
More than half of syndactyly cases involve the long and ring fingers.

250. **Poland syndrome includes syndactyly and what other congenital defect?**
In Poland syndrome, there is absence of the ipsilateral sternal head of the pectoralis major muscle. The syndactyly typically involves multiple fingers but is simple (skin or soft tissue bridges) and incomplete.

251. **What is Apert syndrome?**
Apert syndrome is a rare genetic syndrome characterized by multiple complex hand syndactylies and abnormal facies. The syndactylies create a spoon-shaped hand. These patients have a broad forehead, flat occiput, wide-set sloping eyes, and a prominent mandible. Mental retardation is also common in patients with Apert syndrome.

252. **What considerations are important in preparing for surgical separation of syndactyly?**
It is important to consider skin coverage and shared structures. Nerves, vessels, tendons, and fingernails may all be shared between the syndactylous digits. These may need to be divided so that the separated fingers do not become insensate, dysvascular, or

dysfunctional. Recreation of the web space can be particularly difficult to perform and will impact abduction of the fingers.

253. **What is polydactyly?**
Polydactyly is digit duplication. It may be preaxial (bifid thumb), postaxial (small finger duplication), or central. The duplication may occur at the metacarpal level or any of the phalanges. The tendons, muscles, neurovascular structures, and fingernails may or may not be duplicated. The collateral ligaments typically are not duplicated.

254. **Which digit should be removed in preaxial polydactyly?**
If one of the thumbs is more dominant or well-formed, this digit should be maintained. If they are structurally and functionally equal, the radial thumb should usually be removed to preserve the ulnar collateral ligament for pinch. For distal duplications, the central portion of each digit can be removed with fusion of the remaining portions (Bilhaut–Cloquet procedure).

255. **What demographic group is most affected by postaxial polydactyly?**
Postaxial polydactyly is common in the black population, occurring in approximately 1 in 300 births.

256. **What are the three types of postaxial polydactyly?**
Type I postaxial polydactyly involves only a rudimentary skin and soft-tissue tag. The practice of removing these with suture ligature at the base of the digit is discouraged due to the potential for significant hemorrhage. Type II involves a well-formed supernumary digit that should be surgically excised. Type III involves duplication of the entire ray, including the metacarpal.

257. **What is macrodactyly?**
Macrodactyly is congenital enlargement of a digit due to a localized deregulation of growth. It may occur as an enlargement that is present at birth and grows proportionally to the remaining digits (static macrodactyly), or a progressively enlarging digit that exceeds the normal growth of the remaining digits (progressive macrodactyly). Progressive macrodactyly frequently develops an angular deformity. The index finger is most commonly involved.

258. **What are the treatment options for macrodactyly?**
Debulking procedures can be done for progressive macrodacyly, and include removal of excessive soft tissues, and often epiphysiodesis of the involved bones. When a digit is to be debulked, a staged approach is utilized to reduce the risks of devascularization. Digital shortening procedures involve resecting portions of one or more phalanges to achieve a more normal length. Wedge osteotomies may be used to correct angular deformities. Recurrence is the most common complication of surgical treatment for macrodactyly, and surgical treatment may be followed by rebound growth as this is a biologic problem. Many patients ultimately require an amputation to control the disease process.

259. **What are the six types of hypoplastic thumbs?**
The six types of hypoplastic thumbs are absent thumb, short thumb, adducted thumb, abducted thumb, clasped thumb, and floating thumb. Absent thumb is usually associated with radial longitudinal deficiency and may be treated with pollicization of the index finger or recession of the index finger to allow for lateral pinch between the index and long fingers. A short thumb is one that does not reach the PIP joint of the index finger. It is often associated with a syndrome. An adducted thumb usually results from hypoplasia of the thenar muscles, and limits thumb opposition. An abducted thumb results from anomalous insertion of a radially-displaced flexor pollicus longus muscle into the extensor pollicus longus. Clasped thumb refers to a deformity of adduction and flexion of the thumb due to an imbalance in thumb flexors and extensors. The extensor pollicis longus and/or brevis may be absent altogether. Milder cases may respond to splinting, whereas more severe cases usually require muscle transfer. Floating thumb is a deformity caused by absence of the first metacarpal and sometimes the trapezium and scaphoid bones of the wrist, leaving a thumb that extends from the radial hand without any bony articulation. The floating thumb does not have any intrinsic or extrinsic muscle function. It is usually treated with amputation and pollicization of the index finger.

260. **Brachymetacarpia (shortening of the metacarpal) affects what type of hand function?**

    More than 1 cm of shortening of a metacarpal bone affects the normal arch created by the metacarpal bones, which weakens grip strength.

261. **What is camptodactyly?**

    Camptodactyly is a flexion deformity of the PIP joint that is often progressive. The small finger is most commonly involved. If serial casting or splinting fails, surgical intervention may be warranted for functionally limiting cases, though outcomes are unpredictable (Fig. 6.38).

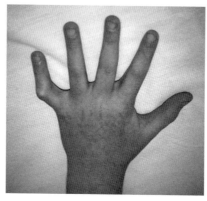

Figure 6.38. Campodactyly (flexion deformity of proximal interphalangeal joint) involving the little finger only. *(From Jobe MT: Campbell's Operative Orthopaedics, pp. 3713–3794.e6. Copyright © 2013 by Mosby, Elsevier Inc.)*

262. **What is clinodactyly?**

    Clinodactyly is an angular deformity of the digit in the radial or ulnar direction (coronal plane) distal to the metacarpophalangeal joint. Clinodactyly most often affects the small finger with a radial angulation. A delta phalanx is a common cause of clinically significant clinodactyly (Fig. 6.39).

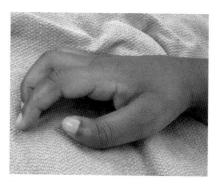

Figure 6.39. Clinodactyly of the thumb. *(From Carrigan RB: Nelson Textbook of Pediatrics, pp. 2383–2387.e1. Saunders, Copyright © 2011 Elsevier Inc.)*

263. **What is a delta phalanx?**

    A delta phalanx is an abnormally shaped phalanx that appears as a triangle on x-ray, though it is actually trapezoidal in shape. The epiphysis is J-shaped or C-shaped, influencing the progressive, abnormal growth of the phalanx. Delta phalanx usually occurs in association with other hand deformities.

264. **What are trigger digits?**
A trigger digit is a term used to describe abnormal gliding of the flexor tendon within its sheath. In adults, the tendon catches in a relatively stenotic region of the sheath, but can be actively or passively extended after it catches. In contrast, the congenital or pediatric trigger digit tends to present as a fixed flexion deformity of the digit. The cause of the abnormal gliding can be a thickened and narrowed section of the tendon sheath, an intratendinous nodule or ganglion cyst, chronic inflammation, or a combination of these.

265. **What digit is most commonly involved in congenital trigger digit?**
The thumb is most commonly involved in congenital trigger digit.

266. **What percentage of patients with congenital trigger digit has bilateral involvement?**
Twenty-five percent of patients with trigger digits have bilateral involvement.

267. **What is the most appropriate initial treatment for patients with congenital trigger digit who present in the first year of life?**
This group of patients deserves a trial of observation as spontaneous resolution of the trigger digit has been noted to occur in approximately 30% of such cases. Gentle manipulation and splinting may be attempted as well.

268. **If non-operative treatment is not successful, at what age should surgical intervention be considered?**
Cases that fail to resolve with non-operative management should be treated surgically before age 3 to prevent the development of flexion contractures.

269. **What structure is released in surgical treatment of trigger digit?**
The first annular pulley (A1) is released in trigger digit surgery. If tendon gliding is still abnormal after complete release of the A1 pulley, the A3 pulley should be inspected and released if it is a source of triggering.

270. **What is congenital constriction band syndrome?**
Congenital constriction band syndrome, also referred to as early amniotic rupture sequence or Streeter's dysplasia, is a condition involving superficial or deep circumferential skin creases around a limb or digit. These give the appearance of the tissue being strangulated by a tight band. It is thought to result from torn shreds of amniotic membrane that form around the limb in utero. The bands are usually transverse, and may cause a congenital amputation in the most severe cases. The digit or limb distal to the band may have chronic venous congestion or lymphedema.

271. **How is congenital constriction band syndrome treated?**
Deep creases that cause lymphedema, impaired circulation, or significant deformity should be surgically excised and closed via Z-plasty method to prevent scar contracture. Complete circumferential bands are often excised in two stages (half each time) to make sure that the limb will not be devascularized.

272. **What is a Madelung deformity?**
Madelung deformity is a deformity of the distal radius that results from an abnormality of the volar ulnar physis that results in a progressively worsening volar and ulnar tilt to the distal radius. While the true cause of Madelung deformity has not been established, there are multiple different processes that can lead to this appearance – trauma, skeletal dysplasias, and genetic syndromes (Fig. 6.40).

BRACHIAL PLEXUS PALSY

CASE 6-18

You are called to the newborn nursery to evaluate a 1-day-old baby girl for a suspected right arm injury. She was the result of a full-term pregnancy complicated by gestational diabetes of the mother. She was 10 lbs, 7oz at birth. The delivery itself was long but otherwise uncomplicated. The baby is holding her right arm close to her body with the elbow fully extended and the hand pronated. Passively, her range of motion is normal and seems to be painless. There is no tenderness to palpation over the clavicle or humerus, and she moves her left arm and both legs spontaneously.

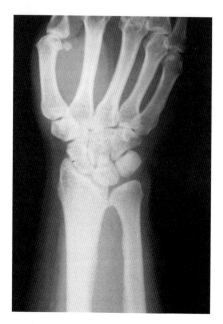

Figure 6.40. Radiographic appearance of Madelung deformity. Note abnormalities of radius, ulna, and carpal bones. (*From Jobe MT, Campbell's Operative Orthopaedics, pp. 3713–3794.e6. Copyright © 2013 by Mosby, Elsevier Inc.*)

273. **What is brachial plexus birth palsy?**
Brachial plexus birth palsy is a traction injury of the brachial plexus caused by complicated delivery of the infant during birth. It results in a varying degree of paralysis of the upper extremity, depending on the extent of the injury.

274. **What are the risk factors for brachial plexus birth palsy?**
Risk factors for brachial plexus birth palsy include high birth weight, difficult delivery (e.g., shoulder dystocia, breech positioning), prolonged labor, forceps delivery, and a maternal history of brachial plexus birth palsy with prior births.

275. **What are the three general categories of nerve lesions?**
The three categories of nerve lesions are neurapraxia, axonotmesis, and neurotmesis. Neurapraxia is paralysis of the nerve without peripheral degeneration. Axonotmesis involves damage to the nerve with peripheral degeneration, but regeneration is possible. Neurotmesis describes damage to the nerve itself and the supporting tissues in which continuity is lost, so full recovery is not possible. This is known as the Seddon classification.

276. **What are the four types of brachial plexus birth palsy according to the Narakas classification?**
Type I describes upper plexus (C5–C6) injuries, known as an Erb's palsy. In the classic form, the child's shoulder is adducted and internally rotated, the elbow extended, the forearm pronated, and wrist flexed ("waiter's tip" position). Type II injuries affect the C5–C7 roots. Type III injuries involve the entire brachial plexus (C5–T1) and leave a paralyzed, insensate upper extremity. Type IV palsies involve the lower plexus (C8–T1) and are known as Klumpke palsies. These patients have elbow flexion, wrist extension and supination deformities from the unopposed action of the biceps and wrist extensors.

277. **What type of brachial plexus birth palsy has the best prognosis? What type has the worst prognosis?**
Type I injuries have the best prognosis. Type III injuries have the worst prognosis. Overall, spontaneous recovery of brachial plexus birth palsy may be seen in as many as 90% of cases.

278. **What is Horner's syndrome?**

The features of Horner's syndrome are ptosis (eyelid drooping), miosis (pupillary constriction), and anhydrosis (decreased perspiration), which occur on the same side of the face as the lesion. The nerve lesion that causes Horner's syndrome is the T1 cervical sympathetic chain. The presence of a Horner's syndrome in association with brachial plexus birth palsy portends a worse prognosis.

279. **What other diagnoses should be considered in the setting of apparent paralysis of the upper extremity in a newborn?**

Clavicle fractures, proximal humerus or humeral shaft fractures, and septic shoulder can cause a pseudoparalysis of the upper extremity and should be considered as alternative diagnoses.

280. **What is the natural history of persistent brachial plexus birth palsy?**

In cases that do not spontaneously resolve, persistent muscle imbalance results in progressive contractures. Weak shoulder external rotators and abductors are overpowered by the unaffected internal rotators and adductors. The contracture may result in progressive posterior subluxation, glenoid erosion, and even dislocation of the humerus over time. These children tend to have difficulty bringing the hand to the face or over the head.

281. **Function of which muscle is used to determine which cases can be managed non-operatively and which cases should undergo surgical exploration?**

The return of biceps function against gravity by 3 months of age suggests an excellent prognosis.

282. **What treatments are available for brachial plexus birth palsy?**

In the early stages, a stretching regimen is crucial to minimize the development of contractures. Occupational therapy and bracing, especially at night, can be particularly helpful. Surgical strategies are evolving, and the timing and specifics continue to be debated. Options for surgery focusing on enhancing neurologic recovery of function include exploration of the brachial plexus with microsurgical repair or grafting, or nerve transfers. With regard to secondary musculoskeletal deformities, a combination of soft-tissue releases and tendon transfers, with or without osteotomy, may help to restore motion and improve function.

HAND INJURIES

CASE 6-19

A 12-year-old boy presents to the Emergency Department with his father with a swollen, painful left hand after his dirt bike fell over onto his hand. He felt an intense pain when his hand was crushed, and it swelled almost immediately. Now the hand is throbbing around the knuckles of his small and ring fingers. The hand is moderately swollen, especially on the ulnar side, and some bruising is evident. He has exquisite tenderness to palpation along the ulnar hand and the small and ring fingers. X-rays of his hand are shown in Figure 6.41.

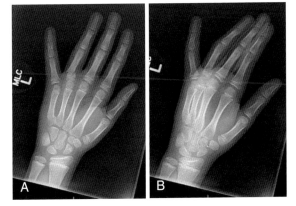

Figure 6.41. X-rays of the left hand show a Salter–Harris II fracture of the proximal phalanx of the small finger, a transverse shaft fracture of the proximal phalanx of the ring finger, and a 5th metacarpal base fracture.

283. **What difference does the thick periosteum of children's bones make in relation to hand fractures?**

The thick periosteum can act as a sleeve or hinge to facilitate reduction of fractures that would otherwise be unstable. However, it can also make fracture reduction more difficult if the periosteum is torn and becomes incarcerated in the fracture site.

284. **Repeated attempts at reduction of finger fractures risk what complication?**

Iatrogenic injury to the physis is a risk that increases with multiple attempts at reduction of finger fractures, particularly in fractures that are more than 5 days old.

285. **Small lacerations over joints in the hand should be presumed to be caused by what mechanism?**

These lacerations should be treated as bite wounds unless proven otherwise. They require thorough irrigation and treatment with antibiotics active against oral flora.

286. **What is the "wrinkle test?"**

Detecting nerve injuries in children can be difficult because it requires a high level of cooperation. The "wrinkle test" is an alternative to the standard two-point discrimination. The child's hand is submerged in sterile water for 5 minutes. Denervated digits will not exhibit the typical wrinkling of the volar fingertip.

287. **How are pediatric nailbed injuries treated?**

Pediatric nailbed injuries are treated very similarly to adult nailbed injuries. Under appropriate anesthesia, the nail is removed, the wound is irrigated, the nailbed is repaired with absorbable suture (typically 5-0 or smaller chromic gut suture), and the removed nail is placed back under the nailfold to protect the nailbed and germinal matrix. Children are often placed in a cast that covers the entire hand and goes above the elbow, known as a "mitten cast," to prevent them from removing the dressing while the wound is healing.

288. **Where are the physes located in the phalanges? Where are the physes located in the metacarpals?**

The physes are located in the proximal end of the phalanges. The metacarpal physes are located distally, except in the thumb, where the physis is located proximally.

289. **Fractures in the pediatric hand most often fall into which Salter–Harris type?**

Salter–Harris type II fractures are most common in the pediatric hand. The proximal phalanx is the most frequently fractured bone in children. At the interphalangeal joints, the collateral ligaments insert into both the phalangeal epiphysis and metaphysis. At the metacarpophalangeal joints, the collateral ligaments insert almost exclusively into the epiphysis, so Salter–Harris type III fractures are more common.

290. **Where do the deep flexor tendons insert? Where do the extensor tendons insert?**

The deep flexor tendons insert into the epiphysis and metaphysis of the volar distal phalanx. The extensor tendons insert into the epiphysis of the dorsal distal phalanx. Therefore, distal phalanx Salter–Harris I fractures through the physis result in an apex–dorsal angulation due to volar displacement of the distal fragment.

291. **A Salter–Harris III fracture of the distal phalanx is equivalent to what type of adult fracture?**

A Salter–Harris III fracture of the distal phalanx mimics an adult mallet finger. The epiphyseal fragment is displaced dorsally by the extensor tendon, and the rest of the distal phalanx is pulled volarly by the unopposed flexor tendon.

292. **What is a Seymour's fracture?**

A Seymour's fracture occurs at the physis of the distal phalanx, and is associated with a nail bed laceration. These are technically open fractures, and the germinal matrix or other soft tissue may be interposed in the fracture site. Treatment should consist of irrigation and débridement, removal of any interposed tissue, fracture fixation, and nailbed repair.

293. **What are the indications for surgical intervention of phalangeal head fractures?**
Articular surface displacement of more than 1–2 mm and angulation of more than 5–10°
are indications for surgery.

294. **What is the typical alignment of a phalangeal shaft fracture distal to the insertion of the flexor digitorum superficialis?**
These fractures typically have an apex–volar angulation due to the pull of the extensor
mechanism on the distal fragments.

295. **What is an "extra-octave" fracture?**
The "extra-octave" fracture describes a physeal fracture of the 5th proximal phalanx. The
angulation of the fracture gives the appearance that the small finger could abduct further
to reach the next octave on a piano.

296. **What are the acceptable amounts of angulation in pediatric metacarpal fractures?**
In fractures at the metacarpal neck, up to 15° of angulation for the 2nd and 3rd
metacarpals and up to 45° of angulation for the 4th and 5th metacarpals is acceptable. For
fractures of the metacarpal shaft, dorsal angulation less than 10° for the 2nd and 3rd
metacarpals and less than 20° for the 4th and 5th metacarpals is acceptable. For 1st
metacarpal base fractures distal to the physis, up to 30° of angulation can be accepted in
young children. Any degree of rotational deformity is unacceptable, because no significant
remodeling can be expected.

297. **How is rotational deformity of the fingers assessed?**
Rotational deformities are easiest to see with the fingers flexed as if making a loose fist.
Disruptions in the alignment or normal cascade tend to be pronounced. In an uncooperative
child, gentle wrist extension facilitates this gesture due to the tenodesis effect.

298. **In what position are metacarpal fractures typically casted?**
The intrinsic-plus position, with the metacarpophalangeal joints flexed to 70–90° and the
interphalangeal joints fully extended, is the safest cast position to prevent extension
contractures of the metacarpophalangeal joints. Fractures of the 1st metacarpal are casted
in a thumb spica cast.

NEUROMUSCULAR DISORDERS IN PEDIATRIC ORTHOPEDICS

CEREBRAL PALSY

CASE 6-20

A 10-year-old child comes to your office in a wheelchair, and he has a history of anoxia as an infant.

299. **What is the definition of cerebral palsy?**
Cerebral palsy (CP) is a non-progressive disorder of movement and posture resulting from
injury to the immature brain. By definition the onset of CP must be prior to 2 years of age.
CP is a *non-progressive* neurologic disturbance; however, musculoskeletal problems may
progress throughout growth and development. Patients are most often diagnosed by
documenting a delay in neurologic maturation or motor development, identifying evidence
of central nervous system involvement (hyperreflexia, clonus), and ruling out other causes.

300. **What are the different types of neurologic disorders observed in CP?**
The physiologic classification of CP includes several major types. The majority of
patients have more than one physiologic type identified on close examination ("mixed"),
but usually one will predominate. *Spasticity* ("pyramidal" involvement) describes an
increase in muscle tone which varies with the rate of stretching and may lead to the
development and progression of musculoskeletal deformities. A variety of terms have
been used to characterize extrapyramidal involvement, which is often related to damage to
the basal ganglia and cerebellum. *Athetosis* represents slow, writhing movements which can
be observed in the fingers, resulting from damage to the basal ganglia. *Ataxic* is
characterized by wide-based gait, and difficulty with coordination, typically due to
problems with the cerebellum or spinocerebellar system. *Mixed* contains elements of the
above three.

CASE 6-20 continued

You notice that the child has total body involvement. His mother states that the child is unable to ambulate and is incontinent. He has never been able to sit independently. He is fed through a gastrostomy tube. His arms are in a flexion posture at the elbow and wrist. The child can look at you and is interactive.

301. **What is the geographic classification in CP?**
     Quadriplegic: Total body involvement, wheelchair bound
     Diplegic: Lower extremities involved more than upper extremities, cognitively usually closer to normal
     Hemiplegic: Arms more than legs on one side of the body
     Triplegic: Both legs and one arm.

302. **What is the classification system for function that is commonly used for patients with CP?**
     The *Gross Motor Function Classification system* is the most commonly used. The definition of each level varies by the age of the child. There are five levels ranked from 1 to 5 with higher levels representing higher levels of neurologic involvement and disability. At maturity, GMCS 5 children are totally dependent for mobility, even with a power wheelchair. GMCS 4 children are generally able to independently locomote with a power wheelchair. GMCS 3 children are able to ambulate with a device short distances, and can often maneuver a manual wheelchair independently. They may require transport for long distances or uneven surfaces. GMCS 2 children are able to ambulate without a device, though they may require assistance or a rail for steps. They may have trouble in crowds or uneven surfaces. GMCS 1 children are essentially normal children, though they have difficulty with coordination, speed, and balance.

303. **What are some non-orthopedic surgical treatment options for spastic CP?**
     Physical and occupational therapies are commonly used in CP to promote neuromuscular development, to treat or prevent muscle contractures, to strengthen muscles, and to help with training for activities of daily living. A variety of treatment options are available for spasticity, with the goal of reducing or eliminating dynamic muscle contractures and preventing the development of muscle contractures. Intramuscular injection with:
     Botulinum toxin A (Botox) results in a reversible denervation at the neuromuscular junction by competitively inhibiting acetylcholine at presynaptic receptors. The effects last for 3–8 months after which reinnervation is observed.
     Oral Baclofen (GABA agonist) may reduce muscle tone, but the dosages required will often result in sedation which may interfere with daily activities and school. In non-ambulators, an intrathecal baclofen pump may be implanted to reduce spasticity, without the side effect of sedation.
     Intrathecal baclofen may unmask muscle weakness and have a negative impact on ambulation. Baclofen pumps are rarely appropriate in the ambulatory population.
     Rhizotomy involves selective or nonselective resection of posterior sensory rootlets, resulting in a permanent reduction in spasticity. The indications for this procedure are narrow, and it is typically performed in diplegic children (4–8 years) who have adequate underlying muscle strength, adequate selective motor control, and minimal soft-tissue contractures or bony deformities. Rhizotomy has been unsuccessful in non-ambulatory patients and those with extrapyramidal disease.

CASE 6-20 continued

The mother is curious about what types of problems she should expect from an orthopedic standpoint, and what can be done about them.

304. **Describe the spine problems encountered in CP.**
     Scoliosis is encountered more commonly in non-ambulatory patients with quadriplegic CP (Fig. 6.42), and results from global weakness of the trunk, often associated with asymmetric spasticity. Once curves progress beyond 40–60°, they will continue to progress

even after skeletal maturity, resulting in loss of sitting balance and hinderance of pulmonary and gastrointestinal function. These curves are usually in the thoracolumbar or lumbar region, and are associated with pelvic obliquity. Bracing can help to achieve positional curve control, and may slow down progression, but will not alter the natural history of scoliosis. Spinal fusion from the upper thoracic spine (T2) to the pelvis with segmental instrumentation is most commonly performed. While the risks are significant, especially infection and medical complications, the majority of patients benefit with regards to quality of life (Fig. 6.43).

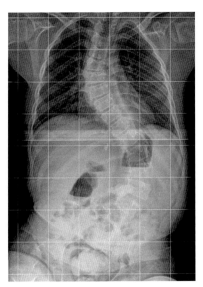

Figure 6.42. Spinal deformity with pelvic obliquity in cerebral palsy.

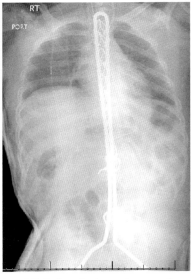

Figure 6.43. Radiograph of unit rod construct for neuromuscular scoliosis.

305. Describe the hip problems encountered in CP.

Neuromuscular hip dysplasia develops gradually in response to persistent spasticity and muscle imbalance, as the muscles of flexion and adduction overpower the muscles of extension and abduction. An adduction contracture develops, and then the femoral head is gradually displaced laterally and proximally. This displacement also contributes to a progressive dysplasia of the acetabulum, which is typically deficient globally or posterolaterally. Some hips will progress to complete dislocation, 50% of which may become chronically painful. Abnormalities in proximal femoral morphology include persistent fetal anteversion (normally 40° at birth and remodels to 15° in adults) and sometimes a proximal femoral valgus deformity. The neck shaft angle is normally 135°, but in patients with cerebral palsy it ranges from normal to 150° or more of valgus. The neck-shaft angle may be difficult to assess on standard images due to the excessive anteversion, so either an anteroposterior radiograph in maximum internal rotation or an exam under fluoroscopy at the time of surgery, is required to obtain a true anteroposterior view.

306. What are the stages of hip instability in CP and how are they typically measured? What is the treatment?

Patients progress from normally stable hips to a *hip at risk*, which may be defined clinically as less than 45° of passive abduction assessed with the hips in full extension and defined radiographically as an increase in the Reimer's migration percentage (uncovering of the femoral head by the acetabulum) beyond approximately 30%. Preventive soft-tissue releases are considered in patients with these at risk signs, and the best results are achieved in patients with lesser overall degrees of neurologic involvement and no subluxation on radiographs. The soft tissue release involves the adductor longus, the gracilis, and fibers of the adductor brevis. Some authors also release the psoas tendon. A neurectomy of the anterior branch of the obturator nerve should be avoided due to the risk of a disabling extension and abduction contracture. This preventative surgery has been shown to be effective in eliminating the need for bony surgery in 25–60% of patients at midterm follow-up.

When the hip has progressed to subluxation, the migration percentage is more than 30%, Shenton's line may be broken, and there may be signs of acetabular dysplasia (Fig. 6.44). Hips with a migration percentage above 66% will all become dislocated over time, and those with a migration percentage between 40% and 66% have approximately a 25% chance of being progressive. At this stage in which the hip is significantly subluxated, surgical treatment involves a soft-tissue release, proximal femoral varus derotational osteotomy, and often a volume reducing pelvic osteotomy (Fig. 6.45). An open reduction may need to be performed when the hip is completely dislocated. In the *chronically painful* and dislocated hip, resection of the femoral head and neck, coupled with a valgus osteotomy, may be necessary to relieve pain.

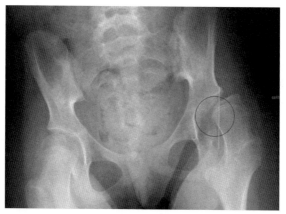

Figure 6.44. CP hip subluxation showing a migration percentage greater than 70%. Note the black circle is where the hip would be reduced, the white line is perpendicular to the sourcil.

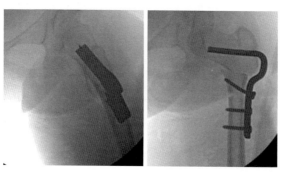

Figure 6.45. Intraop pictures of a varus derotational osteotomy (VDRO), showing reduction of the femoral head.

307. **What are the two most common foot deformities in CP? How are they treated?**
Equinovarus foot is due to muscle imbalance and spasticity of the tibialis anterior or posterior (or both) and gastrocsoleus. It is characterized by inversion of the foot during the gait cycle, and the patient lands on the outer border of the foot which rolls inward. In early stages, when the deformity is relatively flexible, treatment may include a recession of the gastrocsoleus along with a split tendon transfer. The split transfer helps to balance the forces, as transfer of an entire tendon may result in production of the opposite deformity. A dynamic EMG test is often utilized to determine which muscle is creating the deformity. Options include transfer of tibialis posterior to the peroneus brevis, and/or transfer of the tibialis anterior to the cuboid. Rigid deformities require soft-tissue releases and/or osteotomies to restore mobility prior to tendon transfer. Severe deformities in older patients are treated by bony osteotomies or triple arthrodesis.

Planovalgus is the opposite problem. The foot appears as a rigid flatfoot. The hindfoot is in valgus, the peroneal muscles are often contracted and also contribute dynamically to the deformity, and the subtalar joint is permanently unlocked resulting in poor propulsion at the start of the gait cycle. This problem may be associated with external tibial torsion. Flexible deformities are treated by gastrocsoleus recession and lateral column lengthening (calcaneal osteotomy with insertion of a bone graft). Severe and rigid deformities are treated by triple arthrodesis, especially in older adolescents.

CASE 6-21

A 15-year-old spastic diplegic patient comes to your office. He had numerous orthopedic surgeries as a child. He is a community ambulator, but recently has begun to have more difficulty walking. You watch him walk, and notice that his knees remain bent throughout the gait cycle. He complains of anterior knee pain and has popliteal angles of 70°. His lateral x-ray is shown in Figure 6.46.

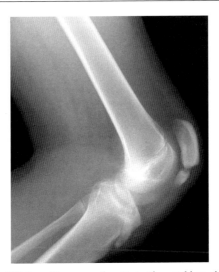

Figure 6.46. Lateral knee x-ray of a patient with a painful crouch gait.

308. **Name the common gait disorders in CP and their treatment.**
a. *Toe walking*: This gait pattern can be caused by spasticity of the gastrocsoleus and often contracture of the muscle. Treatment includes botulinum toxin injection for spasticity, stretching and/or serial casting, use of an ankle-foot orthosis (if no significant contracture), and surgical lengthening. Surgical treatment consists of selective gastrocnemius recession rather than a percutaneous non-selective technique to reduce the risk of overlengthening and iatrogenic calcaneus deformity.

b. *Crouched gait*: This gait pattern is generally mutifactorial, and related to both bone and soft-tissue problems. Soft-tissue contractures include flexion deformity of the hip and/or knee, and equinus contracture at the ankle. Bony lever arm problems may be contributory factors, usually internal femoral torsion and external tibial torsion. Crouched gait may be secondary to soleus insufficiency, usually following surgical lengthening of the tendo Achilles. Surgical treatment consists of multilevel soft-tissue and bony procedures (Figs 6.46 and 6.47).

c. *Stiff knee gait*: This gait pattern is characterized by inadequate knee flexion during swing phase and is due to inappropriate activity of the rectus femoris during swing phase. Treatment involves either removing a section of rectus femoris or transferring it to the sartorius, gracilis, or semitendinosus.

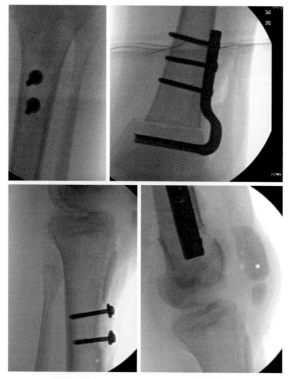

Figure 6.47. Intraoperative fluoroscopy of single event multilevel surgery (SEMLS) performed for adolescent crouch gait. This patient underwent a distal femoral osteotomy and patellar ligament advancement.

309. **What are the upper extremity problems found in CP, how are they treated?**
Treatment of upper extremity problems in CP is largely dependent on the function of the patient. If the patient has severe involvement and the hand is functionless, then surgical releases may be considered to improve hygiene. In contrast, for the hemiplegic patient who exhibits some degree of function and adequate rehabilitation potential, surgical treatment is directed towards improving function. Common contractures include elbow flexion, forearm pronation, wrist and finger flexion, and thumb adduction. Non-operative treatment includes stretching, splinting, and botulinum toxin injection to address spasticity. Botulinum toxin injections often help to predict the response to selected

surgical procedures. Surgical treatment usually includes fractional lengthening of muscles or tendon transfers such as flexor superficialis to profundus and FCU to ECRB.

SPINA BIFIDA (MYELOMENINGOCELE)

CASE 6-22

Your distraught friend calls you on the phone. Her infant has been diagnosed with spina bifida at the L4 level. She knows that you are on a pediatric rotation, and would like some advice and expert help.

310. **What is myelomeningocele? What are the orthopedic manifestations? What are the common medical issues involved?**
Myelomeningocele or spina bifida is failure of closure of the *neural tube* during development. This entity may be due to *folate deficiency* during pregnancy, hence many cases are preventable. Folate supplementation during pregnancy has significantly reduced the number of infants born with this problem. Spina bifida is truly a central nervous system disease, and all patients have a Chiari II malformation, most have hydrocephalus (many require shunting), and many will have coexisting intraspinal anomalies and tethering of the spinal cord. The orthopedic manifestations are secondary and are often compounded by the effects of growth and development. Orthopedic problems which result involve the feet, knees, hips, and spine. Additionally, these patients have a high rate of *latex allergy* which can result in anaphylaxis, so latex allergy is assumed in spina bifida. A rapid decline in function can indicate tethering of the cord with normal growth and should be imaged and treated urgently. Fractures can often be mistaken for infection/cellulitis.

311. **What are the functional levels of the lower extremity in spina bifida?**
S1–4: Normal ambulatory – has bowel and bladder dysfunction
L5: Community ambulatory – has intact toe dorsiflexion, hip extension, and hip abduction
L4: Household ambulatory – has intact quadriceps, ankle dorsiflexors and inverters
L3: Transfers plus limited household ambulatory – has intact hip flexors and hip adductors (high rate of dislocation because of unbalanced flexors and adductors)
L2 and above: non-ambulator.

312. **Describe the scoliosis in spina bifida.**
Scoliosis may result from co-existing congenital vertebral anomalies, or progressive spinal collapse due to muscle weakness or imbalance. Scoliosis is more prevalent with higher level defects. If the scoliosis begins to progress rapidly, a neurologic etiology such as shunt malfunction, tethered cord, or Chiari malformation/syrinx must be ruled out. Bracing will not impact the natural history, but may be considered to improve sitting balance and slow progression of the curve. Spinal instrumentation and fusion is considered for progressive and symptomatic curves beyond 40–60°, although complications are frequent, especially wound infection (10–15%) and pseudarthrosis. Many surgeons will do an antero-posterior fusion in these children, and non-ambulatory patients must be fused at the pelvis. Plastic surgery may be consulted to assist with soft-tissue coverage. Similarly, a progressive kyphosis (congenital or neuromuscular) can occur and in selected cases surgical stabilization is recommended.

313. **What is the most common level for hip disorder in myelodysplasia? What is the treatment?**
L3 level is the most common level of deficit in children with myelodysplasia. This is primarily due to unopposed hip flexion and adduction causing progressive subluxation and dislocation. The treatment is largely non-operative. Procedures to reduce and contain the hip (pelvic and femoral osteotomies) are generally only considered for patients with *active quadriceps* function (L4 and below) and unilateral disease, owing to the high risk of complications such as recurrent subluxation or dislocation and stiffness. These patients may also develop hip flexion and abduction contractures that may lead to sitting difficulties. One can consider an *Ober–Yount* procedure, which is proximal and distal division of the tensor fascia lata.

314. **What are common knee problems in spina bifida, and how are they addressed?**
Weak quadriceps may be addressed with orthotics (knee-ankle-foot orthosis, or KAFO).
Flexion or extension contractures may be treated with physical therapy, serial casting,
soft-tissue release or lengthening (including posterior capsule), or by osteotomy.

315. **What are some common foot problems with spina bifida? What are the treatments?**
Spina bifida is commonly associated with a clubfoot or congenital vertical talus (less
common), which is typically rigid and less likely to respond to casting or to the minimally
invasive Ponseti method. While casting is still the initial treatment of choice, care must
be taken to minimize the risks of pressure sores as the feet are insensate. Many patients
will require surgical soft-tissue releases with or without osteotomies to achieve a
plantigrade foot to facilitate bracing. These patients can also develop *calcaneus
(dorsiflexion) deformity (L5)* due to a strong tibialis anterior that is unopposed by a
paralyzed gastrocsoleus. This usually requires release of the tibialis anterior with or without
a calcaneal osteotomy. Arthrodesis is avoided because it is often complicated by pressure
sores and infection. Retaining mobility helps to distribute stresses and limit the risks of
these skin complications. Many ambulatory patients will require an amputation by their
fourth decade for skin complications or chronic osteomyelitis.

CHARCOT–MARIE–TOOTH

316. **What is Charcot–Marie–Tooth (CMT)? What are the causes? Which muscles are involved?**
CMT is an autosomal dominant defect in *peripheral myelin protein 22*. It is a Hereditary
Sensory Motor Neuropathy (HSMN) type I (type II generally occurs in adults). The
disorder affects the *tibialis anterior, peroneus brevis*, intrinsic muscles of the hands and feet,
and sometimes the peroneus longus. The most common manifestations of this disease are
pes cavovarus and hammer toes, though it has been associated with scoliosis and hip
dysplasia as well.

317. **What is the pathophysiology of the deformity in CMT?**
The muscle imbalance between the tibialis anterior (weak) and the peroneus longus
(strong) results in forefoot valgus, or *plantarflexion of the first ray*. The soft tissues on the
plantar surface of the foot become contracted, resulting in a fixed cavus deformity.
Hindfoot varus develops to compensate for the forefoot deformity, so that the foot stays flat
on the ground. This hindfoot deformity is initially flexible, but becomes rigid over time
(Fig. 6.48).

318. **What is the surgical treatment of foot disorders in CMT?**
Physical therapy is initially recommended. Most patients benefit from the use of an
ankle–foot orthosis. Surgical intervention is commonly required to make the feet
braceable. Flexible deformities are treated by soft-tissue release (plantar fascia) and transfer
of the tibialis posterior tendon to the dorsum of the foot, sometimes combined with a
Jones transfer (EHL to metatarsal neck). More rigid deformities will also require bony
realignment, usually a dorsiflexion osteotomy of the medial cuneiform or first metatarsal to
correct the plantarflexion of the 1st ray, and sometimes a calcaneal osteotomy (valgus
producing or lateral slide) for the hindfoot varus. The disease is marked by gradual
progression of weakness, so recurrence of deformities is common, and many adults
ultimately require a triple arthrodesis (hind foot fusion between the talus, the calcaneus,
and the cuboid) to maintain adequate alignment.

OTHER NEUROMUSCULAR DISORDERS

319. **What are the orthopedic and medical disorders associated with Friedrich's ataxia?**
Friedrich's ataxia is an autosomal recessive disorder involving the *frataxin* gene, which is
involved in iron metabolism. The most devastating condition associated with Friedrich's

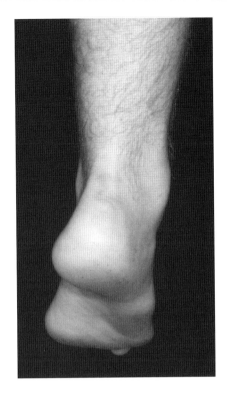

Figure 6.48. 18-year-old man with Charcot–Marie–Tooth disease with fixed hindfoot varus, marked forefoot equinus, plantar flexed first ray, forefoot pronation during weight bearing, tight plantar fascia, and contracted Achilles tendon but no palpable contraction of peroneus longus. (*From Richardson EG: Campbell's Operative Orthopaedics, pp. 4079–4116.e2. Copyright © 2013 by Mosby, Elsevier Inc.*)

ataxia is a *cardiomyopathy*, which results in premature death in middle age. Orthopedic complications include a cavus foot, and scoliosis. The *spinocerebellar* system is heavily involved, and thus patients present with a wide-based, clumsy gait. Many patients will become non-ambulatory depending on the severity of disease. The cavus foot is rigid and should be treated early with soft tissue and bony procedures. Progressive scoliotic deformities are treated with spinal instrumentation and fusion.

320. **What is the etiology of spinal muscular atrophy (SMA), what are the orthopedic manifestations?**
Spinal muscular atrophy is caused by loss of alpha-motor neurons in the anterior horn of the spinal cord. It is autosomal recessive and related to cell apoptosis mechanisms. Common orthopedic problems related to SMA are scoliosis and hip subluxation. *Deep tendon reflexes are absent* which is a distinguishing physical exam finding from Duchenne muscular dystrophy. Muscle biopsy or DNA analysis can provide a diagnosis. Treatment of hip subluxation or dislocation is non-operative, as children with flaccid paralysis are less prone to the development of fixed contractures and also tend to have minimal symptoms (pain, sitting imbalance) in comparison with those who have spastic hip disease. Recurrence is common after surgical treatment for hip instability. Operative management is favored for spinal disorders. Bracing may be considered, but may add to pulmonary impairment by restricting expansion of the chest wall. A posterior spinal fusion is the definitive treatment for progressive curvatures, but should be delayed until the lungs have matured and trunk height has ideally been maximized. Early onset scoliosis is sometimes treated by growing rods or vertical expandable prosthetic titanium rib (VEPTR), both of which achieve and maintain some correction while allowing for further growth of the thorax. They require regular lengthening and occasional revision of the implants as the patient grows.

321. **What is the etiology of Duchenne muscular dystrophy? Becker's? How are they diagnosed?**

Duchenne muscular dystrophy (DMD) is characterized by progressive muscle weakness which is most pronounced in proximal muscle groups. Children will rise up from the floor by walking their hands up their legs and thighs to compensate for proximal lower extremity weakness (*Gower's sign*). Patients are typically delayed in achieving independent ambulation until approximately 18 months, and initially begin to walk with a normal heel–toe gait but then develop toe walking from contracture of the Achilles tendon. Patients have normal deep tendon reflexes, and typically have pseudohypertrophy of the calf muscles. Muscle tissue is gradually replaced by fibrous tissue. Duchenne and Becker's muscular dystrophy are both X-linked recessive. Duchenne muscular dystrophy is associated with an absent *dystrophin* protein and is more severe than Becker's which is associated with an abnormal dystrophin. These diseases were traditionally diagnosed by muscle biopsy; however, there are now laboratory tests which allow the diagnosis to be established.

322. **What are the treatment goals for DMD?**

The prognosis for Duchenne muscular dystrophy is poor and most patients succumb to the disease in the 3rd decade due to respiratory problems. Patients usually lose the ability to ambulate in late childhood, although treatment with steroids has been shown to prolong ambulation and delay the development of scoliosis. All children will require bracing (ankle–foot orthosis) for ambulation, and in some cases, tendon lengthenings and transfers are performed with the goal of prolonging ambulation. Flexion and abduction contractures at the hip may be treated by soft-tissue release in the rare case that these interfere with sitting or wheelchair use. Progressive and rigid equinovarus deformities may require soft-tissue releases to facilitate shoe wear.

323. **What are the treatment principles of scoliosis in DMD?**

Scoliosis is seen in more than 90% of patients, and the natural history is rapid progression with a negative impact on sitting balance and pulmonary function. As a result, an instrumented posterior spinal fusion is offered as soon as progression is documented, typically when curvatures are in the range of 20–30°. The procedure is much safer from a medical perspective when done early, before the predictable decline in cardiopulmonary function has been observed.

PEDIATRIC HIP DISORDERS

DEVELOPMENTAL DYSPLASIA OF THE HIP (DDH)

CASE 6-23

The parents of a newborn bring her to your office for an examination. They are concerned because their pediatrician heard a "click" when examining their daughter's hips.

---

324. **What is DDH?**

DDH is the most common hip disorder in children. The term describes a spectrum of abnormalities, from neonatal instability (subluxation or dislocation) to acetabular dysplasia (flattening or underdevelopment of the acetabulum).

325. **What is the incidence of DDH?**

The incidence is approximately 1 per 100 births. Frank dislocation is approximately 10 times less common.

326. **What are risk factors for DDH?**

While family history and breech presentation are the most important factors, others include female gender, first born, and oligohydramnios. DDH is also associated with torticollis and metatarsus adductus, as well as other significant musculoskeletal abnormalities.

327. **How is DDH detected on exam?**

In neonates the problem is usually instability, often associated with ligamentous hyperlaxity. The physical examination centers on the Ortolani and Barlow maneuvers.

Both are performed with the child supine. The Barlow maneuver attempts to dislocate a hip that is reduced; the hip is flexed and adducted, and posterior pressure is exerted in an attempt to push the hip out of joint. A Barlow positive involves feeling the femoral head clunk out of the acetabulum.

The Ortolani maneuver attempts to reduce a hip that is dislocated. The hip is abducted and the examiner elevates the trochanter with several fingers while cupping the knee in the same hand. A hip that is dislocated will be pushed back into the joint, causing a palpable "clunk" of reduction (positive Ortolani sign) (Fig. 6.49).

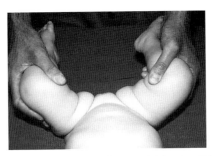

Figure 6.49. Ortolani maneuver for routine screening of congenital dislocation of hip. Examiner gently stabilizes infant's left hip and lower extremity and places left hand round right thigh and index and middle fingers over greater trochanter. (*From Kelly DM, Campbell's Operative Orthopaedics, pp. 1079–1118.e4. Copyright © 2013 by Mosby, an imprint of Elsevier Inc.*)

328. What imaging is used to evaluate DDH?

Ultrasound is the preferred imaging modality during the first few months of life, and plain radiographs are usefully once the ossific nuclei have formed, typically from 4 to 6 months of age. The ultrasound can be used to perform a static examination of the hips to assess anatomy, and a dynamic examination to assess stability. Two angles are relevant in the static exam. The alpha angle reflects the depth of the acetabulum, and is the angle subtended by a line through the iliac bone and tangential to the acetabular roof. It should be greater than 60° at 4–6 weeks. The beta angle is subtended by a line through the labrum that intersects a line through the iliac bone, and indirectly represents the position of the femoral head. It should be less than 55°. The dynamic exam assesses the stability of the hip with stress (Fig. 6.50A and B). Plain radiographs are utilized in older infants and children, and variables to assess include the size and symmetry of the ossific nuclei, Shenton's line, and the acetabular index.

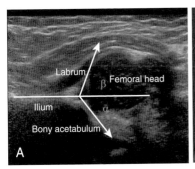
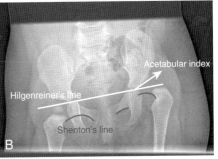

Figure 6.50. (A and B) Ultrasound and antero-posterior pelvis radiograph showing developmental dysplasia of the hip.

329. **How is DDH treated in a newborn?**

DDH may be treated in a Pavlik harness in patients up to 6 months of age, and this device actively positions the hip in flexion, while avoiding adduction. The child is kept in the harness until ultrasound parameters normalize, and is then weaned out of the harness over a period of weeks. The success rate is approximately 80%. If the hip cannot be stabilized in the harness, the next treatment option is an arthrogram, closed reduction (with or without percutaneous or open adductor release), and a spica cast. If successful, the duration in the cast is typically 3–4 months. Risks include avascular necrosis and recurrent hip subluxation. If these treatments fail the patient often requires an open reduction.

330. **How is DDH treated in older children?**

In children between 6 and 18 months of age, closed reduction and spica casting is the initial treatment of choice. If this is unsuccessful, open reduction is warranted. In children older than 2 years of age, secondary bony procedures are often required. These include femoral osteotomy (shortening and derotation) and a pelvic osteotomy to redirect or reshape the acetabulum and achieve better anterolateral coverage of the femoral head.

331. **What are the different types of pelvic osteotomies?**

Reshaping osteotomies such as the Pemberton or Dega involve an incomplete cut through the ilium, and the acetabular fragment is hinged downward through the triradiate cartilage. A bone graft is placed to maintain the correction. These osteotomies decrease the volume of the acetabulum.

Redirectional osteotomies, such as the Salter and Steele (triple) osteotomies, involve complete cuts through the ilium (the triple also involves pubic and ischial cuts), and the acetabulum is rotated anteriorly and laterally.

Salvage procedures are indicated when a congruent reduction cannot be obtained and the patient has disabling pain from degenerative changes in the hip. Options include the Chiari and the shelf. The Chiari osteotomy is a medial displacement osteotomy which moves the entire hip joint towards the patient's midline. It has been criticized because it limits the size of the acetabular roof laterally. The shelf procedure essentially builds an extension on the deficient acetabulum to provide better coverage for the femoral head. Bone grafts are used as a buttress. Loads are then distributed over a greater surface area. The capsule underneath the bone graft undergoes metaplasia into fibrocartilage, which is less durable than normal hyaline articular cartilage (Fig. 6.51).

SLIPPED CAPITAL FEMORAL EPIPHYSIS (SCFE)

CASE 6-24

An obese 14-year-old patient presents to your office. He has been limping for several months, and recently has been unable to walk without significant pain. Initially he had complained about knee pain. Knee x-rays are unremarkable.

332. **What is SCFE?**

Slipped capital femoral epiphysis is the most common hip problem in adolescents. SCFE represents displacement of the femoral head relative to the femoral shaft, occurring through the physis. It is the slippage of the femoral head posterior and inferior to the femoral neck, usually through the hypertophic zone of the physis and analogous to a Salter–Harris type 1 fracture.

333. **What is the incidence of SCFE?**

The incidence is between 2 and 13 per 100 000.

334. **What are risk factors for SCFE?**

Most patients are above the 95th percentile for weight. Boys are more likely to develop SCFE than girls, and African-American and Polynesian children are also at greater risk. Various endocrinopathies, including panhypopituitarism, hypo- or hyperthyroidism, or renal osteodystrophy, may lead to SCFE. Treatment with growth hormone is also a risk.

335. **How is SCFE diagnosed?**

Antero-posterior pelvis and frog lateral radiographs are usually diagnostic (Fig. 6.52). On the antero-posterior view, Klein's line should be drawn. This is a line along the lateral

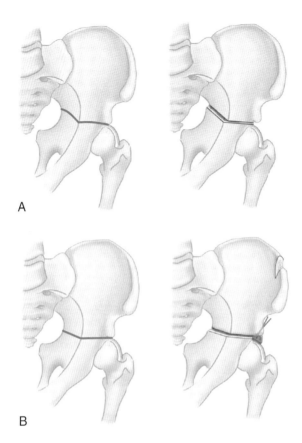

Figure 6.51. (A) Ideal Chiari osteotomy with 15° upslope to obtain coverage in mild hip dysplasia. (B) Chiari osteotomy with supplemental graft and shelf for severely dysplastic hip. *(From Canale ST: Campbell's Operative Orthopaedics, pp. 1133–1199.e10. Copyright © 2013 by Mosby, Elsevier Inc.)*

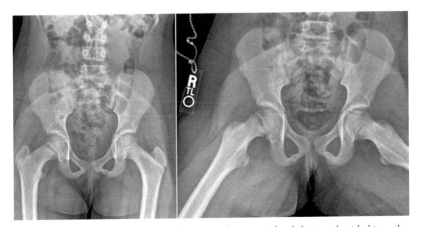

Figure 6.52. Antero-posterior (AP) and lateral projections showing a widened physis on the right hip on the AP, the frog lateral shows the slipped epiphysis.

aspect of the superior femoral neck and should normally intersect a portion of the femoral head. The slip is easier to identify on the frog lateral as there is posterior displacement of the femoral head relative to the neck, and there may be some rounding or prominence along the anterior femoral neck from remodeling. Subtle cases may show only widening of the physis. At the earliest stage of the disease, edema within the physis may be observed on an MRI (pre-slip). On physical examination, patients will have pain, especially with internal rotation, and the hip will externally rotate while brought into greater degrees of flexion.

336. **Why do patients with SCFE sometimes complain of knee pain?**
This is likely referred pain in the distribution of the femoral and obturator nerves. Failure to suspect a hip etiology for this pain can lead to delays in diagnosis and even unnecessary knee procedures. A careful hip exam should always be performed in patients with knee pain.

337. **How is SCFE classified?**
Traditionally SCFE had been classified as acute or chronic based on the length of symptoms – more or less than 3 weeks. The additional classification of stable vs. unstable is also valuable, based on whether the patient is able to bear weight (with or without crutches) on the affected side. Unstable SCFE is associated with a high (20–47%) risk of avascular necrosis.

338. **How is SCFE treated?**
Stable SCFE is treated by in situ fixation with a single cannulated screw. Unstable SCFE is usually treated emergently by in situ fixation with one or two cannulated screws, and the joint is often decompressed to reduce risks of avascular necrosis from tamponade by the effusion. While controversial, some surgeons advocate a gentle reduction maneuver prior to stabilization. More recently, there has been interest in acute open reduction and fixation of the slip using the technique of surgical dislocation. Further study will be required to clarify the indications for this approach. Patients with restricted motion or hip impingement following in situ fixation may be treated by realignment osteotomy after physeal closure.

339. **What are the indications for prophylactic pinning of the contralateral hip?**
Indications are controversial, but typically younger age (boys <12 years of age, girls <10 years of age), open triradiate cartilage, presence of an endocrinopathy, and treatment with growth hormone.

FEMORAL ACETABULAR IMPINGEMENT (FAI)
CASE 6-25

A 16-year-old girl presents to your office complaining of hip pain. She is a ballerina, and points to her anterior groin as the source of her pain, which is reproduced when you flex and internally rotate her hip. A radial MRI image is shown in Figure 6.53.

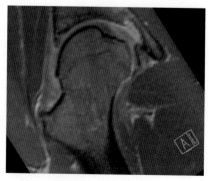

Figure 6.53. Radial sequence MRI showing a cam lesion and an anterosuperior labral tear.

340. **What is femoroacetabular impingement (FAI)?**
FAI involves structural abnormalities of the hip joint leading to limitations in range of motion.

341. **What are the types of FAI?**
Cam impingement occurs when a prominence along the femoral neck abuts against the acetabulum, limiting motion. Typically this is at the anterolateral head–neck junction. *Pincer impingement* involves retroversion of the acetabulum, causing "overcoverage" of the femoral head and abutment against the femoral neck. Both of these can cause labral damage (Fig. 6.54).

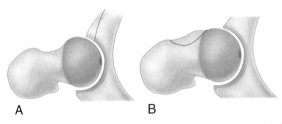

A   **B**

Figure 6.54. (A) Pincer impingement occurs when acetabulum has localized or there is global overcoverage leading to contact of acetabular rim with femoral head–neck junction during normal hip motion. (B) Cam impingement occurs when prominent head–neck junction contacts acetabular rim during hip flexion. (*From Guyton JL, Campbell's Operative Orthopaedics, pp. 333–373.e6. Copyright © 2013 by Mosby, Elsevier Inc.*)

342. **What are risk factors for developing FAI?**
Athletes, dancers especially, seem to be at risk for FAI, which also occurs more commonly in girls than boys. Impingement may also be identified in patients with DDH and slipped capital femoral epiphysis.

343. **How is FAI diagnosed?**
The impingement test is suggestive of intra-articular hip pathology, including FAI. The patient is supine, and the examiner flexes, adducts, and internally rotates the hip, and a positive test will reproduce the patient's symptoms. Radiographs are performed to assess femoral and acetabular morphology, including an antero-posterior, true lateral, and often a false profile view. An MRI can assist in the diagnosis as well, particularly in demonstrating labral tears.

344. **What is the treatment for FAI?**
Initial treatment is usually conservative, involving activity modification and physical therapy. If the pain persists, surgical treatment options include hip arthroscopy, open surgical dislocation with osteoplasty (removal of impingement lesions) and sometimes labral repair, and a redirectional pelvic osteotomy if the primary cause is acetabular retroversion.

PEDIATRIC SPORTS

SHOULDER

CASE 6-26

A football player comes to your office after sustaining an injury to his shoulder. He felt his shoulder "pop out;" it was put back into place by the trainer at his game.

345. **What are common shoulder injuries in young athletes?**
Young overhead athletes may develop glenohumeral instability. This may be classified as traumatic or atraumatic/multidirectional shoulder instability (MDI). Traumatic dislocations most often involve anterior instability and are caused by an event, such as a collision,

while the arm is abducted and externally rotated. An MDI is often a result of ligamentous laxity.

Another condition encountered in young throwers is "little leaguer's shoulder," in which repeated microtrauma across the proximal humeral physis results in a chronic stress injury (epiphysiolysis). This is most commonly seen in ages 11–13 (at maximal physeal growth). Other shoulder problems include GIRD (glenohumeral internal rotation deficit), SLAP (superior labrum anterior to posterior) lesions, and rotator cuff tendinitis.

346. What are the treatment options?

Acute shoulder dislocations should be reduced, and sedation is frequently required. Recurrence correlates with age at first dislocation (may approach 100% in patients with open physes), leading to an increased interest in early surgical intervention. Capsulorraphy (tightening of the lax capsule, usually anteriorly) and repair of a Bankart lesion (capsulolabral detachment) may both be performed arthroscopically or as an open procedure. Non-surgical management includes a period of immobilization followed by dynamic shoulder stabilization. MDI should first be approached non-operatively.

Treatment of little leaguer's shoulder involves a period of rest, 2–3 months, followed by a progressive throwing program. GIRD is treated by an aggressive posterior capsular stretching program. SLAP treatment begins with rest followed by stretching and strengthening, with possible arthroscopic repair if conservative management fails. Rotator cuff pathology is similarly treated first with rest and physical therapy, with progression to surgery only after failure of conservative management. Rotator cuff surgery is very uncommon in young athletes.

CONCUSSION

CASE 6-26 continued

His mother is concerned about concussions in football players.

347. What is a concussion?

Concussion is a complex pathophysiologic process affecting the brain. It is induced by trauma during which force is transmitted to the head. The symptoms, often short-lived neurologic impairment, are generally functional and without structural abnormality. Loss of consciousness is not necessary for the diagnosis of concussion.

348. What is the risk for young athletes?

Because their brains are still developing, concussions are particularly dangerous for young athletes. Girls are reported to have higher rates of concussions for similar sports than boys; the reason for this has not been clearly elucidated. Football is particularly prone to concussions, as well as girls' soccer and basketball, rugby, ice hockey, and lacrosse.

349. How should concussion be treated?

Recognition is the first step in concussion management. Players, coaches, and trainers must be prepared to remove an athlete from play if a concussion is suspected. Several sideline assessment tools exist to assist in this determination. Once recognized, rest is the essential component of treatment for a concussion. Athletes must refrain from cognitive as well as physical tasks while they are recovering. Second-impact syndrome – a second head injury before the symptoms of the first have cleared – is a potentially devastating and even fatal occurrence.

ELBOW

CASE 6-27

A pitcher presents to your office with persistent pain in his elbow. He plays on a school team as well as a travel team; his parents report that they believe that each of his coaches monitors his pitch count.

350. What are common elbow injuries in young athletes?

Acutely, high valgus stresses and contraction of the flexor-pronator mass can lead to medial epicondyle avulsion fractures; however, elbow problems in the young athlete more commonly result from repetitive/chronic stress. Chronic injuries include "little leaguer's elbow," medial epicondylar apophysitis, ulnar collateral ligament injuries/valgus instability (less common in young pitchers), osteochondritis dessicans (most commonly in the capitellum), lateral epicondylitis/apophysitis (often associated with racquet sports), and posterior compartment injuries such as valgus extension overload from repetitive throwing (leading to posteromedial impingement and olecranon osteophyte formation).

351. **What are preventative measures for young pitchers?**
Young athletes consistently demonstrate poorer pitching mechanics than older players, including inadequate synchronized coordination. Instruction on proper pitching mechanics as early as possible is essential. Intensity of training is also an issue – young pitchers who throw more pitches per game or per season, pitch more months during the year, throw higher-velocity pitches, or pitch with arm fatigue are more likely to be injured. Guidelines for little league players mandating pitch counts and rest days should be carefully followed.

352. **What are treatment options for these injuries?**
Medial epicondyle avulsion fractures are increasingly treated operatively, particularly when displaced more than ~5 mm and/or in throwers' dominant arm. Treatment of overuse injuries generally involves a period of rest and physical therapy. Failure of conservative treatment may mandate surgery. The ulnar collateral ligament may be reconstructed; posteromedial osteophytes may be removed (open or arthroscopically); and OCD lesions may be drilled, fixed, or replaced with autologous osteochondral transplantation.

KNEE

CASE 6-28

A soccer player comes to your office after a twisting injury to her knee during a game. She was unable to continue playing, and several hours later noticed significant swelling in her knee.

353. **What are common knee injuries in young athletes?**
Anterior cruciate ligament (ACL) tears are increasingly common amongst young athletes; these often occur after twisting or varus/valgus forces about the knee, sometimes producing an audible popping and often resulting in significant swelling and inability to continue to play. Female athletes are particularly susceptible to this injury. Other problems include torn menisci, tibial tubercle avulsions, patellar instability, OCD lesions, and tendinitis/osteochondroses.

354. **What are preventative measures?**
Significant recent attention has been focused on ACL injury prevention. Neuromuscular exercise training programs have been developed and may be incorporated into athletes' practice regimens to improve strength, kinematics, and dynamic balance.

355. **How are ACL tears diagnosed?**
Classic exam findings include anterior laxity with the anterior drawer and Lachman tests, as the tibia moves forward relative to the femur when an anterior stress is applied. MRI is the imaging modality of choice for ligamentous and meniscal injuries to the knee.

356. **What are treatment options for young athletes with injured knees?**
Particularly for athletes who wish to return to play, ACL reconstruction is a reasonable option. Significant delay in reconstruction (>12 weeks) may result in further damage, particularly to the medial meniscus and lateral articular cartilage. For patients with open physes, physeal-sparing techniques may be employed. Most meniscal tears will require surgical treatment (either repair or partial meniscectomy) as well. Stable OCD lesions – those without fractured cartilage or separation of the underlying subchondral bone – should be initially treated non-operatively, usually with bracing and activity modification. Lesions refractory to conservative management and unstable lesions warrant surgical treatment (drilling, fixation, or if necessary, a salvage procedure such as autologous chondrocyte implantation or osteochondral autologous transplantation). Tibial tubercle avulsions are treated with internal fixation if significantly displaced. These injuries must be monitored carefully for development of compartment syndrome. Tendinitis/osteochondroses such as Osgood–Schlatter and Sinding–Larsen–Johansson disease (pain at the tibial tuberosity or inferior pole of the patella, respectively) and patellar tendinitis are treated conservatively, with activity modification, NSAIDs, physical therapy, and ice.

Treatment of patellar instability is usually non-operative with activity restriction and quadriceps strengthening. Surgical treatment for patellar subluxation includes reconstruction of the medial patellofemoral ligament (acute injuries, controversial) or patellar realignment procedures. Skeletal realignment, such as tibial tubercle transfer, should be reserved for skeletally mature patients with an abnormal tibial tubercle-trochlear groove interval.

BIBLIOGRAPHY

1. Abel MF, Blanco JS, Pavlovich L, et al. Assymetric hip deformity and subluxation in cerebral palsy: an analysis of surgical treatment. J Pediatr Orthop 1999;19:479–85.
2. Abel MF, Damiano DL, Pannunzio M, et al. Muscle-tendon surgery in diplegic cerebral palsy: Functional and mechanical changes. J Pediatr Orthop 1999;19:366–75.
3. Auerbach JD, Spiegel DA, Zgonis MH, et al. The correction of pelvic obliquity in patients with cerebral palsy and neuromuscular scoliosis: is there a benefit of anterior release prior to posterior spinal arthrodesis? Spine (Phila Pa 1976) 2009;34(21):E766–74.
4. Baldwin K, Hsu JE, Hosalkar HS, et al. Treatment of femur fractures in school aged children using elastic stable intramedullary nailing: a systematic review. J Paediatr Orthop B 2011;20:303–8.
5. Baldwin K, Pandya N, Hosalkar H, et al. Femur fractures in children: accident or abuse? Clin Orthop Rel Res 2011;469:798–804.
6. Baldwin K, Obatunde D, Hosalkar H, et al. Open fractures of the tibia in the pediatric population: a systematic review. J Child Orthop 2009;3:199–208.
7. Bautista SR, Flynn JM. Trauma prevention in children. Pediatr Ann 2006;35:85–91.
8. Bednar MS, James MA, Light TR. Congenital longitudinal deficiency. J Hand Surg [Am] 2009;34:1739–47.
9. Brooks H, Azen S, Gerberg E, et al. Scoliosis: A prospective epidemiologic study. J Bone Joint Surg Am 1975;57:968–72.
10. Bulman WA, Dormans JP, Ecker ML, et al. Posterior spinal fusion for scoliosis in patients with cerebral palsy: A comparison of Luque rod and unit rod instrumentation. J Pediatr Orthop 1996;16:314–23.
11. Caird MS, Flynn JM, Leung YL, et al. Factors distinguishing septic arthritis from transient synovitis of the hip in children. A prospective study. J Bone Joint Surg Am 2006;88:1251–7.
12. Canale ST, Beaty JH, editors. Campbell's Operative Orthopaedics. 11th ed. Philadelphia: Mosby Elsevier; 2008.
13. Cavalier R, Herman MJ, Cheung EV, et al. Spondylolysis and spondylolisthesis in children and adolescents: I. Diagnosis, natural history, and nonsurgical management. J Am Acad Orthop Surg 2006;14:417–24.
14. Chambers H, Lauer A, Kaufman K, et al. Prediction of outcome after rectus femoris surgery in cerebral palsy: the role of cocontraction of the rectus femoris and vastus lateralis. J Pediatr Orthop 1998;18:703–11.
15. Cheung EV, Herman MJ, Cavalier R, et al. Spondylolysis and spondylolisthesis in children and adolescents: II. Surgical management. J Am Acad Orthop Surg 2006;14(8):488–98.
16. Davids JR, Rowan F, Davis RB. Indications for orthoses to improve gait in children with cerebral palsy. J Am Acad Orthop Surg 2007;15:178–88.
17. Dormans JP. Pediatric orthopaedics: core knowledge in orthopaedics. Philadelphia: Elsevier Mosby; 2005. p. 237–44.
18. Flynn JM, Sarwark JF, Waters PM, et al. The surgical management of pediatric fractures of the upper extremity. Instr Course Lect 2003;52:635–45.
19. Flynn JM, Skaggs DL, Sponseller PD, et al. The surgical management of pediatric fractures of the lower extremity. Instr Course Lect 2003;52:647–59.
20. Gage JR, Deluca PA, Renshaw TS. Gait analysis: principle and applications. Emphasis on its use in cerebral palsy. J Bone Joint Surg Am 1995;77:1607–23.
21. Gage JR, editor. Gait Analhysis in Cerebral Palsy. London, England: MacKeith Press; 1991.
22. Goldfarb CA. Congenital hand differences. J Hand Surg [Am] 2009;34:1351–6.
23. Hale HB, Bae DS, Waters PM. Current concepts in the management of brachial plexus birth palsy. J Hand Surg [Am] 2010;35:322–31.
24. Halsey MF, Finzel KC, Carrion WV, et al. Toddler's fracture: presumptive diagnosis and treatment. J Pediatr Orthop 2001;21:152–6.
25. Harrington P. The etiology of idiopathic scoliosis. Clin Orthop Rel Res 1977;126:17–25.
26. Herkowitz HN, Garfin SR, Eismont FJ, et al., editors. Rothman-Simeone. The Spine. 5th ed. Philadelphia: Saunders Elsevier; 2006.
27. Hotchkiss RN, Pederson WC, Wolfe SW. Green's Operative Hand Surgery. 5th ed. Philadelphia: Elsevier Churchill Livingstone; 2005.
28. Jaramillo D. Infection: musculoskeletal. Pediatr Radiol 2011;41(Suppl. 1):S127–34. [Epub 2011 Apr 27].
29. Jobe MT. Congenital anomalies of the hand. In: Canale ST, Beaty JH, editors. Campbell's Operative Orthopaedics. 11th ed. Philadelphia: Mosby Elsevier; 2008.
30. Kamath A, Baldwin K, Horneff J, et al. Operative versus non operative management of medial epicondyle fractures: a systematic review. J Child Orthop 2009;3:345–57.

31. Kim HK. Legg–Calvé–Perthes disease. J Am Acad Orthop Surg 2010;18:676–86.
32. Kocher MS, Mandiga Zurakowski D, Barnewolt C, et al. Validation of a clinical prediction rule for the differentiation between septic arthritis and transient synovitis of the hip in children. J Bone Joint Surg Am 2004;86:1629–35.
33. Koval KJ, Zuckerman JD. Handbook of Fractures. 3rd ed. Philadelphia: Lippincott, Williams and Wilkins; 2006.
34. Lenke LG, Betz RR, Harms J, et al. Adolescent idiopathic scoliosis: a new classification to determine extent of spinal arthrodesis. J Bone Joint Surg Am 2001;83-A:1169–81.
35. Lincoln TL, Suen PW. Common rotational variations in children. J Am Acad Orthop Surg 2003;11:312–20.
36. Lowe TG, Line BG. Evidence based medicine: analysis of Scheuermann kyphosis. Spine 2007;32(19 Suppl.):S115–19.
37. Namdari S, Ganley T, Baldwin K, et al. Fixation of displaced midshaft clavicle fractures in skeletally immature patients. J Pediatr Orthop 2011;1:507–11.
38. Maschke SD, Seitz W, Lawton J. Radial longitudinal deficiency. J Am Acad Orthop Surg 2007;15:41–52.
39. Morrissy RT, Weinstein SL, editors. Lovell and Winter's pediatric orthopaedics. 6th ed. Lippincott: Williams and Wilkins; 2006.
40. Ogon M, Giesinger K, Behensky H, et al. Interobserver and intraobserver reliability of Lenke's new scoliosis classification system. Spine 2002;27:858–62.
41. Palavan S, Baldwin K, Pandya N, et al. Proximal humerus fractures in the pediatric population: a systematic review. J Child Orthop 2011;5:187–94.
42. Pandya NK, Baldwin K, Kamath AF, et al. Unexplained fractures: child abuse or bone disease? A systematic review. Clin Orthop Rel Res 2011;469:805–12.
43. Pandya N, Baldwin K, Wolfgruber H, et al. Humerus fractures in young children, an algorithm to identify abuse. J Pediatr Orthop B 2010;19:535–41.
44. Pandya N, Baldwin K, Wolfgruber H, et al. A comparison of characteristics of accidental and non accidental orthopaedic trauma a 15 year experience at a level I pediatric trauma center. J Pediatr Orthop (Am) 2009;29:618–25.
45. Park MJ, Baldwin K, Weiss-Lexer M, et al. Composite playground safety measure to correlate the rate of supracondylar humerus fractures with safety: an ecologic study. J Pediatr Orthop (Am) 2010;30:101–5.
46. Pearl ML. Shoulder problems in children with brachial plexus birth palsy: evaluation and management. J Am Acad Orthop Surg 2009;17:242–54.
47. Punaro M. Rheumatologic conditions in children who may present to the orthopaedic surgeon. J Am Acad Orthop Surg 2011;19:163–9.
48. Rosenthal RE, Levine DB. Fragmentation of the distal pole of the patella in spastic cerebral palsy. J Bone Joint Surg 1977;59A:934.
49. Ruchelsman DE, Pettrone S, Price AE, et al. Brachial plexus birth palsy: an overview of early treatment considerations. Bull NYU Hosp Jt Dis 2009;67:83–9.
50. Sankar WN, Hebela NM, Skaggs DL, et al. Loss of pin fixation in displaced supracondylar humeral fractures in children: causes and prevention. J Bone Joint Surg Am 2007;89:713–17.
51. Sankar WN, Spiegel DA, Gregg JR, et al. Long term follow up after one stage reconstruction of dislocated hips in patients with cerebral palsy. J Pediatr Orthop 2006;26:1–7.
52. Schwend RM, Drennan JC. Cavus foot deformity in children. J Am Acad Orthop Surg 2003;11:201–11.
53. Skaggs DL, Friend L, Alman B, et al. The effect of surgical delay on acute infection following 554 open fractures in children. J Bone Joint Surg Am 2005;87:8–12.
54. Smith BG, Cruz AI Jr, Milewski MD, et al. Lyme disease and the orthopaedic implications of lyme arthritis. J Am Acad Orthop Surg 2011;19:91–100.
55. Spiegel DA, Flynn JM. Evaluation and treatment of hip dysplasia in cerebral palsy. Orthop Clin North Am 2006;37:185–96.
56. Spiegel DA, Loder RT, Alley KA, et al. Spinal deformity following selective dorsal rhizotomy. J Pediatr Orthop 2004;24:30–6.
57. Sponseller PD, editor. OKU2 Pediatrics. Rosemont, IL: AAOS; 2002.
58. Tracy MR, Dormans JP, Kusumi K. Klippel–Feil syndrome: clinical features and current understanding of etiology. Clin Orthop Relat Res 2004;424:183–90.
59. Van Heest AE, House JH, Cariello C. Upper extremity surgical treatment of cerebral palsy. J Hand Surg Am 1999;24:323–30.
60. Waters PM. Update on management of pediatric brachial plexus palsy. J Pediatr Orthop B 2005;14:233–44.
61. Weinstein SL, Ponseti I. Curve progression in idiopathic scoliosis: Long-term follow-up. J Bone Joint Surg Am 1983;65:447–55.
62. Wills BP, Dormans JP. Nontraumatic upper cervical spine instability in children. J Am Acad Orthop Surg 2006;14:233–45.

CHAPTER 7

REHABILITATION AND NEURO-ORTHOPEDIC SURGERY

Keith D. Baldwin, Alberto Esquenazi and Mary Ann Keenan

GENERAL PRINCIPLES

1. What are the different types of actions a muscle can take a joint through?
   a. *Concentric*: The muscle contracts to become shorter and move the joint through a range of motion.
   b. *Eccentric*: The muscle contracts to prevent a force from lengthening it.
   c. *Isokinetic*: This requires a machine to guide and produce constant force.
   d. *Isometric*: The muscle contracts, but creates no joint motion.
   e. *Isotonic*: Tension remains unchanged throughout the range of motion.

2. How is strength graded by manual muscle testing?
   Strength is graded on a 0–5 scale. Change in strength must be substantial before differences in the higher end (4–5) can be detected.
   - 0/5 indicates no force, and no voluntary palpable twitch.
   - 1/5 indicates palpable twitch on a voluntary basis, but no joint motion.
   - 2/5 indicates that the muscle is able to provide force to produce a full range of motion in a gravity eliminated position.
   - 3/5 indicates that the muscle can provide strength to produce a full range of motion against gravity but not against resistance.
   - 4/5 indicates the examiner is able to overcome the patient's strength with effort during testing.
   - 5/5 indicates that the patient has strength that cannot be overcome with manual muscle testing.

   Note that single leg calf raises are the best way to assess plantar flexion strength, requiring 20 repetitions to be considered normal, or 5/5.

3. How is range of motion tested?
   Range of motion is tested clinically with goniometry. The error of measurement is reported to be 6–8°. There are more sophisticated methods of joint motion analysis, but goniometry is the most widely used and clinically useful method (Fig. 7.1).

4. Who are the members of the rehabilitation team other than the surgeon?
   Physical medicine and Rehabilitation physician (Physiatrist or PM & R): These specialists deal with inpatient and outpatient rehabilitation issues, wheelchair prescriptions, prosthesis fitting and design, diagnostic EMG, and gait analysis. Physiatrists provide non-operative ongoing musculoskeletal medical care in collaboration with the surgeon.
   Physical therapist (PT): Provides exercise therapy, gait training, various physical modalities to deal with disorders of motion, gait, balance, and muscle strength. They provide physiotherapy care under the supervision of a physician.
   Occupational therapist (OT): Provides upper extremity exercise therapy, and assistance in the ability to perform instrumental activities of daily living (IADLs). These activities include fine motor tasks and activities of daily living (ADLs), such as eating, grooming, and bathing.
   PT and OT assistants (PTA/OTA): Provide PT and OT care following assessment by a therapist.
   Speech therapist: Assists patients with issues of speech and swallowing disorders.

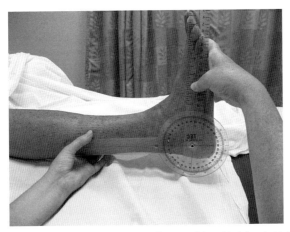

Figure 7.1. A therapist measures the range of motion of the ankle (tibiotalar) joint.

Case manager/Social worker: Can provide assistance in obtaining placement, and durable medical equipment such as wheel chairs, walkers, shower chairs, and other essential items.

5. **What are some of the physical therapy modalities and what are their purposes?**
   Exercise therapy: This is the cornerstone of physical therapy, and can be used to increase the range of motion (ROM) of joints, or strength and endurance of muscles. Often physical therapy is designed to bring balance to the forces around a joint through a well-designed combination of stretching and strengthening.
   Heat: Heat is used to relieve muscle spasm and encourage local blood flow, which is thought to increase the removal of harmful waste products of injury, and bring in nutrients to the area. Heat is available in the superficial form, through moist hot packs, paraffin baths, and warm water immersion. Heat is also available in the deep form, such as ultrasound therapy and diathermy.
   Cold: Cold is used to decrease inflammation, and slow metabolic processes which are thought to be counterproductive or too robust. As such, this modality is generally used in acute phases of injury or surgery, or following a therapy session in order to settle irritated tissues, and decrease swelling and inflammation.
   Electrical stimulation: Several different protocols of electrical stimulation are available. Their purposes range from biofeedback to preferential training of muscle groups, stimulation to physically cause muscle contraction for strength or motor control, or protocols to interrupt pain nerve signals to the spinal cord (TENS).
   Aquatherapy: Aquatherapy is used to produce aerobic activity, or muscle strengthening in a gravity-supported environment. It is generally helpful for patients with arthritis and other conditions that make weight bearing painful.
   Manual therapy: Joint mobilization and massage are manual therapies used to soothe aching muscles, and stretch joints in non-physiologic ways, such as providing a stretch to a joint capsule in a translatory fashion.
   Traction: Mechanized or manual traction is a special type of treatment for spinal disorders that is thought to allow decompression to the spinal canal, and relieve stress that disk herniations and other disorders can cause.

6. **From a rehabilitation standpoint, what is the generalized flow of surgical patients from an inpatient to outpatient setting?**
   Generally, patients who have orthopedic surgery are either discharged home or admitted to an inpatient orthopedic service. Patients who are discharged are generally seen in the office by their surgeon and started on a specific outpatient rehabilitation protocol. For some conditions,

like frozen shoulder, rehabilitation is initiated on the first day after surgery. These patients will be given a prescription for physical therapy in their discharge orders. Inpatients generally see physical therapists on an inpatient basis for exercises, gait training, and ADL training. If patients are deemed safe, they are discharged home with either home therapy or outpatient rehabilitation, depending on the situation. If the patient needs more rehabilitation prior to discharge, they are sent to either an inpatient rehabilitation unit, or a skilled nursing facility. If patients are able to tolerate intensive rehabilitation (3 hours per day), they are sent to inpatient rehabilitation. If patients cannot tolerate intensive rehabilitation or if insurance will not approve inpatient rehabilitation they go to a skilled nursing facility, which provides approximately half the amount of rehabilitation training per day.

SPORTS REHAB
CASE 7-1

A running back on a high school football team is tackled, and is slow to get up. He can bear weight on his leg, but his knee is visibly swollen, and he struggles back to the sideline, the athletic trainers immediately provide attention.

7. **What is the RICE principle?**
RICE stands for rest, ice, compression, and elevation. It is a method of decreasing inflammation. This would be the initial treatment for the patient described in Case 7-1.

8. **What is glenohumeral internal rotation deficit? How is it generally treated?**
Glenohumeral internal rotation deficit generally occurs in throwing athletes. It occurs as a result of a lax anterior glenohumeral joint capsule and a tight posterior capsule. This results in a significant side to side difference in internal rotation relative to external rotation. Generally this is treated with extensive therapy focused on posterior capsular stretching and muscle force balance. Surgical treatment is controversial with anterior capsular tightening vs. posterior capsular release being described in the literature.

9. **What is chondromalacia patellae? What are the typical thoughts as far as non-operative treatment?**
Chonromalacia patella, commonly referred to as patellofemoral pain syndrome or anterior knee pain, is softening or degeneration of the cartilage on the undersurface of the patellofemoral joint. Patients present with pain under the knee cap that is worsened when rising from a chair or climbing steps. Occasionally, patients will develop a knee effusion. Multiple theories regarding the etiology of chondromalacia patellae include uneven pull of the vastus medialis and vastus lateralis, core instability, or other sources of biomechanical disadvantage (ex. quadriceps weakness) across the knee. This condition is commonly treated with physical therapy focused on core stabilization, hamstring stretching, heel cord stretching and vastus medialis strength training.

10. **What are the non-operative treatment options of patellar tendonitis?**
Patellar tendonitis is commonly referred to as jumper's knee. It is an overuse syndrome resulting from the pull of the patellar tendon on the tibial tubercle. Early, the treatment course involves resting the knee, with ice used liberally. When the inflammation remits, restoration of strength by physical therapy is employed. Eccentric exercise is thought to be helpful for patellar tendonitis in the strengthening phase. An infrapatellar strap can be used to alter the pull of the patellar tendon on the tibial tubercle. When strength is regained, sport-specific training is begun. Surgery is rarely necessary, and involves tendon debridement.

11. **What are the principles of lower back rehabilitation?**
Physical therapy is the first-line treatment for most adult spinal problems. Physical therapy for back problems has several goals. The first focus is symptom alleviation through the use of modalities such as ultrasound, heat, electrical stimulation, and joint mobilization. Patient education is utilized to teach proper biomechanics, posture, and lifting/ergonomic techniques. Core stability is emphasized through abdominal wall and thoracolumbar muscle

strengthening. Specific programs have been designed around specific pathologies, such as Mackenzie stretching exercises for herniated nucleus pulposus.

12. **What are the principles of ankle rehabilitation?**

Ankle rehabilitation focuses on stretching of tight muscles, notably the gastroc-soleus complex, along with retraining proprioception and complex ankle motions. Balance training activities and higher level closed chain and sport-specific activities are added in a sequential manner as symptomology and patient strength allows. Strengthening of the calf muscles cannot be overemphasized.

13. **What are the principles of anterior cruciate ligament (ACL) reconstruction rehabilitation?**

Though rehabilitation protocols after ACL reconstruction are surgeon-specific, there are a few guiding principles. In general when an athlete injures their ACL, the patient initiates a series of pre-operative range of motion exercises to ensure that the knee regains normal, or near normal, range of motion before surgery. Following surgery, the patient is often placed in a hinged knee brace and range of motion exercises and light quad strengthening are initiated. As the patient progresses, closed chain exercises and isokinetic exercises are added. As the ACL graft utilized during the reconstruction matures over the weeks and months that follow, a running program is added, which begins with in-line running followed by cutting and directional challenges. Some surgeons use a "hop test" to determine when side-to-side strength is approximately equal enough to allow directional running (cutting, zig zags, circle running). In older patients and those who elect to undergo non-operative treatment of an ACL tear, hamstring rehabilitation is undertaken because the hamstrings act as a restraint to tibial translation. Although their role as a secondary stabilizer is incomplete and has not been shown to be helpful in preventing secondary meniscus tears, hamstring strengthening can be useful in non-operatively treated patients. ACL prevention programs have been shown, in some studies, to decrease the rate of ACL tears in high-risk athletes. These programs generally consist of plyometric exercises and neuromuscular retraining. Brace wear is controversial and has not been shown to be helpful with the notable exception of downhill skiers.

NORMAL AND PATHOLOGIC GAIT

14. **What are the components of normal gait (walking)?**

Gait is an important consideration in the daily lives of all people. It allows people the ability to travel to the bathroom, to their refrigerator, to their car, from their car to work, and countless other activities during the day. An injury, disease, or other pathologic process that interferes with gait will disrupt almost every other everyday activity in the patient's life.

Normal gait involves a "stance" phase for each lower limb which comprises about 60% of the gait cycle, and a "swing" phase, which comprises about 40% of the gait cycle. Of note, the 60–40 division is for normal walking speed. For about 20% of the normal gait cycle, there is double limb support (i.e., both feet are contacting the ground). The major difference between walking and running, in terms of the gait cycle, is that there is no double limb support during running. This is sometimes referred to as "double float".

15. **What is the gait cycle?**

A gait cycle begins with foot contact of one limb, and ends with foot contact of the *same* limb (i.e., the progression of one limb through space from one point in the cycle to the same point), also known as a *stride*.

16. **What differentiates a step from a stride?**

Step length is the *distance between heel contact of the opposite feet* (i.e., right step length is the distance between the right heel strike and the left heel strike.). In normal gait, right step length is equal to left step length, but the step lengths may (and probably will) be different in various pathologic states. *Stride length* is the distance between heel strikes of the same foot (2 steps). The *walking base* or *base of support* is the distance between the heels of opposite feet during gait. This base may be wide if the patient has poor balance, or may even be negative if the patient's legs scissor during gait.

17. **What is cadence? How can walking performance be measured?**

Cadence will impact walking speed and is measured by the *number of steps per minute*. Walking performance can be measured with a stopwatch and the person walking 10 meters (normal range of velocity is 1.2 to 1.5 m/s with some variability with gender and age).

A more complex assessment is the *timed up and go test*. During this test, a patient begins seated in a chair, and is asked to get up, walk 3 meters, and return to the chair to sit down. The patient is allowed to use any walking aids including any orthotics that they normally use. Less than 10 seconds is considered normal for an elderly patient. Greater than 14 seconds is suggestive of high fall risk, and greater than 30 seconds is suggestive of requiring dependence in ADLs.

18. **What are the components of the "stance" and "swing" phases, and what muscles act during these phases?**

Initial contact: In normal gait, the heel of the leading foot touches the floor and the ground reaction force is posterior to the ankle and knee joint. The hip extensors, ankle dorsiflexors, and toe extensors are active to absorb the impact force and prevent plantar flexion of the ankle from occurring too quickly. At this moment, the contralateral limb is in pre-swing (period of double limb support).

Loading response: This phase is characterized by the foot touching the floor, and the opposite limb leaving the floor. This phase involves loading the limb to accept weight. The weight shift during this phase is known as the first rocker and involves a fulcrum at the heel (heel rocker). The ankle dorsiflexors are active in eccentric contraction. The vastus muscles also provide an eccentric contraction while the hip extensors and abductors are active at the hip in a concentric contraction.

Mid-stance: This is the period of the second rocker (ankle rocker) in which the fulcrum of rotation has moved to the ankle. The plantar flexors slow the forward angular motion of the tibia. Meanwhile, the action of the hip extensors stops midway through midstance, and the hip capsule and ligamentous structures become a passive restraint to further hip extension.

Terminal stance: This period is referred to as the third rocker (forefoot rocker). The ankle plantar flexors change their mode of action from eccentric to concentric, and the rocker moves anterior to the metatarsal heads. Tibialis posterior and peroneal tendons prevent inversion and eversion of the ankle.

Pre-swing: The contralateral swinging foot now touches the ground. The plantar flexors are contracting concentrically, and the hip flexors (other than the rectus femoris) and long adductors are contracting to flex the femur. The knee is being bent by the ground reaction force which is now posterior to its axis.

Initial swing: The foot begins to swing forward like a pendulum, with motion, in part, generated by the hip flexors. The activity is largely passive, except for the tibialis anterior, which must dorsiflex the ankle to prevent toe drag.

Mid swing: The tibialis anterior maintains its activity to keep the ankle in neutral and prevent toe drag.

Terminal swing: The swinging leg needs to decelerate to contact the ground. This is accomplished by the hip and knee flexors, the former of which slows the swing while the latter serves to dampen the extension moment caused by initial contact. As the foot strikes, the dorsiflexors change from concentric to eccentric contraction to slow the acceleration of the foot and prevent foot slap.

19. **Where is the center of gravity (mass) located?**

The center of mass (COM) is located midway *between the hips and anterior to S2*. The least energy consuming locomotion occurs when the COM travels in a straight line. It should be noted that in the coronal plane, the COM travels in a smooth sinusoidal rhythm because of the transfer of weight between hips. The highest point of COM is in midstance, and the lowest point is in double limb support.

If the center of mass is displaced in an individual in any direction away from its normal position, the individual will attempt to compensate to prevent a fall. For example if a patient has a hip flexion contracture, which causes the body to bend at the hip and translate the center of mass anteriorly, then the patient will assume a lordotic posture to accommodate the hip flexion contracture. Accommodating for COM is expensive to the patient metabolically and will result in decreased cadence and endurance.

CASE 7-2

A 13-year-old boy with spastic diplegic from cerebral palsy presents to the outpatient clinic. He is a bright, interactive young man. He has been having increasing difficulty ambulating over the past several months. He has a history of having a percutaneous tendo-achilles lengthening 5 years ago. You send him for instrumented gait analysis as part of his preoperative assessment.

20. **What are the six determinants of normal gait?**
    - *Pelvic rotation*: The pelvis rotates 8° forward on the swing side. This enables a longer step length while minimizing the amount the hip needs to flex/extend. This results in a more efficient gait by decreasing the amount the COM needs to move up and down.
    - *Pelvic tilt*: This is a 5° dip of the pelvis on the swinging side. This reduces the height of the apex of the COM during gait.
    - *Stance phase knee flexion*: Functionally shortens the stance leg during stance phase to minimize the height of the apex of the COM.
    - *Ankle dorsiflexion at initial contact*: Functionally lengthens the leg at heel contact, which prevents excessive lowering of the COM at this point in gait.
    - *Ankle plantar flexion at push off*: Functionally lengthens the leg at push-off which prevents excessive lowering of the COM at this point in gait.
    - *Narrow base of support*: Prevents excessive lateral translation of the body and allows for efficient gait.

21. **What is "antalgic" gait? What are some common causes?**
    Antalgic, or *painful* gait, presents with shortening of the stance phase on the involved side. This is typically thought of as a "limp". This type of gait pattern is non-specific, and can have many causes and presentations. Osteoarthritis, fractures, radiculopathy or sprains are among the many possible causes of antalgic gait in an adult. In a child, one can consider slipped capital femoral epiphysis, osteomyelitis, fracture, or Legg–Calve–Perthes disease as possible causes.

22. **What is a "Trendelenberg" gait? What are some causes?**
    Trendelenberg gait is described as a *lateral trunk lean* when the involved leg is in stance phase. The gait is a result of weak hip abductors. The body compensates by leaning the COM further over the involved limb to prevent pelvic drop. Though the gait has many causes (neurologic, osteoarthritis, post-surgical) the final common pathway is weakness of the hip abductors. A cane can be used on the side opposite the weakness for support in stance phase. Bilateral trendelenberg gait is referred to as a "waddling" gait.

23. **What are four ways a patient can compensate for a leg-length inequality (either functional or anatomical)?**
    A limb can be *actually* too long or short, due to malunion, surgery (such as hip arthroplasty, or amputation), congenital leg-length discrepancy, or degenerative deformity. Alternatively, the limb can be *functionally* short or long due to spasticity, limitation in joint range of motion, scoliosis, deformity, or muscular weakness. One of four gait patterns will emerge. *Circumduction* occurs when the long limb will make a laterally based arc trajectory in swing phase to accommodate the relatively shorter stance limb. *Hip hiking* occurs when the relatively longer swing leg cannot clear the floor, so the pelvis displaces superiorly to clear the leg. *Vaulting gait* occurs when the stance limb plantar flexes early in stance phase to help clear a functionally longer swing limb. *Steppage gait* is an exaggerated hip and knee flexion during the swing phase.

24. **What are some causes of increased walking base of support?**
    Normal walking base (recall: heel of one foot to heel of the other foot) measures between 5 and 10 cm. Widened base of support can occur in deformity (ex. valgus deformity of the knee). More commonly, an increased walking base results from a balance issue that is

caused either centrally (cerebellar ataxia) or peripherally (ex. diabetic neuropathy). A widened base of support in these cases is due to the body's attempt to create a more stable walking pattern.

25. **What are the causes of toe drag or foot slap?**

Toe drag and foot slap are both caused by inadequate dorsiflexion control. This can be the result of weak dorsiflexors (as the result of peroneal nerve palsy, or peripheral nerve injury), or spastic plantar flexors as the result of central nervous system damage. The leg is functionally long in swing phase (because of lack of dorsiflexor activity, and so, the foot is held in plantar flexion). Additionally, initial contact occurs at foot strike or toe strike, as opposed to at heel strike. As such, the first rocker, and the mechanical advantage that it provides, is absent.

26. **What is the cause of stiff knee gait?**

Stiff knee gait, in the setting of central nervous system injury, is generally caused by persistent activity of the *rectus femoris* muscle or lack of hip flexion in the swing phase. The rectus femoris is a quadriceps muscle that crosses the hip and knee joint. During pathologic gait, it may have inappropriate activity. If this is the case, the involved limb becomes functionally longer due to knee stiffness and a "stiff knee gait" ensues. Stiff knee gait in the absence of upper motor neuron disease can result from joint stiffness (either from effusion, arthritis, or contracture), ankle plantar flexor or knee extensor muscle weakness, or overactivity of the quadriceps muscles (i.e., as a splinting response from pain).

This particular type of gait should be distinguished from *back knee* gait in which the knee hyperextends during midstance. This back knee gait can be the result of equinus ankle foot posture, over lengthened hamstrings in cerebral palsy, or a poorly balanced total knee replacement. Additionally, if the quadriceps are weak, the patient will tend to maintain knee extension during stance to provide limb stability and compensate for the lack of muscle power. This produces a penalty of gait inefficiency, higher energy cost, and ultimately, limited walking capacity.

27. **What is crouch gait? What are the causes?**

Crouch gait generally occurs in the patient with cerebral palsy. Crouch gait is the result of bilateral knee flexion posture. The etiology of crouch gait is incompletely understood. It generally becomes worse in adolescence. Many patients have a history of a tendo Achilles lengthening (TAL). Some experts believe that patients with a TAL have insufficient gastro-soleus complexes; as a result, this causes excessive dorsiflexion of the foot during weight bearing. In order to keep the base of support under the center of gravity, the knees flex. Over time, this results in a fixed knee flexion attitude, resulting in knee flexion throughout the gait cycle. This gait pattern is extremely energy inefficient and generally requires either treatment with surgery and braces or wheelchair use for mobility.

28. **What is lever arm dysfunction?**

The normal orientation of the foot is pointing straight forward so that the tibial tubercle (and patella) are in line with the second metatarsal, which points in the direction of forward progression. In the setting of tibial torsion, the lower extremity is either excessively internally or externally rotated. This can be exacerbated by foot deformities such as planus or cavus. When this occurs, the push-off surface is shorter and displaced from normal, which decreases the efficiency of the third rocker. Gait becomes more inefficient, and decreased walking tolerance ensues.

ORTHOTICS AND GAIT AIDS

CASE 7-3

An 83-year-old female presents with difficulty in ambulation. She has spinal stenosis, and has found walking without assistance to be progressively more difficult. Her caregivers express concern that she is at an increased risk of falling. You perform the timed up and go test, and it takes her 1 minute to perform. She does not currently use an assistive device.

29. **What are different types of gait aids, from least restrictive to most restrictive, and their uses?**

    Single point cane: A single point cane is the least restrictive gait aid. It is a standard cane. Single point canes are useful for hip abductor dysfunction or for antalgic gait where removing some load from the involved joint is useful. They cause minimal disruption of the normal gait cycle and are generally used opposite the weak limb (as a stance aid). They are of limited help in the setting of significant balance disturbances (Fig. 7.2).

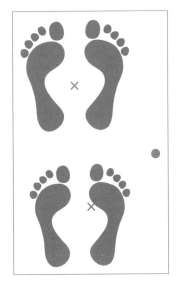

Figure 7.2. Diagram of where the center of pressure (COP) falls during standing with (below) and without (above) a cane.

    Quad cane: Quad canes are more restrictive than single point canes but provide more balance assistance than a single point cane. They come in *narrow-based* and *wide-based* varieties. They are useful when one limb is more severely disabled, and a single-point cane does not offer enough support. Generally, one limb is either minimally affected or not affected, allowing for usage of a single-arm device. They provide the advantage that the cane stands on its own and is available at all times. They are otherwise used similarly to a single-point cane.

    A *frame walker:* Also referred to as a hemi-walker, this device is a fold out device that has four points of contact with the floor, but allows the patient to lean into it. These devices are more restrictive than quad canes but provide more support when lateral trunk stability is an issue. These are generally reserved for hemiparetic patients with a trunk lean that would otherwise preclude ambulation.

    Crutches: Crutches come in several varieties. The most common are *axillary crutches*, which are generally intended for short term use with a "*swing through*" or "*step through*" gait. This often occurs when one limb has limited weight bearing status from surgery or injury. They are not intended for long-term use because they can cause pressure on the axillary nerve, which can result in neuropathy. *Canadian* or *Lofstrand* crutches are more suitable for long-term ambulation assistance and have handles with forearm clasps. These are most often used by patients with chronic lower limb weakness, but enough coordination to use them.

    Walkers: Walkers also come in different varieties. *Standard walkers* consist of an H-shaped frame connected in the middle. The patient stands in the center, advances the walker, then advances their limbs one at a time. *Rollators*, or rolling walkers, have wheels in the front, and may be fitted with tennis balls or pontoons in the rear to allow for easy transport across carpets and rough surfaces. Walkers are used for patients with more severe weakness/motor control issues. They are also more restrictive because they cannot be used on stairs and may be more difficult for uneven surfaces.

Knee Scooters: These devices are relatively new assistive devices. They are generally used by a young person with a unilateral lower extremity injury (generally distal tibia or lower) and limited allowable weight bearing. These scooters allow for full speed locomotion, but require good balance and strength. Patients must be able to bear weight through their knee and femur and not have any breakdown or skin issues on their knee or anterior tibia.

Parallel bars, partial weight bearing systems, parapodiums, standers: These are all rehabilitation tools. None of these are efficient enough to be thought of as gait aids, but are used by therapists to train gait during rehabilitation. *Parapodiums* and *standers* are often used in patients who are unable to stand independently for strength training. *Parallel bars* are bars that are fixed to the floor. During use, a patient stands in between the bars, a therapist stands in front of the patient, and a wheelchair is placed behind the patient to allow for safe gait training in the very weak patient. Lite gait is a brand name for *partial weight-bearing systems* intended to support the patient's weight while allowing for the reciprocating pattern of gait.

30. **What are the gait patterns available with crutches and other assistive devices?**
Four point gait: In this pattern, the patient advances the left crutch, right foot, then right crutch, then left foot, and repeats. This gait pattern is used for patients with weakness or restricted weight bearing in both limbs or with poor lower extremity coordination. There are three points of contact at all times, so this type of gait provides excellent stability, but it comes at a cost of slow speed and high learning curve.

Three point gait: In this gait pattern, the patient moves both crutches and the weaker limb forward simultaneously. Then the patient bears all the weight through the crutches as the strong leg steps through. This gait pattern is indicated for limited weight bearing status on one limb. It requires excellent balance and can be difficult on uneven surfaces.

Two point gait: This gait pattern is with two canes or two crutches. The patient advances the right aid and left foot followed by the left aid and right foot. This gait pattern is indicated when there is weakness in both lower extremities. This pattern promotes reciprocal motion, but is difficult to learn, and is less stable than four point gait.

Swing to gait: In this gait pattern, both crutches are advanced followed by both feet to a point slightly behind the advancement of the crutches. This gait is indicated with weakness of bilateral lower extremities. Advantages are that it is easy to learn, but it requires excellent upper body strength.

Swing through gait: This gait pattern is indicated when there is inability to bear weight fully on both legs. Both crutches are advanced together followed by swinging the feet to a point beyond the crutches. This is the fastest assistive device gait, and is, in fact, faster than normal walking. It is also the least stable assistive device gait, and requires excellent upper body strength and coordination.

31. **Name some shoe modifications and their usages.**
Shoes can be considered to be foot based orthoses. The following are some of the more common shoe modifications that are useful:

Extra depth shoe: These shoes can be custom made or made from a regular shoe by removing inlays. This type of shoe can be useful for accommodating foot deformities. It can also be useful in the setting of diabetes to avoid irritation of soft tissues by relieving pressure over bony prominences or pressure sensitive areas. In general, rigid deformities should be accommodated whereas flexible deformities can be managed with stiffer shoes to support a more normal foot shape.

Flare: This modification is a medial or lateral based extension of the weight bearing surface of the shoe to accommodate for medio-lateral instability or decreased balance.

Extended shank: This modification is a piece of metal or carbon fiber that is placed in the entire sole of the shoe to support the foot. It maintains the continuity of the rocker bottom, and is useful in patients with limited ankle motion, or an inefficient or absent (such as midfoot amputation) third rocker.

Rocker bottom: This modification makes the sole of the shoe into an arc shape. This shape eases the amount of work that needs to be done by the rocker mechanisms of the foot. It is useful in patients where the rocker mechanisms are disrupted by deformity or surgery (such as a tibiotalar fusion).

32. **What is an Orthosis?**

Orthoses are devices applied to the external surface of the body to achieve one or more of the following: relieve pain, immobilize musculoskeletal segments, prevent or correct deformity, and improve function. Orthotic devices are named by the joints they encompass in correct sequence followed by the word orthosis. For example, an orthosis that crosses the ankle and the foot is named an ankle–foot orthosis (AFO). One that crosses the knee, ankle, and foot is called a knee–ankle–foot orthosis (KAFO).

33. **What is a UCBL brace? What is it used for?**

A UCBL brace is a foot orthosis; "University of California Biomechanics Lab" (at Berkley) brace. It is placed inside the shoe. The brace is useful to control motions of the subtalar and midtarsal joints. It is most commonly used as a first-line orthotic in the setting of adult or pediatric flat foot. It is useful in posterior tibialis tendon dysfunction when the deformity is flexible (Fig. 7.3).

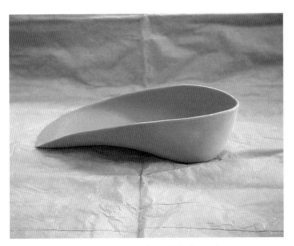

Figure 7.3. Photograph of an UCBL foot orthrosis.

34. **How are ankle foot orthoses (AFOs) used?**

An AFO can substitute for weak muscles by holding joints in alignment. An AFO can be a plastic device, or a device that fits in a shoe with metal uprights and straps. AFOs are usually only helpful during walking on level ground. Because they limit motion at the subtalar and midtarsal joints, they may hinder ambulation on uneven surfaces. They also come at the cost of extra weight during the swing phase of gait. Springs may provide dorsiflexion assistance when the pre-tibial muscles are weak. AFOs can also substitute for weak calf muscles by limiting dorsiflexion when the center of gravity falls anterior to the ankle. An AFO can also be designed with a plantar flexion stop to limit plantar flexion and prevent toe drag and foot slap (Fig. 7.4).

35. **What are the indications for various types of AFOs?**

Free ankle joint (free plantar flexion/dorsiflexion): Indicated for medial/lateral instability

Free plantar flexion, dorsiflexion assist: Indicated for foot drop (such as in cases of peripheral nerve injury)

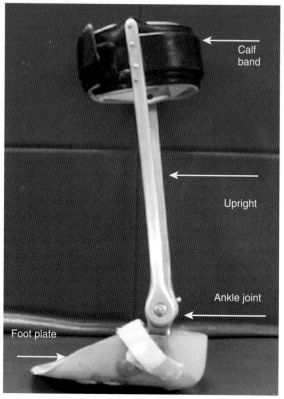

Figure 7.4. Photograph of an ankle foot orthosis, with identification of the major components of the orthosis.

Dorsiflexion assist, plantar flexion stop: Indicated for foot drop and recurvatum of the knee (weak pretibial muscles and a back knee gait)

Free plantar flexion, limited dorsiflexion: Indicated for weak gastroc-soleus complex or weak quadriceps, to prevent the ankle from falling into dorsiflexion or the knee from falling into recurvatum

Locked ankle (solid AFO): Indicated for ankle instability or pain.

36. **What are different types of knee joints employed for knee–ankle–foot orthoses (KAFOs)?**

A KAFO (knee–ankle–foot orthosis) is a brace that controls motion of the knee, ankle and foot joints. They can be all metal and leather or made from a combination of plastic, metal and Velcro. They differ from an ankle–foot orthosis by the presence of a knee joint:

Single axis: The axis is aligned with the rotational axis of the knee joint. Useful for medial/lateral stabilization. Can have a stop to prevent hyperextension (back knee gait).

Posterior offset: This offset shifts the weight bearing axis anterior to the anatomic knee joint. This provides an extension moment in early stance, but allows for free flexion during swing.

Polycentric: Allows for limited multiplanar motion during flexion and extension and is considered in patients with arthritic knees.

Drop locks: This is a knee joint which prevents knee flexion during gait. It has rings that lock the knee joint in extension, resulting in a stiff but stable gait. These orthoses are useful with severe weakness or instability and often have a manual control to unlock the orthosis and allow for flexion for the purpose of sitting.

Bail locks: Have a semicircular extension (the bail) in the back of the knee. The knee is normally locked as soon as full extension is reached, but can be unlocked by pulling on the bail or backing up to a chair. Care is required, because the bail can result in knee flexion at unexpected times if the patient bumps into something.

37. **What are the indications for a KAFO?**

Indications for a KAFO include knee instability due to weakness, injury, or paralysis that is too severe to be controlled by an AFO alone.

38. **What are the purposes of orthoses which go to the hip or higher?**

HKAFO: This orthosis provides stability to the hip and pelvis. It can be used in patients with spina bifida, spinal cord injury, and patients at risk for hip dislocation.

Reciprocating gait orthosis (RGO): This orthosis is used in similar types of patients to the HKAFO but is used more in pediatric patients. As the forward leg flexes, the RGO causes the contralateral limb to extend.

Parapodium and standers: This is a rehab tool to promote upright positioning. It is does not allow locomotion.

NEURO-ORTHOPEDICS

CASE 7-4

A 25-year-old patient presents to the outpatient clinic. He was involved in a motor vehicle collision 2 years ago, and sustained a traumatic brain injury. He now has left-sided spastic hemiplegia. His left upper extremity is held in shoulder adduction, elbow flexion, forearm pronation, and wrist flexion. He has some volitional control of the extremity. He is able to walk, but reports that it is becoming more difficult. He wears a solid AFO. On examination his foot and ankle are in equinus and varus.

39. **What are the principles of neuro-orthopedics and the orthopedic surgery of rehabilitation?**

Neuro-orthopedics is a discipline within orthopedics that deals specifically with the sequelae of neurologic injury on the musculoskeletal system. Neuro-orthopedic surgery can be used to optimize the lever system of the musculoskeletal system by lengthening tight muscles, releasing non-functional muscles, correcting contractures, transferring the tendons of working muscles to areas in which the muscles no longer work, and correcting skeletal deformities:

Operate early: Operating early results in superior results, because the deformities have not become severe and fixed. Surgical or non-surgical modalities should be selected based on which is predicted to produce optimal patient outcomes.

Better motor control = better function for the extremity: Orthopedic surgery can only optimize whatever function the injured nervous system is able to impart to the muscles. This motor control, or lack thereof, is subsequently transferred through the muscles to the bones and joints.

Distinguish the function of the individual from the function of the limb: If a patient is cognitively intact, surgical release of a contracted limb may impart independence in dressing, and maneuvering in public.

Consider the cost of not intervening: If greater independence can be imparted to a patient with diagnostic EMG analysis and surgery, the overall cost may be less than the cost of attendant care and other non-operative therapy associated with not intervening.

40. **What is the treatment for painful inferior shoulder subluxation in a paretic arm?**

This condition occurs in patients with flaccid upper extremity paralysis. They complain of pain when the limb is dependent. Physical exam reveals pain which is exacerbated by dependent positioning of the limb and is relieved by supporting the limb. Patients also commonly exhibit a sulcus sign when the limb is unsupported. These patients may be treated with a biceps suspension procedure. In this procedure, the long head of the biceps is disconnected from its muscle belly distally, and looped through bone tunnels in the proximal humerus. The humeral head is then reduced and the tendon sewed to itself.

Adduction and internal rotation contractures are often comorbid and can be treated by tendon lengthening or release at the time of suspension surgery.

41. **What is the cause of the spastic adducted internally rotated shoulder? What is the treatment?**

Spastic pectoralis major, latissimus dorsi, teres major, and subscapularis are responsible for this deformity. These muscles can be selectively lengthened through a deltopectoral incision by incising the tendon where it overlies the muscle belly. The patient is allowed active and active assistive ROM immediately after surgery. If the limb is completely non-functional, releases, rather than lengthenings, of the tendons may be performed for ease of hygiene and pain relief.

42. **What is the cause of a spastic abduction shoulder deformity? What is the treatment?**

A spastic abduction deformity most often results from an increase in tone in the supraspinatus muscle. Patients will often complain of difficulty with ambulation because they knock things over or bump into people. A *supraspinatus slide* procedure may be performed. This procedure involves surgically lengthening the supraspinatus muscle/tendon unit to allow for decreased upper extremity abduction during physical activity.

43. **When tendons are fractionally lengthened (the tendon is cut where is overlies the muscle belly) in surgery, what happens to the tendon long term?**

A new tendon forms in the lengthened area in approximately 3 weeks.

44. **What is the treatment of the spastic flexed elbow? The spastic extended elbow?**

Lengthenings of the short and long heads of the biceps are performed through an incision in the proximal, anterior arm. Next the brachialis is lengthened by transecting the tendon overlying the muscle belly on the lateral aspect of the elbow. Finally, the brachioradialis is lengthened in the upper radial forearm. Releases may be performed in the functionless arm with real or impending breakdown in the antecubital fossa. Spastic elbow extension is uncommon; it generally is a result of a brainstem level injury. A selective lengthening of the triceps distally allows for increased range of motion and ability to perform ADLs.

45. **What is the treatment of the spastic pronated forearm?**

Spastic pronation makes instrumental activities of daily living (IADL), such as feeding and grooming, difficult. The pronator quadratus and the pronator teres are responsible to a large extent. Dynamic EMG is often helpful to determine the extent to which each muscle influences the deformity observed. The pronator quadratus is found in the interval between the mobile wad and the flexor carpi radialis (FCR). The muscle is fractionally lengthened by cutting the tendon overlying the muscle belly. The pronator quadratus is found in the interval between the FCR and radial artery distally. The muscle is lengthened as described above. The arm is supinated to allow the muscle to lengthen.

46. **What is the treatment for a spastic wrist flexion contracture?**

Wrist flexion contracture is often found following brain injury or stroke. Although EMG can be used to detect the extent to which each contributes, flexor carpi radialis (FCR), flexor carpi ulnaris (FCU), palmaris longus (PL), flexor digitorum sublimis (FDS) and flexor digitorum profundus (FDP) are potential culprits. If the EMG shows volitional control of the flexors, selective lengthenings are performed in order to preserve motor control. If the goal is simply for hygiene in a non-functional limb, a wrist fusion and proximal row carpectomy with tendon releases may be performed. A superficialis to profundus transfer can be performed at the same time if a clenched fist co-exists.

47. **What are some problems associated with spastic hip adduction contracture? What is the treatment?**

Spastic hip adductors presdispose patients to a scissoring gait. Non-ambulatory patients have hygiene, positioning and skin breakdown problems. Children may have progressive hip instability due to spastic adductor muscles. In the ambulatory patient, the anterior branches of the obturator nerve can be transected. In a patient with a fixed myostatic contracture, adductor release is often needed.

48. **What are some problems associated with hip flexion contracture, how is it treated?**
A hip flexion contracture can be either a primary problem or a secondary problem that results from knee flexion contractures or incompetent triceps surae (ex. crouch gait in cerebral palsy). If the problem is secondary, the primary problem should be addressed and the hip flexion contracture reassessed and treated if still significant. The iliopsoas may be either lengthened at the pelvic brim, or at the lesser trochanter. It is possible to release the tendon distally without completely releasing the tendon due to hip capsular attachments. Some authors prefer to do the lengthening at the pelvic brim, although less correction can be expected. In the case of a non-ambulatory patient, a more extensive release of the sartorius, rectus, and iliopsoas may be performed through a Smith-Peterson anterior approach.

49. **What treatments are available for a spastic knee flexion deformity?**
Knee flexion contractures are typically due to overactivity of the hamstring muscles. If the patient has volitional control of the hamstrings, lengthening procedures are performed of both muscle groups through medial and lateral incisions. In children, a selective lengthening of the medial hamstrings may be performed for mild, dynamic contractures. On the lateral side, the iliotibial (IT) band that is posterior to the knee axis should be divided as well. In contractures over 60° or in non-ambulators, hamstring release should be performed. A knee posterior capsulotomy can be performed at the time of surgery as well. Approximately 50% of the correction can be expected at the time of initial surgery. The remainder of the correction is obtained over a period of weeks with serial weekly casting. Care must be taken to protect the neurovascular structures which are in particular risk during correction of long-standing and severe contractures.

50. **What causes spastic stiff knee gait? What is the treatment?**
Overactivity of the rectus femoris during swing phase causes the knee to inappropriately remain in an extended position throughout the gait cycle. This effectively lengthens the limb and leads to tertiary coping mechanisms such as hip hiking or circumduction. A fractional lengthening of the vastus muscles and transfer of the rectus tendon to the gracilis may be performed to transform the rectus femoris from a deforming to a correcting force.

51. **What are a group of surgeries that can be used to correct spastic equinovarus in a foot that is not in rigidly fixed equinus?**
If the foot is in rigid equinovarus or if there is underlying bony deformity, an arthrodesis procedure may be required to correct the deformity. Otherwise there is a group of procedures that can reliably produce a plantigrade foot in flexible spastic equinovarus:
Split anterior tibial tendon transfer: If the EMG reveals overactivity in the tibialis anterior muscle, it can contribute to varus positioning of the forefoot. The tendon is split, and the lateral half is transferred to the lateral side of the foot and secured in the cuboid.
Gastroc-soleus lengthening: Contracture of the Achilles tendon is often responsible for equinus position of the ankle. A Silverskold test may be used to determine if the contracture is due to the gastrocnemius alone. If this is the case, a Strayer intramuscular lengthening of the gastrocnemius is indicated. If both the gastrocnemius and the soleus are implicated in deformity, a Hoke tendo Achilles lengthening is indicated.
EHL to midfoot: Spastic equinovarus feet often are accompanied by hyperextension of the great toe. Additionally, because the tendon is on the medial foot, it can contribute to the varus position of the foot. To correct this, the tendon is disconnected distally and placed through a bone tunnel into the middle cuneiform.
Posterior tibial tendon lengthening: If the EMG reveals overactivity in the tibialis posterior muscle, it can contribute to varus positioning of the hindfoot. The tendon is lengthened.
Toe flexor releases: Following correction of the equinovarus, the toes often assume an obligate flexion position because of tenodesis effect. The toe flexors can be tenotomized distally via small plantar incisions for each toe.
Plantar fascia release: This procedure is performed through a medial incision on the midfoot and corrects cavus due to tight plantar fascia.

FDL to os calcis: In patients with the ability to ambulate, push off strength is decreased. The strength can be partially augmented by transferring the FDL tendon, which has been released, to the os calcis to augment the power of the triceps surae.

WHEELCHAIR PRESCRIPTION

CASE 7-5

A 30-year-old male who sustained a C7 spinal cord injury 4 months ago presents for a custom wheelchair prescription. He is able to transfer independently and can perform most activities of daily living. He is in a rehabilitation hospital but is about to be discharged home.

52. **What is the purpose of a custom wheelchair prescription?**
    A wheelchair prescription ensures custom seating for patients who spend a significant proportion of their day in the wheelchair. A proper wheelchair prescription promotes comfort, prevents complications such as pressure sores, and provides access to the individual who uses it.

53. **What are the different weights of manual wheelchairs available?**
    Standard weight: These wheelchairs are 40–45 pounds, provide a stable base, but allow for limited seating options and are generally a fixed frame. These wheelchairs are the typical wheelchairs found in hospitals or outpatient settings.
    Lightweight: These commercially available wheelchairs weigh between 25 and 35 pounds. They generally include some frame options, ability to adjust seat height, and enhanced seating options.
    Ultralight weight: These wheel chairs weigh between 20 and 30 pounds. These chairs are ideal for patients with spinal cord injury but normal upper body function. Ultralight weight chairs optimize self-mobilization. These chairs come in folding and rigid varieties and have a variety of seating options.
    Notably, bariatric- and pediatric-sized wheelchairs are also available, as are an array of custom and motorized chairs.

54. **What are the components of a wheelchair that may be modified in a wheelchair prescription?**
    Seat: A simple sling seat is standard in most wheelchairs. The sling seat is not optimal for *long-term* wheelchair use for a variety of reasons. These seats lead to adduction and internal rotation of the hips that can lead to pressure sores and contractures. A variety of commercially available seating systems are available to relieve pressure using air cells, or gel or foam cushions. Additionally, custom seats may be built to accommodate an individual patient's specific anatomy.
    Back: Similar to the seat, the default seat back is a sling back. This seating system is also not ideal for chronic users because it induces a kyphotic posture. Seat backs also come in a flat back, or in a standard contour to accommodate lumbar lordosis. Patients with significant orthopedic deformities or trunk control issues may require a molded seat back.
    Secondary supports: These supports are used for patients with muscle control problems. They may be placed laterally to prevent trunk listing or anteriorly to prevent flexion. Additionally, a neck support may be placed to prevent the head from falling forward.
    Leg rests: Leg rests can be standard or extendable. Extendable leg rests are helpful when it is desirable for the patient's knee to be in full extension, such as post injury (Fig. 7.5).

55. **What are some features of a wheelchair that can be addressed during wheelchair prescription?**
    Tilt in space vs. reclining: Tilt in space is often used as a permanent feature of a wheelchair (where the whole chair tilts) for the purpose of fatigue and pressure management. In reclining wheelchairs, only the seat back lowers. This feature can facilitate hygiene and is useful when the patient is post orthopedic surgery and has hip motion restrictions.
    Manual vs. power: Manual wheelchairs promote muscle usage and are not as heavy as power chairs. It is often difficult to transport a power wheelchair without a custom van or bus.

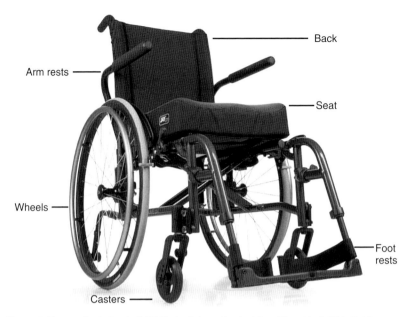

Figure 7.5. Photograph of a Quickie® QXi™ ultra lightweight wheelchair. *(Copyright © 2014, Quickie-Wheelchairs.com. All rights reserved.)*

Manual chairs can have special brakes installed, along with handle grips, to increase propulsion. Power chairs are appropriate when the patient does not have the motor control, strength, or endurance to use a manual chair.

56. **What are some important considerations about the patient's home environment that the physician must consider?**
It is important to know the general dimensions of the patient's home space. It is important to know how wide the doorways are – a wheelchair is of no use to a patient if they can't get it into their house. Additionally important questions include: how many levels are in the patient's house? Is it accessible? On which floor does the patient live? All of these questions must be addressed in order to adequately treat a patient's mobility issues with a wheelchair prescription.

AMPUTATIONS AND PROSTHETICS

CASE 7-6

A 26-year-old man was involved in a motor vehicle collision and sustained a severe open distal femur fracture with vascular injury and segmental bone loss that resulted in an above the knee amputation. He is presenting following rehabilitation for a definitive prosthetic prescription. He is athletically built and very motivated.

57. **What are some indications for amputations in children and adults?**
Amputations can be performed for a variety of reasons. In children, indications for amputations are generally congenital anomalies, trauma, and malignant tumors. In adults, peripheral vascular disease, trauma, and malignant tumors predominate, though patients with chronically infected arthroplasties or other failed reconstructive procedures may also be candidates for amputation. Amputation is a reconstructive procedure and should be thought of as such. A well-functioning amputation may perform as well, if not better, than limb salvage in select circumstances.

58. What are the levels of lower extremity amputation?
    Hemipelvectomy
    Hip disarticulation
    Trans femoral*
    Knee disarticulation
    Trans tibial*
    Ankle disarticulation*
    Partial calcanectomy
    Pirigoff
    Boyd
    Symes
    Chopart
    Trans metatarsal*
    Ray resection*
    *most common levels of amputation.

59. What are some features of hemipelvectomy and hip disarticulation?
    Hemipelvectomy is performed most often in the setting of a malignant tumor or severe trauma. Hemipelvectomies can be *internal*, in which the bony pelvis is resected but the limb remains intact. A fusion or saddle prosthesis is often utilized to stabilize the remaining limb. Hemipelvectomies can also be *external*, during which the bony pelvis is resected along with the limb attached to it. Special seating systems are necessary because of the bony imbalance that results. Hip disarticulation can be performed for vascular disease, trauma, or tumor. Patients who require hip disarticulation as a result of vascular disease have a mortality that exceeds 50%. Ambulation is generally does not require a prosthesis but utilizes crutches and a "swing-through" gait pattern.

60. What are some features of trans femoral amputations and knee disarticulations?
    Trans femoral amputations typically allow for ambulation using a prosthesis. Younger patients are better able to tolerate this amputation level than older patients because of the increased energy cost of ambulation using a prosthesis. The flexion and abduction muscular forces must be balanced during surgery to prevent subcutaneous migration of the femur (Fig. 7.6). This is done by attaching the adductors to the distal end of the residual limb using heavy suture.

    Knee disarticulations are more common in the pediatric population. In adults, knee disarticulations are performed in a setting where a trans tibial level is not possible; however, it would be beneficial to maintain length of the limb. This level makes prosthetic fitting more challenging because the knee joint is positioned on different levels compared to the other limb. Knee disarticulations may also be performed in the non-ambulatory patient with severe contractures.

61. What are some features of trans tibial amputations?
    Trans tibial amputations are the most common level of amputation for the lower extremity and can be performed for all the indications listed above. Trans tibial amputations have far less energy consumption during locomotion than more proximal amputations. A wide variety of prosthetic options are available. In the early phases of rehabilitation, it is critical to guard against knee flexion contracture. Patients must be casted or immobilized in extension soon after surgery to avoid this complication. Surgery is performed with creation of a long musculocutaneous posterior flap (Fig. 7.7) and the posterior calf muscles are myodesed to the distal end of the tibia.

62. What are some features of trans metatarsal amputations?
    Trans metatarsal amputations are one of the more common amputations performed. Often these are performed for diabetic foot wounds, infections, or vascular insufficiency. The bony cuts are made through the metatarsals or Lisfranc joints. A gastrocsoleus lengthening should be considered to prevent equinus contracture.

63. What are some complications associated with amputation surgery?
    a. *Wound breakdown*: Meticulous soft-tissue technique is necessary, nutrition should be optimized, and an assessment of vascular status is important.

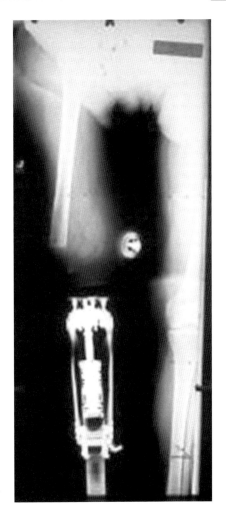

Figure 7.6. A patient status post trans femoral amputation with subcutaneous migration of the distal femur secondary to failure to perform adductor myodesis during the index surgery.

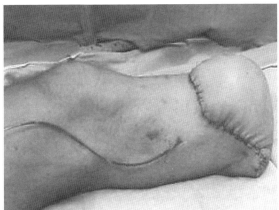

Figure 7.7. Photograph of postoperative trans tibial amputation. Note the long posterior flap and the tension free closure of the wound.

b. *Hematoma*: Large surgical drains are placed following surgery and are often maintained until dry.

c. *Swelling*: Compressive dressings are used to shrink the residual limb in order to allow it to ultimately accept a prosthesis.

d. *Joint contracture*: The residual limb is at risk to develop a contracture of the non-amputated joints, interfering with prosthetic management and gait.

e. *Phantom limb pain*: Physical modalities and medications are available to help symptomatic treatment of this complication.

f. *Residual limb breakdown*: This is generally a prosthetic issue, and the socket must be adjusted by the prosthetist.

g. *Gait problems*: Typically due to prosthetic issues, a prosthetist should be consulted to help evaluate and correct these problems.

64. **What are the general components of a prosthesis?**

a. *Socket*: The socket protects and cushions the residual limb, and transmits forces from the prosthesis to the limb.

b. *Sock or gel liner*: These devices provide extra cushioning for the residual limb and can be added or subtracted for fine tuning the fit of the prosthesis.

c. *Suspension system*: The suspension system is the way that the prosthesis is connected to the limb. It can be connected via suction fit, belt, or silicone sleeve.

d. *Articulating joint* (for trans femoral or above): The prosthesis may be polycentric or single axis. It must provide support during stance, but also smooth motion during swing and allow for flexion during sitting.

e. *Pylon*: A tube or structure that connects the socket to the terminal device.

f. *Terminal device*: This is the foot or the terminal extent of the prosthesis. It can be simple or energy storing to allow for high performance.

65. **What are some different terminal devices?**

SACH (solid-ankle/cushioned heel): This device has soft spots that allow mimicking of the normal rockers of gait. It is good for every day walking, but is not as good for uneven surfaces.

Multiaxis: This foot adds ankle motion in all planes including inversion and eversion, and is better on uneven surfaces. These feet are good for a patient with a moderate activity level.

Energy storing foot: This foot is beneficial for higher level of function and athletic endeavors.

66. **What are the energy requirements compared to normal by amputation level?**

Trans tibial: increased 10–20%
Bilateral trans tibial: increased 20–60%
Trans femoral unilateral: increased 60–70%
Bilateral trans femoral: >200%

HETEROTOPIC OSSIFICATION

CASE 7-7

A 50-year-old male is in the ICU. He has been in a coma for several weeks following a rollover motor vehicle accident. He has been receiving passive range-of-motion exercises at bedside with physical therapy. His right elbow recently became swollen and warm to the touch. His x-rays were negative. He was started on empiric antibiotics. His therapists have noticed that he has lost range of motion in the last few sessions.

67. **What is heterotopic ossification, what are some common etiologies?**

Clinically significant heterotopic ossification (HO) is the *inappropriate formation of new bone around a joint* that results in loss of range of motion. Patients at risk for heterotopic ossification are patients with traumatic brain or spinal cord injuries, direct trauma (or surgery), or burns.

68. What are some clinical signs of heterotopic bone formation?

    Patients present with pain, redness, swelling, and loss of joint motion. The clinical presentation of HO formation often leads clinicians to confuse this process with thromboembolic disease or infection.

69. What is the relationship between neurologic injury and direct trauma as it relates to heterotopic bone formation?

    Patients who receive both a traumatic neurologic insult and direct trauma are far more likely to develop heterotopic ossification. For example elbow heterotopic ossification occurs in 4% of patients with traumatic brain injury (TBI) only, but in 89% with TBI and direct elbow trauma (fracture or dislocation).

70. What is the relationship between heterotopic ossification and spasticity?

    Heterotopic ossification typically follows lines of stress. Spastic muscles produce more stress, and the heterotopic bone forms along the lines of that spastic muscle.

71. What are the most common locations of heterotopic ossification in brain injury?

    Hips and elbows are the most common sites, followed by shoulders and knees.

72. What are the most common locations of heterotopic bone in spinal cord injury?

    Hips and knees are most commonly affected.

73. What is the utility of heterotopic bone prophylaxis?

    Heterotopic ossification can be prophylaxed against with either radiation or medication. The two categories of medications that have been proposed are Diphosphonates (didronel) or NSAIDs (indomethacin). Radiation has also been proposed. Studies regarding prophylaxis have not consistently shown efficacy. Prophylaxis may still be considered in select high-risk patients (i.e., spastic TBI with an elbow dislocation).

74. What are some early diagnostic tests that can be useful in the diagnosis of heterotopic ossification?

    Radiographs may show early calcification. Technetium bone scan or ultrasound may be able to detect HO earlier, but it is unclear if the natural history of this process can be altered with currently available treatment modalities. As a result, it is questionable whether it is useful to perform earlier tests. Serum alkaline phosphatase is elevated in patients who are developing HO, though as noted, it is unclear if early intervention is helpful. Serum alkaline phosphatase is suggested to gauge "maturity" of heterotopic bone in terms of timing of excision, though in joints such as the elbow, maturity may be less important than intervening prior to the onset of stiffness. Most authors recommend obtaining plain films. If the plain films show a clear cortical margin then excision can be safely performed; however, the timing of excision of HO remains controversial.

75. Where does heterotopic bone form in the hip?

    Anterior: The HO typically follows the iliopsoas muscle, often involving neurovascular structures (femoral nerve/artery, profunda femoris). The femoral nerve is most often involved in the heterotopic bone, but any vital structure can be encased.

    Lateral: HO typically is found adjacent to the abductor muscles. Care must be taken to preserve the abductors, if possible, during excision.

    Medial: HO is often found from the pubis to the anteromedial femoral shaft, following the abductor musculature. A medial approach to the hip is used to excise the HO.

    Posterior: HO is often found from the ilium to the posterior shaft of the femur, often encasing the sciatic nerve. The sciatic nerve is freed from the heterotopic bone and then more aggressive resection can be pursued (Fig. 7.8).

76. What is the indication to resect heterotopic bone about the knee?

    Heterotopic bone about the knee is resected if it causes pain or limits motion. Occasionally heterotopic bone will form in the setting of an MCL injury (Pellegrini–Steida lesion). Care must be taken to protect the stability of the knee postoperatively with a hinged knee brace.

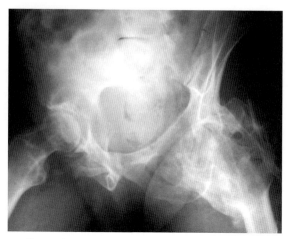

Figure 7.8. Obturator oblique Judet view of the left hip/hemipelvis demonstrating extensive heterotopic ossification around the hip joint, causing ankylosis.

77. **When is heterotopic bone about the elbow resected?**

Elbow HO is resected early if the patient's medical condition allows. Outcome studies favor resection before the elbow gets stiff. Improved range of motion can be expected in most patients, though in patients with compromised motor control, range of motion gains are less reliable.

SPINAL CORD INJURY

CASE 7-8

You are called to see an intubated patient in the trauma bay. She is an 18-year-old female who attempted suicide earlier that night. She crashed her car into a brick wall. She has multiple long bone fractures, as well as a C6 spinal facet dislocation. Her distraught parents are inquiring about prognosis.

78. **What is "spinal shock," how can one tell when spinal shock has ended?**

Spinal shock is the complete loss of motor and sensory level below the level of the injury in spinal cord injury. Polysynaptic reflexes such as the bulbocavernosus reflex are the first to return. The return of these reflexes indicates the end of spinal shock. At this point in time, the maximum ability of the level of the spinal cord injury will become apparent (i.e., the strength of the muscles below the level of the injury zone). Monosynaptic reflexes will return at a later time and will be hyper-reflexive because they have been released from the control of the central nervous system.

79. **What is the definition of "level" of spinal cord injury?**

The level of the spinal cord injury is the most caudal level that has normal motor and sensory function.

80. **Describe the ASIA classification.**

The ASIA classification is a descriptor of the completeness of a spinal cord injury:

ASIA A: Complete injury with no motor or sensory below the injury and no sacral sparing

ASIA B: Sensory incomplete; preservation of sensation below the level of the injury

ASIA C: Motor incomplete; voluntary anal sphincter contraction, motor grade 3 or less below

ASIA D: Motor incomplete; voluntary anal sphincter contraction, motor grade 3 or greater below

ASIA E: Normal; may have hyperreflexia.

81. What are the functional levels of spinal cord injury?

    C1–4: These patients are dependent for activities of daily living (ADLs). They are ventilator dependent and need total care, but may use sip and puff power wheelchair for mobility.

    C5: These patients have intact elbow flexion. With special modifications, they may be able to self-feed and groom and can use a power chair with hand controls. Driving is possible for the motivated individual with specialized hand controls

    C6: These patients have intact wrist extension. Extension of the wrist allows for a limited tenodesis grip. It is technically possible for a C6 tetraplegic individual to function without assistance, though this is not common. Elbows can be locked in extension which can allow for independent sliding board transfers. Wheelchair mobility is possible with a power chair with hand controls. These individuals can assist with dressing and some can dress their upper bodies independently. With assistive technology, they can answer the phone and turn pages.

    C7: These patients have intact elbow extension. The ability to extend the elbow greatly enhances the patient's ability to perform ADLs. Active extension allows for independent transfers, bed mobility, feeding, and upper body dressing. They may use a manual wheelchair, but will not be able to go over curbs. This level is the highest level that patients can be functionally independent in any reliable sense.

    C8: These patients have intact finger flexion. The ability to flex the fingers allows for increased dexterity and the ability to use a manual wheelchair on even and uneven surfaces. These patients are independent with most ADLs, bed mobility transfers, and bowel and bladder care.

    Thoracic level: These patients are usually independent with ADLs. Lower thoracic levels may occasionally be able to use KAFOs, crutches, and swing through gait for ambulation. Unfortunately, the energy expenditure required for this type of ambulation causes most of these patients to rely on wheelchairs for mobility.

    Lumbar level: Function varies by the level injured, but in general, these patients may be independent community ambulators. They may require gait aids, such as crutches, or orthotics, such as AFOs or KAFOs.

82. What are common purposes of orthopedic surgery in spinal cord injury?

    Orthopedic surgery can assist by transferring working muscles to replace the function of non-working muscles. One must note that when transferring a tendon, the muscle associated with that tendon loses one grade of strength. The most high-yield transfers give C5 spinal-cord-injured patients wrist and elbow extension, give C6 spinal cord injured patients elbow extension, and give C7 patients increased dexterity in their hand. These techniques require a motivated patient and an experienced surgeon.

BIBLIOGRAPHY

1. Akbar M, Balean G, Brunner M, et al. Prevalence of rotator cuff tear in paraplegic patients compared with controls. J Bone Joint Surg Am 2010;92:23–30.
2. Baldwin K, Hosalkar H, Donegan D, et al. Surgical resection of elbow heterotopic ossification: outcomes in post-traumatic and brain injured patients. J Hand Surg [Am] 2011;36:798–803.
3. Botte MJ, Keenan MA, Abrams RA, et al. Heterotopic ossification in neuromuscular disorders. Orthopedics 1997;20:335–41, 342–3.
4. Botte MJ, Keenan MA, Gellman H, et al. Surgical management of spastic thumb-in-palm deformity in adults with brain injury. J Hand Surg [Am] 1989;14:174–82.
5. Botte MJ, Keenan MA, Korchek JI, et al. Modified technique for the superficialis-to-profundus transfer in the treatment of adults with spastic clenched fist deformity. J Hand Surg [Am] 1987;12: 639–40.
6. Chae J, Mascarenhas D, Yu DT, et al. Post stroke shoulder pain: its relationship to motor impairment, activity limitation, and quality of life. Arch Phys Med Rehabil 2007;88:298–301.
7. Chan KT. Heterotopic ossification in traumatic brain injury. Am J Phys Med Rehabil 2005; 84:145–6.
8. Cipriano CA, Pill SG, Keenan MA. Heterotopic ossification following traumatic brain injury and spinal cord injury. J Am Acad Orthop Surg 2009;17:689–97.
9. Esquenazi A, Mayer NH, Keenan MA. Dynamic polyelectromyography, neurolysis, and chemodenervation with botulinum toxin A for assessment and treatment of gait dysfunction. Adv Neurol 2001; 87:321–31.

10. Fuller DA, Keenan MA, Esquenazi A, et al. The impact of instrumented gait analysis on surgical planning: treatment of spastic equinovarus deformity of the foot and ankle. Foot Ankle Int 2002;23:738–43.

11. Garland DE, Keenan MA. Orthopedic strategies in the management of the adult head-injured patient. Phys Ther 1983;63:2004–9.

12. Hebela N, Keenan MA. Neuro-orthopedic management of the dysfunctional extremity in upper motor neuron syndromes. Eura Medicophys 2004;40:145–56.

13. Horstmann HM, Hosalkar H, Keenan MA. Orthopaedic issues in the musculoskeletal care of adults with cerebral palsy. Dev Med Child Neurol 2009;51(Suppl. 4):99–105.

14. Keenan MA. The management of spastic equinovarus deformity following stroke and head injury. Foot Ankle Clin 2011;16:499–514.

15. Keenan MA. Surgical decision making for residual limb deformities following traumatic brain injury. Orthop Rev 1988;17:1185–92.

16. Keenan MA. Management of the spastic upper extremity in the neurologically impaired adult. Clin Orthop Relat Res 1988;233:116–25.

17. Keenan MA, Esquenazi A, Mayer NH. Surgical treatment of common patterns of lower limb deformities resulting from upper motoneuron syndrome. Adv Neurol 2001;87:333–46.

18. Keenan MA, Haider TT, Stone LR. Dynamic electromyography to assess elbow spasticity. J Hand Surg 1990;15:607–14.

19. Keenan MA, Kauffman DL, Garland DE, et al. Late ulnar neuropathy in the brain-injured adult. J Hand Surg 1988;13:120–4.

20. Keenan MA, Korchek JI, Botte MJ, et al. Results of transfer of the flexor digitorum superficialis tendons to the flexor digitorum profundus tendons in adults with acquired spasticity of the hand. J Bone Joint Surg Am 1987;69:1127–32.

21. Keenan MA, Lee GA, Tuckman AS, et al. Improving calf muscle strength in patients with spastic equinovarus deformity by transfer of the long toe flexors to the os calcis. J Head Trauma Rehabil 1999;14(2):163–75.

22. Keenan MA, Mehta S. Neuro-orthopedic management of shoulder deformity and dysfunction in brain-injured patients: a novel approach. J Head Trauma Rehabil 2004;19:143–54.

23. Keenan MA, Ure K, Smith CW, et al. Hamstring release for knee flexion contracture in spastic adults. Clin Orthop Relat Res 1988;236:221–6.

24. Kozin SH, Keenan MA. Using dynamic electromyography to guide surgical treatment of the spastic upper extremity in the brain-injured patient. Clin Orthop Relat Res 1993;288:109–17.

25. Lusskin R, Grynbaum BB, Dhir RS. Rehabilitation surgery in adult spastic hemiplegia. Clin Orthop Relat Res 1959;63:132–41.

26. Namdari S, Alosh H, Baldwin K, et al. Outcomes of tendon fractional lengthenings to improve shoulder function in patients with spastic hemiparesis. J Shoulder Elbow Surg. E-publish ahead of print available: <http://www.jshoulderelbow.org/inpress>.

27. Namdari S, Alosh H, Baldwin K, et al. Shoulder tenotomies to improve passive motion and relieve pain in patients with spastic hemiparesis after upper motor neuron injury. J Shoulder Elbow Surg 2011;20:802–6.

28. Namdari S, Horneff JG, Baldwin K, et al. Muscle releases to improve passive motion and relieve pain in patients with spastic hemiplegia and elbow flexion contractures. J Shoulder Elbow Surg. E-published ahead of print available: <http://www.jshoulderelbow.org/inpress>.

29. Namdari S, Keenan MA. Treatment of glenohumeral arthrosis and inferior shoulder subluxation in an adult with cerebral palsy: a case report. J Bone Joint Surg Am 2011;93:e1401–5.

30. Namdari S, Keenan MA. Outcomes of the biceps suspension procedure for painful inferior glenohumeral subluxation in hemiplegic patients. J Bone Joint Surg Am 2010;92:2589–97.

31. Namdari S, Park MJ, Baldwin K, et al. Correcting spastic equinovarus foot in patients with hemiparetic stroke: do age, sex, and timing matter? Foot Ankle Int 2009;30:923–7.

32. Namdari S, Pill SG, Makani A, et al. Rectus femoris to gracilis muscle transfer with fractional lengthening of the vastus muscles: a treatment for adults with stiff knee gait. Phys Ther 2010;90:261–8. [Epub 2009, Dec 18].

33. Namdari S, Yagnik G, Ebaugh DD, et al. Defining functional shoulder range of motion for activities of daily living. J Shoulder Elbow Surg 2012;21:1177–83.

34. Pappas N, Baldwin K, Keenan MA. Efficacy of median nerve recurrent branch neurectomy as an adjunct to ulnar motor nerve neurectomy and wrist arthrodesis at the time of superficialis to profundus transfer in prevention of intrinsic spastic thumb-in-palm deformity. J Hand Surg [Am] 2010;35:1310–16.

35. Patrick JH, Keenan MA. Gait analysis to assist walking after stroke. Lancet 2007; 369:256–7.

36. Pill SG, Keenan MA. Neuro-orthpaedic management of extremity dysfunction in patients with spasticity from upper motor neuron syndromes. In: Brashear A, Mayer NH, editors. Spasticity and other forms of muscle overactivity in the upper motor neuron syndrome. We Move; 2008. p. 119–41.

37. Pomerance JF, Keenan MA. Correction of severe spastic flexion contractures in the nonfunctional hand. J Hand Surg 1996;21:828–33.

38. Rayan GM, Young BT. Arthrodesis of the spastic wrist. J Hand Surg [Am] 1999;24:944–52.

39. Reddy S, Kusuma S, Hosalkar H, et al. Surgery can reduce the nonoperative care associated with an equinovarus foot deformity. Clin Orthop Relat Res 2008;466:1683–7.

40. Rubertone J, Baldwin K, Bucknum J, et al. Reliability analysis of the Wisconsin gait scale for novice evaluators. Phys Ther 2000;80:(published abstract).

41. Sciascia A, Thigpen C, Namdari S, et al. Kinetic chain abnormalities in the athletic shoulder. Sports Med Arthrosc 2012;20:16–21.

42. Yarkony GM, Roth E, Lovell L, et al. Rehabilitation outcomes in complete C5 quadriplegia. Am J Phys Med Rehabil 1988;67:73–6.

43. Yarkony GM, Roth EJ, Heinemann AW, et al. Rehabilitation outcomes in C6 tetraplegia. Paraplegia 1988;26:177–85.

44. Young S, Keenan MA, Stone LR. The treatment of spastic planovalgus foot deformity in the neurologically impaired adult. Foot Ankle 1990;10:317–24.

CHAPTER 8

SHOULDER AND ELBOW

Surena Namdari and Jason E. Hsu

SUBACROMIAL SYNDROMES

CASE 8-1

A 65-year-old male presents to the office with a chief of complaint of persistent right shoulder pain for 4 months. He denies any trauma or specific injury that preceded the pain. He notes that pain is on the lateral aspect of the shoulder and is aggravated by overhead activities and he has been unable to swim recreationally for several months. The patient denies fevers, chills, or other constitutional symptoms. On physical examination, he has full range of motion but notes pain with active forward elevation and abduction beyond 90°. He has full strength, but pain with resisted forward elevation and abduction.

1. What are the most common differential diagnoses of exertional shoulder pain?
   - Subacromial syndromes (rotator cuff tears, tendinitis, impingement)
   - Shoulder instability
   - Cervical radiculitis
   - Acromioclavicular degenerative disease
   - Glenohumeral arthrosis
   - Suprascapular nerve entrapment
   - Thoracic outlet syndrome.

2. What are the causes of subacromial syndromes?
   - Repetitive overhead use
   - Trauma
   - Forward sloping acromion or hooked or curved acromion
   - Os acromiale
   - Shoulder instability
   - Technique errors during overhead shoulder sports.

3. What is subacromial impingement syndrome?
   Subacromial impingement syndrome is believed to result from external compression on the rotator cuff from the anterior acromion, coracoacromial ligament (CAL), and acromioclavicular joint. Secondary causes of impingement include tuberosity fracture nonunion or malunion, a mobile os acromiale, calcific tendinitis, instability, and iatrogenic factors.

4. What two physical examination maneuvers have been classically described for impingement syndrome?
   Neer impingement test: pain with passive forward elevation with the shoulder in internal rotation
   Hawkins impingement test: pain with passive forward elevation to 90°, cross-body adduction, and internal rotation.

5. What are some possible etiologies of shoulder pain that are related to subacromial impingement syndrome?
   1. Subacromial bursitis
   2. Rotator cuff tendinopathy
   3. Partial- and full-thickness rotator cuff tear.

6. Describe the treatment of subacromial syndromes.
   - Modification of activities, avoiding repetitive overhead use or technique errors
   - Ice and non-steroidal antiinflammatory drugs (NSAIDs)
   - Therapeutic exercises and stretching
   - Subacromial injections
   - Surgical decompression and repair of rotator cuff tears.

7. What are the different types of acromial morphology and how do they relate to rotator cuff disease?
   1. Acromial morphology is classified into three types based on acromial shape on a scapular Y radiograph or sagittal CT or MRI images (Fig. 8.1):
      Type I = flat
      Type II = curved
      Type III = hooked
   2. A hook-shaped acromion has been associated, in some studies, with rotator cuff degeneration and tears.

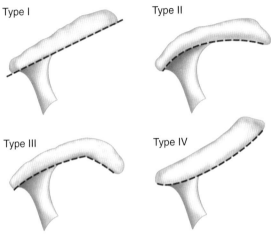

Type I Type II Type III Type IV

Figure 8.1. Acromial configuration. The acromial type is determined by the configuration of the undersurface of the acromion. Acromial types II (gentle undersurface curvature) and III (anterior hook) place an individual at an increased risk for the clinical syndrome of impingement. (*Reprinted from Morrison W, Sanders T: Problem Solving in Musculoskeletal Imaging, 1st ed, pp. 327–407. Copyright © 2008, with permission from Mosby, Elsevier Inc.*)

8. Do all rotator cuff tears result from subacromial impingement syndrome?
   No. The cause of rotator cuff tears is likely multifactorial and includes various degrees of external compression, age-related degeneration, trauma, and vascular compromise.

9. What four muscles make up the rotator cuff? What nerve innervates each muscle? What is the function of each muscle? Where does it insert? (Fig. 8.2) (Table 8.1)

10. What is the anatomy of the rotator cuff footprint?
    1. Supraspinatus: Triangular in shape, with an average maximum medial-to-lateral length of 6.9 mm and an average maximum anteroposterior width of 12.6 mm
    2. Infraspinatus: Trapezoidal in shape, with an average maximum medial-to-lateral length of 10.2 mm and an average maximum anteroposterior width of 32.7 mm
    3. Teres minor: Triangular in shape, with an average maximum medial-to-lateral length of 29 mm and an average maximum width of 21 mm
    4. Subscapularis: Comma-shaped insertion, with an average maximum medial-to-lateral length of 40 mm and an average maximum width of 20 mm.

11. What is the spectrum of rotator cuff pathology?
    1. No tear:
       a. Tendinopathy: degenerative process with little evidence of inflammation:
          i. Macroscopic studies show disorganized, soft, yellow-brown tendons with loss of the normal, tightly bundled appearance. Microscopically, there is increased collagen fiber turnover, fibrosis, and neovascularization. The proliferation of fibroblastic and vascular tissue found in damaged tendons is referred to as angiofibroblastic hyperplasia.

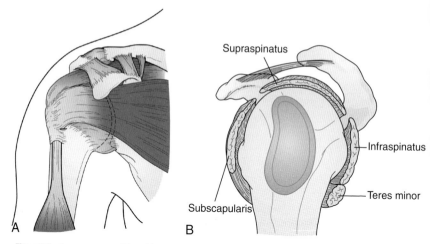

Figure 8.2. Anteroposterior (A) and lateral cross-sectional (B) drawings of the shoulder demonstrate the relationship of the rotator cuff muscles (supraspinatus, infraspinatus, teres minor, and subscapularis) to the bony structure of the shoulder. (*From Rakel RE, Rakel DP, [eds] Textbook of Family Medicine, 8th ed, pp. 601–630. Copyright © 2011, with permission from Saunders, Elsevier Inc.*)

Table 8.1. Rotator Cuff Anatomy

MUSCLE	NERVE	SHOULDER FUNCTION	INSERTION
Supraspinatus	Suprascapular	Primary initiator of elevation	Greater tuberosity
Infraspinatus	Suprascapular	External rotation	Greater tuberosity
Teres minor	Axillary	External rotation	Greater tuberosity
Subscapularis	Upper and lower subscapular	Internal rotation	Lesser tuberosity

   b. Tendonitis/bursitis: inflammatory condition that is generally acute in nature and affects the rotator cuff tendons and potential space between the rotator cuff and the acromion

2. Partial-thickness tear: tear that does not extend through the entire width of the tendon
   a. Can be articular sided, bursal sided, intratendinous, or a combination of these patterns

3. Full-thickness tear: tear that extends through the entire width of the tendon
   a. Traumatic: acute, generally with immediate weakness and pain
      i. Accounts for only 8% of those who present with symptomatic rotator cuff tears
   b. Degenerative: chronic, generally with poorer tendon and muscle quality

12. **What is typically found in the history and physical examination of a patient with a rotator cuff tear?**
Patients typically present complaining of pain that is exacerbated by overhead activity. Night discomfort, weakness, and loss of motion are also common complaints.
    On inspection, atrophy of the supraspinatus and infraspinatus may indicate a large, chronic tear. Passive shoulder motion is often preserved with rotator cuff tearing; however, active motion is often limited due to pain or weakness. Muscle strength should be utilized to test strength, but it is important to remember that strength can be limited by pain. The supraspinatus is tested with the shoulder abducted to 90°, flexed 30°, and then maximally

internally rotated. Downward pressure exerted by the examiner is resisted primarily by the supraspinatus. The infraspinatus is tested with the shoulder adducted at the side while the elbows are fixed 90°. The examiner resists active external rotation.

13. **What are the changes that can be seen on a plain radiograph in the setting of chronic rotator cuff pathology?**
    1. Sclerosis at the undersurface of the acromion
    2. Calcification within the coracoacromial ligament
    3. Cystic changes in the greater tuberosity
    4. Proximal humeral migration with large-sized tears

14. **What is the classification system for fatty degeneration of the rotator cuff?**
    The Goutallier classification is used to determine fatty degeneration. It was initially described using CT scans; however, most orthopedists today utilize MRI:
    Stage 0: Normal muscle
    Stage 1: Some fatty streaks
    Stage 2: Less than 50% fatty muscle atrophy
    Stage 3: 50% fatty muscle atrophy
    Stage 4: Greater than 50% fatty muscle atrophy

15. **On what MRI/CT view is this classification done?**
    The measurement is made on a sagittal cut at level of the medial border of the spine of the scapula. The T1 sagittal series is typically used to determine muscle quality (Fig. 8.3).

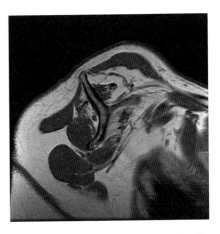

Figure 8.3. Sagittal magnetic resonance image of the shoulder showing fatty infiltration of the supraspinatus, infraspinatus, and subscapularis muscles. *(From DeLee JC, et al. [eds], DeLee and Drez's Orthopaedic Sports Medicine, 3rd ed, pp. 769–115. Copyright © 2010, with permission from Saunders, Elsevier Inc.)*

16. **a) On what orthogonal MRI view is level of tendon retraction best determined?**
    b) Medial–lateral width of the tear? c) Anterior–posterior width of the tear?
    d) Presence of a subscapularis tear?
    a. Coronal
    b. Coronal
    c. Sagittal
    d. Axial.

17. **What is the relationship between age and rotator cuff tear? How common are bilateral rotator cuff tears?**
    There is a high correlation between the onset of rotator cuff tears (either partial or full thickness) and increasing age. Twenty-eight percent of those over 60 years of age have a full-thickness tear, while 65% of patients older than 70 years have a full-thickness tear. Bilateral rotator cuff disease, either symptomatic or asymptomatic, is common in patients who present with unilateral symptomatic disease. There is a 50% likelihood of a bilateral tear after the age of 66 years, and patients who present with a full-thickness symptomatic tear have a 35.5% prevalence of a full-thickness tear on the contralateral side.

18. When should one be concerned about tear progression in a patient with an asymptomatic rotator cuff tear?

Pain development in shoulders with an asymptomatic rotator cuff tear is associated with an increase in tear size.

19. How are partial-thickness rotator cuff tears treated?

Partial-thickness tears can be articular sided, bursal sided, intratendinous, or a combination. If non-operative treatment is unsuccessful, surgical treatment is considered. Though this is controversial; in general, when tears involve <50% of the tendon, they are debrided and when tears involve >50% of the tendon they are repaired. Further controversy exists regarding how to repair a partial tear, with some advocating repair in situ while others recommending completion of the tear to a full-thickness tear followed by repair.

CASE 8-1 continued

The patient undergoes an MRI of the right shoulder that demonstrates a small, full-thickness tear of the supraspinatus. The patient elects to undergo non-operative treatment with physical therapy and a corticosteroid injection. After 8 weeks, the patient's pain is improved and she is satisfied with her treatment. Six months later, the patient presents with complaint of worsening shoulder pain and weakness for 1 week after a fall. A repeat MRI is obtained that demonstrates a large, full-thickness tear involving the entire supraspinatus and half of the infraspinatus (Fig. 8.4). The tendons are retracted to the level of the level of the glenoid. Muscle quality is assessed and noted to be Goutallier stage 1. Treatment options are discussed and the patient elects to undergo an attempted rotator cuff repair.

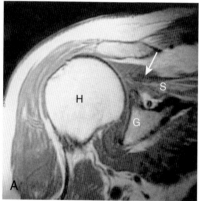 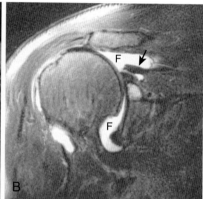

Figure 8.4. Rotator cuff tear with retraction. (A) T1-weighted oblique coronal MR image of the shoulder shows elevation of the humeral head (H) in relation to the glenoid (G). There is narrowing of the distance between the humeral head and the acromion. The supraspinatus (S) is atrophic and infiltrated with fat. The dark tendon (arrow) is seen retracted proximally. (B) Oblique coronal T2-weighted image is better at showing the torn, retracted edge of the supraspinatus tendon (arrow). The joint fluid (F) is bright on this sequence and communicates through the rotator cuff defect with the subacromial subdeltoid bursal fluid. (*From Firestein GS, et al. [eds], Kelley's Textbook of Rheumatology: 8th ed, pp. 753–769.e4. Copyright © Saunders, Elsevier Inc., 2009.*)

20. What are the healing rates for rotator cuff repairs?

Failure of rotator cuff healing after surgical repair remains one of the most common and well-known complications, and recent studies have reported structural failure rates can range from 30% to 94%.

21. Does rotator cuff repair reverse fatty infiltration of muscle or tendon atrophy?

A successful repair does not necessarily lead to improvement or reversal of muscle degeneration and a failed repair often results in significantly more progression. In general, healed repairs demonstrate minimal progression. As a result, many believe that repairs should be performed, if possible, before more significant deterioration in the cuff musculature in order to optimize outcomes.

22. **How has the operative approach to rotator cuff repair evolved?**
    1. Open repair: Traditionally, rotator cuff repair was conducted via an open approach. Open repair involves elevation of the anterior deltoid off of the anterior acromion and lateral clavicle. Disadvantages of the open approach included need for deltoid detachment, large incision size, difficulty in visualizing the glenohumeral joint, and a potentially higher infection rate.
    2. Mini-open repair: With the advent of arthroscopy, rotator cuff repair evolved to a mini-open approach. In this technique, the glenohumeral joint is evaluated with an arthroscope and the subacromial space is decompressed using arthroscopic techniques. The rotator cuff tear is identified and traction sutures are often placed into the tear edges. Once this is complete and the tear has been mobilized, the deltoid is split in a limited-open approach, the cuff tear is identified, and fixation is completed.
    3. All-arthroscopic repair: The trend today is for all-arthroscopic rotator cuff repair. Specific arthroscopic rotator cuff repair techniques are beyond the scope of this text; however, it is important for the reader to know that a recent systematic review demonstrated that there is no statistically significant difference in postoperative ASES, UCLA, or pain scores or incidence of recurrent rotator cuff tears in rotator cuffs repaired all-arthroscopically versus using the mini-open technique. However, there might be decreased short-term pain in patients who undergo arthroscopic repairs.

23. **What are the different rotator cuff repair constructs? How do they compare?**
    - *Transosseous* repairs refer to the repairs that are often performed by using open and mini-open techniques in which sutures are placed directly through transosseous tunnels for soft-tissue fixation.
    - *Single-row* repairs are performed by placing bone anchors in a linear fashion (usually 1 to 2 anchors placed laterally).
    - *Double-row* repairs include techniques that use some configuration of a medial row of suture anchors placed at the articular cartilage margin of the anatomic neck and a second more laterally placed row along the lateral edge of the rotator cuff footprint along the tuberosity. Transosseous equivalent repairs use suture anchors to achieve what is considered to resemble biomechanically traditional open transosseous repair.

      Transosseous repairs are shown to have the highest ultimate load resistance and the lowest gap formation. Double-row repairs, especially using a "transosseous-equivalent technique," are designed to achieve initial fixation strength comparable to that of open or mini-open transosseous repair. Biomechanical studies comparing single-row repair and double-row repair show increased load to failure, improved contact at the tendon–bone interface, and decreased gap formation with the latter. It is unknown whether double-row repairs lead to better healing rates or better clinical outcomes.

24. **What variables are associated with failed rotator cuff repair?**
    Advanced patient age and two or more torn rotator cuff tendons correlate with failure of repair. Additionally, failed rotator cuff repair is associated with advanced muscle atrophy and fatty degeneration. Intrinsic patient factors such as medical comorbidities may impede rotator cuff healing. Clinically, diabetic patients have worse results and higher rates of infection and failure than non-diabetic patients. Smoking has also been shown to increase the failure rate and worsen clinical results.

25. **What is the most common mechanism of injury in acute subscapularis tears?**
    The mechanism is a forced external rotation with or without abduction.

26. **What physical examination maneuvers, when positive, may indicate a tear of the subscapularis?**
    Lift-off test (Fig. 8.5a): Inability to maintain active maximal internal rotation with the hand away from the lumbar spine without extending the elbow. This test activates the lower subscapularis muscle.
    Belly-press test (Fig. 8.5b): Inability to maintain maximal internal rotation without the elbow moving posterior to the sagittal plane of the trunk. This test activates the upper subscapularis muscle.

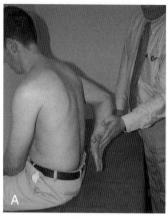
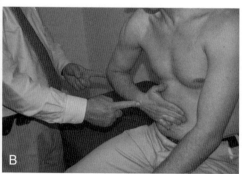

Figure 8.5. Tests for evaluating rotator cuff integrity. (A) Lift-off test. (B) Belly press test. *(From Canale ST, Beaty JH [eds], Campbell's Operative Orthopaedics, 12th ed, pp. 2364–2377.e1. Copyright © 2013, Mosby Elsevier Inc.)*

27. **What physical examination maneuver, when positive, may indicate a tear of the teres minor?**
    Hornblower test: Weakness or inability to achieve full external rotation with the shoulder in an abducted position.

28. **What is suprascapular nerve entrapment? How is it diagnosed?**
    Suprascapular nerve entrapment may cause symptoms that mimic the findings associated with rotator cuff tear. Suprascapular nerve entrapment can also co-exist with rotator cuff tear. Symptoms include posterior shoulder pain and rotator cuff weakness. The diagnosis is established with electromyographic testing.

29. **What is the anatomy of the suprascapular nerve and where is the suprascapular nerve usually entrapped?**
    The suprascapular nerve arises from the *upper trunk* of the brachial plexus and travels posteriorly through the suprascapular notch just medial to the base of the coracoid. The nerve can be compressed in two locations: in the suprascapular notch and along the neck of the spine of the scapula at the spinoglenoid notch. The nerve is most often compressed at the suprascapular notch by a thickened or ossified transverse scapular ligament. Traction injury to the nerve has been described with cases of massive retracted rotator cuff tears and compression in the spinoglenoid notch has been associated with labral cysts. Compression at the suprascapular notch presents with dull pain in the posterior-lateral shoulder and can lead to *atrophy of the supraspinatus and infraspinatus*. In contrast, compression at the spinoglenoid notch can be pain-free and *atrophy is limited to the infraspinatus*.

30. **What is the treatment of suprascapular nerve entrapment?**
    The initial treatment, in the absence of a space-occupying lesion, should involve symptom management with analgesics and physical therapy. Surgical treatment is indicated when non-operative management is not successful after 6–12 months. Surgery involves decompression of the nerve at the spinoglenoid or suprascapular notch by open or arthroscopic approaches.

31. **What are treatment options for massive irreparable rotator cuff tears?**
    Treatment for this entity is controversial. Some authors advocate arthroscopic subacromial decompression and wide debridement of the cuff tear as a means of affording pain relief. Latissimus dorsi tendon transfer to the greater tuberosity can be used to treat irreparable posterosuperior tears (supraspinatus/infraspinatus/teres minor). Pectoralis major transfer to the lesser tuberosity can be used to treat irreparable subscapularis tears. Ideal patients for these transfers are young, with good deltoid function, and have not undergone prior surgery.

ACROMIOCLAVICULAR AND STERNOCLAVICULAR INJURIES

CASE 8-2

A 22-year-old male presents to the office after a fall from a bicycle 2 days ago in which he suffered a direct blow to the shoulder. He complains of pain, difficulty elevating the shoulder, and a prominence on the superior aspect of the shoulder. He is neurovascularly intact and denies other symptoms. He initially presented to the Emergency Department where he was placed in a sling.

32. **What is the anatomy of the acromioclavicular (AC) joint?**
    The medial aspect of the acromion and the lateral aspect of the clavicle meet to form a diarthrodial joint with hyaline articular cartilage and a synovial-lined joint capsule. At this articulation is a small, fibrocartilaginous disc.

33. **What provides stability to the AC joint?**
    The AC ligaments, the coracoclavicular ligaments (conoid and trapezoid), the coracoacromial ligament (CA), the joint capsule, and the attachments of the deltoid and trapezius provide stability. The acromioclavicular ligaments are the primary restraint to anterior–posterior forces and the coracoclavicular ligaments are the primary restraints to superiorly directed forces. The trapezoid attaches to the undersurface of the clavicle at an anterolateral position and the conoid attaches to the undersurface of the clavicle at a posteromedial position (Fig. 8.6).

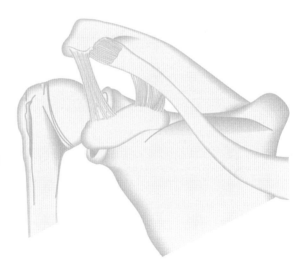

Figure 8.6. Normal anatomy of the acromioclavicular joint. (From Rockwood CA Jr, et al., Disorders of the Acromioclavicular Joint, In: Rockwood CA Jr, Matsen FA III, Wirth MA, Lippitt SB [eds]: The Shoulder, 3rd ed, pp. 453–526. Philadelphia, Saunders, Copyright © 2004.)

34. **Why can pain related to the AC joint be difficult to distinguish from pain related to the glenohumeral joint?**
    There is a dual innervation of the AC joint by the lateral pectoral nerve and the suprascapular nerve.

35. **Describe the most common mechanism of injury to the AC joint.**
    The AC joint is most commonly injured by a direct fall onto the point of the shoulder with the arm adducted.

36. **What physical examination maneuvers can isolate the AC joint?**
    - Direct tenderness to palpation at the AC joint
    - Pain at the AC joint with AC joint compression test (movement of the AC joint while isolating the glenohumeral joint)
    - Pain at the AC joint with cross-body adduction.

37. **What shoulder radiographic views are typically used to assess an AC joint injury?**
A standard anteroposterior, axillary, scapular Y, and Zanca view are recommended and are usually sufficient to distinguish the type of injury. A *Zanca view* is created by tilting the x-ray beam 15° in a cephalad direction. The axillary view is important to determine anterior–posterior translation of the clavicle with respect to the acromion.

38. **How are AC joint injuries classified? (See Table 8.2.)**

Table 8.2. Rockwood Classification of Acromioclavicular Joint Injuries

TYPE	AC LIGAMENTS	CC LIGAMENTS	DELTOPECTORAL FASCIA	INCREASE IN CC DISTANCE	RADIOGRAPHIC APPEARANCE	REDUCIBLE
I	Sprained	Intact	Intact	Normal	Normal	N/A
II	Disrupted	Sprained	Intact	<25%	Widened	Yes
III	Disrupted	Disrupted	Disrupted	25–100%	Widened	Yes
IV	Disrupted	Disrupted	Disrupted	Increased	Posterior displacement	No
V	Disrupted	Disrupted	Disrupted	100–300%	N/A	No
VI	Disrupted	Intact	Disrupted	Decreased	N/A	

(Adapted from Simovitch et al. J Am Acad Orthop Surg 2009 Apr;17(4):207–19).

CASE 8-2 continued

The patient is seen in the office and physical examination demonstrates a prominence of the clavicle at the AC joint. The patient undergoes standard AC joint radiographs and is noted to have a type V AC joint separation. He discusses treatment options and elects to undergo AC joint reconstruction.

39. **How is an acute type I or type II acromioclavicular injury treated?**
Ice and immobilization are needed initially. Patients are usually most comfortable in an arm sling. Early introduction of range-of-motion exercises is recommended.

40. **What type of treatment is recommended for acute type IV through type VI injuries?**
Type IV injuries often require operative treatment because the clavicle is buttonholed through the trapezius and remains painful, especially with overhead activities. Operative treatment is recommended for open injuries, type VI injuries, and when the clavicle is subcutaneous and in danger of eroding through the skin (type V). Operative treatment consists of repair or reconstruction of the coracoclavicular structures. Multiple methods of open and arthroscopic reconstruction have been described, ranging from anatomic suture fixation to coracoacromial ligament transfer to anatomic coracoclavicular ligament reconstruction using allograft or autograft tendon. In general, pins or wires placed across the acromioclavicular joint are avoided due to risk of migration.

41. **What type of treatment is recommended for acute type III AC joint injuries?**
Treatment of type III AC joint injuries is controversial. Several studies have demonstrated equal outcomes in patients with type III injuries who are treated surgically and non-surgically. In general, decision-making includes consideration of multiple factors including activity level, hand-dominance, occupation, and a patient's goals and expectations of treatment. One commonly used approach is to treat type III injuries non-operatively for 3 months and to consider surgical intervention if treatment is not successful.

42. **What procedure is often included in the treatment of chronically painful acromioclavicular separations?**
Excision of the distal clavicle is often warranted.

43. **What are other causes of AC joint pain without an acute injury? What are the radiographic hallmarks of each?**
   - Primary osteoarthritis and post-traumatic arthritis (AC joint injury, distal clavicle fracture)
     - Osteophyte formation, sclerosis, subchondral cysts
   - Rheumatoid arthritis
     - Periarticular erosions, osteopenia
   - Distal clavicle osteolysis: often seen in weight-lifters
     - Widened joint space, cystic changes in distal clavicle, osteopenia

44. **Are radiographic signs of AC joint arthritis an indication for treatment?**
No. AC joint degeneration is a frequent finding on shoulder radiographs; however, symptomatic arthritis is not common. Edema in the AC joint seen on MRI often correlates with symptoms.

45. **What is the initial management of AC joint arthritis?**
Activity modification, ice/heat, physical therapy, NSAIDs, and a corticosteroid injection are the hallmarks of initial management. An AC joint injection can serve a diagnostic and a therapeutic purpose as it can confirm the clinical suspicion that pain is, in fact, coming from the AC joint. If patients fail conservative treatment of 3 to 6 months duration, operative intervention is considered.

46. **What is the operative treatment of AC joint arthritis?**
Surgical treatment involves a distal clavicle resection. This can be completed via both open and arthroscopic approaches. Though there is some controversy regarding the amount of distal clavicular bone to resect, most surgeons resect approximately 8 mm to 10 mm of the distal clavicle. Care should be taken to preserve the AC ligaments and the superior capsule to prevent iatrogenic instability.

CASE 8-3

A 17-year-old male is involved in a high-speed motor vehicle crash. He is noted to have a concussion and a blunt liver injury. He also complains of central chest pain and mild shortness of breath. He is noted to have tenderness to palpation at the left SC joint during the secondary trauma survey. On his chest CT scan, a left posterior sternoclavicular (SC) joint dislocation is noted (Fig. 8.7).

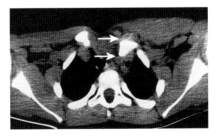

Figure 8.7. Computed tomographic scan of an adolescent with a left posterior sternoclavicular dislocation (arrows). Note the impingement on the posterior structures. (*Reprinted from Mooney J, Webb LX, In: Green NE, Swiontkowski M [eds]: Skeletal Trauma in Children, 4th ed, pp. 283–311. Copyright © 2009, with permission from Saunders, Elsevier Inc.*)

47. **What type of joint is the sternoclavicular joint?**
The sternoclavicular joint, similar to the acromioclavicular joint, is a diarthroidal (synovial) joint with a fibrocartilaginous disc between the clavicle and sternum.

48. Name the important ligaments around the sternoclavicular joint.

Intra-articular disc ligament: from the synchondral junction of the first rib and the sternum, through the SC joint, and attaches to the superior and medial clavicle
   - Resists medial displacement of the clavicle

Costoclavicular ligaments: attach upper part of first rib to the inferior surface of the medial clavicle
   - Anterior fibers that resist upward rotation of the clavicle
   - Posterior fibers that resist downward rotation of the clavicle

Interclavicular ligament: attach superomedial aspect of each clavicle to the capsular ligaments and upper sternum
   - Hold up the lateral aspect of the clavicle

Capsular (sternoclavicular) ligaments: cover the anterior-superior and posterior aspects of the joint
   - Resist upward displacement of the medial clavicle

49. What is the usual mechanism of injury to the sternoclavicular joint?

The most common mechanism of injury is a motor vehicle accident. Significant forces are necessary to cause dislocation of the sternoclavicular joint. A direct blow to the clavicle most commonly causes a posterior dislocation of the sternoclavicular joint. An indirect force to the anterolateral aspect of the clavicle can cause an anterior dislocation of the sternoclavicular joint, whereas an indirect force to the posterolateral aspect of the shoulder will cause a posterior dislocation of the sternoclavicular joint.

50. What are the common findings on physical examination of a dislocated sternoclavicular joint?
   - With anterior sternoclavicular dislocation, the medial aspect of the clavicle is prominent. It is important to look for symmetry between the right and left sides of the body.
   - With a posterior sternoclavicular dislocation, the findings are subtle. The medial end of the clavicle may be less palpable, but more tender when compared with the other side. Patients also may complain of shortness of breath or have difficulty swallowing.

51. Describe the best way to evaluate the sternoclavicular joint radiographically.

AP views of the sternoclavicular joint are often difficult to interpret. Special projections include the serendipity view, which involves a 40° cephalic tilt of the x-ray beam. The medial aspect of both clavicles is seen on this view. Superior displacement of the clavicle represents an anterior dislocation, whereas inferior displacement represents a posterior dislocation. CT scans easily delineate the position of the medial clavicle compared to the sternum. MRI also can be used to provide the same information as the CT scan, but it also shows the soft tissue anatomy and associated mediastinal structures. It is important to look for signs of tracheal or vascular compression in the setting of a posterior dislocation.

CASE 8-3   continued

The thoracic surgeon on-call is made aware of the case and is present in the hospital. The patient is taken to the operating room by the orthopedic team and a closed reduction is attempted. The clavicle is able to be reduced with a towel clamp, but is unstable and quickly returns to its dislocated position. As a result, an open reduction and ligament reconstruction is performed.

52. What are the treatment recommendations for acute sternoclavicular sprains? Dislocations?
   - With mild sprains that are not dislocated, patients are treated symptomatically with a sling until they are comfortable, followed by early rehabilitation.
   - Anterior dislocation of the sternoclavicular joint is treated with closed reduction done under either intravenous sedation or general anesthesia. Unfortunately, many anterior dislocations are unstable after closed reduction. In general, these become asymptomatic over time and open reduction is generally not necessary.
   - Acute posterior dislocation is reduced with closed reduction and usually performed under general anesthesia. A towel clip may be required to manually assist reduction of the sternoclavicular joint.
   - An open reduction may be needed for a posterior dislocation in the event that it is irreducible by closed means or is unstable after closed reduction. Ligament repair or

reconstruction can be selected based on the chronicity of the injury and the quality of the ligaments. Such injuries should be reduced to avoid complications – erosion into the underlying mediastinal structures, thoracic outlet syndrome, or vascular compromise. It is important to have a thoracic surgeon on-call and available in the hospital in the event that a complication arises.

53. What is the treatment recommended for chronically dislocated sternoclavicular joints?

For chronic anterior sternoclavicular dislocation, non-operative treatment is generally preferred. Patients are usually minimally symptomatic and the condition is primarily a cosmetic problem. For chronic posterior dislocation of the sternoclavicular joint, operative treatment may be necessary to prevent potential complications (erosion of the clavicle into the underlying mediastinal structures). Treatment often involves resection of the medial aspect of the clavicle and ligament reconstruction.

SHOULDER STIFFNESS

CASE 8-4

A 47-year-old female with a past medical history of diabetes mellitus (insulin-controlled) and hypothyroidism presents to the office complaining of 3 months of shoulder pain and progressively worsening stiffness. She notes that pain is exacerbated by any attempt at shoulder motion and she has difficulty sleeping. Her primary care physician had obtained plain radiographs and an MRI which were both normal. She denies trauma, fevers/chills, or other constitutional symptoms.

54. What are causes of shoulder stiffness?

Shoulder stiffness can result from intra-articular adhesions, capsular contracture, subacromial adhesions, and subdeltoid adhesions. These can have an idiopathic, post-surgical, or post-traumatic etiology.

55. Is shoulder stiffness another term for adhesive capsulitis? What is adhesive capsulitis?

No. Shoulder stiffness can result from the anatomic causes noted above. Adhesive capsulitis is a specific pathologic entity in which chronic inflammation of the capsule subsynovial layer produces capsular thickening, fibrosis, and adherence of the capsule to itself and to the anatomic neck of the humerus. The contracted, adherent capsule causes pain, especially when it is stretched suddenly, and produces a mechanical restraint to motion. Characteristics of adhesive capsulitis include a global limitation of glenohumeral motion, with a loss of compliance of the shoulder capsule, with a normal x-ray, and no specific underlying cause.

56. What demographic variables are commonly seen in patients with adhesive capsulitis? Adhesive capsulitis is most often associated with what conditions?

Adhesive capsulitis is more common in middle-aged females. The non-dominant shoulder is often affected and there are associations with diabetes, thyroid dysfunction (commonly hypothyroidism), cardiovascular diseases, and trauma. Diabetes is associated with a significantly worse prognosis, greater need for surgery, and suboptimal results.

CASE 8-4 continued

Your physical examination reveals that passive external rotation is limited to 20° with significant pain at the end-range. Forward elevation is similarly limited and painful beyond 60°. You diagnose her with adhesive capsulitis and recommend non-operative treatment with physical therapy for stretching and NSAIDs for pain control. After 3 months of physical therapy, 2 months of home stretching exercise, and two corticosteroid injections, her motion is near normal and her pain is resolved.

57. What plane of motion is most often limited in adhesive capsulitis?

External rotation.

58. What are the clinical stages of adhesive capsulitis?

- Painful: gradual onset of diffuse pain
- Stiff: decreased range of motion; affects daily activities
- Thawing: gradual return of motion

59. **What are the arthroscopic stages of adhesive capsulitis?**
   Stage 1: Fibrinous inflammatory synovitic reaction, typically with full motion but pain
   Stage 2: Proliferative synovitis, which is hypertrophic, typically with motion loss and pain
   Stage 3: Maturation of the capsule, with reduced vascularity, slow improvement in pain but motion still limited
   Stage 4: Burnt out synovium with a dense scar appearance, shoulder motion gradually resolves.

60. **What is the treatment for adhesive capsulitis?**
   - Non-operative treatment is generally effective if initiated in the first 4–6 months and involves physical therapy focused on active-assisted motion and capsular stretching. NSAIDs are used for pain relief. An intra-articular corticosteroid injection can be important in the early stages to relieve pain.
   - Operative treatment is generally reserved for cases that are unresponsive to non-operative treatment or chronic cases. Described treatments include a manipulation of the shoulder under general anesthesia or arthroscopic capsular release to restore motion. Physical therapy remains critical even after surgical treatment in order to maintain motion.

61. **What is calcific tendonitis?**
   Calcific tendonitis is a condition that primarily affects the supraspinatus tendon. It is more frequent in women and is often self-limiting. The etiology is unknown, but radiographs demonstrate calcifications within the tendon. Treatment is most often non-operative in nature and consists of physical therapy, NSAIDs, and corticosteroid injections. Removal of the deposits, either via open or arthroscopic surgery, is sometimes necessary, but care should be taken to repair rotator cuff tears that often exist after excision of calcific bodies from within the tendon.

GLENOHUMERAL ARTHRITIS

CASE 8-5

A 65-year-old, right-hand-dominant homemaker complains of 10 years of progressively worsening right shoulder pain. She had slowly begun to primarily use her left arm for housework. Her primary care physician had prescribed NSAIDs several years ago, but these medications ceased being effective approximately a year ago. She attended physical therapy for 3 months before discontinuing it because the activity seemed to aggravate her condition further. She is referred to your office for consultation. She describes the pain as a constant dull, throbbing ache that is "deep" within the shoulder. Pain worsens with activity and interferes with sleeping. She also experiences pain and stiffness with attempted shoulder elevation and daily activities, such as washing her back and putting on a coat.

A focused examination demonstrates active range of motion is 60° of forward elevation, 50° of abduction, 0° of external rotation; internal rotation is to the L5 vertebral level. Passive motion is 90° of forward elevation, 80° of abduction, and 5° of external rotation with pain and crepitus. Rotator cuff muscle strength testing is 5/5 in all planes. She has negative belly press and negative lift-off tests.

Three radiographic views of the right shoulder were obtained and showed glenohumeral joint space narrowing, subchondral sclerosis and large inferior humeral osteophytes. She is educated regarding her diagnosis of glenohumeral osteoarthritis and treatment options are discussed.

62. **What is glenohumeral arthritis?**
   Glenohumeral arthritis refers to loss of glenohumeral joint articular cartilage, leading to shoulder pain and stiffness.

63. **What are the etiologies of glenohumeral arthritis?**
   - Idiopathic osteoarthritis
   - Rheumatoid arthritis
   - Post-traumatic arthritis
   - Post-surgical/post-capsulorrhaphy arthropathy
   - Avascular necrosis
   - Crystalline arthropathy (gout, pseuodogout)
   - Septic arthritis.

64. What is the common history and physical examination noted with glenohumeral arthritis?

Shoulder pain and stiffness are the primary presenting complaints. The history will often determine the etiology of glenohumeral arthritis and place it in one of the categories noted above. Patients often exhibit shoulder pain at rest that is worsened with attempted active or passive range of motion. Range of motion is often limited by pain and/or osteophytes. Passive external rotation is most often limited as a result of arthritis. This is because the anterior and inferior capsular ligaments become contracted.

65. What is the classification system for shoulder avascular necrosis? What surgical treatment options exist based on stage?

Cruess classification:
  Stage I: Visible on MRI, not visible on x-ray
  Stage II: Sclerotic bone, osteopenia on x-ray
  Stage III: Subchondral fracture (crescent sign)
  Stage IV: Collapse/incongruity/flattening not affecting the glenoid
  Stage V: Arthritic changes in glenoid

66. Describe the radiographic appearance of glenohumeral arthritis secondary to rheumatologic disease.

Radiographs often demonstrate a central erosion pattern with periarticular erosions and cystic changes due to the inflammatory nature of the disease. Osteophytes seen in osteoarthritis are uncommon in rheumatoid arthritis. Bone loss on either side of the glenohumeral joint may occur (Fig. 8.8).

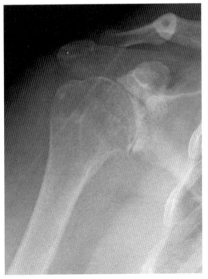

Figure 8.8. Rheumatoid arthritis – concentric medial migration of the humeral head. (*From DeLee JC, DeLee & Drez's Orthopaedic Sports Medicine: Principles and Practice, pp. 769–1155. Copyright © 2010, with permission from Saunders, Elsevier Inc.*)

67. Describe the radiographic appearance of glenohumeral osteoarthritis.

In glenohumeral osteoarthritis, humeral head articular surface wear typically begins centrally and is accentuated by peripheral osteophyte formation. This is referred to as the "Friar Tuck" sign. With progression, an inferior humeral head "goat-beard" osteophyte develops as the head flattens. Glenoid articular surface wear typically occurs posteriorly as anterior soft-tissue structures tighten, creating obligate posterior translation, glenoid wear and erosion. One may often note posterior glenoid erosion on the essential axillary radiograph (Fig. 8.9).

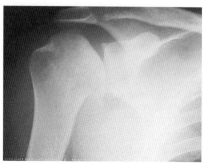

Figure 8.9. Radiograph typical of glenohumeral osteoarthritis. *(Reprinted from Frontera WR: Essentials of Physical Medicine and Rehabilitation, 2nd ed, pp. 91–95. Copyright © 2008, with permission from Saunders, Elsevier Inc.)*

68. **When should a CT scan be obtained to evaluate glenohumeral arthritis? MRI?**
    While some surgeons will obtain a CT scan in all cases of glenohumeral arthritis, many will obtain this study to better delineate glenoid wear and version that is insufficiently determined on plain radiographs. MRI should be obtained in cases where there is concern for a rotator cuff tear. This is most common in patients with inflammatory arthritides.

69. **What is normal glenoid version? What is normal humeral version?**
    • Glenoid = 3° of retroversion
    • Humerus = 20–30° retroversion.

70. **What is the classification system for glenoid deformity in osteoarthritis?**
    Walch classification (Fig. 8.10):
    Type A: Centered
    Type B: B1- posteriorly subluxed
          B2- posteriorly subluxed with posterior erosion
    Type C: Posteriorly subluxed with increased retroversion (hypoplasia).

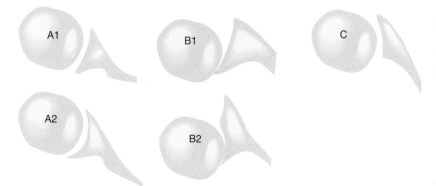

Figure 8.10. Walch classification. *(From Walch G, Badet R, Boulahia A, Hhoury A: Morphologic study of the glenoid in primary osteoarthritis. J Arthroplasty 14:756–760, 1999.)*

71. To what does a "biconcave glenoid" refer?

In glenohumeral osteoarthritis, varying amounts of anterior glenoid articular surface remain when posterior erosion is present. Posterior erosion, due to tightness of anterior soft tissues and obligate posterior translation of the humeral head, is manifested by a posterior glenoid concavity where the existing humeral head articulates. This leaves a vertical ridge in the glenoid that separates the posterior concavity from the original glenoid concavity that is made up of remaining anterior glenoid articular surface. Glenoid morphology is noted on an axillary radiograph and is commonly referred to as a biconcave glenoid if two concavities exist. Glenoid concavity and morphology have very important implications in glenohumeral arthroplasty. Bi-concave glenoids are also commonly seen in those with post-capsulorraphy arthropathy. Glenoid morphology can be difficult to quantify based on an axillary radiograph (because of factors such as projection) and is often underestimated.

72. What is capsulorraphy arthropathy?

Capsulorraphy arthropathy is a glenohumeral arthritic condition that results from previous anterior shoulder capsular surgery. Anterior structures are often tightened in surgery for anterior dislocations. As a result, with external rotation affected, shoulders develop obligate posterior translation and subsequent wear. Capsulorraphy arthropathy often leads to some of the most severe cases of posterior erosion.

73. How often is idiopathic osteoarthritis associated with a full-thickness rotator cuff tear? Rheumatoid arthritis?
- 5–10%
- 25–40%.

CASE 8-5 continued

The patient is given a corticosteroid injection as she is hoping to avoid surgical intervention. This injection provides approximately 2 weeks of relief, at which point the pain returns. She notes that over the past 2 to 3 months, the pain has become progressively worse, and the patient can no longer reach even her bottom kitchen shelves. She is ready to consider surgical treatment at this time.

Given her long-standing disease and your concerns regarding medialization of her glenoid, you obtain a CT scan that demonstrates adequate glenoid bone stock for a total shoulder arthroplasty. Understanding that her most reliable surgical solution for pain relief and restoration of function is a total shoulder arthroplasty, she agrees to undergo the procedure.

At 6 months after surgery, the patient reports excellent control of her pain and improved function due to dramatically improved range of motion. On examination, her incision was well-healed, and her active motion had improved to 165° of elevation, 155° of abduction and 60° of external rotation.

74. What are non-operative treatments of glenohumeral arthritis?

Similar to other joints, non-operative treatment for arthritis of the glenohumeral joint includes activity modification, NSAIDs, and corticosteroid injections.

75. When is non-prosthetic surgical intervention considered for glenohumeral arthritis?

Arthoscopic or open debridement is considered when patients are too young and/or active for prosthetic replacement.

76. What anatomic variable is most important to consider when determining surgical treatment options for glenohumeral arthritis?

Results of surgical treatment are dictated by the status of the rotator cuff. If a rotator cuff tear is present, it must be determined whether the tear is reparable.

77. In the setting of glenohumeral arthritis and an intact rotator cuff, what are prosthetic options for treatment?
- Hemiarthroplasty
- Hemiarthroplasty with biologic glenoid resurfacing
- Total shoulder arthroplasty.

78. **What is the difference between shoulder hemiarthroplasty and total shoulder arthroplasty?**
    - Shoulder hemiarthroplasty is the surgical resurfacing of the humeral head only with a metallic prosthetic implant. Anatomic resurfacing is the goal. Humeral component fixation may be achieved with a press-fit uncemented humeral prosthesis or with a cemented humeral prosthesis. More recently, humeral head replacements have been created that achieve fixation in the metaphysis and do not violate the diaphysis of the humerus.
    - Total shoulder arthroplasty refers to resurfacing the humeral head *and* glenoid surfaces. Glenoid resurfacing is typically performed with a polyethylene prosthesis. After appropriate concentric glenoid reaming, the glenoid component is typically implanted with the aid of methylmethacrylate. Various forms of keeled and pegged polyethylene glenoid components exist. Uncemented metal-backed glenoid components also exist.

79. **Which treatment option provides the most reliable pain relief and restoration of function?**
    Total shoulder arthroplasty with a polyethylene glenoid component.

80. **If total shoulder arthroplasty provides the most reliable pain relief and restoration of function, why are all cases of glenohumeral arthritis that are treated surgically not treated this way?**
    The most common cause of aseptic failure of total shoulder arthroplasty is progressive polyethylene wear and loosening of the glenoid component.

81. **What is the rocking horse phenomenon?**
    The rocking horse phenomenon refers to cyclic, eccentric loading of the humeral head on the glenoid. This induces a torque about the fixation surface thereby increasing tensile stresses at the implant–cement and bone–cement interfaces. Repetitive eccentric loading may ultimately lead to glenoid failure by disassociation.

82. **When is a total shoulder arthroplasty considered as a treatment for glenohumeral arthritis?**
    Total shoulder arthroplasty is used for sedentary or moderate activity level, adequate glenoid bone. There is substantial controversy regarding whether to treat the young patient (less than 50 to 55 years of age) with end-stage shoulder arthritis with total shoulder arthroplasty or hemiarthroplasty.

83. **When is hemiarthroplasty considered as a treatment option for glenohumeral arthritis?**
    Hemiarthroplasty is used for patients with normal or minimally involved glenoids, occupation or activity that involves heavy labor or weight lifting, and inadequate glenoid bone.

84. **What is biologic glenoid resurfacing?**
    Biologic resurfacing employs a means of biologic interposition with a variety of graft materials. Techniques have been described using autograft anterior capsule, autograft fascia lata, tendo Achilles allograft, lateral meniscal allograft, and a variety of commercially available grafts/scaffolds. Biologic resurfacing provides an interposition between the native glenoid and the humerus with a decreased risk of violating the native glenoid bone stock.

85. **Is hemiarthroplasty with biologic glenoid resurfacing more effective than hemiarthroplasty alone?**
    While hemiarthroplasty with biologic glenoid resurfacing has demonstrated good results at short-term follow-up, there is a significant risk of reoperation to a total shoulder arthroplasty. To date, there are no comparative studies of hemiarthroplasty alone and hemiarthroplasty with biologic glenoid resurfacing.

86. **When performing a hemiarthroplasty of the glenohumeral joint what consideration should be given to the glenoid?**
    The glenoid should be assessed for concentricity. In the case of a biconcave glenoid, establishment of a concentric glenoid is necessary. Often the anterior concavity is preferentially reamed to achieve one concavity for eventual glenoid component placement or for a smooth articulation with the prosthetic humeral component. Posterior bone-grafting is a potential option when there is difficulty establishing concentricity.

87. What are the two possible surgical approaches for shoulder arthroplasty?

Deltopectoral approach (most common): uses the internervous plane between the deltoid (axillary nerve) and the pectoralis major (medial and lateral pectoral nerves).

Anterosuperior approach: access to the shoulder by reflecting the anterior deltoid from the acromion.

88. How is the subscapularis managed during shoulder arthroplasty through a deltopectoral approach?

It is necessary to reflect the subscapularis in order to obtain adequate access to the glenoid for resurfacing. Subscapularis can be managed with a tenotomy followed by surgical repair with heavy suture and bone tunnels. Alternatively, the subscapularis can be managed with a lesser tuberosity osteotomy. There is currently no gold standard and no study has shown a direct benefit between these two approaches.

89. What is "overstuffing" in reference to shoulder arthroplasty?

Overstuffing refers to placing components that are too large for the capsular volume of the shoulder. This is a frequent mistake in shoulder arthroplasty, often made in an attempt to obtain stability. Unfortunately, overstuffing sacrifices motion by tightening soft tissues. This leads to postoperative stiffness, which is often painful, as well as excessive glenoid loads. Thus, anatomic restoration should be the goal with appropriate releases and lengthenings.

90. What are the complications of shoulder arthroplasty?

- Stiffness: Probably the most frequent complication suffered by patients.
- Component malposition: This can frequently lead to stiffness. Excessive retroversion of the humeral component, excessive humeral head height, "overstuffing," and insufficient glenoid preparation and fixation are common errors.
- Infection: The infection rate of shoulder arthroplasty (0.5–3%) is consistent with that in other joints. Rates are higher in patients with rheumatoid arthritis because of their immunocompromised state.
- Instability: Instability results from soft-tissue imbalance, muscle atrophy, or malposition of components.

91. What are the contraindications to shoulder arthroplasty?

The only absolute contraindication is active infection. Relative contraindications include patients with a neuropathic joint and young, heavy laborers who are unwilling or unable to alter their lifestyle.

92. What are outcomes of shoulder arthroplasty?

Pain relief is the major result. Studies with 15-year follow-up report relief of pain in 90–95% of patients with osteoarthritis who undergo total shoulder arthroplasty. Hemiarthroplasty yields pain relief in 85–90% of patients, but pain worsens with time due to glenoid arthritis. Pain relief with hemiarthroplasty is much lower in those with biconcave glenoids. For hemiarthroplasty, the best functional results are obtained in patients with concentric glenoids and intact rotator cuffs. Generally those younger than 50 will have less well-perceived results than those older than 50, regardless of whether they have had a hemiarthroplasty or a total shoulder arthroplasty. Survivorship of total shoulder arthroplasty in patients with an intact and reparable rotator cuff is 84% to 88% at 15 years.

93. How is revision shoulder arthroplasty approached in the setting of aseptic glenoid loosening?

The glenoid component must be removed with care taken to preserve as much glenoid bone stock as possible. At the time of glenoid component resection for symptomatic loosening, sometimes enough bone does not remain to accept a new glenoid prosthesis. Hemiarthroplasty with resection of the loose glenoid component and cement can reasonably improve pain without re-implantation of a glenoid component. Bone grafting of the defect with eventual return to resurface the glenoid in patients with persistent pain is a reasonable treatment strategy.

94. **What is the concavity compression?**
    Concavity compression provides stability to the glenohumeral joint. This is accomplished by the rotator cuff muscles' ability to compress the humeral head into the glenoid.

95. **What is cuff tear arthropathy?**
    Cuff tear arthropathy refers to arthritic glenohumeral changes due to rotator cuff insufficiency and, therefore, loss of the concavity compression mechanism that the cuff provides. Humeral head proximal migration, with respect to the glenoid, is typical due to the pull of the deltoid muscle. The unprotected humeral head is abraded by the undersurface of the coracoacromial arch, leading to arthrosis. Surgical reconstruction is difficult because of the almost complete loss of the constraining force of the rotator cuff.

96. **What is pseudoparalysis?**
    Pseudoparalysis is the inability of a functioning deltoid to create active elevation of the arm due to loss of concavity compression.

97. **What are the radiographic hallmarks of cuff tear arthropathy?**
    1. Decreased acromiohumeral distance
    2. "Femoralization" of the proximal humerus: humeral head appears round and the contour of the tuberosities is lost due to chronic abrasion
    3. "Acetabularization" of the acromion: sclerosis and concavity of the undersurface of the acromion to match the shape of the humeral head.

98. **What are non-operative treatment options for cuff tear arthropathy?**
    Given the chronic nature of the rotator cuff tear and the presence of glenohumeral joint arthritis, options are limited to activity modification, physical therapy for stretching, NSAIDs, and occasional corticosteroid injections.

99. **What are operative treatment options for cuff tear arthropathy?**
    • Hemiarthroplasty: Most often surgeons elect to use designs that are specifically manufactured for cuff tear arthropathy. In these designs, the implants have a larger head in order to provide an arc of surface area >180° to allow articulation with the lateral aspect of the humeral head against the acromion. Results from this procedure have been reliable in terms of pain-relief, but somewhat unpredictable in terms of restoration of function. This procedure should not be performed if there is evidence of incompetence of the coracoacromial arch, as anterosuperior instability of the prosthesis can result.
    • Reverse shoulder arthroplasty: A reverse total shoulder involves a hemisphere ball placed onto the glenoid and an articulating cup placed on the humerus. This reverse ball-and-socket prosthesis increases the efficiency of the deltoid muscle for abduction by lengthening the lever arm upon which it operates, thereby allowing it to generate more torque for a given force. This, in effect, allows the deltoid to compensate for the incompetent rotator cuff. Additionally, the semi-constrained design prevents superior migration and instability seen with hemiarthroplasty (Fig. 8.11).

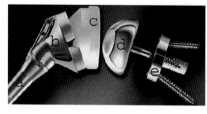

Figure 8.11. Components of reverse shoulder prosthesis: shaft (a), epiphysis (b), polyethylene inlay (c), glenosphere (d), and baseplate (e). (*From Werner CM, Steinmann PA, Gilbart M, et al.: Treatment of painful pseudoparesis due to irreparable rotator cuff dysfunction with the Delta III reverse-ball-and-socket total shoulder prosthesis. J Bone Joint Surg 87A:1476, 2005.*)

100. **What is the complication rate with reverse shoulder arthroplasty?**
    The complication rate is approximately 25%. The most common complications are scapular notching, hematoma formation, glenoid dissociation such as baseplate failure or aseptic loosening, glenohumeral dislocation, acromial and/or scapular spine fracture, infection, and nerve injury. Studies have shown as low as a 30% survival rate at 8 years postoperatively; however, more recent studies have indicated lower complication rates and higher survivorship. This may be an indication of the learning curve associated with reverse arthroplasty.

101. What is scapular notching?

Scapular notching is a mechanical complication caused by direct impingement between the humeral component and the inferior glenoid. Progressive abutment between the prosthesis and bone leads to polyethylene wear, histologic osteolysis, and the subsequent radiographic appearance of a notch. The rate of notching has been quoted as high as 96%. Although the clinical relevance of scapular notching remains controversial, inferior scapular notching has been associated with lower functional outcome scores, polyethylene wear, osteolysis as a result of polyethylene wear debris, and glenoid failure. Newer glenosphere designs have moved the center of rotation from the center of the glenoid to a more distal and/or lateral position in an effort to address this potential problem (Fig. 8.12).

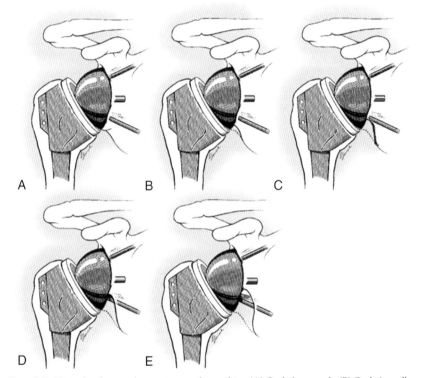

Figure 8.12. Nerot classification of progressive scapular notching. (A) Grade 0, no notch. (B) Grade 1, small notch. (C) Grade 2, notch with condensation (stable). (D) Grade 3, evolutive notch (erosion of inferior screw). (E) Grade 4, first glenoid loosening. (*From McFarland EG, Sanguanjit P, Tasaki A, et al.: The reverse shoulder prosthesis: a review of imaging features and complications. Skeletal Radiol 35:488, 2006.*)

102. What is shoulder arthrodesis? What are the surgical indications?

Shoulder arthrodesis is surgical resection of the glenohumeral surfaces and fusion with the aid of internal fixation. Relative indications for shoulder arthrodesis include young heavy laborers with osteoarthritis who are unwilling or unable to alter their lifestyle. Arthrodesis is occasionally recommended because of the fear of rapid mechanical loosening of an overused shoulder arthroplasty. Other indications include uncontrolled joint sepsis, recurrent shoulder instability, complete loss of the rotator cuff and deltoid musculature, brachial plexopathies with functional trapezial and rhomboid musculature, and salvage for failed total shoulder arthroplasty.

103. **In what position should the shoulder be fused?**
Shoulder arthrodesis should be performed so that the arm rests comfortably at the side without scapular winging and the hand can be brought easily to the mouth and the perineum. Twenty degrees of flexion, 30° of abduction, and 40° of internal rotation have been generally recommended. Because of problems with periscapular muscle fatigue and pain, some authors recommend a position with much less flexion and abduction.

104. **What is resection arthroplasty? What are the surgical indications?**
Resection arthroplasty is resection of the humeral head. One of the original techniques for treatment of intractable pain due to shoulder arthritis, this procedure is now rarely indicated because it renders a flail shoulder. Resection arthroplasty is most often used for intractable joint infection, infected non-union of shoulder arthrodesis, and neoplastic processes of the shoulder.

NERVE AND MUSCLE DISORDERS

105. **What is the thoracic outlet space? What is thoracic outlet syndrome?**
The thoracic outlet space is created by the clavicle, first rib, subclavius muscle, costoclavicular ligament, and anterior scalene muscle. Thoracic outlet syndrome is a compression of the nerves and blood vessels that pass through thoracic outlet space. It most often affects the subclavian artery, vein, and lower trunk (C8/T1) of the brachial plexus. Patients often note pain and ulnar paresthesias (ring and small finger). Pulse examination may demonstrate obliteration of radial pulse and recreation of symptoms with the arm placed in a variety of positions. For example, Wright test involves extension, abduction, and external rotation of the arm with the neck rotated away from the affected side leading to obliteration of the radial pulse and reproduction of symptoms.

106. **What radiographs should be obtained?**
If thoracic outlet syndrome is suspected, a standard shoulder series should be obtained as well as a chest x-ray. Chest x-ray is important to rule out cervical ribs that could be causing compression. Additionally, a chest x-ray is important in ruling out a Pancoast tumor that can masquerade as shoulder pain.

107. **What is the surgical treatment of thoracic outlet syndrome?**
Surgical intervention most often involves resection of the first rib, although supraclavicular neuroplasty has also been described.

108. **What is the quadrilateral space? What is quadrilateral space syndrome?**
The quadrilateral space is defined as the region bordered by the long head of the triceps medially, the humeral shaft laterally, the teres minor superiorly, and the teres major inferiorly. The axillary nerve and the posterior humeral circumflex artery exit through this space.
Quadrilateral space syndrome often presents with complaints of shoulder/arm pain and paresthesias with overhead activity. Most often, this is seen in throwing athletes and is most notable at the late cocking and acceleration phases of throwing in which the arm is in an abducted, extended, and externally rotated position. The diagnosis is confirmed by an arteriogram demonstrating compression of the posterior humeral circumflex artery.
Treatment should begin with a non-operative approach, including analgesics, physical therapy, and avoidance of athletic activities. Surgery is usually reserved for those suffering acute or chronic symptoms not responding to conservative care. Surgery involves a posterior approach to expose the quadrilateral space and to undertake a lysis of fibrous tissue (Fig. 8.13).

109. **What is "snapping scapular syndrome"?**
Also known as scapulothoracic crepitus, "snapping scapular syndrome" is painful crepitus at the scapulothoracic joint upon elevation of the arm. Many believe this syndrome to be associated with scapular dyskinesis or altered mechanics leading to maltracking. Other causes include atrophied or fibrotic muscle, anomalous muscle insertions, elastofibroma dorsi (a rare soft-tissue tumor on the chest wall), osteochondroma, or malunited rib fractures. There is also some suggestion that a hooked superomedial scapula can cause altered biomechanics and impingement.

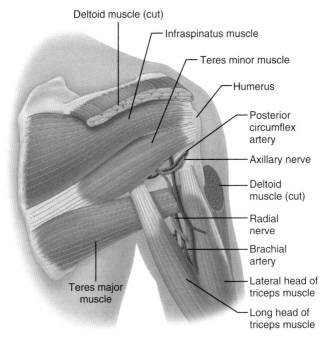

Deltoid muscle (cut)

Infraspinatus muscle

Teres minor muscle

Humerus

Posterior circumflex artery

Axillary nerve

Deltoid muscle (cut)

Radial nerve

Brachial artery

Lateral head of triceps muscle

Teres major muscle

Long head of triceps muscle

Figure 8.13. Drawing of quadrilateral space viewed from behind. (*From Canale & Beaty [eds], Campbell's Operative Orthopaedics, 12th ed. Copyright © 2013, Mosby Elsevier Inc.*)

110. What comprises the scapulothoracic articulation?

The scapulothoracic articulation is cushioned by the subscapularis and the serratus anterior. Additionally, there are two major and four minor bursae:

Major: Infraserratus – between serratus anterior muscle and chest wall
Supraserratus – between serratus anterior and subscapularis
Minor: Two at the superomedial angle of the scapula
One at the inferior angle of the scapula
One at the medial base of the spine of the scapula

111. What are typical physical examination findings and treatment options?

On physical examination, the pain is generally relieved with scapular stabilization. Occasionally, there may be palpable or audible crepitus over the scapulothoracic region. Physical therapy for periscapular strengthening and stabilization is paramount in the treatment algorithm. Some patients obtain pain relief from NSAIDs, taping or bracing, and corticosteroid injections in the scapulothoracic bursa. An injection can also serve a diagnostic purpose. Occasionally, patients may require open or arthroscopic bursectomy and/or resection of the superomedial portion of the scapula.

112. What imaging should be obtained?

At minimum, tangential views of the scapula should be obtained to rule out a bony anomaly. If there is a question regarding the bony architecture, a CT scan can be obtained and an MRI can be used to determine the extent of bursitis or co-existing soft-tissue pathology.

113. What is pseudowinging?

Sometime in the case of scapulothoracic crepitus, fullness in the involved area and pain may result in altered scapulothoracic mechanics that give the impression of winging. However, there is no neurologic cause.

114. What is scapular winging?

Scapular winging is a rare disorder often caused by neuromuscular imbalance in the scapulothoracic stabilizer muscles that leads to abnormal scapulothoracic posture and motion. Lesions of the *long thoracic* and *spinal accessory* nerves are the most common causes. The serratus anterior muscle is innervated by the long thoracic nerve, originating from the 5th, 6th, and 7th cervical nerve roots. As a unit, the serratus anterior muscle acts to protract and stabilize the scapula, orienting the glenoid for effective use of the upper extremity. The trapezius is a large muscle innervated by the spinal accessory nerve that has a broad origin from the external occipital protuberance, the medial one-third of the nuchal line (i.e., the ligamentum nuchae), and the spines of the 7th cervical and 12th thoracic vertebrae.

115. **What causes scapular winging and how can the cause be determined on physical examination?**
   1. Long thoracic nerve palsy: *medial* scapular winging
      a. The most common cause of primary scapular winging is paralysis of the serratus anterior muscle after insult or injury to the long thoracic nerve. Injury to this nerve includes compression, traction, and laceration.
      b. The scapula assumes a superior translation, with the inferior pole rotated medially.
   2. Cranial nerve XI (trapezius) palsy: *lateral* scapular winging
      a. Injury can occur iatrogenically from surgical dissections around the neck, from trauma, from infection (viral), or from other causes.
      b. Patients often complain of radiating arm pain that is thought to result from the drooping posture of the scapula leading to traction on the brachial plexus.

116. **How is scapular winging treated?**
   - Long thoracic nerve palsy
      - Non-operative: Most cases of scapular winging are the result of neuropraxic injury. Neuropraxic injury commonly resolves within 6 to 9 months. Once diagnosis is made, non-surgical therapies should be initiated to maintain shoulder motion and prevent stiffness. In the absence of penetrating trauma or previous surgery, many authors recommend a course of non-surgical treatment of 12 to 24 months to observe for nerve recovery.
      - Operative: Recent results of long thoracic nerve neurolysis and nerve transfer for scapular winging have been favorable. In general, however, scapular winging resulting from spontaneous neuromuscular palsy, traction injury, or contusion that does not resolve within 12 to 24 months is an indication for dynamic muscle transfer. Chronic serratus anterior muscle palsy is effectively addressed with *transfer of the sternal head of the pectoralis major muscle to the inferior angle of the scapula.*
   - Cranial nerve XI palsy
      - Non-operative: If nerve injury is not detected for >6 months, nerve repair is not recommended and a >12 month period of non-operative treatment is often recommended. Pain relief can sometimes be achieved with non-operative treatment, but functional limitations often persist.
      - Operative: If nerve injury is detected early (<6 months), nerve repair or reconstruction can be considered. If nerve repair is unsuccessful or patients are not satisfied with their outcome after a period of non-operative treatment, *an Eden–Lange procedure* is often the treatment of choice.

117. **What is the Eden–Lange procedure?**
   The Eden–Lange procedure involves lateral transfer of the levator scapulae, rhomboid major, and rhomboid minor to substitute for the deficient parts (superior, middle, and inferior) of the trapezius. The transfer allows for stabilization of the scapula and improved biomechanics at the scapulothoracic articulation.

118. **What is Milwaukee shoulder?**
   Milwaukee shoulder is a rapidly destructive arthritis of the shoulder. This condition has been described with various names in the literature, including: hemorrhagic shoulder of the elderly. It predominantly occurs in elderly female patients. Unilateral, dominant shoulder joint involvement is most common. A long history of shoulder pain with loss of motion is a typical presentation. Radiographic changes include degenerative changes in the glenohumeral joint with rupture of the rotator cuff. *A synovial fluid aspirate is typically bloody, non-inflammatory and positive for calcium apatite crystals.* Patients often have damage to the rotator cuff and exacerbation of pain by acute episodes of inflammation that occur with shedding of crystals.

ELBOW

ELBOW DISLOCATIONS AND INSTABILITY

CASE 8-6

A 23-year-old male presents to the Emergency Department after a fall from his bicycle onto his outstretched right hand. He complains of elbow pain, swelling, and notes some tingling in his small and ring finger. On examination, the patient holds his right elbow in slight flexion and supported by his left hand. The elbow is notably swollen and the patient complains of baseline pain that is exacerbated by any attempt at active or passive movement. He has 2+ radial and ulnar pulses and sensation is intact to light touch in the radial, ulnar, and median nerve distributions, though the patient notes subjective numbness in the ulnar nerve distribution. Muscle strength is 5/5 in the medial, radial, ulnar, anterior interosseous, and posterior interosseous nerve distributions.

119. **What are the static and dynamic restraints to elbow dislocation?**
   - Primary static constraints:
     - Bony = ulnohumeral articulation
     - Ligamentous = anterior bundle of the medial collateral ligament (MCL), lateral ulnar collateral ligament (LUCL)
   - Secondary static constraints: capsule, radiocapitellar articulation, common flexor and extensor tendon origins
   - Dynamic constraints: muscles that cross elbow joint (anconeus, triceps, brachialis) apply compressive forces

120. **What is an elbow dislocation?**
   An elbow dislocation is a disassociation of the joint that connects the humerus with the radius and the ulna.

121. **How common are dislocations of the elbow?**
   Although the elbow is one of the most highly constrained or stabilized joints, dislocations of the elbow are not rare. Only dislocation of the shoulder and the proximal interphalangeal (PIP) joints of the fingers are more common.

122. **How do most elbow dislocations occur?**
   Most occur in young people aged 15–25 years during sports participation. Elbow dislocations also may occur in high-speed motor vehicle or motorcycle accidents.

123. **What is the mechanism of injury in most elbow dislocations?**
   The usual mechanism of injury is a fall on an extended or hyperextended elbow.

124. **How are elbow dislocations described?**
   - Classification: elbow dislocations can be considered simple or complex
     - Simple: without osseous injury
     - Complex: with osseous injury
   - Direction: Like all dislocations, elbow dislocations are described by the position of the distal segment in relation to the proximal segment. In 90% of cases, the dislocation is posterior or posterolateral (i.e., the ulna is posterior to the humerus in a posterior elbow dislocation). Although the most common dislocation is posterior, elbow dislocations also may be anterior, medial, lateral, or divergent. Anterior dislocations are rare and are associated with a high degree of soft-tissue disruption. In a divergent dislocation, which is also rare, but very serious, the radius and the ulna dislocate from the humerus in different directions. For a divergent dislocation to occur, the strong musculotendinous complex that binds the ulna and radius together must be completely disrupted.

125. **What is posterolateral rotatory instability?**
   Posterolateral rotatory instability is a proposed mechanism for elbow injury that leads to dislocation, ligament disruption, and fractures. It results from a combination of supination and valgus forces leading to posterolateral instability and possibly complete dislocation of the elbow. The force begins laterally and results in disruption of the LUCL and then progresses medially with disruption of the posterior and anterior capsules. If the force is strong enough, it can then result in disruption of the MCL. This is believed to be the mechanism for a *terrible triad injury*.

126. What is the lateral pivot shift test of the elbow for posterolateral instability of the elbow?

The lateral pivot shift test is a clinical examination maneuver that reproduces the injury pattern of a posterolateral dislocation. A symptomatic elbow demonstrates instability with the maneuver of axial compression, valgus stress, and supination. The test is best performed with the patient in a supine position with the arm positioned over the head. The examiner stands at the head of the table. One hand holds the wrist with the forearm in full supination. The other hand is positioned on the proximal forearm. The arm is held in full extension. To perform the test, slowly flex the elbow while simultaneously applying axial compression and a valgus force to the elbow. At approximately 40° of flexion the patient either experiences an audible "clunk" or has such apprehension that he or she aborts the test because the test will reproduce the feeling of instability.

127. What is a terrible triad injury?

A terrible triad injury is a fracture of the radial head, a fracture of the coronoid process, and a lateral ulnar collateral ligament tear (Fig. 8.14).

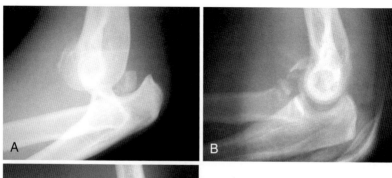

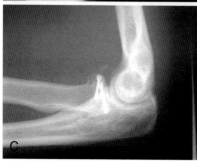

Figure 8.14. (A) Lateral radiograph of the "terrible triad" of the elbow consisting of elbow dislocation, a radial head fracture, and a coronoid fracture. (B) After closed reduction, the radial head is not concentrically reduced, the ulnohumeral joint space is increased, and the coronoid fragment remains displaced. (C) These injuries are inherently unstable after closed reduction because of the limited soft tissue or bony constraint to posterior translation. (*Reprinted from Browner BD et al.: Skeletal Trauma, 4th ed, pp. 1503–1592. Copyright © 2009, with permission from Saunders, Elsevier Inc.*)

128. What is the classification system for radial head fractures?

Mason classification (Fig. 8.15):

Type 1: Small or marginal fracture with minimal displacement

Type 2: Marginal fracture with displacement

Type 3: Comminuted fracture of the head or neck.

129. What is the classification system for coronoid fractures?

Reagan and Morrey classification:

Type 1: Tip fracture

Type 2: Less than 50% of coronoid

Type 3: Greater than 50% of coronoid.

130. What is posteromedial rotatory instability?

This is commonly the mechanism of injury in an elbow dislocation that results in a LUCL disruption and a medial coronoid facet fracture *without* a fracture of the radial head.

Type I

Type II

Type III

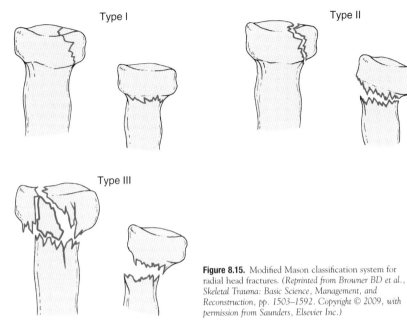

Figure 8.15. Modified Mason classification system for radial head fractures. (*Reprinted from Browner BD et al., Skeletal Trauma: Basic Science, Management, and Reconstruction, pp. 1503–1592. Copyright © 2009, with permission from Saunders, Elsevier Inc.*)

131. **What are the physical findings in an elbow dislocation?**
Pain is a typical symptom associated with any dislocation. On inspection, patients often hold the affected forearm with the opposite hand. The elbow is usually held in slight flexion. The forearm appears slightly foreshortened compared with the normal forearm. The olecranon is usually palpable and prominent posteriorly. Swelling of the elbow is usually present and increases with time.

132. **How does one check the neurovascular function?**
First, check the sensation to light touch in the medial, ulnar, and radial nerve distribution. Test the median, ulnar, radial, anterior interosseous, and posterior interosseous nerves for muscle strength distal to the elbow. Ask the patient to touch the thumb to the fifth finger to assess median nerve function. Anterior interosseous nerve function can be tested by asking the patient to flex the DIP joint of the thumb or index finger (often done by asking the patient to make an "ok" sign). Ulnar nerve function can be assessed by testing the interosseous muscles, all of which are innervated by the ulnar nerve. Have the patient spread the fingers apart to test for interosseous function. The radial nerve can be assessed by having the patient extend the wrist. Posterior interosseus nerve function can be tested by asking the patient to extend the thumb. The ulnar and radial arteries should be palpated at the wrist. All findings should be documented.

133. **What neurovascular injuries are common in elbow dislocations?**
Most nerve injuries are neuropraxias and are not permanent. The ulnar nerve is most commonly affected, although any nerve that crosses the joint can be injured with an elbow dislocation.

134. **What should be done if neurovascular injury is present?**
After documentation of the injury, an attempt should be made promptly to reduce the dislocation. Often neurovascular injuries resolve with reduction. Carefully check the neurovascular status after relocation. An arteriogram should be obtained promptly if vascular injury is suspected.

CASE 8-6 continued

Radiographs are obtained immediately upon presentation and a clear posterior elbow dislocation is noted. There is also a bony fragment noted anteriorly and concern for a fracture of the radial head. The patient is consented and prepared for an attempted closed reduction in the Emergency Department.

135. **Describe the procedure for reducing a dislocation of the elbow.**
Elbow dislocations should be reduced as soon as possible. Team physicians covering sports with a high incidence of elbow dislocations are able to quickly and easily reduce the elbow shortly after the injury. If time has elapsed since the injury occurred and soft-tissue swelling is present, reduction is best accomplished under regional or general anesthesia. As noted previously, before any reduction maneuver, the neurovascular status *must* be documented. If radiographs have been obtained, they should be examined carefully, looking for any associated fractures, especially at the coronoid process of the proximal ulna and the radial head. In most cases, the ulna is posterior to the humerus.

Many methods have been described for reduction of elbow dislocations. Logistically, the reduction maneuver is most often conducted with the patient in the supine position. The easiest and most reliable method involves gentle traction applied to the forearm with counter traction applied to the distal aspect of the humerus by an assistant. As the elbow is gently extended, any medial or lateral displacement of the ulna can be corrected by a counterforce applied to the side of the displacement. Then, the elbow is carefully flexed, while maintaining gentle traction to accomplish the reduction. In a posterior dislocation, it is often helpful to push the distal humerus posteriorly with one hand while flexing and pulling the forearm anteriorly. If no assistant is available, a closed reduction of the elbow with the patient in a prone position may be useful. The gravity method of reduction described by Parvin is a gentle method that can be used by the sole practitioner. The patient lies prone on the stretcher while gentle downward traction is applied with one hand to his or her wrist. After a few minutes of traction, the muscle spasm should subside. With your opposite hand apply a gentle upward pressure on the anterior distal humerus, lifting the arm as traction continues to be applied downward. The reduction should occur with an audible "clunk."

After reduction, carefully reassess neurovascular function and gently flex and extend the elbow to ensure that the reduction is complete and to determine the range of stability. A well-padded posterior splint with the elbow held at approximately 90° of flexion is applied, though the degree of flexion and forearm rotation should be decided based on the range of stability. Obtain post-reduction radiographs to ensure complete reduction of the dislocation and to rule out any new fractures. It is important to critically assess the ulnohumeral and radiocapitellar articulations for congruency. Additionally, a valgus stress view can be helpful to determine the competence of the MCL. Alternatively, an MRI can be obtained to diagnose a ligament tear.

136. **What should be done if the elbow dislocation cannot be reduced?**
The usual cause of an irreducible dislocation is entrapped fragments within the joint space, most often the fractured medial epicondyle. If the dislocation has not reduced after two gentle attempts under intravenous anesthesia, closed reduction under general anesthesia should be attempted. If the elbow is not reducible even after general anesthesia, open reduction is necessary.

137. **When should a CT scan be acquired for an elbow dislocation?**
In general, CT scans are not necessary for simple dislocations. CT scans can be helpful for complex dislocations to accurately identify fracture fragments and displacement of the articular surface in order to guide surgical decision-making. Additionally, CT scans can be helpful in identifying loose bodies or fracture fragments within the joint space. We do not recommend obtaining CT scans before the elbow joint is reduced, as comminuted and displaced fracture fragments are often difficult to define anatomically when the joint is not reduced properly.

138. **What is the treatment for a simple elbow dislocation?**
In general, simple elbow dislocations do not require surgical treatment. The elbow is immobilized in a posterior splint or a sling for 3 to 5 days. The goal is to start gentle elbow range of motion and stretching exercises through the stable arc of motion in order to prevent stiffness. If instability is present at less than 30° of flexion, a hinged orthosis that prevents extension and controls rotation is often utilized for the first 6 weeks to allow for protected range of motion. If instability persists despite use of an orthosis, surgical treatment with ligamentous repair or reconstruction is considered.

139. **How does one approach surgical fixation of a simple elbow dislocation?**
The LUCL is considered to be the essential lesion, and so, it is addressed first. The LUCL most commonly avulses from the humeral origin (isometric point on the lateral capitellum). In the acute setting, it can be secured back to bone using bone tunnels or other bone anchoring devices. In the chronic setting, reconstruction may be necessary using either autograft or allograft. Once the LUCL is repaired, elbow stability is assessed, as restoration of the LUCL is often sufficient to confer elbow stability even in the setting of an MCL injury.

140. **What are late complications of elbow dislocation?**
1. Recurrent dislocation of the elbow is extremely rare, but when it occurs, it is disabling.
2. Mild loss of terminal extension
    • Loss of motion can be minimized through an early range-of-motion program.
3. Heterotopic ossification may occur after dislocation of the elbow.
4. Neurovascular injury

CASE 8-6 continued

A reduction is completed and the elbow feels most stable in neutral forearm rotation and 85° of flexion. A well-padded posterior splint is placed in this position and post-reduction x-rays are obtained. Radiographs demonstrate a reduced elbow joint with evidence of a displaced radial head fracture and a coronoid fracture. A CT scan is obtained to better delineate the fractures. CT scan demonstrated a type II radial head fracture and a type III coronoid fracture. After discussing the risks and benefits of surgery, the patient undergoes open reduction and internal fixation of the coronoid and radial head fractures and repair of the LUCL. The patient's elbow is noted to be stable at 30–130° of motion. Postoperatively, he is placed in a hinged elbow brace for 6 weeks and early motion is initiated. At 12 weeks follow-up, the patient's fractures are healed and motion has improved to 5–130°.

141. **Why is operative treatment often selected for complex dislocations?**
A major goal of treatment is to allow early range of motion in an effort to prevent stiffness. Surgical treatment conferring stability by ligament repair (or reconstructions) and fracture fixation allows for early motion to be initiated before bony or ligamentous healing is complete.

142. **What is the treatment algorithm for operative fixation of complex elbow dislocations?**
In general surgical dissection is begun on the lateral side of the elbow. Through this exposure, fixation proceeds from deep within the elbow to more superficial as it is difficult to access the deep structures when the superficial structures are intact or repaired. The coronoid fracture should first be reduced and fixed. Attention should then be turned to the radial head which should be fixed or replaced, depending on the level of comminution and fracture pattern. More superficially, the LUCL should be repaired or reconstructed. At this point, elbow stability should be assessed with a goal of obtaining stable motion in the range of 30–130°. If stability is not achieved, attention should be turned towards the medial side where the MCL is repaired or reconstructed. When working on the medial side of the elbow it is important to identify and protect the ulnar nerve. Stability is again assessed and if the elbow remains unstable, an external fixator is applied.

143. **What is the problem with radial head excision *acutely* after dislocation?**
Excision of the radial head in the acute setting of an elbow dislocation is associated with proximal migration of the radius and is not recommended. In the acute setting, the radial head should be reduced and internally fixed or replaced.

ELBOW ARTHRITIS/STIFFNESS

CASE 8-7

A 74-year-old right-hand dominant female with a long-standing history of rheumatoid arthritis presents with complaint of left elbow pain for over 20 years. She notes that she has been managed medically with antiinflammatory and disease-modifying antirheumatic drugs. She notes that pain has progressively worsened and she has lost elbow motion. She notes that pain is constant and exacerbated by lifting or stretching. On physical examination, elbow range of motion is from 35° to 110° with crepitus and pain. She has a mild effusion and tenderness to palpation at the radiocapitellar joint. Her elbow joint is grossly unstable to varus and valgus stress. She is otherwise neurovascularly intact.

144. **What are the major types of arthritis that involve the elbow?**
    In order of frequency, the most common types of elbow arthritis are
    1. Rheumatoid: Between 20% and 50% of patients with rheumatoid arthritis will demonstrate elbow involvement, usually within 5 years of disease onset. Approximately 90% of patients also have hand and wrist involvement, and 80% also have shoulder involvement.
    2. Posttraumatic
    3. Osteoarthritis: Approximately 2% of the population is affected by symptomatic primary osteoarthritis of the elbow.

145. **Describe the typical presenting history of elbow arthritis.**
    Patients with rheumatoid arthritis generally present to their primary physician or rheumatologist with a painful, stiff elbow and a previous diagnosis of rheumatoid arthritis. Patients that do not have rheumatoid arthritis typically present between the 3rd and 8th decades of life with a history of a previous fracture or dislocation of the elbow, repetitive elbow trauma, or an occupation that requires heavy upper extremity physical labor.

146. **What are the physical examination findings of a patient with elbow osteoarthritis?**
    Stiffness is quite common with elbow arthritis, especially loss of extension. Crepitus is often noted with flexion/extension and pronation/supination. Pain is often elicited with extension and flexion, especially at the extremes of motion.

147. **Describe the radiographic appearance of osteoarthrosis of the elbow.**
    Anteroposterior and lateral radiographs typically reveal osteophytes of the olecranon and coronoid processes as well as osteophytes in the coronoid and olecranon fossae. Loose bodies may be present. Anteroposterior radiographs are difficult to obtain in elbows with flexion contractures. An anteroposterior view of the distal humerus as well as an anteroposterior view of the proximal radius and ulna should be obtained separately to gain a true appreciation of the anatomy of each distinct side of the joint.

148. **What is functional range of motion of the elbow?**
    Traditionally, functional range of motion has been defined as 30–130° of extension/flexion and 50° of pronation and supination in order to perform activities of daily living. More recent study indicates that more motion (approximately 27–149° of flexion/extension, and 65° of pronation and 77° of pronation) may be necessary to perform modern activities of daily living (computer mouse, keyboard, cell phone use).

149. **What are the non-operative treatments options for elbow osteoarthritis?**
    Non-operative treatment of elbow arthritis centers on pain relief and maintenance of motion. NSAIDs, gentle stretching programs, and occasional corticosteroid injections may help provide satisfactory elbow comfort and function for many patients.

150. **What are indications for surgical treatment of elbow osteoarthritis?**
    Failure of non-operative treatment, loss of motion that affects activities of daily living, and mechanical symptoms (locking, catching, or buckling that is painful) are indications for surgery.

151. **What are surgical treatment options for elbow osteoarthritis?**
    Elbow capsular releases, loose body removal, and osteophyte excision: open or arthroscopic:
       Combinations of these three parts are generally performed. Increased motion and decreased mechanical pain are often attainable; however, elimination of rest pain and

need for future surgery are unlikely. Ulnar nerve symptoms should be recognized preoperatively with a low threshold for transposition, especially when correcting for significant flexion contractures.

Interposition/distraction arthroplasty:

This procedure may be considered for osteoarthritis, but is generally reserved for young, active patients with post-traumatic elbow arthritis without other reasonable options. It is often combined with the above procedures; however, the durability and long-term outcomes of this procedure are unclear. Simply stated, the procedure involves the resection of the diseased articulating surfaces and resurfacing the joint with interposed biologic materials (muscle flaps, fascia, synthetic scaffolds, allograft, amongst others). An external fixator is sometimes placed on either side of the elbow to allow joint distraction as healing occurs. The technique has the disadvantages of unpredictable pain relief and unpredictable stability and its role in the treatment algorithm for elbow arthritis is unclear.

Total elbow arthroplasty:

Total elbow arthroplasty may be performed for elbow osteoarthritis but has led to early failures, due to high demand and resultant early loosening. As a result, age less than 65 is generally considered a relative contraindication to total elbow arthroplasty.

152. **How can osteoarthritis be treated arthroscopically?**
Arthroscopy can allow excision of osteophytes from the olecranon, coronoid, and olecranon and coronoid fossa. Loose bodies are excised; however, this alone is not believed to be effective for treating arthritis. If the arthritis is associated with capsular contracture, some advocate arthroscopic capsular release. If indicated, the radial head can be excised arthroscopically.

153. **What risk is associated with excision of osteophytes?**
Damage to articular cartilage and neural structures are risks of osteophyte excision. The posteromedial osteophyte is close to the ulnar nerve. The ulnar nerve is also close to the prominence of the osteophyte on the trochlea and, therefore, removal of osteophytes from this region should be done with care.

154. **What are relative contraindications to arthroscopic treatment of elbow osteoarthritis?**
Arthrofibrosis, previous elbow surgery, and need for ulnar nerve transposition are relative contraindications to arthroscopic treatment.

155. **What are the physical examination findings of a patient with elbow inflammatory arthritis (RA)?**
Stiffness is common with elbow inflammatory arthritis. However, more commonly than in primary osteoarthritis, soft-tissue attenuation in inflammatory arthritides can lead to varus or valgus instability. Crepitus is often noted with flexion/extension and pronation/supination. Pain is often elicited with extension and flexion, especially at the extremes of motion and ulnar neuropathy is sometimes present.

156. **Describe the typical radiographic presentation of rheumatoid arthritis.**
In general, the disease progresses from soft-tissue inflammation and damage to articular damage and, finally, to periarticular or subchondral erosions and destruction.

Mayo classification of the rheumatoid elbow:

Grade I: No radiographic abnormalities except periarticular osteopenia with accompanying soft-tissue swelling. Mild to moderate synovitis is generally present.

Grade II: Mild to moderate joint space reduction with minimal or no architectural distortion. Recalcitrant synovitis that cannot be managed with NSAIDs alone.

Grade III: Variable reduction in joint space with or without cyst formation. Architectural alteration, such as thinning of the olecranon, or resorption of the trochlea or capitellum. Synovitis is variable and may be quiescent.

Grade IV: Extensive articular damage with loss of subchondral bone and subluxation or ankylosis of the joint. Synovitis may be minimal.

157. **What is the natural history of rheumatoid arthritis in the elbow?**
    1. Synovitis is the first, prominent pathologic process. Biomechanics remain normal. Osteoporosis is present but without gross articular destruction.
    2. Joint narrowing generally occurs with progressive osteoporosis.
    3. Joint architecture becomes distorted. Osteoporosis worsens, subchondral cysts form, and clinical complaints of instability begin, distinguishing rheumatoid arthritis from osteoarthritis.
    4. Finally, gross destruction results in loss of articular surfaces and gross instability. Instability often results from soft-tissue inflammation and damage that leads to ligament destruction and incompetence.

158. **What are the non-operative treatments options for elbow inflammatory arthritis?**
    Non-operative treatment centers on medical management and use of disease modifying drugs to prevent joint destructions and other systemic effects of the disease. Splinting and pain relief with NSAIDs, gentle stretching, and corticosteroid injections can be helpful in providing temporary pain relief.

159. **What are the surgical options for treatment of rheumatoid arthritis of the elbow?**
    Stage, age, and other joint involvement determine one of two choices:
    - Synovectomy with or without radial head excision is considered in Mayo grade I or II cases. Synovectomy can be accomplished via open or arthroscopic approaches, depending on surgeon preference, degree of synovitis, and need for additional procedures.
    - Total elbow arthroplasty is considered in Mayo grade III and IV cases (Fig. 8.16).

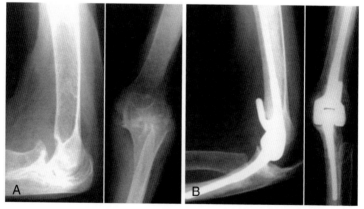

Figure 8.16. Total elbow arthroplasty for rheumatoid arthritis. (A) Advanced disease in the elbow of a 66-year-old woman with rheumatoid arthritis. (B) After total elbow arthroplasty. *(From Canale ST, Beaty JH [eds], Campbell's Operative Orthopaedics, 11th ed, p. 996. Copyright © 2008, Mosby Elsevier Inc.)*

160. **What are the indications, advantages, and disadvantages of radial head resection?**
    Resection is recommended for pain relief when the radiocapitellar joint is involved and the ulnohumeral involvement is relatively mild or moderate. This procedure is recommended for pain relief, not for increased motion. Radial head resection is not offered as a long-term solution to the patient with rheumatoid arthritis because the disease most likely will progress to involve the ulnohumeral joint.

161. **What is total elbow arthroplasty?**
    Total elbow arthroplasty involves replacement of the articulating surfaces of the distal humerus and the proximal ulna. There are currently two types of elbow implant designs:

1. Linked implants: These implants are connected by a "sloppy hinge" that allows for flexion/extension as well as some limited varus/valgus laxity. Early loosening is a concern due to the forces placed across the hinge.
2. Unlinked implants: These implants do not involve a connection between the humeral and ulnar components. These components articulate as they would in a native elbow. Instability is a concern with these implants as they rely on soft-tissue restraints to maintain joint stability:
   - These implants are oftentimes not suitable for cases of inflammatory arthritis due to the soft-tissue attenuation that is often encountered.

162. **When is total elbow arthroplasty indicated?**
Most surgeons agree that the indications for total elbow arthroplasty are narrow. The primary indication is for advanced elbow arthritis in patients with rheumatoid arthritis or other inflammatory arthritides that render the elbow functional demands as low. There may also be some select cases of elbow osteoarthritis and post-traumatic arthritis in low-demand patients in whom total elbow arthroplasty may be considered. Acutely, total elbow arthroplasty may also be used in cases of severe supracondylar and intracondylar fractures of the elbow in elderly patients with osteoporotic bone. In addition, it may be indicated for intracondylar and supracondylar non-unions of the distal humerus in elderly patients.

163. **What are the contraindications to total elbow arthroplasty?**
Active infection in the joint is an absolute contraindication. Relative contraindications are young patients with an active lifestyle or heavy laborers unwilling or unable to alter their lifestyle.

164. **List the major complications of total elbow arthroplasty.**
- Wound problems and infection:
  - Risk factors include previous elbow surgery, previous elbow infection, severe rheumatoid arthritis, wound drainage, or reoperation
  - *A two-stage revision with initial resection and placement of an antibiotic spacer is recommended for infected total elbow arthroplasties.*
- Component loosening
- Instability, including dislocations, subluxations, or maltracking (all primarily with the unconstrained designs)
- Ulnar nerve injury
- Triceps insufficiency

165. **Identify the main technical considerations in elbow arthroplasty.**
- Arthroplasty is usually performed through a posterior approach. The ulnar nerve must be explored and may be transposed anteriorly. The triceps may be "peeled" from the olecranon, split, or preserved. Preservation is more technically challenging but may allow for better triceps function, an important detail in patients with rheumatoid arthritis that use their arms to push themselves out of bed and chairs. Meticulous soft-tissue handling is paramount.
- Careful attention must be given to soft-tissue balancing and elbow axis restoration and component rotational alignment. Soft-tissue reconstruction is especially important with the unconstrained design where ligamentous and capsular reconstructions may be difficult due to the poor tissue often found in patients with rheumatoid arthritis.
- Careful handling, reaming, and preservation of bone are essential.

166. **What are the results of total elbow arthroplasty?**
Elbow arthroplasty provides reliable pain relief and restoration of motion. Survivorship is often dependent on implant type and indication. For rheumatoid arthritis, survival studies have demonstrated 10-year survival in the range of 75–90%. One study demonstrated that the cumulative survival for total elbow arthroplasty performed for post-traumatic arthritis, fractures, or supracondylar nonunion was 73% at 3 years and 53% at 5 years. These are significantly worse than the cumulative 3–5-year survivals of 92% and 90%, respectively, for patients with inflammatory arthritis. Further studies are necessary to determine long-term survivorship of elbow arthroplasty for post-traumatic arthritis and osteoarthritis.

167. **Other than arthritis, what are causes of elbow stiffness?**
Congenital abnormalities, paralytic deformities, burn contractures, sequelae of joint infections, and, most commonly, trauma to the elbow can result in elbow stiffness.

168. **How is post-traumatic elbow stiffness classified?**
1. Extrinsic (extra-articular):
   - Skin, subcutaneous tissues, capsule, collateral ligament contractures, myostatic contractures, heterotopic ossification, ulnar neuropathy
2. Intrinsic (intra-articular):
   - Articular deformity or adhesions, osteophytes, fibrosis, loose bodies
3. Mixed

169. **What are non-operative treatments of elbow stiffness?**
The major goal is to prevent stiffness by allowing for range of motion after traumatic injuries or injuries that create pain and limit a patient's ability to move the elbow. Once stiffness occurs, non-operative treatment must be tailored to the etiology. However, NSAIDs, ice/heat, corticosteroid injections, and physical therapy can help to reduce pain and increase/maintain motion. Static progressive splinting (turnbuckle splints) or custom molded splints with articulating hinges can be used to gently progress maximal levels of extension and/or flexion. The success of these splints is often influenced by patient compliance with wear and instructions.

170. **What are operative treatments of elbow stiffness in the absence of arthritis?**
When stiffness is not associated with significant joint arthrosis, soft-tissue releases, including anterior/posterior capsulectomy, brachialis muscle slide, and debridement of all encroaching soft tissue in the fossae of the distal humerus are indicated. If the brachialis muscle is shortened, it should be released or recessed off the humerus. If the triceps or biceps muscle is shortened, a tenolysis or a tendon lengthening can be considered. Bridging or impinging heterotopic ossification should be excised. If the radial head has been fractured and is blocking pronation, supination, or flexion secondary to malunion or global enlargement, it should be excised at the head–neck junction, with care taken to preserve the annular ligament. Ulnar nerve neurolysis and transposition should be included in the operative plan of patients with preoperative ulnar nerve symptoms or those in which the nerve is visibly tethered or under tension after releases are complete.

TENDON INJURIES
CASE 8-8

A 50-year-old male presents to clinic after an injury 3 days ago during which he was lifting a couch and felt a sudden tearing sensation in his dominant arm. He experienced pain and mild swelling in the anterior elbow. He noticed that the next day his elbow was bruised and he noted a lump in his arm. On physical examination, he had ecchymosis in his antecubital fossa and above the elbow. Additionally, he was significantly weak in elbow supination and had mild weakness with elbow flexion. He had a positive "hook" test. Surgery was performed 3 days later to repair the tendon. After 3 months he had regained approximately 80% of his strength and after 5 months he was completely normal and was doing all activities with his arm.

171. **What is the mechanism of injury for a distal biceps tendon rupture? Who is most commonly affected?**
The mechanism of injury is generally an unexpected extension force applied to the elbow that is approximately 90° flexed. This force is followed by an eccentric contraction of the biceps with a resulting tearing sensation in the antecubital fossa. The distal biceps tendon most commonly avulses from its insertion on the radial tuberosity. Men in their 40s to 60s are most commonly affected and typically notice ecchymosis in the antecubital fossa and weakness (most commonly in supination).

172. **Do symptoms usually precede acute biceps rupture at the elbow?**
Yes. Athletes commonly report preexisting chronic tendinitis. Degenerative changes in the tendon may make it more susceptible to a tear from a traumatic event.

173. **What are common physical examination findings with a distal biceps rupture?**
A loss of the normal biceps contour and an obvious deformity may be present. Important to note, an intact lacertus fibrosus may tether the torn biceps tendon and prevent more

proximal retraction, thereby making deformity more subtle. The biceps "squeeze" test may be positive. With this test, the biceps brachii is squeezed to elicit forearm supination if the tendon is intact. The "hook" test is often positive in a complete tendon rupture. This test is performed by inserting the finger under the lateral edge of the biceps tendon between the brachialis and biceps tendons and hooking the finger under the cord-like structure spanning the antecubital fossa with the patient's elbow flexed 90°. Weakness is most often noted in supination. This is because the biceps tendon's primary role is as a supinator as well as its role as a secondary elbow flexor.

174. **What is seen on imaging after a distal biceps rupture?**
Radiographs of the elbow may show enlargement and irregularity at the radial tuberosity or an avulsion of the radial tuberosity itself. Magnetic resonance imaging can be useful to confirm the diagnosis, distinguish between full-thickness and partial-thickness tears, demonstrate the amount of tendon retraction, and to determine tendon quality. MRI is not considered necessary for diagnosis (Fig. 8.17).

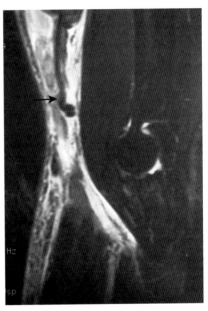

Figure 8.17. Rupture of distal biceps tendon. Sagittal inversion recovery image of elbow shows ruptured distal biceps tendon. Proximal tendon (arrow) has retracted several centimeters, and edema is present in tissues anterior to brachialis muscle. (*From Canale ST, Beaty JH [eds], Campbell's Operative Orthopaedics, 11th ed, p.150. Copyright © 2008, Mosby Elsevier Inc.*)

175. **What is the treatment of distal biceps rupture?**
- Non-operative treatment is an option for patients who do not require restoration of full elbow flexion and supination strength. Often, this cohort is limited to elderly, low-demand patients. Additionally, non-operative treatment is employed for patients who are not medically fit for operative treatment. Non-operative treatment consists of temporary immobilization, pain control, and physical therapy.
- Operative treatment is considered in active patients who require restoration of strength or for patients with partial tears that fail to respond to nonsurgical treatment. Multiple techniques for surgical fixation have been described, including single and double incision techniques with anatomic (repair to the radial tuberosity) and non-anatomic (repair to the brachialis muscle) repairs using suture anchors, bone tunnels, interference screws, cortical buttons, or other methods of bony fixation. Important to note, chronic ruptures with tendon retraction and/or poor tendon quality may require grafting procedures or tenodesis to the brachialis muscle.

176. **What patient population is at risk for triceps rupture?**
Rupture of the triceps is a rare diagnosis that is sometimes seen in debilitated patients or body builders. Patients who have had previous injections for olecranon bursitis,

those with inflammatory arthritides, or those that use anabolic steroid are at heightened risk.

177. **What is the common mechanism of injury?**

The mechanism of injury is usually an eccentric load on a triceps muscle that is contracting. Ruptures typically occur at the triceps insertion and are less commonly seen through the muscle belly or musculotendinous junction.

178. **What physical examination findings are typically seen with a triceps rupture?**

Acutely, ecchymosis, swelling, and pain are typical findings. Weakness in elbow extension and a palpable gap on the posterior aspect of the arm can be seen. Similar to biceps tears, MRI is not necessary for diagnosis, but can be used to distinguish partial and full-thickness tears, to determine the extent of tendon retraction, and the quality of the tendon.

179. **What is the treatment of a triceps rupture?**

Similar to a biceps rupture, non-operative treatment is reserved for patients who do not require elbow extension strength and often have medical comorbidities that preclude surgery. Operative treatment is considered in all other patients in order to restore strength. Repair generally involves sutures placed through the triceps tendon and secured to the olecranon through drill holes.

180. **What is tennis elbow? What causes it?**

Tennis elbow or lateral epicondylitis is an overuse syndrome due to repetitive tension overloading of the wrist extensor origins at the lateral epicondyle. The problem is common in racquet sport athletes and golfers. Other wrist dorsiflexion and supination activities, such as hammering and using a screwdriver, are also common causes.

181. **What are the risk factors associated with tennis elbow in tennis players?**

Inappropriate grip size, high string tension, poor swing technique, and a heavy racquet are all risk factors for lateral epicondylitis.

182. **What tendon origin is most often affected in tennis elbow?**

The extensor carpi radialis brevis is most commonly involved and pain is increased by resisted wrist dorsiflexion, long finger extension, gripping, and tenderness to palpation just below the lateral epicondyle. The extensor digitorum communis can also be involved. The histopathologic change at the tendon origin is angiofibroblastic hyperplasia.

183. **Is imaging necessary for diagnosis?**

Imaging is often obtained to rule out concomitant pathology; however, plain radiographs are often normal and MRI may show increased signal intensity and/or degeneration in the ECRB tendon origin.

184. **What are nonsurgical treatment options?**

As is typical with non-operative management in orthopedics, rest, activity modification, NSAIDs, bracing, and corticosteroid injections can be helpful. Physical therapy should be included in the treatment plan and includes extensor stretching and strengthening. Bracing generally involves using a tennis elbow strap which is applied to the forearm just distal to the lateral epicondyle. It is thought that compressive force applied just distal to the origin of the ECRB reduces force transmission across the inflamed portion of the muscle tendon unit.

185. **When is surgery indicated? What surgical options exist?**

Surgery is indicated only after a compliant patient has failed non-operative treatment (often for over 6 months). Most described surgical techniques involve debridement of the extensor carpi radialis brevis tendon with removal of the degenerated portions. The healthy tendon that remains is repaired. Arthroscopic methods of extensor carpi radialis brevis debridement or release have been described.

186. **What is golfer's elbow?**

Golfer's elbow, or medial epicondylitis, is an overuse syndrome due to repetitive tension overloading of the flexor-pronator muscle at or near its insertion on the medial epicondyle. Symptoms often result from repetitive gripping activities, and with resisted forearm pronation or wrist flexion.

187. **What are the likely symptoms and findings in patients with golfer's elbow?**
Athletes complain of medial and proximal forearm pain aggravated by activities that require repetitive wrist flexion or forearm pronation. Diagnosis can be confirmed by reproducing the pain with resisted wrist flexion and forearm pronation.

188. **What tendon origin is most often affected in golfer's elbow?**
The pronator teres and the flexor carpi radialis are most commonly affected.

189. **What are the treatment options for golfer's elbow?**
Treatment options are similar between tennis elbow and golfer's elbow. The mainstay of treatment involves physical therapy, activity modification, counterforce bracing, and NSAIDs. Surgery is not indicated in patients who are non-compliant with non-operative treatment. However, those who fail non-operative treatment can undergo surgical treatment to excise the degenerated portions of the flexor-pronator mass and reattachment of healthy tendon back to the origin. The ulnar nerve is sometimes compressed or irritated with golfer's elbow due to its close proximity to the area.

BIBLIOGRAPHY

1. Arkkila PE, Kantola IM, Viikari JS, et al. Shoulder capsulitis in type I and II diabetic patients: association with diabetic complications and related diseases. Ann Rheum Dis 1996;55:907–14.
2. Bassett RW, Cofield RH. Acute tears of the rotator cuff. The timing of surgical repair. Clin Orthop Relat Res 1983;175:18–24.
3. Bigliani LU, Morrison DS, April EW. The morphology of the acromion and its relationship to rotator cuff tears. Orthop Trans 1986;10:228.
4. Bohsali KI, Wirth MA, Rockwood CA Jr. Complications of total shoulder arthroplasty. J Bone Joint Surg Am 2006;88:2279–92.
5. Bruno RJ, Lee ML, Strauch RJ, et al. Posttraumatic elbow stiffness: evaluation and management. J Am Acad Orthop Surg 2002;10:106–16.
6. Chen AL, Shapiro JA, Ahn AK, et al. Rotator cuff repair in patients with type I diabetes mellitus. J Shoulder Elbow Surg 2003;12:416–21.
7. Cho NS, Yi JW, Lee BG, et al. Retear patterns after arthroscopic rotator cuff repair: single-row versus suture bridge technique. Am J Sports Med 2010;38:664–71.
8. Clement ND, Hallett A, MacDonald D, et al. Does diabetes affect outcome after arthroscopic repair of the rotator cuff? J Bone Joint Surg Br 2010;92:1112–17.
9. Cole BJ, ElAttrache NS, Anbari A. Arthroscopic rotator cuff repairs: an anatomic and biomechanical rationale for different suture-anchor repair configurations. Arthroscopy 2007;23:662–9.
10. Cruess RL. Experience with steroid-induced avascular necrosis of the shoulder and etiologic considerations regarding osteonecrosis of the hip. Clin Orthop Relat Res 1978;130:86–93.
11. Curtis AS, Burbank KM, Tierney JJ, et al. The insertional footprint of the rotator cuff: an anatomic study. Arthroscopy 2006;22(609):e1.
12. Deshmukh AV, Koris M, Zurakowski D, et al. Total shoulder arthroplasty: long-term survivorship, functional outcome, and quality of life. J Shoulder Elbow Surg 2005;14:471–9.
13. Deutsch A, Kroll DG, Hasapes J, et al. Repair integrity and clinical outcome after arthroscopic rotator cuff repair using single-row anchor fixation: a prospective study of single-tendon and two-tendon tears. J Shoulder Elbow Surg 2008;17:845–52.
14. Epstein RE, Schweitzer ME, Frieman BG, et al. Hooked acromion: prevalence on MR images of painful shoulders. Radiology 1993;187:479–81.
15. Fealy S, Kingham TP, Altchek DW. Mini-open rotator cuff repair using a two-row fixation technique: outcomes analysis in patients with small, moderate, and large rotator cuff tears. Arthroscopy 2002;18:665–70.
16. Galatz LM, Ball CM, Teefey SA, et al. The outcome and repair integrity of completely arthroscopically repaired large and massive rotator cuff tears. J Bone Joint Surg Am 2004;86-A:219–24.
17. Gill DR, Morrey BF. The Coonrad–Morrey total elbow arthroplasty in patients who have rheumatoid arthritis. A ten to fifteen-year follow-up study. J Bone Joint Surg Am 1998;80:1327–35.
18. Gladstone JN, Bishop JY, Lo IK, et al. Fatty infiltration and atrophy of the rotator cuff do not improve after rotator cuff repair and correlate with poor functional outcome. Am J Sports Med 2007;35:719–28.
19. Goutallier D, Postel JM, Bernageau J, et al. Fatty muscle degeneration in cuff ruptures. Pre- and postoperative evaluation by CT scan. Clin Orthop Relat Res 1994;304:78–83.
20. Kauffman JI, Chen AL, Stuchin S, et al. Surgical management of the rheumatoid elbow. J Am Acad Orthop Surg 2003;11:100–8.
21. Keener JD, Wei AS, Kim HM, et al. Revision arthroscopic rotator cuff repair: repair integrity and clinical outcome. J Bone Joint Surg Am 2010;92:590–8.
22. Kraay MJ, Figgie MP, Inglis AE, et al. Primary semiconstrained total elbow arthroplasty. Survival analysis of 113 consecutive cases. J Bone Joint Surg Br 1994;76:636–40.

23. Lindley K, Jones GL. Outcomes of arthroscopic versus open rotator cuff repair: a systematic review of the literature. Am J Orthop (Belle Mead NJ) 2010;39:592–600.
24. Little CP, Graham AJ, Karatzas G, et al. Outcomes of total elbow arthroplasty for rheumatoid arthritis: comparative study of three implants. J Bone Joint Surg Am 2005;87:2439–48.
25. Lo IK, Burkhart SS. Double-row arthroscopic rotator cuff repair: re-establishing the footprint of the rotator cuff. Arthroscopy 2003;19:1035–42.
26. Mall NA, Kim HM, Keener JD, et al. Symptomatic progression of asymptomatic rotator cuff tears: a prospective study of clinical and sonographic variables. J Bone Joint Surg Am 2010;92:2623–33.
27. Mallon WJ, Misamore G, Snead DS, et al. The impact of preoperative smoking habits on the results of rotator cuff repair. J Shoulder Elbow Surg 2004;13:129–32.
28. Mason M. Some observations on fractures of the head of the radius with a review of one hundred cases. Br J Surg 1954;42:123–32.
29. Meier SW, Meier JD. Rotator cuff repair: the effect of double-row fixation on three-dimensional repair site. J Shoulder Elbow Surg 2006;15:691–6.
30. Meininger AK, Figuerres BF, Goldberg BA. Scapular winging: an update. J Am Acad Orthop Surg 2011;19:453–62.
31. Milgrom C, Schaffler M, Gilbert S, et al. Rotator-cuff changes in asymptomatic adults. The effect of age, hand dominance and gender. J Bone Joint Surg Br 1995;77:296–8.
32. Mochizuki T, Sugaya H, Uomizu M, et al. Humeral insertion of the supraspinatus and infraspinatus. New anatomical findings regarding the footprint of the rotator cuff. J Bone Joint Surg Am 2008;90:962–9.
33. Morrey BF, Adams RA. Semiconstrained arthroplasty for the treatment of rheumatoid arthritis of the elbow. J Bone Joint Surg Am 1992;74:479–90.
34. Morrey BF, Askew LJ, Chao EY. A biomechanical study of normal functional elbow motion. J Bone Joint Surg Am 1981;63:872–7.
35. Neviaser RJ. Painful conditions affecting the shoulder. Clin Orthop Relat Res 1983;173:63–9.
36. Neviaser AS, Neviaser RJ. Adhesive capsulitis of the shoulder. J Am Acad Orthop Surg 2011;19:536–42.
37. O'Driscoll SW, Bell DF, Morrey BF. Posterolateral rotatory instability of the elbow. J Bone Joint Surg Am 1991;73:440–6.
38. Phillips AM, Smart C, Groom AF. Acromioclavicular dislocation. Conservative or surgical therapy. Clin Orthop Relat Res 1998;353:10–17.
39. Prasad N, Dent C. Outcome of total elbow replacement for rheumatoid arthritis: single surgeon's series with Souter–Strathclyde and Coonrad–Morrey prosthesis. J Shoulder Elbow Surg 2010;19:376–83.
40. Regan W, Morrey B. Fractures of the coronoid process of the ulna. J Bone Joint Surg Am 1989;71:1348–54.
41. Sardelli M, Tashjian RZ, MacWilliams BA. Functional elbow range of motion for contemporary tasks. J Bone Joint Surg Am 2011;93:471–7.
42. Sher JS, Uribe JW, Posada A, et al. Abnormal findings on magnetic resonance images of asymptomatic shoulders. J Bone Joint Surg Am 1995;77:10–15.
43. Shubin Stein BE, Ahmad CS, Pfaff CH, et al. A comparison of magnetic resonance imaging findings of the acromioclavicular joint in symptomatic versus asymptomatic patients. J Shoulder Elbow Surg 2006;15:56–9.
44. Simovitch R, Sanders B, Ozbaydar M, et al. Acromioclavicular joint injuries: diagnosis and management. J Am Acad Orthop Surg 2009;17:207–19.
45. Sirveaux F, Favard L, Oudet D, et al. Grammont inverted total shoulder arthroplasty in the treatment of glenohumeral osteoarthritis with massive rupture of the cuff. Results of a multicentre study of 80 shoulders. J Bone Joint Surg Br 2004;86:388–95.
46. Skytta ET, Eskelinen A, Paavolainen P, et al. Total elbow arthroplasty in rheumatoid arthritis: a population-based study from the Finnish Arthroplasty Register. Acta Orthop 2009;80:472–7.
47. Sperling JW, Cofield RH, Rowland CM. Neer hemiarthroplasty and Neer total shoulder arthroplasty in patients fifty years old or less. Long-term results. J Bone Joint Surg Am 1998;80:464–73.
48. Thomas BJ, Amstutz HC, Cracchiolo A. Shoulder arthroplasty for rheumatoid arthritis. Clin Orthop Relat Res 1991;265:125–8.
49. Toivonen DA, Tuite MJ, Orwin JF. Acromial structure and tears of the rotator cuff. J Shoulder Elbow Surg 1995;4:376–83.
50. Tuoheti Y, Itoi E, Yamamoto N, et al. Contact area, contact pressure, and pressure patterns of the tendon–bone interface after rotator cuff repair. Am J Sports Med 2005;33:1869–74.
51. Walch G, Badet R, Boulahia A, et al. Morphologic study of the glenoid in primary glenohumeral osteoarthritis. J Arthroplasty 1999;14:756–60.
52. Yamaguchi K, Ditsios K, Middleton WD, et al. The demographic and morphological features of rotator cuff disease. A comparison of asymptomatic and symptomatic shoulders. J Bone Joint Surg Am 2006;88(8):1699–704.

CHAPTER 9

SPINE

Andrew H. Milby, Jonathan B. Slaughter and Nader M. Hebela

ANATOMY AND EXAMINATION

1. **How many vertebrae does the human body have?**
   The human body has a total of 33 vertebrae.

2. **What are the names of the different spinal regions?**
   The spine is divided into five different regions. From top to bottom they are: *cervical spine, thoracic spine, lumbar spine, sacrum, and coccyx* (Fig. 9.1).

3. **How many vertebrae make up the cervical spine?**
   The cervical spine consists of the first seven vertebrae of the spinal column.

4. **How many vertebrae make up the thoracic spine?**
   The thoracic spine consists of 12 vertebrae.

5. **How many vertebrae make up the lumbar spine?**
   The lumbar spine consists of five vertebrae.

6. **How many vertebrae make up the sacrum?**
   The sacrum consists of five vertebrae, and they are fused together.

7. **How many vertebrae make up the coccyx?**
   The coccyx consists of the last four vertebrae, and they are also fused together.

8. **What are the normal spinal curves?**
   The spine has four normal curves: cervical lordosis, thoracic kyphosis, lumbar lordosis, and sacral kyphosis. The thoracic and sacral kyphosis are primary curves due to the bony architecture of the vertebrae. Cervical lordosis is due to the posterior tension band of the paraspinal muscles, ligaments, and tendons. Lumbar lordosis results from the intervertebral disc anatomy, where the anterior disc heights are greater than they are posteriorly (see Fig. 9.1).

9. **What are the first two cervical vertebrae called?**
   Atlas (C1) and *Axis* (C2).

10. **Which cervical vertebra has no vertebral body and no spinous process?**
    Atlas (C1).

11. **Which elements of the cervical spine are responsible for its mobility?**
    The elements primarily responsible for the mobility of the spine are the *discs* and the facet joints. Each of these elements provides a relative contribution to degree and pattern of motion, such as flexion–extension and rotation.

12. **Which cervical level provides the majority of neck rotation?**
    The *C1–C2* (atlantoaxial) articulation provides 50% of the total neck rotation.

13. **Which vertebrae are responsible for flexion–extension?**
    Primary flexion of the cervical spine is determined from C3–C7 with the primary movement coming from the C2–C3, C3–C4, and C4–C5 vertebral spaces.

14. **Is the atlantoaxial joint (C1, C2) a stable or unstable joint?**
    The atlantoaxial joint is unstable because of its opposed convexity with a small contact area between the joint surfaces. This configuration is necessary for the joint to perform movements in all directions; flexion–extension, lateral flexion, and rotation. Stability between the atlas and axis depends on the transverse ligament, alar ligaments, and apical ligament of the dens (Fig. 9.2).

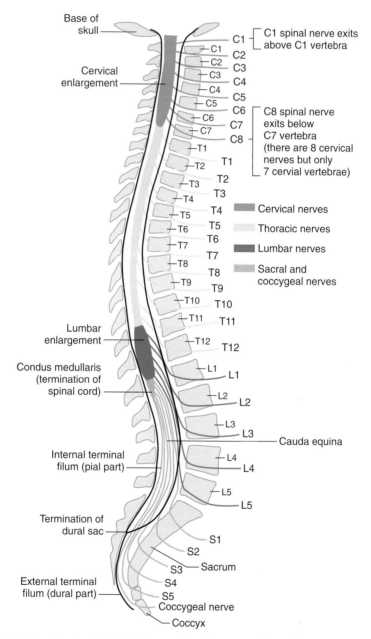

Figure 9.1. View of the spine showing the different regions of the spine as well as the four normal curvatures of the spine. (*From Goldman L, Schafer AI, [eds], Goldman's Cecil Medicine, 24th ed., Copyright © 2012, Saunders, Elsevier.*)

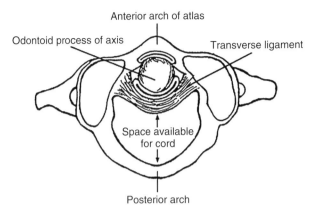

Figure 9.2. Axial anatomy of the atlantoaxial articulation. *(From Atlee JL, et al., [eds], Complications in Anesthesia, 2nd ed., Copyright © 2007, Saunders, Elsevier.)*

15. **What is the transverse ligament?**
A strong, thick ligament that connects to both sides of the atlas ring, holding the odontoid process (dens) in contact with the anterior arch of the atlas (C1).

16. **What is the odontoid process?**
It is also known as the dens, and is an upward projection from the axis (C2) that articulates with the anterior arch of the atlas (C1). It is surrounded by the transverse ligament, providing stability.

17. **The articulations between the posterior vertebral arches of the cervical spine are maintained by what anatomic structures?**
The articulations between the vertebral arches are maintained by (1) the *supraspinous ligaments*, which in the cervical spine have evolved into the ligamentum nuchae; (2) the *interspinous* ligaments; (3) the *ligamentum flavum* at each level; and (4) the *synovial facet joints*.

18. **What artery has an intimate relationship with the cervical spine and serves as the major source of blood to the cervical cord and cervical spine?**
The *vertebral artery* is the major source of blood for the cervical cord and cervical spine. The vertebral arches originate from the subclavian artery on each side and are usually the first and largest branches of the subclavian artery. The vertebral artery travels in the transverse foramina of C1–C6, but not of C7.

19. **What is the first step in evaluating back pain?**
A thorough history and physical exam.

20. **What does localized pain suggest?**
Tumor, infection, or fracture.

21. **What does mechanical pain suggest?**
Instability, degenerative disc disease, or arthritis.

22. **What does radicular pain suggest?**
Herniated disc, stenosis or, processes that result in compression of the neural elements.

23. **What does night pain suggest?**
Tumor or ankylosing spondylitis.

24. **What do systemic symptoms (fever, weight loss) suggest?**
Infection or tumor.

25. **What should the physical exam include?**
Physical exam should include inspection of spinal column including overall alignment, assessment of gait, palpation, inspection of extremities, range of motion, provocative tests, and a thorough neurological exam testing muscle strength, sensation to light touch, and reflexes.

26. **What are provocative tests for cervical spine pathology?**
Hoffman's sign, hyperreflexia, Babinski reflex, Spurling's test, and Lhermitte's sign.

27. **What is Spurling's test?**
The patient will have reproduction of their symptoms when an axial load is applied to their head with lateral flexion of their neck toward their involved side (Fig. 9.3). Radiation of pain may indicate nerve root compression.

28. **What is Lhermitte's sign?**
The patient will have shock-like sensations radiating into the person's arms or legs with extreme flexion or extension, causing stretch and compression of the spinal cord. This sign is classic for multiple sclerosis but is not specific.

29. **What is Hoffman's sign?**
While extending the metacarpophalangeal (MCP) joint of the long finger, the examiner can flick the distal interphalangeal (DIP) joint of the same long finger. Involuntary flexion of the index finger proximal interphalangeal (PIP) and DIP joints and the thumb IP joint is a positive Hoffman's sign and strongly, but not invariably, associated with upper motor neuron problems (Fig. 9.4).

30. **What is the distraction test?**
The patient will get relief of symptoms when an upward distracting force is applied to their neck. Relief of symptoms indicates foraminal compression of the nerve root.

31. **What is the shoulder abduction relief test?**
The patient will get relief of symptoms when their involved arm is abducted away from their body. Relief of symptoms indicates compression of the nerve root.

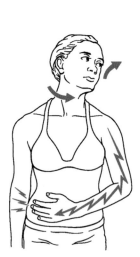

Figure 9.3. Illustration of positive Spurling's test and resulting symptoms. (*From Vaccaro AR [ed], Core Knowledge in Orthopaedics: Spine, 1st ed., Copyright © 2005, Mosby, Elsevier.*)

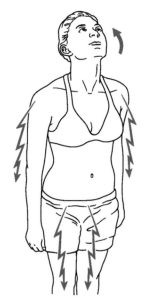

Figure 9.4. Illustration of positive Lhermitte's sign and resulting symptoms. (*From Vaccaro AR [ed], Core Knowledge in Orthopaedics – Spine, 1st ed., Copyright © 2005, Mosby, Elsevier.*)

32. **What are provocative tests for lumbar spine pathology?**
    Lasegue sign (straight-leg raise), contralateral straight-leg raise, bowstring test, femoral stretch test, or sitting root (flip sign).

33. **What is Lasegue sign?**
    It is the straight-leg raise. With the patient supine, flex their hip with their knee straight and dorsiflex the foot (Fig. 9.5). If they have pain radiating below the knee, it is indicative of nerve root compression.

34. **What is the contralateral straight-leg raise?**
    Passive flexion of the contralateral leg produces pain in the affected leg (Fig. 9.6). This test is sensitive and specific for a herniated disc.

35. **What is the bowstring test?**
    With the patient supine, flex their hip with approximately 20° knee flexion and apply pressure to the popliteal fossa. Reproduction of pain is suggestive of sciatic nerve etiology.

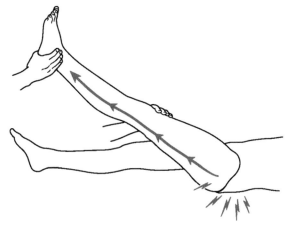

Figure 9.5. Illustration of positive straight-leg raise test and resulting symptoms. *(From Vaccaro AR [ed], Core Knowledge in Orthopaedics – Spine, 1st ed., Copyright © 2005, Mosby, Elsevier.)*

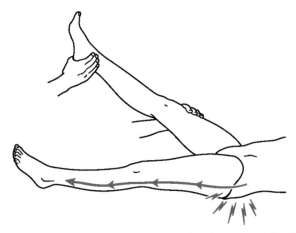

Figure 9.6. Illustration of positive crossed straight-leg raise test and resulting symptoms. *(From Vaccaro AR [ed], Core Knowledge in Orthopaedics – Spine, 1st ed., Copyright © 2005, Mosby, Elsevier.)*

36. **What is the femoral stretch test?**
    With the patient prone, extend the hip. Pain in the anterior thigh (L2–L3) or medial leg (L4) is suggestive of a herniated disc at those levels.

37. **What are two tests for sacroiliitis?**
    Gaenslen maneuver and FABER test.

38. **What is the Gaenslen maneuver?**
    With the patient supine, let one leg hang off the side of the table and extend the hip and flex the opposite hip at the same time. This flexes both sacroiliac joints. Pain is suggestive of sacroiliitis.

39. **What is the FABER test?**
    Flexion Abduction External Rotation of the hip. With the patient supine, have the patient flex their knee resting their foot on their opposite knee. Slowly apply pressure to the flexed knee causing external rotation of the hip. At the same time, apply pressure to the contralateral iliac crest. Pain in the sacroiliac area is suggestive of sacroiliitis.

40. **What are Waddell signs?**
    Overreaction/exaggerated response, pain to light touch, pain or numbness in non-anatomic distribution, negative flip sign with positive straight-leg test, producing back pain by pushing on the head. These are highly suggestive of non-organic pathology/pain.

41. **What should the neurological examination incude?**
    Muscle strength and examination for wasting, sensation, gait, balance, coordination, reflexes, and provocative tests.

42. **What sensory levels are commonly tested? (Table 9.1)**
    See Figure 9.7 for illustration.

Table 9.1. Sensory Dermatomes and Corresponding Anatomic Landmarks	
LEVEL(s)	**CORRESPONDING ANATOMIC REGION**
C5	Clavicles
C5,6,7	Lateral aspect of upper extremities
C8, T1	Medial aspect of upper extremities
C6	Thumb
C6,7,8	Hand
C8	Ring and little fingers
T4	Nipples
T10	Umbilicus
L1	Inguinal/groin
L1,2,3,4	Anterior and inner surfaces of lower extremities
L4,5,S1	Foot
L4	Medial aspect of foot
L5	1st webspace of foot
S1	Lateral aspect of foot
L5,S1,2	Posterior and outer surfaces of lower extremities
S2,3,4	Perineum

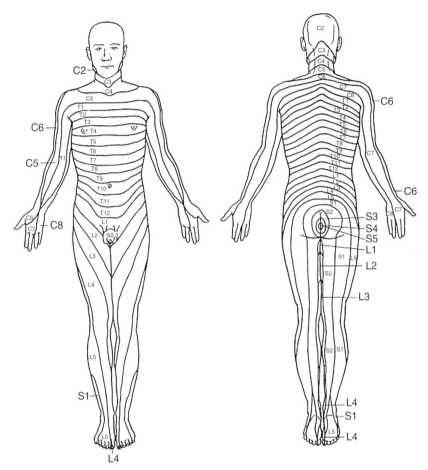

Figure 9.7. Illustration showing the sensory dermatomes. *(From Leventhal MR: Fractures, Dislocations, and Fracture-dislocations of Spine. In: Canale ST, Beaty JH [eds], Campbell's Operative Orthopaedics, 10th ed., Philadelphia: Mosby; 2003.)*

43. In cervical nerve root compression, list each disc level as well as the nerve root typically affected by a paracentral disc herniation at each level, as well as the motor, sensory, and reflex deficit associated with compression of each nerve root. Please refer to Table 9.2.

44. Which cervical level is the most commonly affected by nerve root compression?
    C5–C6 affecting the C6 nerve root.

45. In lumbar/sacral nerve root compression, list each disc level as well as the nerve root for each level, the motor loss from each level, the sensory loss from each level, as well as the reflex for each level.
    Refer to Table 9.3.

46. Which lumbar level is the most commonly affected?
    L4–L5, affecting the L5 nerve root.

Table 9.2. Cervical Radiculopathy Syndromes by Disc Level and Affected Exiting Nerve Root

DISC LEVEL	NERVE ROOT	MUSCLES AFFECTED	SENSORY LOSS	REFLEX
C3–C4	C4	Scapular, diaphragm	Lateral neck, shoulder	None
C4–C5	C5	Deltoid, biceps	Lateral shoulder and arm	Biceps
C5–C6	C6	Wrist ext., bi/triceps	Radial forearm and thumb	Brachioradialis
C6–C7	C7	Triceps, wrist flexors	Post. forearm, mid. finger	Triceps
C7–T1	C8	Finger flex., interossei	Ulnar forearm and hand	None
T1–T2	T1	Interossei	Ulnar forearm	None

Table 9.3. Lumbar Radiculopathy Syndromes by Disc Level and Affected Traversing Nerve Root

DISC LEVEL	NERVE ROOT	MUSCLES AFFECTED	SENSORY LOSS	REFLEX
L1–L2	L2	Psoas	Upper anterior thigh	None
L2–L3	L3	Quadriceps	Anteromedial thigh	None
L3–L4	L4	Tibialis anterior	Medial leg, ankle, foot	Patellar
L4–L5	L5	Ext. hallucis longus	Dorsal foot, 1st webspace	None
L5–S1	S1	Gastroc/soleus	Posterior leg and lateral foot	Achilles
S2–S5	S2–S4	Bowel/bladder sphincter	Perianal	Cremasteric/wink

47. **At what sites do disc herniations occur, and how do they differ in terms of clinical presentation?**

    Disc herniations may occur in any of four anatomic zones, which have implications as to which nerve roots may be affected at a given level.

    A straight posterior herniation causes compression in the central canal zone. This may result in central canal stenosis, and, depending on level, may contribute to cervical myelopathy or lumbar stenosis. An acute posterior herniation in the lumbosacral region may also result in cauda equina syndrome.

    A paracentral herniation causes compression in the subarticular zone, also referred to as the lateral recess. This is the most common site of herniation due to the thinning of the posterior longitudinal ligament and relative weakness of the annulus fibrosus in this region. In the cervical spine, a herniation at this location typically causes compression of the exiting nerve root at this level (e.g., C4–C5 disc herniation resulting in C5 radiculopathy). In contrast, a lumbar paracentral disc herniation typically causes compression of the traversing nerve root before it exits at the level below (e.g., L4–L5 paracentral disc herniation resulting in L5 radiculopathy).

    Foraminal disc herniations are uncommon, but may be exquisitely painful due to direct compression of the affected exiting nerve root and dorsal root ganglion. Extraforaminal or far-lateral disc herniations are also less common, and can have varied presentations depending on exact sites of compression. Extraforaminal disc herniations may even result in compression of the superiorly exiting nerve root and ganglion (e.g., L4–L5 extraforaminal disc herniation resulting in L4 radiculopathy) (Fig. 9.8).

48. **What imaging techniques and diagnostic tests are used in evaluation of the spine (vertebral bodies, intervertebral discs, spinal cord and canal, nerve roots, and nerves)?**

    Radiography (x-ray), computed tomography (CT), myelography, magnetic resonance imaging (MRI), nuclear medicine bone scan, and electromyography (EMG).

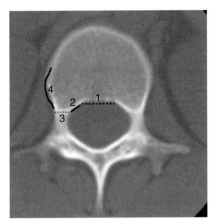

Figure 9.8. Anatomic zones of disc herniation (1: central canal zone, 2: subarticular zone or lateral recess; 3: foraminal or pedicle zone, 4: extraforaminal or far-lateral zone). (*From Wiltse LL, Berger PE, McCulloch JA: A system for reporting the size and location of lesions in the spine. Spine 1997;22:1534–1537.*)

49. **What is radiography (x-ray) and when is it most effective?**
   X-rays are radiographic images obtained by projecting x-ray beams through the body onto an image detector. The more radiodense an object is (bone or metal) the more radiation it absorbs creating a white image. The more radiolucent an object is (air), the less radiation is absorbed creating a black image. X-rays are fast to obtain and relatively inexpensive, which is why they are the most commonly used medical imaging modality. X-rays show bony detail, making them useful to evaluate for fractures, degenerative or arthritic changes, malalignment, scoliosis, spondylolisthesis, and spondylolysis. X-rays are not effective for imaging soft tissue due to poor contrast resolution.

50. **What is myelography?**
   Myelography consists of injecting a contrast material into the spinal sac, followed by serial x-rays, CT scan, or MRI. Water-soluble contrasts are the most popular contrast agents because the body will absorb them over time. Indications include suspicion of an intraspinal lesion or questionable diagnosis resulting from conflicting clinical findings in other studies. Myelography has value in previously operated spines and in spinal stenosis, especially in conjunction with CT. Because myelography is an invasive study, reactions may occur, including headache, pain, nausea, vomiting, meningitis, and localized infection. Myelography has largely been replaced by MRIs.

51. **What is computed tomography (CT)?**
   CT uses x-ray beams to create tomographic images (slices) of an object. These images are reassembled to create a 3-D image of the object. The advantages of CT over myelography include better visualization of lateral lesions, such as foraminal stenosis and lateral disc herniations, lower radiation dose, and absence of adverse reactions. CT generally allows discrimination between neural compression caused by soft tissue and that caused by bone. CT is extremely useful in the diagnosis of lateral or foraminal herniations of the lumbar disc. The disadvantages are higher doses of radiation compared to x-ray and MRI, metal distorts the image by creating artefact, obese patients may be too large for the scanner, and does not show anatomic detail of neural elements. Prior to the use of MRI scans, CT myelography was the study of choice for evaluating the contents of the spinal canal, albeit indirectly.

52. **What is magnetic resonance imaging (MRI)?**
   MRI is non-radiation based, and uses strong magnets that send and receive radio frequency signals. These signals cause all protons to line up, and then relax back to their natural alignment. The detectors pick up the weak signal produced by the protons relaxation and

create a 3-D image. The advantage of MRI over a CT scan includes the ability to demonstrate intraspinal tumors, to examine the entire spine, and to identify degenerative discs. Anatomic detail of neural elements is much better than CT, but MRI does not demonstrate bone anatomy as well as CT. MRIs are contraindicated for patients with pacemakers, defibrillators, and metal implants.

53. **What is a nuclear medicine bone scan?**
Bone scans use a radioactive tracer that is given to the patient to serve as a marker of biologic activity. The radioactive tracer collects in areas of highest biologic activity. Bone scans can be used when physicians suspect diseases other than lumbar disc disease or spinal stenosis. Bone scan confirms neoplastic, infectious, traumatic, or arthritic problems of the spine.

54. **What is electromyography (EMG)?**
EMG is used to evaluate electrical activity produced by skeletal muscle. It involves placing needle electrodes into skeletal muscle and recording the electrical activity. They are often performed to evaluate for denervation, which can be caused by nerve compression (slipped disc, spinal stenosis). Spontaneous electrical activity will be measured if a muscle has lost its normal innervation.

55. **Is electromyography useful in patients with lumbar disc disease?**
Electromyography is commonly used to help in differentiating radicular symptoms from peripheral neuropathy or upper motor neuron lesions and in determining the presence or absence of generalized myopathy.

56. **What radiographic examinations are important in the diagnosis of spinal stenosis?**
MRI is the study of choice for evaluating spinal stenosis. CT myelograms are reserved usually for patients with contraindications to MRI (aneurysm clips, pacemakers) or in patients where stainless steel metal artefact makes MRI difficult to interpret. True stenosis is considered absolute with a 10–12 mm sagittal diameter. Both studies show the neural foramina, facet joints, ligamentum flavum, and any compression on the spinal canal. Other abnormalities, including post-traumatic deformities, overgrowth of spinal fusions, Paget's disease, vertebral ligament hypertrophy, and intraspinal masses also can be identified.

57. **If you are concerned for a possible c-spine fracture, what imaging study should be obtained first?**
A scout lateral radiograph of the cervical spine with evaluation from the base of the skull to the top of T1.

58. **What other radiographs are helpful in determining cervical fractures or dislocations?**
A full four-view cervical-spine series, consisting of anterior and posterior, lateral, oblique, and odontoid radiographs of the spine should be obtained to evaluate for fractures and spinal alignment. The oblique views are essential in evaluation of the apophyseal joints, which indicate either unilateral or bilateral facet dislocation. Tomograms are also helpful in determining odontoid fractures.

59. **What radiographic parameter may be useful in determining the presence of an occult fracture?**
Prevertebral soft-tissue swelling often accompanies fractures of the cervical spine. If there is no obvious evidence of fracture on plain radiographs of the cervical spine, the thickness of prevertebral soft tissues should be assessed. The prevertebral soft tissues should be within the following normal limits of thickness by level: C3 = 3.5 mm; C4 = 5.0 mm; C5–C7 = approximately 15–20 mm increasing distally. If abnormal widening is noted at any area along the anterior cervical spine, fracture should be suspected.

60. **What type of radiographs should be obtained if cervical spinal instability is suspected?**
Flexion–extension radiographs.

61. Are routine radiographs helpful in evaluation of lumbar spine disease?

They are usually of low yield. Only 1–2% of the spine radiographs in patients with back pain between 20 and 50 years of age have unsuspected findings. Most studies have found some disc space narrowing or osteophyte formation in this age group. Spondylolisthesis and spondylolysis may be seen on radiographs, along with some disc space narrowing at the affected level. Such findings, however, are also present in patients with no back pain and no clinically significant pathology.

62. What are some of the various MRI findings that may be found in patients with spinal cord injuries?

Myelomalacia, or edema within the spinal cord is seen as fusiform enlargement of the cord with increased signal intensity on T2-weighted images. Hematoma is characterized by increased signal intensity on T2 images acutely and is often surrounded by a halo of T2 enhancement from adjacent edema. Extrinsic cord compression by osseous elements, disc material, soft tissue, or fluid may be present, with or without resultant signal change in the cord. Significant soft-tissue edema is also common, especially in the cervical spine when the posterior tension band is disrupted after hyperflexion injuries.

63. What are "red flags" in the history or evaluation of a patient with neck or back pain?

There are numerous potential causes of isolated neck or back pain. In the majority of cases, the pain is self-limiting and symptoms will resolve with activity modification and analgesia within 4–6 weeks. Further diagnostic evaluation in these cases is typically of low-yield; however, the possibility exists that certain serious etiologies of back or neck pain may be missed with an indiscriminate approach. The Agency for Healthcare Policy and Research (AHCPR) has formulated guidelines to identify "red flags" that may indicate the presence of conditions that can result in permanent impairment or death. Such conditions as malignancy, infection, fractures, and cauda equina syndrome require additional workup and/or prompt intervention, and must be excluded during initial evaluation. For cancer or infection, red flags are: history of cancer, unexplained weight loss, immunosuppression, urinary infection, intravenous drug use, prolonged use of corticosteroids, back pain not improved with rest, and age of patient over 50.

For spinal fracture, red flags are: history of significant trauma (for example, a fall from a height, motor vehicle accident, or direct blow to the back for a young adult, or a minor fall or heavy lift in a potentially osteoporotic or elderly individual), prolonged use of steroids, and age over 70.

For cauda equina syndrome or severe neurologic compromise, red flags are: medical history or physical examination findings of acute onset of urinary retention or overflow incontinence, loss of anal sphincter tone or fecal incontinence, saddle anesthesia (about the anus, perineum, and genitals), and global or progressive motor weakness in the lower limbs.

64. What types of infections may occur in the spine?

Spinal infections may be broadly grouped into pyogenic (i.e., bacterial) and non-pyogenic (i.e., mycobacterial or fungal).

Pyogenic infections may be spontaneous in children or patients with risk factors as described above, or may occur postoperatively. The most common pathogen is *Staphylococcus aureus*. Presentations may range from spondylodiscitis (infection of the disc space and/or vertebral body) to epidural abscess or meningitis. The goals of intervention are to eradicate the infection, maintain spinal stability, and prevent neurologic deterioration. Life-threatening sepsis may occur if untreated, and both antibiotic therapy and surgical debridement are frequently required for successful treatment. The treatment course is often complicated by the presence of instrumentation and the need for suppression of infection until fusion can occur.

Non-pyogenic infection most frequently refers to mycobacterial disease of the spine. Spinal tuberculosis, or Pott's disease, may have an indolent course, and is an important cause of spinal deformity in the developing world especially in areas with a high prevalence of HIV. Other organisms, such as *Brucella*, *Aspergillus*, *Candida*, and

Cryptococcus are possible causes of non-pyogenic infections in endemic areas or in immunocompromised hosts. Non-pyogenic infections are less likely to cause generalized sepsis in the competent host, but are challenging to eradicate. Given the duration and toxicity of pharmacologic treatment needed to treat such infections, image-guided or open biopsies are often required for accurate diagnosis and determination of sensitivities. Surgical intervention may need to be staged depending on the extent of deformity and required reconstruction.

65. **What types of tumor may occur in the spine? (Tables 9.4 and 9.5)**

Table 9.4. Diagnosis According to Age

10 TO 30 Years	30 TO 50 YEARS	OLDER THAN 50 YEARS
Aneurysmal bone cyst	Chondrosarcoma	Metastatic
Ewing sarcoma	Chordoma	Myeloma
Giant cell carcinoma	Hodgkin disease	
Histiocytosis X	Hemangioma	
Osteoblastoma		
Osteoid osteoma		
Osteochondroma		
Osteosarcoma		

Table 9.5. Diagnosis According to Location

Vertebral body	Posterior elements	Adjacent vertebrae	Multiple vertebrae
Chordoma	Aneurysmal bone cyst	Aneurysmal bone cyst	Metastatic
Giant cell carcinoma	Osteoblastoma	Chondrosarcoma	Myeloma
Hemangioma	Osteoid osteoma	Chordoma	Histiocytosis X
Histiocytosis X	Osteochondroma		
Metastatic disease			
Myeloma			

(From Charbot JNC, et al. Spine tumors: Patient evaluation. Semin Spine Surg 1995;7:260.)

66. **What are the most common types of metastatic lesions to the spine?**
Metastatic tumors are by far the most common malignant lesions found in bone, present 40 times more frequently than all other primary malignancies of bone combined. Tumor types predisposed to bony metastases include breast, lung, prostate, kidney, thyroid, lymphoma, and multiple myeloma. As cancer survival continues to improve, spinal metastases are becoming an increasingly important entity which may result in significant impairment of quality of life. In patients with metastases, the spine is involved in 50–85 percent of cases, most often affecting the vertebral bodies of the lumbar spine, followed by the thoracic, cervical, and sacral regions. Diagnosis may be made on the basis on a combination of imaging studies, typically including bone scan, MRI or PET/CT. Treatment is highly dependent on symptoms, patient-specific factors, neurologic status, tumor type, and overall prognosis, and may include a combination of chemotherapy, radiation therapy, and/or surgical excision with stabilization depending on the overall clinical picture.

CERVICAL

CASE 9-1

A 17-year-old male presents to a local Emergency Department complaining of neck pain after landing on the back of his flexed head during a failed attempt at performing a backflip. He did not lose consciousness and reports no other injuries, but is complaining of severe neck pain. Neurologic examination reveals no focal motor, sensory, or cranial nerve abnormalities. His cervical spine radiograph is seen in Figure 9.9 below.

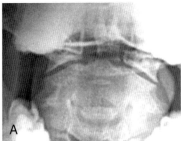
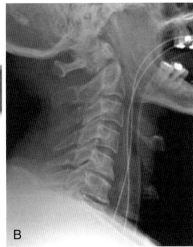

Figure 9.9. Open-mouth antero-posterior and lateral radiographs of the cervical spine. *(From Marx JA, et al., [eds], Rosen's Emergency Medicine, 7th ed., Copyright © 2010, Mosby, Elsevier Inc.)*

67. **What is the diagnosis?**
    The patient has suffered an *odontoid fracture* with posterior and lateral displacement.

68. **What is an odontoid fracture?**
    An odontoid fracture is a fracture of the odontoid process. The odontoid process, also called the dens, is a small vertical projection upwards from C2 (axis). The odontoid articulates with the anterior aspect of C1 (atlas) and allows C1–C2 rotation and is the *primary horizontal stabilizer* of the cervical spine.

69. **What is the mechanism of an odontoid fracture?**
    The majority of odontoid fractures are caused by flexion loading which results in anterior displacement of the odontoid. A minority of odontoid fractures are caused by a posterior force on the forehead (extension loading), which results in posterior displacement of the odontoid.

70. **What is the incidence of neurologic involvement?**
    About 5–10%, ranging from Brown-Séquard syndrome, hemiparesis, and quadriparesis.

71. **How are odontoid fractures diagnosed?**
    Odontoid fractures are usually diagnosed through x-rays, but can be missed due to overlying bone. CT scans are the most sensitive study to diagnose odontoid fractures.

72. **How are odontoid fractures classified?**
    Type I: Fractures through the tip of the odontoid process. Type I fractures are rare and are usually caused by an avulsion of the alar ligament which connects the odontoid to the occiput.

Type II: Fractures through the base of the odontoid neck (junction of the odontoid and body of the C2 vertebra). These are the most common odontoid fractures and have a high nonunion rate.

Type III: Fractures that extend into the cancellous bone of the body of C2. These fractures are unstable because they allow the C1 vertebrae and occiput to move together as a unit (Fig. 9.10).

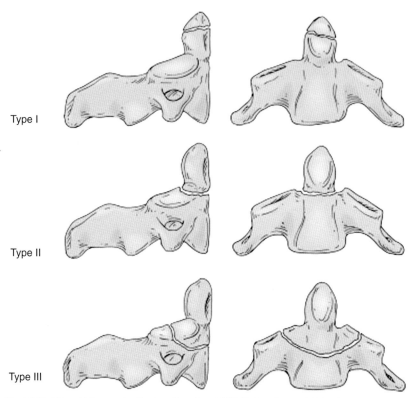

Type I

Type II

Type III

Figure 9.10. Odontoid fracture classification. *(From Benzel EC [ed], Spine Surgery, 3rd ed., Copyright © 2012, Saunders, Elsevier Inc.)*

73. **What potential complication may be seen with Type II odontoid fractures?**
    Type II fractures have a high (~40%) incidence of nonunion. This is due to blood supply compromise as well as lack of periosteum and cancellous bone in the tip of the odontoid process.

74. **What are risk factors for nonunion of a Type II fracture?**
    Age >50, >5 mm displacement and posterior displacement, and fracture older than 2 weeks.

75. **How are odontoid fractures treated?**
    Treatment is dependent on the type of fracture. Type I fractures, if isolated, are stable and are treated with immobilization in a cervical collar. Treatment of Type II fractures is variable, although surgical management has become more common due to the high incidence of nonunion. Non-operative management would consist of halo immobilization. Operative management may consist of anterior screw fixation of the odontoid or a posterior C1–C2 fusion. Type III fractures are treated with halo immobilization and have a high likelihood of union.

CASE 9-2

A 34-year-old male is brought to the trauma bay after a single-vehicle motor vehicle crash. The patient was an unrestrained driver and was ejected out of the car through the windshield. He was found unconscious but breathing spontaneously at the scene. Upon presentation to the trauma bay the patient is still breathing spontaneously, heart rate is 86 bpm, and blood pressure is 108/70 mmHg. He has a 7 cm laceration over his forehead with multiple abrasions around his right eye and cheek but no obvious osseous injury. The primary survey is complete with his airway intact, breathing spontaneous, and heart rate regular with distal pulses intact. He is still in the c-collar placed at the scene. There are no spontaneous movements of his extremities and no reflexes, as well as no bulbocavernosus reflex.

76. **In an unconscious patient with obvious blunt trauma to the forehead, what type of injuries must be ruled out during the secondary survey?**
With obvious head trauma and unconsciousness, one needs to rule out a cervical spine fracture. This is best done with a scout lateral radiograph of the cervical spine.

77. **To evaluate for cervical trauma, which radiograph should be obtained first to evaluate the stability of the cervical spine?**
The initial radiograph should be a *lateral radiograph of the cervical spine*. This is preferably made with the patient still on the transportation stretcher. If possible, all handling should be postponed until the results of the radiographic examination are known. If handling is necessary, the patient should be stabilized by moving "as one piece" by at least four persons to avoid cervical cord injury, especially in the unconscious patient. One person needs to be dedicated to stabilizing the patient's head and neck during any handling and log rolls. In order to be of diagnostic value, the lateral cervical spine radiograph must adequately visualize the cervicothoracic junction (articulation of C7 on T1).

78. **After obtaining the initial lateral radiograph, what radiographic examinations are necessary or useful for patients with suspected spinal cord injury?**
A full four-view cervical-spine series, consisting of anterior and posterior, lateral, oblique and odontoid radiographs of the spine should be obtained to evaluate for fractures and spinal alignment. However, many times these plain radiographs are not obtained and CT scans are obtained instead. CT of the cervical spine visualizes bony detail and can demonstrate bony impingement on the neural canal and assesses stability. Sagittal and coronal reconstructions are advantageous in the evaluation of transverse or axially oriented injuries, horizontal lamina fractures, and some facet injuries. MRI may more precisely demonstrate the status of the spinal canal, spinal cord, intervertebral disc, potential sites of ligamentous injury, and presence of epidural hematoma.

CASE 9-2   continued

The patient's lateral c-spine radiograph and CT c-spine are obtained and shown in Figure 9.11 below.

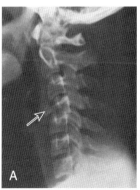
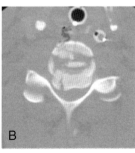

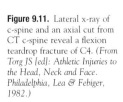

Figure 9.11. Lateral x-ray of c-spine and an axial cut from CT c-spine reveal a flexion teardrop fracture of C4. (*From Torg JS [ed]: Athletic Injuries to the Head, Neck and Face. Philadelphia, Lea & Febiger, 1982.*)

79. **What is seen on the imaging studies?**
A C4 flexion teardrop fracture.

80. **What is a flexion teardrop fracture?**
A flexion teardrop fracture is a fracture of the *anterior and middle bone columns and a disruption of the posterior ligamentous tension band*; fracture fragments may be displaced into the neural canal to a variable extent, often injuring the cord. These fractures are unstable and often associated with significant neurological injury.

81. **What is the mechanism of a cervical burst fracture?**
Axial loading with the neck in neutral or flexed position.

82. **How should flexion-teardrop fractures be managed?**
Immobilization should be maintained as soon as the injury is recognized. Because this is an unstable, three column injury, surgical decompression and fusion is typically the management of choice.

83. **What is the most likely reason for the patient's lack of reflexes?**
The patient is in spinal shock with likely associated spinal cord injury.

84. **What is spinal shock?**
Spinal shock is defined as a dysfunction of the nervous tissue of the spinal cord based on physiologic rather than structural disruption; it occurs after spinal cord injury. It is characterized by loss of sensation and motor (flaccid paralysis with no reflexes). Spinal shock typically resolves within 48 hours.

85. **What physical finding signals the end of spinal shock?**
The bulbocavernosus reflex signals the end of spinal shock.

86. **What is the bulbocavernosus reflex?**
The bulbocavernosus reflex involves the S1, S2, and S3 nerve roots and a spinal cord-mediated reflex arc. It is useful for gaining information about the state of spinal cord injuries and testing for spinal shock. Bulbocavernosus reflexes are tested by compressing the glans penis in males or by applying pressure to the clitoris in females (or tug on an indwelling Foley catheter) and observing contraction of the anal sphincter. Return of this reflex marks the resolution of spinal shock. However, the bulbocavernosus reflex may permanently be interrupted if the spinal injury is at or below the level of the conus medullaris or cauda equina.

CASE 9-2   continued

The patient was initially reduced with traction. When hemodynamically stable, he was taken to the operating room where he underwent decompression and fusion with anterior and posterior instrumentation. After several days in the hospital, the patient has regained consciousness and is able to move his shoulders and flex his elbows, but cannot extend his wrist or move his fingers. He also has no motor or sensation of his torso and legs.

87. **Does this patient have complete or incomplete spinal cord injury?**
Complete spinal cord injury.

88. **What is complete spinal cord injury?**
A complete spinal cord injury is manifested by total motor and sensory loss distal to the injury level (no spared motor or sensory function in the lowest sacral segments). A complete spinal cord injury diagnosis cannot be made until spinal shock is over. This is seen with the return of the bulbocavernosus reflex. If the bulbocavernosus reflex is positive but no sacral sensation or motor function has returned, the paralysis is complete and will likely be permanent in most patients.

89. **What is sacral sparing?**
Sacral sparing is evidenced by perianal sensation, rectal motor function, and great toe flexor activity. Sacral sparing means that an incomplete spinal cord lesion is present, with at least partial structural continuity of the white-matter long tracts, and has the potential for some recovery of function in the extremities.

90. **What is an incomplete spinal cord injury?**
In an incomplete spinal cord injury some motor or sensory function is spared distal to the cord injury. Several types of incomplete spinal cord syndromes have been identified:

Brown-Séquard syndrome, anterior cord syndrome, posterior cord syndrome, and central cord syndrome.

91. **What is Brown-Séquard syndrome?**
Brown-Séquard syndrome is a *spinal cord hemisection*, an injury to either half of the spinal cord. It most frequently results from a penetrating injury, but can also result from a lamina or pedicle fracture. *Symptoms include loss of motor and position sense, vibration on the side of the lesion (ipsilateral paralysis), and contralateral loss of pain and temperature sensation.* Prognosis for recovery is *good*; neurologic improvement often is significant.

92. **What is anterior cord syndrome?**
Anterior cord syndrome has *complete motor loss and loss of pain and temperature discrimination below the level of injury.* Posterior columns, including deep-touch position sense and vibratory sensation, are spared. It is usually caused by a hyperflexion injury in which bone compresses the anterior spinal artery and cord. Prognosis for recovery is **poor**.

93. **What is posterior cord syndrome?**
Posterior cord syndrome involves the dorsal columns of the spinal cord, and is characterized by *loss of proprioceptive vibratory sense with sparing of sensory and motor function.* This syndrome is rare.

94. **What is central cord syndrome?**
Central cord syndrome involves destruction of the central area of spinal cord. It is typically manifested by *weakness affecting the upper extremities more than the lower extremities.* Centrally located arm tracts are most severely affected, whereas the leg tracts are affected to a lesser extent. Sensation is variably spared but often involves a severe burning, neuropathic pain in the distal upper extremities. This usually results from a hyperextension injury in an older person with preexisting spinal stenosis or from flexion injuries in younger patients.

95. **What is the most common type of incomplete spinal cord injury?**
Central cord syndrome.

96. **Which type of incomplete spinal cord injury has the best prognosis for recovery?**
Brown-Séquard syndrome.

97. **What is the three-column concept of the spine?**
The three-column concept of the spine was popularized by Denis, and offers a biomechanical rationale for the patterns of failure observed with differing mechanisms of spinal injury. *The anterior column includes the anterior longitudinal ligament, the anterior portion of the annulus, and the anterior half of the vertebral body. The middle column consists of the posterior longitudinal ligament, the posterior portion of the annulus, and the posterior portion of the vertebral body. The posterior column is made up of the pedicles, facets, lamina, and posterior ligamentous complex, including the interspinal ligaments, ligamentum flavum, and facet joint capsule.* These columns may fail individually or in combination as a result of four basic mechanisms of injury: (1) compression (axial force), (2) distraction, (3) rotation, and (4) shear forces. These forces result in the most common major types of spinal fractures.

98. **What is the most common mechanism of cervical spinal cord injury?**
Motor vehicle accidents account for about half. Other common mechanisms include falls, sports injuries, and acts of violence.

99. **What role do steroids have in the treatment of acute spinal cord injuries?**
The use of steroids in acute spinal cord injury remains a highly controversial topic. A systematic review performed by the Cochrane Group concluded that high-dose methylprednisone therapy improved neurologic recovery if administered within 8 hours of injury. Bracken et al.'s original paper showed neurological improvement with the regimen of 30 mg/kg given within 8 hours of injury, then 5.4 mg/kg for an additional 23 hours. The systematic review found additional improvement in motor recovery and functional status if methylprednisone therapy was extended for another 24 hours (48 hours total). The initiation of therapy after 8 hours from injury has been associated with some improvement

in sensory recovery, but these findings remain controversial. The use of high-dose methylprednisolone is also associated with significant risks, and its use must be considered in the context of the patient's other injuries and comorbidities.

100. **In C4 quadriplegia, with lesion between C4 and C5 vertebrae, what changes in motor function, sensory function, or upper extremity reflexes are expected?**

Motor: In C4 quadriplegia, you expect the patient to breathe spontaneously because C4 innervates the diaphragm. The patient has limited shoulder movement with no flexion or extension of his fingers, wrist, and elbow. They also have complete paralysis of body and legs.

Sensation: Present in the upper anterior chest wall but not in the upper extremities.

Reflexes: Reflexes may be diminished or absent in the acute phase of injury. Following resolution of spinal shock, hyperreflexia is expected due to loss of central inhibition of the reflex arc.

101. **In C5 quadriplegia, what motor, sensation, and upper extremity reflex changes are expected?**

Motor: In C5 quadriplegia, the deltoid muscle and a portion of the biceps muscle are functioning. The patient is able to perform shoulder abduction and flexion–extension as well as some elbow flexion. However, all these functions are weak.

Sensation: Normal over the upper portion of the anterior chest wall and the lateral aspect of the arm from the shoulder to the elbow crease.

Reflexes: Acutely, the biceps and brachioradialis reflexes may be normal or slightly decreased. Following resolution of the acute phase, hyperreflexia would be expected distal to and including the brachioradialis reflex.

102. **In C6 quadriplegia, what motor functions, sensations, and upper extremity reflexes remain intact?**

Motor: Both the biceps and rotator cuff muscles continue to function. The patient has almost full function of the shoulder, full flexion of the elbow, full supination and partial pronation of the forearm, and partial extension of the wrist. The strength of wrist extension is usually normal. Patient can have a passive grip by extending the wrist, but the grip will be weak.

Sensation: The lateral side of the entire upper extremity, as well as the thumb, index, and half of the middle finger, has normal sensory power.

Reflexes: Acutely, the biceps and brachioradialis reflexes should be intact with the triceps reflex being normal or slightly decreased. Following resolution of the acute phase, hyperreflexia would be expected distal to and including the triceps reflex.

103. **In C7 quadriplegia, what motor functions, sensations, and proximal reflexes remain intact?**

Motor: C7 quadriplegia involves the vertebral level of C7, T1.

With the C7 nerve root intact, the triceps, wrist flexors, and long-finger extensors are functional. The patient can hold objects, but the grasp is extremely weak. Although still confined to a wheelchair, the patient may be able to attempt parallel bar and brace function for general exercise because triceps function may be preserved.

Sensation: C7 has little pure sensory representation in the upper extremity. No precise zone for C7 sensation may be mapped.

Reflexes: The biceps, brachioradialis, and triceps reflexes are normal.

104. **Which type of injury is responsible for the majority of cervical spine fractures from C2 to C7: flexion, extension, or axial compression?**

Extreme cervical *compression* is the major cause of cervical spine fractures from C2 to C7. Such compression may occur from diving, American football, trampoline injuries, automobile accidents, and emergency aircraft egress (ejection-seat injuries). Compression forces are responsible for the majority of non-fatal cervical fractures.

105. **What is neurogenic shock?**

Neurogenic shock is defined as *vascular hypotension with bradycardia* as a result of spinal injury. Neurogenic shock is attributed to the traumatic disruption of the sympathetic outflow and unopposed vagal tone. Massive vasodilation is seen. Treatment is with vasopressors.

106. How is neurogenic shock differentiated from hypovolemic shock?
Neurogenic shock is hypotension with bradycardia (loss of sympathetics). Hypovolemic shock is *hypotension with tachycardia* (sympathetic response).

107. What is a flexion–distraction injury?
A flexion–distraction injury, also known as a Chance fracture when it occurs through osseous structures, is common in motor vehicle accidents when the victim is wearing only a lap seatbelt. The fracture involves the anterior, middle, and posterior columns or the posterior ligaments. With a true flexion–distraction injury, neurologic compromise is most likely when a dislocation occurs.

108. What is a fracture–dislocation?
A fracture–dislocation involves disruption of all three columns by a combination of anterior compression with distraction and rotation. On the antero-posterior radiograph, significant translation is seen. This fracture is highly unstable and often associated with significant neurologic deficit, dural tears, and intra-abdominal injuries.

109. What is a unilateral facet dislocation?
A unilateral facet dislocation takes place when the superior facet dislocates upward, forward, and over the tip of the inferior facet, where the superior facet comes to rest in the intervertebral foramen. They are assumed to occur from axial rotation movements as well as flexion movements and distraction. Tearing of the interspinous ligaments and variable amounts of ligamentum flavum and capsule in one of the facet joints leads to facet dislocation.

110. How are unilateral facet dislocations treated?
If there is minimal subluxation, they can be treated in a Philadelphia collar for 6 weeks with follow-up to make sure subluxation does not progress. For complete dislocations, closed reduction should be attempted with skeletal traction with flouroscopy. If closed reduction is successful, treat with halo vest for 3 months. If closed reduction fails or there is still instability after 3 months, surgical intervention is indicated.

111. What is a halo vest?
A halo vest is an external fixation device that encircles the head and provides traction, external support, and immobilization of the cervical spine (Fig. 9.12).

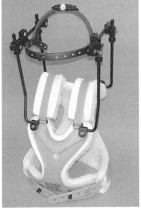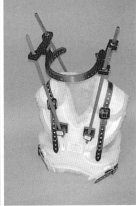

Figure 9.12. A picture of a halo vest. (*From Browner BD, et al. [eds], Skeletal Trauma, 4th ed., Copyright © 2009, Saunders, Elsevier Inc.*)

112. What is a Philadelphia collar?

It is a rigid neck collar that restricts flexion and extension of the cervical spine, but allows minor rotation and lateral bending. It is made of two pieces, a front and a back, that are held together with Velcro straps. This is typically worn following cervical fusion, cervical strain, or certain fractures that are not considered highly unstable (Fig. 9.13).

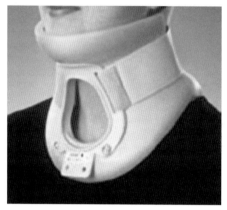

Figure 9.13. A picture of a Philadelphia collar. (*Courtesy of Philadelphia Cervical Collar Company, Thorofare, NJ. In: Roberts JR: Clinical Procedures in Emergency Medicine, 5th edn., Saunders.*)

113. What is a cervicothoracic brace?

A neck brace attached to a two-piece thoracic padded jacket. It is used to restrict neck and upper back movement after cervical spine surgery, or certain injuries including less unstable fractures (Fig. 9.14).

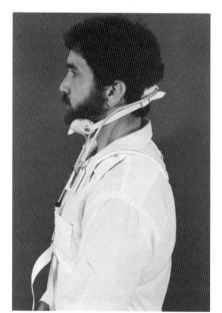

Figure 9.14. A picture of a cervicothoracic brace (sternal occipital mandibular immobilizer type). (*From Hsu JD, et al. [eds], AAOS Atlas of Orthoses and Assistive Devices, 4th ed., Copyright © 2008, Mosby, Elsevier Inc.*)

114. Which cervical orthotic is the most effective in controlling flexion–extension, rotation, and lateral bending?

The halo vest or cast is the most effective in controlling rotation, flexion–extension, and lateral bending. The second most effective device is a rigid cervicothoracic brace, followed by a four-poster brace. The least effective is a soft cervical collar.

115. What is the recommended cervical orthotic device for cervical strain?

Philadelphia collar.

116. What is the most commonly recommended orthotic for most cervical spine fractures?

The halo vest or cast is recognized for most cervical spine fractures. The cervicothoracic brace is used for stable fractures.

117. What is a fracture of the atlas (C1) called?

Jefferson fracture. Axial loading directly downward on the ring of C1 causes multiple fractures of the ring and usually a spreading of the fragments.

118. How is a Jefferson fracture treated?

If the fracture is *stable* (intact transverse ligament), it is treated with a cervical orthotic. If the fracture is *unstable* (ruptured transverse ligament), it is treated with a halo vest or C1–C3 fusion.

119. What is a fracture of the axis (C2) called?

Hangman's fracture. It is scientifically termed a traumatic spondylolisthesis of the axis. The weakest link of the vertebrae is the pars interarticularis of C2, a narrow isthmus located between the superior and inferior facets. This injury usually occurs during rapid deceleration in a motor vehicle accident, when the victim is thrown forward with the head striking the windshield. The accident usually involves a head-on collision with another vehicle or with a fixed object.

120. What are the most common signs and symptoms of a hangman's fracture?

The most common symptoms are frequently vague. The patient often feels marked apprehension and fear with a sense of subjective instability. Pain radiating along the course of the greater occipital nerve (C2), so-called occipital neuralgia, is frequent and leads to marked guarding of neck motion. Another common finding is direct trauma to the top of the forehead of the skull.

121. Where is the most common injury to the cervical spine in children?

Injuries to the cervical spine are rare in children. The most common, however, occur from the occiput to C3. Lesions at the atlantoaxial joint are noted in 70% of children <15 years of age but in only 16% of adults.

122. Athletic injuries to the cervical spine associated with quadriplegia are the result of what mechanism?

Athletic injuries to the cervical spine associated with quadriplegia most commonly occur as a result of *axial loading.* Examples include spearing in football (when a player strikes an opponent with the crown of his helmet), a dive into a shallow body of water with the head striking the bottom, or a hockey player being pushed into the boards headfirst. The fragile cervical spine is compressed between the rapidly decelerated head and the continued momentum of the body.

123. What is meant by the term SCIWORA?

This acronym stands for Spinal Cord Injury WithOut Radiologic Abnormality and describes a phenomenon most commonly observed in pediatric spinal cord injuries. The relative elasticity of the pediatric spine can allow enough elongation under load to injure the neural elements without obvious injury to the bony elements of the spine.

124. What is os odontoideum?

Os odontoideum is a congenital anomaly of the odontoid (dens). The dens is either completely absent, hypoplastic, or incompletely fused to the body of C2 (axis). Most commonly, patients are asymptomatic and it is discovered incidentally. Patients may present clinically with local neck symptoms and transitory episodes of paresthesia after trauma, or frank myelopathy. Clinical manifestations are limited to neck pain and torticollis; depending on the severity, frank brainstem abnormalities may be present (Fig. 9.15).

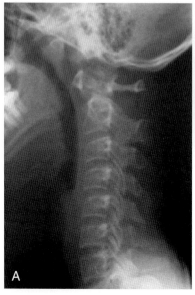

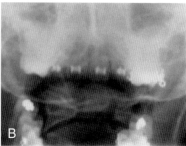

Figure 9.15. Radiographs showing a non-fused os odontoideum. (*From Canale ST, Beaty JH [eds], Campbell's Operative Orthopaedics, 11th ed., p. 1881. Copyright © 2008, Mosby Elsevier Inc.*)

125. **How is os odontoideum treated when patients present with transitory myelopathy?**
Non-operative treatment is sufficient for the patient presenting with a relatively stable os odontoideum and little compromise of the spinal cord. For marked instability, however, a cervical fusion of C1 and C2 is the procedure of choice.

126. **What is the spinal pathology seen in Klippel–Feil syndrome?**
Failure of normal formation of cervical somites, characterized by congenital fusion of any of the seven cervical vertebrae is typically seen (Fig. 9.16).

127. **What are the most common clinical findings in Klippel–Feil syndrome?**
The classic clinical findings are a triad of short neck, a low posterior headline, and limited range of neck motion. However, fewer than 50% of patients have all three elements of the triad.

128. **What are the most common radiographic findings of Klippel–Feil syndrome?**
The most common findings are congenitally fused vertebrae from C2 to C7. The fusions may be multiple-level or single-level.

129. **Do patients with Klippel–Feil syndrome have any auditory abnormalities?**
Yes, *deafness* is a potential auditory abnormality. The incidence of deafness in Klippel–Feil syndrome is approximately 30%.

130. **What other spine abnormality is most commonly associated with Klippel–Feil syndrome?**
Scoliosis is the most commonly associated spinal abnormality in Klippel–Feil syndrome. Approximately 50% of patients report cases of scoliosis, either alone or in combination with *kyphosis*.

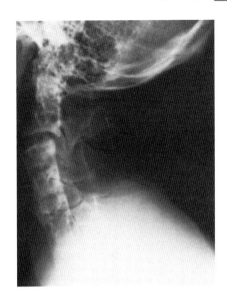

Figure 9.16. A lateral radiograph of the cervical spine demonstrating multiple congenitally fused levels in Klippel–Feil syndrome. (*From Torg JS, Glasgow SG: Criteria for return to contact activities following cervical spine injuries. Clin J Sport Med 1:12–27, 1991.*)

131. **What is the treatment for Klippel–Feil syndrome?**
     The majority of therapy is conservative. Surgery may be indicated if the patient has chronic pain with myelopathy that is associated with instability. *All children should be instructed to avoid collision sports.*

CASE 9-3

A 35-year-old female presents with a 4-month history of right-sided neck, shoulder, and arm pain. She states that the pain radiates down the radial aspect of her forearm to her thumb. She denies any acute trauma. She has recently seen the chiropractor with minimal improvement in symptoms. Exam of her left arm reveals normal strength but decreased biceps reflex and decreased pinprick sensation of the thumb.

132. **What is the likely diagnosis?**
     Cervical radiculopathy caused by a herniated cervical intervertebral disk.

133. **What is cervical radiculopathy?**
     Cervical radiculopathy is a dysfunction of a cervical nerve root. Disc herniation is the most common cause in the younger population. Foraminal narrowing due to degenerative changes (osteophyte formation, uncovertebral hypertrophy, disc narrowing) is the most common cause in the older population.

134. **What is the most common pain pattern of herniated cervical disc?**
     The most common pain pattern for the cervical disc is neck pain with radiation into the scapular area and down the lateral aspect of the arm in to the forearm and hand. The pain is often associated with paresthesias, numbness, or weakness. Symptoms can be intensified with extension or lateral flexion to the herniated side. Valsalva maneuvers can also intensify symptoms.

135. **What is the most common age for a herniated disc?**
     Between 30 and 50 years old.

136. **What are the most commonly affected levels with cervical radiculopathy?**
     C7 (C6–C7 disc herniation) is the most commonly affected nerve root followed by C6 (C5–C6 disc herniation).

137. **What level is most likely involved in the above patient's case?**
C6 radiculopathy caused by a herniation of the C5–C6 disc.

138. **What abnormal findings are expected with a C5–C6 disc herniation?**
Expected findings include decreased sensation in the thumb and index finger, with weakness of the biceps, triceps, and/or wrist extensors, and absence of the brachioradialis reflex.

139. **What abnormalities are expected with a C7 abnormality (e.g., herniated disc at C6–C7)?**
Expected findings include numbness in the long finger and potentially in the index finger, weakness of the triceps, and absence of the triceps reflex.

140. **What abnormality is expected with a C8 nerve abnormality (e.g., herniated disc at the C7–T1 area)?**
Expected findings include numbness in the ulnar nerve distribution of the little finger and ring finger, a claw-hand deformity, weakness of the triceps muscle, and absence of the triceps reflex. Weak thumb extension and wrist ulnar deviation (tested by resisted "thumb's up").

141. **What are the different types of disc herniation?**
The most common type is intraforaminal, which causes predominately sensory changes. The other two types are posterolateral causing predominately motor changes, and central which can cause cervical myelopathy by compressing the spinal cord as well as the nerve root.

142. **What is myelopathy?**
Myelopathy refers to pathology of the spinal cord itself.

143. **How is a herniated disc diagnosed?**
Disc herniation can be suspected through physical exam, and confirmed by radiological testing, usually an MRI scan.

144. **What tests can be done during physical exam that suggest cervical radiculopathy?**
Shoulder abduction relief test, distraction test, and Spurling's test (see previous section for additional detail).

145. **Which radiographic imaging study is the most helpful in determining herniated discs of the cervical spine?**
MRI has become the primary modality to diagnose herniated discs. MRI allows excellent visualization of the spinal cord, nerve roots, and disc material. MRI is also a non-invasive test. The gold standard was once the myelogram with subsequent CT scan. This is a more invasive procedure requiring a lumbar puncture with injection of dye material, and, therefore, is not the primary test used to diagnose herniated discs. A CT scan alone, without contrast or myelogram, is not helpful in diagnosing a disc herniation (Fig. 9.17).

146. **What are the most common methods of conservative treatment of herniated cervical disc?**
The most common methods of treating a herniated cervical disc include physical therapy with cervical traction, a cervical collar, epidural steroid blocks, non-steroidal antiinflammatory drugs (NSAIDs), and time.

147. **What is the rate of success for conservative treatment of herniated cervical discs?**
Conservative treatment of herniated cervical discs is highly successful in 50–60% of cases. A minimum of 3 months of conservative care should be given before considering surgical intervention.

148. **What is the most common surgical treatment for a herniated cervical disc?**
The most common surgical treatment is either an anterior cervical discectomy and fusion (ACDF) with allograft or iliac crest autograft, or a posterior approach with

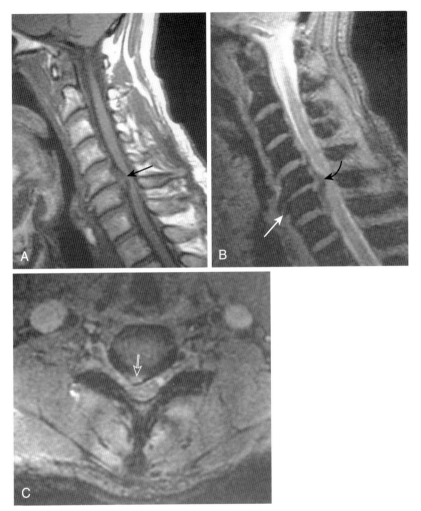

Figure 9.17. MRI showing a herniated C5–C6 disc. *(From Canale ST, Beaty JH [eds], Campbell's Operative Orthopaedics, 11th ed., p.144. Copyright © 2008, Mosby Elsevier Inc.)*

hemilaminectomy, medial facetectomy, and removal of the herniated fragment. The anterior approach is indicated for central or peri-central disc herniation. The posterior approach is indicated for far lateral disc herniation. The posterior approach is a smaller operation and does not necessarily require anterior stabilization or fusion.

CASE 9-4

A 64-year-old male presents with a 2-year history of slowly worsening neck pain that radiates down his left arm into his left radial three fingers. He has no history of neck trauma. He originally saw his family physician, who prescribed NSAIDs and physical therapy. His pain improved with therapy, but started to worsen again after stopping formal physical therapy. He has noticed recently that he is having difficulty holding his coffee mug in his left hand. Physical exam shows weakness of his left wrist extensors and decreased sensation over his left radial three fingers. His grip strength on the left is also decreased from his right.

149. **What is the most likely diagnosis?**
Cervical radiculopathy caused by cervical spondylosis.

150. **What is cervical spondylosis?**
Cervical spondylosis is a combination of *degenerative disk disease* (DDD) and *osteophyte formation* (bone spurs). It is arthritis of the cervical spine. It is most common in people over age 55, and is more common in males. Over time, these arthritic change can press down on one or more of the nerve roots leading to radiculopathy. In advanced cases, the spinal cord can become involved leading to myelopathy.

151. **What are risk factors for cervical spondylosis?**
Age (by age 60, the majority of people show signs of cervical spondylosis on x-ray), male sex, prior neck trauma, prior neck surgery, herniated disc, severe arthritis, repetitive lifting or twisting, being overweight and not exercising, and smoking.

152. **What are symptoms of cervical spondylosis?**
Symptoms usually come on very gradually, but can worsen suddenly. Symptoms are usually not present until the spondylosis progresses to cause radiculopathy and/or myelopathy. Pain or parathesias of the level involved is usually the first symptom. It can progress to weakness in certain muscles, but early on this often is not apparent.

153. **What are the most common levels affected by cervical spondylosis?**
C5–C6 and C6–C7.

154. **How is cervical spondylosis diagnosed?**
Like disc herniation, cervical spondylosis is suspected through physical exam and confirmed with radiological testing.

155. **What physical exam tests suggest radiculopathy from spondylitic changes?**
The shoulder abduction relief test, distraction test, and Spurling's test (see above for definitions).

156. **What radiological test is performed for cervical spondylosis?**
A spine or cervical radiograph will show arthritic changes.

157. **What arthritic changes will be seen on plain radiograph?**
Loss of disc height with subsequent loss of cervical lordosis, osteophytes, instability (subluxation on flexion–extension views). On lateral views, posterior osteophytes will be present. On oblique views, uncovertebral hypertrophy may be noted as well (Fig. 9.18).

158. **What other diagnostic tests can be performed for cervical spondylosis?**
MRI of the cervical spine without contrast will also show arthritic changes, but usually is not performed unless the patient has severe neck/arm pain that is not improved with conservative treatment. MRI is also obtained if the patient has weakness or numbness in their arms/hands. MRI allows cord signal to be examined for possible compression and damage. An EMG can also be performed to examine nerve function. EMGs have a high false-negative rate, but can be useful in differentiating between central nerve root compression and peripheral nerve lesions.

159. **How is cervical spondylosis treated?**
The primary mode of treatment is through conservative measures. Conservative measures include physical therapy, NSAIDs, steroid injections, massage therapy, spinal manipulation, and cold packs or hot packs during acute flare-ups.

160. **When is cervical spondylosis treated with surgery?**
Surgery is considered when conservative treatment fails, the patient has intractable pain, there is a progressive neurological deficit (sensory or motor), or if there is myelopathy.

161. **What is the surgical treatment of cervical spondylosis?**
Cervical spondylosis can be approached through an anterior approach and fusion, or through a posterior approach. The anterior approach involves removing osteophytes, a discectomy, insertion of bone graft between vertebral bodies, and placement of an anterior plate. The posterior approach involves a full decompression procedure (laminectomy or

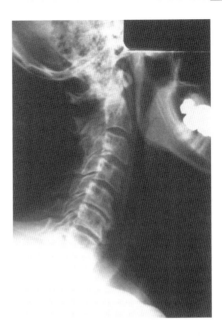

Figure 9.18. A lateral cervical radiograph showing loss of disc height, anterior osteophytes, and loss of cervical lordosis. (*Reprinted with permission from Rosenbaum RB, Campbell SM, Rosenbaum JT, 1996. Clinical Neurology of Rheumatic Disease. Butterworth-Heinemann, Boston.*)

laminoplasty with or without a fusion and instrumentation). The choice of approach may be dictated by the involved levels, the presence of any associated sagittal-plane deformity, and patient-related factors.

THORACOLUMBAR

CASE 9-5

A 78-year-old otherwise healthy female presents to the Emergency Department complaining of back pain after a fall. The patient reports slipping and missing a step while descending a staircase and landing directly on her sacrum. The pain is dull, aching, and unremitting. The patient denies any pre-existing back pain prior to this injury.

162. What is the differential diagnosis?

The case describes acute-onset axial back pain after a fall with a compressive force applied to the base of the spine. The differential diagnosis of axial back pain is quite broad, ranging from degenerative arthritis to infection or malignancy, though the acute onset in this case suggests an injury in the form of muscle and/or ligament strain, or compression fracture. It is important at this point to assess for any neurologic involvement or other factors suggestive of pre-existing pathology that may predispose to such an injury. It is also essential to determine whether an associated head injury occurred, particularly in patients taking anticoagulant medications.

CASE 9-5 continued

Upon further questioning, there has been no associated pain radiation, weakness, numbness, or tingling through either lower extremity, or loss of bowel or bladder control. The patient denies any recent history of fevers, chills, night sweats, or weight loss. There was no head trauma, and the patient does not take aspirin, warfarin, or other anticoagulants. The patient denies any history of fractures, but states that she has yet to undergo a bone-density scan, and does not take calcium or vitamin D supplementation.

163. What is the most likely diagnosis at this point?

The lack of systemic symptoms favors the diagnosis of thoracolumbar compression fracture from the fall. The patient has not undergone bone density evaluation, and should be suspected to be osteopenic until proven otherwise. Osteopenia or osteoporosis greatly increases the risk of compression fractures in the setting of an otherwise low-energy mechanism.

164. **What should be assessed on physical examination?**

Prior to direct examination of the back or extremities, it is important to assess the patient's mental status, balance, and coordination to rule out central causes of disequilibrium that may have predisposed to the fall. The presence of palpitations or syncopal symptoms should prompt further cardiac evaluation. The patient should undergo a complete neurologic examination, including cranial nerves, motor, sensation, and reflexes, to assess for any deficits or localizing signs. The back should be inspected or palpated throughout the entire spine to assess for step-offs or spinous process or paraspinal muscle tenderness. If the patient reports any history or has physical examination findings localizing to the spinal cord or lower extremities, a rectal examination must be performed to assess for tone and sacral reflexes.

CASE 9-5 continued

On examination, the patient is awake, alert, and oriented to person, place, and time with an appropriate affect. Neurologic examination reveals full and intact strength, sensation, and reflexes. The patient is unable to stand for gait examination due to back pain, but cerebellar examination reveals otherwise normal coordination. There is exquisite midline tenderness to palpation in the upper lumbar spine with no palpable step-off.

165. **What further testing or imaging should be performed?**

If there are any symptoms or signs suggestive of altered mental status or other underlying medical causes for disequilibrium, laboratory examination may be performed to rule out metabolic or electrolyte imbalances, or toxin ingestion. Imaging begins with antero-posterior (AP), lateral, and oblique plain radiographs of the lumbar spine in this case, with imaging of the other regions of the spine as dictated by the symptoms and physical examination findings.

CASE 9-5 continued

Laboratory testing reveals no abnormalities. Plain radiographs of the lumbar spine are below (Fig. 9.19):

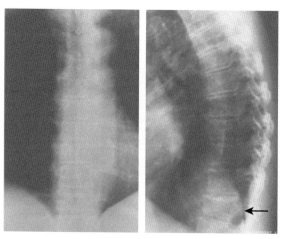

Figure 9.19. Antero-posterior and lateral radiographs of the thoracic spine demonstrating diffuse osteopenia, as well as deformity of the T11 vertebral body with anterior wedging without overt evidence of retropulsion or narrowing of the neural canal. (*Courtesy of Kent R. Theilen, MD, Assistant Professor of Radiology, Mayo Clinic, Rochester, Minn. In: Frontera WR, et al., [eds], Essentials of Physical Medicine and Rehabilitation, 2nd ed., Copyrgith © 2008, Saunders, Elsevier Inc.*)

166. **What other imaging options are available?**
In any case of compression fracture with associated neurologic symptoms or signs, MRI examination must be performed to assess for impingement on the neural canal or nerve roots. CT examination may also be performed to provide fine bony detail in cases of suspected retropulsion of bony fragments, or to assist in preoperative planning. Either of these imaging modalities may also be used if there are additional findings suggestive of pathologic fracture in the setting of suspected malignancy. While not used in the acute setting, DEXA scanning is an important component of bone-density screening for the long-term prevention of insufficiency fractures.

167. **What treatment options are available?**
Compression fractures can be extremely painful, and may be a challenging entity for both the patient and treating physician. For an osteoporotic spinal compression fracture with correlating clinical signs and symptoms in the absence of neurologic compromise, treatment primarily consists of analgesia and activity modification until healing occurs. Moderate evidence exists to suggest that calcitonin (200 IU) daily reduces pain in patients of varying activity levels from 1 to 4 weeks after initial injury. Bisphosphonates may be of benefit in the long-term for prevention of additional compression fractures. For fractures of L3 or L4, the use of L2 nerve blocks has been described, but provides only transient pain relief. No consensus exists on activity modification, exercise, electrical stimulation, alternative therapies, or bracing protocols, and these modalities may be tailored to the benefit of the individual patient.

168. **What are vertebroplasty and kyphoplasty, and do they play a role in the treatment osteoporotic spinal compression fractures?**
Vertebroplasty involves insertion of a needle through the soft tissues of the back into the affected vertebral body, followed by injection of polymethylmethacrylate cement into the vertebral body in an effort to stabilize the fracture. Current guidelines do not support the use of this technique due to the lack of benefit demonstrated in trials comparing vertebroplasty to sham procedures. Kyphoplasty is a similar technique, but additionally involves use of an inflatable balloon to first expand the fractured vertebra in order to restore vertebral body height and spinal alignment. While kyphoplasty may be of benefit in certain patients, considerable controversy exists regarding its use, and the risks of complications with this procedure must be weighed carefully against those of conservative treatment.

CASE 9-6

A 47-year-old male construction worker is brought to the trauma bay after a fall from a 10 foot scaffold complaining of low-back pain and bilateral lower extremity weakness. Airway, breathing, and circulation are intact; Glasgow Coma Scale = 15; and upper extremity function is normal. The patient is subsequently found to have weakness of foot plantar flexion and decreased sensibility to the inner thigh region bilaterally. Rectal examination reveals diminished rectal tone.

169. **What is the differential?**
This case describes acute-onset low-back pain and lower extremity weakness with saddle anesthesia, concerning for a compressive lesion in the region of the lumbar plexus, also known as cauda equina syndrome. In acute cases, this may be the result of extruded intervertebral disc material or fracture fragments, or may have a more subacute progressive presentation in cases of infection or malignancy.

170. **What is the pathophysiology of cauda equina syndrome?**
The cauda equina, or "horse's tail," refers to the bundle of nerve roots contained within the thecal sac inferior to the level of the termination of the spinal cord at the conus medullaris. This typically occurs at approximately the level of the L1 vertebra. A mass lesion at, or inferior to this level may cause some or all of the findings associated with cauda equina syndrome depending on its exact location and the presence of any pre-existing sites of stenosis in the region. In order to manifest in bowel or bladder dysfunction, the compression must affect the sacral nerve roots bilaterally.

171. **What are the other findings associated with cauda equina syndrome?**

Other signs and symptoms may include bilateral leg pain, diminished lower extremity deep-tendon reflexes, fecal and/or urinary incontinence (overflow incontinence secondary to retention), sexual dysfunction, and loss of perineal sensation. These symptoms may be present in varying combinations. If untreated, cauda equina syndrome can lead to permanent neurologic impairment including lower-extremity dysfunction and incontinence of bowel and bladder.

CASE 9-6   continued

Plain radiographs of the spine and CT of the chest, abdomen, and pelvis reveal no evidence of fracture or dislocation.

172. **What is the next appropriate diagnostic step?**

If no apparent bony lesion is identified as a cause of the patient's neurologic compromise, MRI should be performed to look for disc herniation, hematoma, or abscess that may not be visualized on plain radiography or CT (Fig. 9.20).

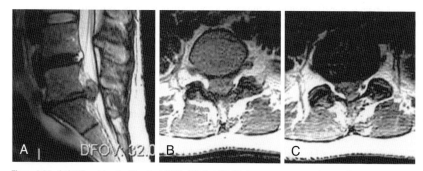

Figure 9.20. (A) T2-weighted midsagittal MRI. (B) Axial MRI demonstrating complete occlusion of the spinal canal at L5–S1. (C) Axial MRI caudal to area of maximal compression (B) demonstrating displacement of the S1 roots and compression of the central sacral roots. (*From Benzel EC [ed], Spine Surgery, 3rd ed., Copyright © 2012, Saunders, Elsevier Inc.*)

173. **What is the appropriate treatment?**

Acute-onset cauda equina necessitates urgent surgical decompression within 48 hours to optimize neurologic recovery. Depending on the etiology, a variety of surgical approaches may be employed, with the most common being a posterior laminectomy to allow for decompression of the nerve roots and excision of extruded disc or fracture fragments. This may be combined with additional internal fixation or fusion procedures if associated with unstable fracture patterns.

CASE 9-7

A 14-year-old female presents for evaluation of her spine after undergoing a routine school screening examination. She feels well and has no complaints at this time. Her mother has noted mild prominence of her right shoulder but is unable to say how long this has been present or whether it has progressed. On examination, the patient demonstrates age-appropriate development and has a normal neurologic examination. The shoulders and pelvis are level and the shoulders are centered over the pelvis when standing. Curvature of the spine is noted with the spinous processes deviating toward the right side in the thoracic region and toward the left in the lumbar region. Forward bending reveals prominence of the right chest wall.

174. **What is the differential diagnosis?**

Spinal deformity may be the result of a specific injury, tumor, or neuromuscular disorder, but in a young adolescent, it is most frequently idiopathic in nature. This patient has what is referred to as *adolescent idiopathic scoliosis* (AIS), with combined coronal and rotational deformity. Kyphoscoliosis refers to the presence of sagittal plane imbalance in addition to coronal and/or rotational deformity.

175. **What is the characteristic curve of adolescent idiopathic scoliosis?**
A convex right-thoracic, left-lumbar curve is typical of AIS. Curves that do not fit this pattern should prompt further evaluation for other associated disorders that may alter the evaluation, management, and prognosis of the deformity.

176. **What disorders may be associated with scoliosis?**
Neurofibromatosis, traumatic injuries including spinal cord injury, connective tissue disorders (Marfan syndrome, Ehlers–Danlos syndrome, neurologic disorders (cerebral palsy, spinal muscular atrophy), metabolic disorders, tumors, and osteochondrodystrophy (dwarfism).

177. **What conditions may cause lateral (coronal) curvature of the spine not associated with rotation (i.e., not true scoliosis)?**
Lateral (coronal) curvature of the spine without rotation can be seen with leg-length discrepancy, posterior element tumors such as osteoid osteomas and osteoblastomas, and psychiatric conditions such as hysterical scoliosis.

178. **What is the incidence of idiopathic scoliosis?**
The incidence of scoliosis has been reported to range from 3% to 5%, with a slightly higher female predominance.

179. **What parameters are used for monitoring of spinal deformity?**
The most commonly used clinical tool to measure spinal rotation is the scoliometer, which is drawn over the spinous processes of the patient while he or she bends at the waist with straight knees and dangling arms. The rotations (in degrees) are recorded at each spinal level. Another important measure is the Cobb angle, which is calculated from standing postero-anterior radiographs.

180. **What is the Cobb angle and how is it calculated?**
The Cobb angle is the term for the angle subtended by the first and last vertebral bodies for each of the respective curve segments (thoracic, lumbar). A postero-anterior 3-ft standing radiograph is taken of the entire spine, including the iliac crests from a 6-ft distance. The superior and inferior vertebrae of each curve are located. The superior and inferior surfaces of the vertebrae tilt maximally into the concavity of the curve. Perpendicular lines are then constructed from the superior end plate of the superior end vertebra and the inferior endplate of the inferior end vertebra. The angle subtended by the intersection of these two lines is the magnitude of the curve. Normal variation includes Cobb angles of up to 10°.

181. **How is skeletal maturity estimated from scoliosis radiographs?**
The Risser classification of skeletal maturity is based on the ossification pattern of the iliac crest epiphysis. Ossification occurs from the anterior superior iliac spine to the posterior superior iliac spine.
   Excursion of ossification is divided into four stages (Fig. 9.21):
Risser 1: 25% excursion
Risser 2: 50% excursion
Risser 3: 75% excursion
Risser 4: 100% (complete) excursion
Risser 5: fusion of the epiphysis to the ilium, representing the end of spinal growth.

182. **What is the minimal amount of lateral (coronal) curvature necessary to qualify as scoliosis?**
Lateral (coronal) curvatures less than 10° are generally not referred to as scoliosis.

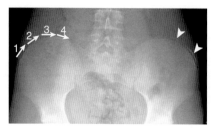

Figure 9.21. Plain radiograph demonstrating iliac crest ossification centers as characterized by the Risser classification. This patient is a Risser stage 2. (*From Manaster BJ, et al., [eds] Musculoskeletal Imaging – The Requisites, 3rd ed., Copyright © 2007, Mosby, Elsevier Inc.*)

CASE 9-7 continued

Further examination reveals no evidence of café au lait spots or sacral dimpling, normal abdominal reflexes, and the absence of cavovarus foot deformity. Maximal thoracic rotational deformity is 7° via scoliometer. The thoracic Cobb angle is 40° (Fig. 9.22).

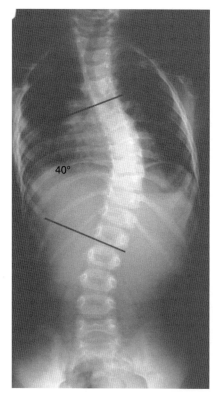

Figure 9.22. Postero-anterior standing scoliosis radiograph demonstrating a right-thoracic curve with a 40° Cobb angle.

183. **How much spinal rotation should be present in order for a patient to be referred to an orthopedic surgeon from a school nurse or primary care physician?**
Under the guidelines of the Scoliosis Research Society, spinal rotations of greater than 7–8° are appropriate for referral to an orthopedic surgeon. This amount of rotation corresponds to approximately 20° of coronal curvature on radiographs. At 5° of rotation, the false-positive rate for scoliosis referral (curves less than 10°) was 36%.

184. **What are the risk factors for progression of curvature in adolescent idiopathic scoliosis?**
The risk factors for progression are curve magnitude (the larger the curve, the greater the risk), growth potential of the patient (the more growth remaining, the greater the risk), and the curve type (double curves have a greater risk of progression). Female gender has not been statistically proven to increase the risk of progression because of the small numbers of males in reported series.

185. **When is non-surgical treatment of adolescent idiopathic scoliosis appropriate?**
No treatment is generally required for patients with curves measuring less than 20°. Non-surgical treatment with bracing is indicated for curves measuring between 20° and 40–45° in skeletally immature patients.

186. **What non-surgical treatment of adolescent idiopathic scoliosis has been shown to alter the natural history of the disease?**
The only nonsurgical treatment of adolescent idiopathic scoliosis that has been shown to alter the natural history is the use of a spinal orthosis (bracing). Bracing is indicated in the skeletally immature patient (Risser stage less than or equal to 3) who presents with a curve of 25–45°, or who presents with a curve of less than 25° with a history of documented progression. Electrical stimulation, exercises, manipulation, and biofeedback have not been shown to alter the natural history.

187. **What are the three most common types of braces used for adolescent idiopathic scoliosis, and how are they most effectively used?**
The three most common types of spinal braces are the Milwaukee (apex T8 and above), TLSO or Boston (apex below T8), and the Charleston bending brace (night-time use only).

188. **What are the indications for operative treatment of adolescent idiopathic scoliosis?**
Operative treatment of adolescent idiopathic scoliosis is recommended for curves greater than 40–45° in the skeletally immature patient, curves that progress despite bracing, or curves greater than 50–60° in the mature adolescent.

189. **What are the goals of surgical intervention in spinal deformity?**
In general, surgical intervention is undertaken to arrest progression of deformity, and if possible, to correct deformity that is already present.

190. **What types of surgical intervention may be performed for spinal deformity in skeletally mature patients?**
In patients approaching skeletal maturity, fusion of affected segments is an effective means of preventing further curve progression. This is typically combined with as much correction of the existing deformity as can be safely achieved at the time of surgery. Depending on the affected levels and types of deformity, this may be undertaken via posterior, anterior, thoracic, or retroperitoneal approaches, with the posterior approach being the most commonly employed for instrumentation and fusion.

191. **What kinds of complications may occur with spinal deformity surgery?**
Spinal deformity correction is a major and highly invasive surgical procedure. As such, it can be associated with *significant blood loss* the potential for *coagulopathy* with prolonged surgical times. *Infection* is also a serious complication in the presence of spinal instrumentation, which may require indefinite suppression or removal of instrumentation once fusion has occurred. *Neurologic complications* including spinal cord injury are also possible, especially with instrumentation at the cervical or thoracic levels. *Blindness* due to ischemic optic neuropathy is a rare, but devastating complication, thought to be due to prolonged prone positioning with periods of hypotension. Over the long term, *failure of fusion with or without failure of the instrumentation* may also occur, resulting in pain, deformity progression, or the need for additional surgical intervention.

192. **What is the crankshaft phenomenon and how can it be avoided?**
The crankshaft phenomenon is the progression of spinal curvature despite solid posterior arthrodesis. It is thought to be related to continued anterior spinal growth against a

posterior tether. This complication can be avoided by fusing both the anterior and posterior columns, or by the use of growth-preserving instrumentation until skeletal maturity is near (Fig. 9.23).

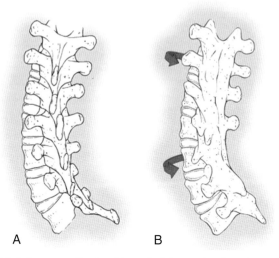

A　　　　　B

Figure 9.23. Crankshaft phenomenon. Despite solid posterior fusion, continued anterior growth may result in progression of deformity in the skeletally immature patient. *(From Warner WC: Juvenile Idiopathic Scoliosis. In: Weinstein SL: Pediatric Spine, Philadelphia, 1994, Raven.)*

193. **What surgical interventions are available for spinal deformity in skeletally immature patients?**
In order to avoid complications associated with continued skeletal growth alongside segmental spinal fusion, a variety of expandable posterior rod-and-screw implants, as well as vertical expandable rib implants in infants, have been employed to counteract spinal deforming forces without requiring fusion. These implants require that patients periodically undergo lengthening procedures or exchange of the implants as their growth continues until definitive fusion may be performed once they near skeletal maturity.

194. **What is kyphosis?**
Kyphosis is a spinal deformity characterized by an increase in the *posterior convex angulation in the sagittal plane*. The normal posterior convex angulation of the thoracic spine is 20–40° measured by the Cobb method.

195. **What is Scheuermann's kyphosis?**
Scheuermann's kyphosis is a disorder of endochondral ossification that affects the vertebral endplates and ring apophyses, resulting in *intravertebral disc herniation, anterior wedging of consecutive vertebrae (>5° in three adjacent thoracic vertebrae), and a fixed thoracolumbar kyphosis*. The exact etiology is unknown. A familial predilection has been theorized. Increased height and repetitive loading may be inciting factors (Fig. 9.24).

196. **What is the prevalence of Scheuermann's kyphosis?**
The prevalence has been estimated to be between 0.4% and 8% of the general population, mainly affecting *adolescents* at puberty.

197. **What are the most common presenting symptoms of Scheuermann's kyphosis?**
The most common presenting symptoms are spinal deformity and pain at the apex of the deformity, which is aggravated by prolonged sitting, standing, and activity. This disorder may account for as much as one-third of the cases of back pain complaint in pediatric patients.

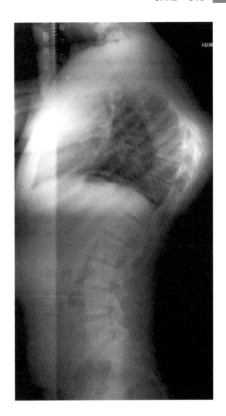

Figure 9.24. Standing lateral radiograph of a 15-year-old male demonstrating Scheuermann kyphosis with anterior wedging of the thoracic vertebrae. (*From Herkowitz HN, et al., [eds], Rothman-Simeone The Spine, 6th ed., Copyright © 2011, Saunders, Elsevier Inc.*)

198. **What is the initial treatment of Scheuermann's kyphosis?**
The initial treatment is nonsurgical, consisting of thoracic extension, abdominal strengthening exercises, and avoidance of heavy lifting. Symptoms usually resolve by the end of growth.

199. **When is bracing recommended for Schuermann's kyphosis?**
Bracing is recommended when the curve exceeds 60° in the skeletally immature patient. A Milwaukee brace is recommended for the thoracic form of the disease and a TLSO can be used for the atypical lumbar form. According to a recent natural history study, patients treated conservatively may have more pain at the apex of the curve as adults, but their overall quality of life should not be affected.

200. **When is surgery recommended for Scheuermann's kyphosis?**
Surgery is recommended if the curve exceeds 75° in a skeletally immature patient, if it exceeds 50–55° in a patient with pain or curve progression refractory to conservative treatment. Restrictive lung disease or neurologic compromise may be seen if the kyphosis exceeds 100°, but these are uncommonly encountered and not typical indications for surgery.

CASE 9-8

A 20-year-old male football player presents complaining of 1 month of progressive low-back pain with intermittent radiation down the back of both thighs. He states that the pain is increased when making tackles, and when seated for prolonged periods of time. He cannot recall a specific time of onset or traumatic injury. His parents have noted that his gait has changed with shorter stride length. He denies systemic symptoms or bowel or bladder dysfunction.

201. **What is the differential diagnosis?**
Low-back pain is common in children, adolescents, and adults, with the majority of cases being idiopathic and self-limited. Persistent pain, night pain, the association with neurologic or systemic symptoms should prompt further evaluation.

CASE 9-8   continued

On examination, the patient is well-developed and stands with the shoulders level and centered over the pelvis. Forward bending is severely limited, and pain is elicited with lumbar hyperextension. There is tenderness to palpation of the lumbar paraspinal muscles. Neurologic examination reveals 4/5 EHL strength bilaterally but is otherwise normal. A lateral radiograph of the lumbar spine is shown below (Fig. 9.25):

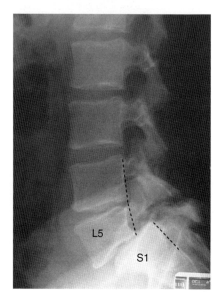

Figure 9.25. Lateral radiograph demonstrating anterolisthesis of L5 on S1 of approximately one-third the width of the vertebral body, associated with a defect in the visible portion of the pars interarticularis. These findings are collectively referred to as L5–S1 spondylolisthesis. (*From Mettler FA, [ed], Essentials of Radiology, 2nd ed., Copyright © 2005, Saunders, Elsevier Inc.*)

202. **What is spondylolysis?**
Spondylolysis describes a defect in the pars interarticularis, usually affecting the lumbar spine.

203. **What is spondylolisthesis?**
Spondylolisthesis describes the slipping forward of an upper vertebral segment on the lower segment, in part due to bilateral pars defects (spondylolysis) at the same level.

204. **How is spondylolisthesis classified?**
The commonly accepted classification system for spondylolisthesis was devised by Meyerding. No anterior slip of the upper vertebral body on the lower is grade 0; 1–25% slippage is grade I; 26–50% slippage is grade II; 51–75% is grade III; and 76–100% is grade IV. Complete anterior dislocation of the upper on lower vertebral body is called spondyloptosis.

205. **What are the five common types of spondylolisthesis?**
Isthmic, degenerative, dysplastic, traumatic, and pathologic.

206. **What is the Scotty dog sign?**
The Scotty dog sign is the radiographic appearance of the pars interarticularis defect seen on oblique films in isthmic spondylolisthesis. The actual defect resembles a collar around the Scotty dog's neck (Fig. 9.26).

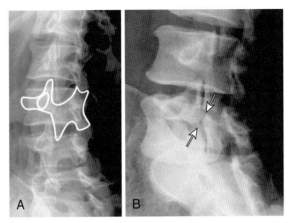

Figure 9.26. (A) The "Scotty dog" (outlined) on an oblique radiograph of the lumbar spine. (B) Fracture of pars interarticularis, the "neck" of the "Scotty dog". *(From Pretorius ES, [ed], Radiology Secrets Plus, 3rd ed., Copyright © 2011, Mosby, Elsevier Inc.)*

207. **What is the incidence of spondylolisthesis in the general population?**
The incidence of spondylolisthesis is 5% for the general population. The incidence in adult Caucasian males is 5–6% and in females is 2–3%. In Eskimos, the incidence has been reported to be 50% and is less than 3% in African-Americans. The incidence increases up to the age of 20 years and then remains constant. This lesion is rarely seen in children less than 5 years of age.

208. **What other adolescent spinal condition is associated with spondylolysis?**
Spondylolysis is seen frequently in association with *Scheuermann's kyphosis*, in which the excessive lumbar lordosis places the L5–S1 articulation under shear. There is a 50% incidence of spondylolysis in patients with Scheuermann's kyphosis and oblique lumbar spine radiographs should be obtained for patients with Scheuermann's kyphosis who develop low-back pain.

209. **What repetitive motion has been postulated as the inciting factor in the development of spondylolysis?**
Repetitive hyperextension activities which cause shear of the posterior elements are thought to be associated with symptomatic spondylosis. As a patient hyperextends, the inferior articular facet of L4 is driven into the pars intra-articularis of L5 and is postulated as another possible cause of spondylosis. Sports with cyclic flexion–extension activity have been positively associated with isthmic spondylolisthesis. An increased incidence has been reported in diving, weightlifting, wrestling, and gymnastics.

210. **What radiographic signs may indicate impending spondylolysis?**
Stress reaction refers to the uptake phase of spondylolysis before the appearance of the actual bony defect. Radiographically, a stress reaction can be associated with sclerosis or elongation of the pars. It is often seen with on the contralateral side of a unilateral spondylolysis.

211. **How long after the onset of symptoms of back pain before a technetium bone scan shows increased uptake at the level of the pars interarticularis?**
A technetium bone scan delineates an acute lesion within 5–7 days of the onset of symptoms.

212. **What is the best study to diagnose spondylolysis in symptomatic patients with normal radiographs and bone scan?**
Single photon emission computed tomography (SPECT) has proven effective in patients with positive symptoms and normal radiographs and bone scans. This test has been shown

to be the most sensitive method of diagnosing stress reactions, allowing early diagnosis and treatment before the development of an established spondylolysis.

213. **Which spinal segments are most commonly affected by spondylolysis/listhesis?**

The most common spondylolisthetic level is L5–S1, followed by L4–L5 and then L3–L4. Slips higher than L5 are usually seen in young adults, not in children or adolescents.

214. **What is the treatment of choice for spondylolysis and grade I spondylolisthesis?**

The treatment of choice for spondylolysis and grade I spondylolisthesis associated with a history of recent injury and short duration of symptoms involves restriction of aggravating activities and a regimen of muscle strengthening for the back and abdomen. Healing may be monitored by the resolution of back pain and hamstring tightness. If symptoms do not resolve and a bone scan shows increased uptake in the area of the pars, a program of rest, NSAIDs, and application of a TLSO or cast with a pantaloon extension down one thigh usually alleviates symptoms. The pantaloon portion of the brace may be removed after pain resolves. If symptoms persist despite immobilization and the bone scan becomes "cold," primary repair of small defects (<2 mm) with internal fixation and bone grafting has been successful for L1–L4 defects in patients younger than 25 years of age.

215. **How are the slip percentage and slip angle determined?**

Slip percentage is measured by representing the distance between the posterior border of the body of L5 and the posterior border of the body of S1 as a percentage of the antero-posterior diameter of S1. The slip angle is measured by drawing a line perpendicular to a line along the posterior border of the sacrum and another line parallel to the inferior endplate of L5. The angle subtended by the intersection of these two lines is the slip angle (Fig. 9.27).

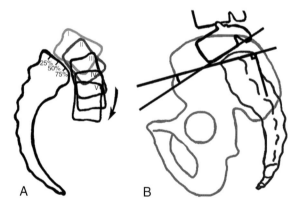

Figure 9.27. (A) Slip percentage. (B) Slip angle. *(Reprinted from Drummond DS, Scott AR: Pediatric Spondylolisthesis. In: Vaccaro AR, et al. [eds], Principles and Practice of Spine Surgery, Philadelphia: Mosby; 2003.)*

216. **What is the Gill procedure and what is its role in the treatment of spondylolysis/listhesis?**

The Gill procedure involves complete removal of the loose laminar fragment and fibrocartilagenous pars defect, and has no role in the treatment of spondylolisthesis because it further destabilizes the spine. This procedure should always be combined with arthrodesis in young patients to prevent further instability.

217. **When is fusion indicated for spondylolysis and spondylolisthesis?**
Patients who have significant back and/or radicular pain are candidates for decompression and possibly fusion if their symptoms do not respond to appropriate conservative care. Patients with spondylolysis without spondylolisthesis have been treated with decompression alone or with simultaneous fusion. Patients with spondylolysis and spondylolisthesis are usually treated with decompression and fusion. The treatment of patients with spinal stenosis and degenerative spondylolisthesis is usually decompression and fusion. Treatment for spondylosis without instability is still being debated. Although some studies have shown improved outcome in patients treated with decompression and fusion, other studies have shown similar results with decompression alone.

218. **What is the treatment of choice for spondylolisthesis of 25–50%?**
Grade II slips in asymptomatic patients should be followed every 4–6 months with spot lateral radiographs of the lumbosacral junction until the end of growth. In-situ posterolateral fusion remains the gold standard for patients with progressive slips, persistent back pain, or neurologic deficits.

219. **What is the treatment of choice for spondylolisthesis of 50–75%?**
In grade III slips, the procedure of choice is in-situ posterolateral fusion. Intertransverse fusion is another option, which may be performed by either a midline incision with two paraspinal fascial incisions or by two paraspinal skin incisions. Anterior interbody fusion techniques are also emerging as potentially viable alternatives to in-situ posterolateral fusion.

220. **What are the current indications for reduction of spondylolisthesis?**
Reduction of spondylolisthesis is currently reserved for high-grade slips (grade III and IV) with a sagittal imbalance that is functionally debilitating or cosmetically unacceptable or in the presence of a neurologic deficit in which a decompressive laminectomy would jeopardize the fusion. Reduction carries a high risk of neurologic injury, and a thorough nerve root decompression must be performed prior to any reduction attempt.

221. **What methods are currently used for slip reduction?**
Current methods for slip reduction include closed reduction by gradual pelvic extension with or without halo-skin traction, followed by segmental posterior instrumentation and postero-lateral bone grafting. The use of anterior column support (either anterior or posterior interbody fusion) may preserve the slip angle correction.

222. **What is the most common neurologic injury seen with spondylolisthesis reduction maneuvers?**
Injury to the L5 nerve root has been described in several studies reporting the results of high-grade spondylolisthesis reductions. The strain per increment of reduction increased rapidly during the second half of reductions in human cadaveric spines. Partial reduction of high-grade slips may be safer than full reduction, as long as the slip angle is improved.

CASE 9-9

A 79-year-old male presents for evaluation of longstanding low-back, buttock, and posterior leg pain. He also reports that he is now able to walk only one or two blocks before his legs feel heavy and he must sit down to rest. He is able to walk longer distances with the use of a rolling walker or shopping cart, and reports no symptoms with the use of a recumbent stationary bicycle. While in your office, he reports that he is currently asymptomatic, and has no apparent abnormality on physical and neurologic examination.

223. **What is the differential diagnosis?**
Low-back pain in adults is common and has an exceedingly broad differential. In this case, the complaint of posterior leg pain which is at least partially activity-related is more specific and suggestive of claudication, which may be either vascular or neurogenic in etiology. In combination with the complaint of low-back pain, lumbar spondylosis with stenosis is the most likely explanation for the patient's symptoms. While most cases of spinal stenosis are degenerative in nature, it is important to rule out other causes of acquired stenosis, such as fracture, tumor, or infection.

224. **How are neurogenic claudication and vascular claudication different?**
Both forms of claudication result in activity-dependent pain or weakness that may limit ambulation. Neurogenic claudication is the result of *stenosis* of the level of the spinal canal and neural foramina causing nerve root compression with repetitive activity in certain postures. This may cause pain or weakness in specific nerve root distributions, as well as non-specific paresthesias or a sensation of "heaviness" that prevents activity. It is frequently relieved at least in part by forward-bending, walking uphill, or sitting down. In contrast, vascular claudication is due to *peripheral vascular disease* causing pain from end-organ ischemia. Vascular claudication is more strictly related to exertion and is typically not posture-dependent. Patients are more likely to have other forms of vascular disease, such as hypertension, chronic kidney disease, or coronary artery disease. Peripheral vascular disease is frequently associated with diminished pulses and skin changes from chronic ischemia, and may be further evaluated with ankle-brachial indices and pulse-volume recordings if clinical suspicion remains high.

225. **What is the next appropriate step in diagnosis of this patient?**
Both CT scan and MRI are able to demonstrate areas of stenosis due to spondylosis with facet hypertrophy or osteophyte formation. MRI is used most commonly due to the ability to visualize the spinal cord and nerve roots, as well as soft tissue causes of stenosis such as ligamentum flavum hypertrophy (Fig. 9.28).

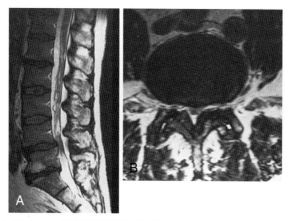

Figure 9.28. Sagittal (A), and axial (B) T2W MRI of the lumbar spine showing a severe spinal canal stenosis at L4–L5 with evidence of compression of the cauda equina, namely obliteration of CSF signal from the thecal sac at the site of compression and some redundant coiling of intrathecal spinal roots above. (*From Adam A, et al., [eds], Grainger & Allison's Diagnostic Radiology: A Textbook of Medical Imaging, 5th ed., Copyright © 2008, Elsevier Ltd.*)

226. **What pathology is involved with degenerative spinal stenosis?**
Spinal stenosis involves the three-joint complex of the facet joints and intervertebral disc. The intervertebral disc usually undergoes significant degenerative changes. Subsequent degeneration leads to collapse of the disc and facet arthritis, which tends to narrow the neural foramina progressively. Narrowing of the spinal canal may result anteriorly from disc protrusion or posteriorly from ligamentum flavum and facet hypertrophy. On a mechanical basis, the neural foramina are then more narrowed with lumbar extension than with lumbar flexion. The site of such compression may either be centrally within the canal or more laterally within the lateral recess or neural foramina.

227. **What other disorders may be associated with spinal stenosis?**
Achondroplasia has a strong association with spinal stenosis due to congenitally short pedicles. Other secondary causes include spondylolisthesis, Paget's disease, ankylosis spondylitis, and diffuse interstitial skeletal hypertrophy.

228. What is the epidemiology of spinal stenosis?

The age at onset of symptoms is variable, but the 5th and 6th decades are common. Spinal stenosis in achondroplasia usually presents in the 4th decade. Degenerative spondylolisthesis is infrequent in patients younger than 50 years. Distribution between men and women is equal. Degenerative spinal stenosis occurs more frequently in workers who have done heavy manual labor.

229. What is the initial treatment for spinal stenosis?

Non-operative treatment involves a physical therapy program emphasizing postural changes, stretching, and strengthening of the tightened lumbar and lower extremity musculature. Biofeedback may be helpful. Transcutaneous electrical nerve stimulator units occasionally have been successful in relieving acute pain. Epidural steroids remain controversial. NSAIDs, particularly aspirin, may reduce leg and back pain. Braces may be used to decrease lumbar lordosis.

230. What are the indications for surgery with spinal stenosis?

Surgery is indicated in patients with severe spinal stenosis and intractable pain who have failed an appropriate non-operative course. Other secondary causes of pain should be ruled out. Surgery is elective, except in the presence of bowel or bladder dysfunction, which is rare.

231. What is the surgical treatment for spinal stenosis?

Typical surgical treatment consists of laminectomy and decompression, with removal of the lamina, ligamentum flavum, spinous process, medial facets, and osteophytes in the lateral recesses. Attempts should be made to leave portions of the facet joints intact. If the spine is destabilized or significant spondylolisthesis or degenerative scoliosis exists, single or multi-level fusion may be required to arrest deformity progression.

232. What complications are seen after decompression for spinal stenosis?

Laminectomy and decompression may result in instability with progressive kyphosis, dural tear, arachnoiditis, nerve root injury, and epidural scarring leading to recurrent stenosis.

CASE 9-10

A 61-year-old female office manager presents in follow-up after a recent Emergency Room visit for severe low-back and right leg pain after twisting while picking up a heavy box. She was given antiinflammatories and muscle-relaxants, and has primarily been resting for the last several days. She states that the pain has partially improved, but she has had several similar, but less-severe, episodes over the past year which have resulted in missed days from work. Currently, she reports pain that radiates from her back down the lateral aspect of her right leg and extends to her great toe. The pain is partially relieved by standing or lying flat.

233. What is the differential diagnosis?

The combination of back and leg pain again points to a lumbar spinal process resulting in radiculopathy. In this case, the acute-onset, episodic nature of the pain renders lumbar stenosis less likely, as this is typically a more chronic process. More likely, the patient is experiencing a recurrent herniation of a lumbar nucleus pulposus, with irritation or compression of one or more nerve roots as they exit the spinal cord.

234. What elements of the physical examination are important in lumbar disc disease?

Patients should be examined in the standing, sitting, and lying positions. A list or limp can be seen with the patient walking. Range of motion of the spine should be examined. Patients with disc herniation frequently complain of leg pain on forward flexion, whereas patients with spinal stenosis often have leg pain on back extension. Muscular atrophy or muscle spasm should be identified with range-of-motion evaluation. Weakness is also determined. A complete neurologic examination is necessary, including testing of motor strengths, reflexes, and sensory deficits. The presence or absence of tension sign is the most important finding in patients suspected of having disc herniation. Evaluation should also include examination for hip and knee pathology.

235. **What are the "tension" signs in lumbar disc herniation?**
Tension signs are maneuvers that tighten the sciatic nerve and in doing so further compress an inflamed nerve root against a herniated lumbar disc. Please refer to Anatomy and Examination for additional details.

236. **What causes some patients with a herniated lumbar disc to "list" or limp?**
Herniation that is lateral to the nerve root produces what is called a list away from the side of the irritated nerve root. Herniation of the disc that is medial to the nerve root, however, in what is called the axillary position, usually produces a list toward the side of the irritated nerve root. When the disc herniation is lateral, patients feel that they must move from the side of the irritated nerve in an attempt to draw the nerve root away from the disc fragment. When the herniation is in the axillary position, medial to the nerve root, the patient lists toward the side of the nerve root in an attempt to decompress the nerve root.

237. **What are the physical findings in a patient with a unilateral paracentral disc herniation at the L3–L4?**
Unilateral paracentral herniation at the L3–L4 disc generally involves compression of the traversing L4 nerve root, with possible sensory deficits in the posterolateral thigh, anterior knee, and medial leg. Motor weakness is variable in the quadriceps and hip adductors. Changes also are apparent in the patellar reflex.

238. **What are the physical findings in a patient with a unilateral paracentral disc herniation at the L4–L5 disc?**
The traversing L5 nerve root is commonly compressed with a paracentral disc herniation at L4–L5. Sensory deficit occurs in the anterolateral leg, dorsum of the foot, and great toe. Motor weakness includes the extensor hallucis longus, gluteus medius, and extensor digitorum longus and brevis. Usually, no reflex changes are present.

239. **What are the physical findings in a patient with a unilateral paracentral disc herniation at the L5–S1 disc?**
Paracentral disc herniation at L5–S1 usually results in compression of the traversing S1 nerve root. Sensory deficits occur in the lateral malleolus, lateral foot, heel, and web of the fourth and fifth toes. Motor weakness involves the peroneus longus and brevis, gastrocnemius-soleus complex, and gluteus maximus. The Achilles reflex is usually diminished.

240. **What other tests should be done in evaluation for lumbar disc disease?**
No spine examination is complete without evaluation of the peripheral circulation. The posterior tibial and dorsal pedis artery should be examined. Vascular claudication is an important cause of leg pain and may mimic lumbar disc disease. The hip and knee also should be evaluated. Limitations in range of motion of the hip, particularly in rotation, along with groin discomfort, are indicative of hip disease. Tenderness over the piriformis muscle in external rotation may implicate piriformis syndrome. Rectal tone should be evaluated in patients suspected of having cauda equina syndrome.

241. **Are plain radiographs helpful in evaluation of lumbar disc disease?**
Only 1–2% of the spine radiographs, in patients with back pain between 20 and 50 years of age, have unsuspected findings. Most studies have found some disc space narrowing or osteophyte formation in this age group. Spondylolisthesis and spondylolysis may be seen on radiographs, along with some disc space narrowing at the affected level. Such findings, however, are also present in patients with no back pain and no clinically significant pathology.

242. **What is the imaging test of choice for evaluation of suspected lumbar disc disease?**
MRI: the primary advantage of which is the ability to visualize the spinal cord, nerve roots, and intervertebral discs, as well as other soft-tissue structures such as fluid collections or tumors. While CT offers better bony visualization, its ability to evaluate the intervertebral discs and neural elements is limited (Fig. 9.29).

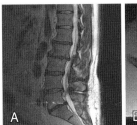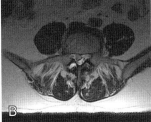

Figure 9.29. A 61-year-old patient with right L5 radiculopathy. (A) T2 sagittal MRI reveals sequestered L4 herniated disc fragment. (B) T2 axial image shows the fragment between L5 pedicles. (*From Canale ST, Beaty JH [eds], Campbell's Operative Orthopaedics, 12th ed., Copyright © 2013, Mosby Elsevier Inc.*)

243. **Is electromyography useful in patients with lumbar disc disease?**
     Electromyography is commonly used to help in differentiating radicular symptoms from peripheral neuropathy or upper motor neuron lesions and in determining the presence or absence of generalized myopathy.

244. **What is the initial treatment for low-back pain with radiculopathy due to an acute lumbar disc herniation?**
     Only about 10% of patients with symptoms and signs ultimately require surgery. Therefore, physicians may expect a 90% relief rate with conservative treatment for patients with lumbar disc disease. Treatment focuses primarily on symptomatic relief, and may include bed rest, NSAIDs, narcotic analgesics, oral or epidural corticosteroids, physical therapy, bracing, traction, manipulation, and techniques such as electrostimulation. Epidural steroids may be beneficial in eliminating acute pain but have limited effectiveness in relieving chronic pain.

245. **What surgical procedure is used for the treatment of lumbar disc disease?**
     Discectomy refers to excision of any herniated disc material that is resulting in nerve root compression or irritation. This historically required a midline incision with a hemilaminectomy or laminectomy for access to the disc at the operative level. The procedure has been progressively refined with the incorporation of magnification for better visualization and to minimize the extent of dissection. Current discectomies may be performed through midline or paramedian incisions, using distractors or tube dilators to gain access through the paraspinous musculature. A window in the ipsilateral lamina is then created with a burr or Kerrison punch to allow for visualization of the disc and affected nerve root. The disc herniation is identified and then removed with careful protection of the nerve root. Early return to activity is encouraged as tolerated. The procedure is typically more successful at relieving the radicular component of the patient's symptoms as opposed to the axial back pain, which may persist following discectomy.

246. **What is lumbar microdiscectomy?**
     Microdiscectomy describes use of an operating microscope with a minimally invasive approach, which limits dissection and lamina excision in order to minimize postoperative pain and allow for earlier mobilization. Surgical results are similar to those of open discectomy, but the procedure requires specialized training and the limited visualization may increase the risk for complications.

247. **What complications may occur with lumbar discectomy?**
     Complications may include dural tear, nerve root injury, discitis, and injury to blood vessels or intra-abdominal viscera.

248. **What is the natural history of conservative and surgical treatment in patients with lumbar disc herniation?**
     In general, the vast majority of patients with radiculopathy due to lumbar disc herniation will experience significant improvement in symptoms with the passage of time, regardless

of the treatment protocol. This finding was confirmed by the Spine Patient Outcomes Research Trial (SPORT), with both non-surgical and surgical treatment groups demonstrating equivalent improvements in the study outcome measures over the long term. This must be considered in light of the greater baseline severity and activity demands in those patients eventually electing to undergo surgical intervention. As a result of the large crossover between non-surgical and surgical treatment groups, subsequent as-treated analyses were performed, with a robust short and long-term surgical treatment effect noted for lumbar discectomy. However, the magnitude of the treatment effect for discectomy is less than that of the other conditions studied in the SPORT trial: degenerative spondylolisthesis and lumbar stenosis. In contrast to disc herniation, these conditions are more frequently progressive in nature, and unlikely to fully resolve without surgical intervention.

249. **When is fusion indicated for recurrent lumbar disc herniations?**
Recurrent lumbar disc herniations may occur in up to 10–15% of patients. Fusion is usually not indicated for the first recurrent disc herniation. However, after the second recurrent disc herniation, fusion is often recommended, especially if the two recurrences occur soon after the original disc herniation.

CASE 9-11

A 51-year-old former construction worker presents for evaluation of chronic low-back pain following a work-related injury sustained 2 years ago. The pain is centered in his low-back and radiates to both buttocks. His pain worsens with forward bending and while picking up heavy objects. He has had an extensive course of conservative treatment, including activity modification, physical therapy, and injections, but has experienced little relief and has required long-acting narcotic analgesia to perform activities of daily living. He appears uncomfortable and is obese, but physical examination is otherwise unremarkable. He is requesting surgical intervention.

250. **What is the differential diagnosis?**
Chronic, isolated low-back pain is common, and represents a final common pathway following many traumatic injuries or surgical procedures, or may be due to worsening spondylosis from repetitive activities or heavy labor. In most cases, it is impossible to isolate a single anatomic source for chronic axial back pain. Potential sources include degenerated intervertebral discs or facet joints, stress fracture, epidural fibrosis, or chronic ligamentous injury or muscle strain. It is often difficult to isolate which findings may be symptomatic as opposed to incidental.

CASE 9-11 continued

To further differentiate between these potential causes of back pain, an MRI of the lumbar spine was obtained (Fig. 9.30).

251. **What are Modic changes?**
The progression of degenerative disc disease on MRI is characterized by a sequential pattern of signal abnormalities in the marrow of the vertebral bodies adjacent to the degenerated disc. First described by Modic in 1988, these changes are correlated with the presence of axial back pain and abnormal histologic findings as detailed below:
Type I: Hypointense T1, hyperintense T2. Due to marrow edema, typically from an acute process. Pathologic examination shows fissuring of the endplate and vascular fibrous tissues in the adjacent marrow.
Type II (most common): Hyperintense T1, isointense or slightly hyperintense signal T2. Representative of fatty degeneration subchondral marrow, typically chronic in nature, with underlying yellow marrow replacement in the adjacent vertebral body.
Type III: Hypointense T1 and T2. Indicative of bony endplate sclerosis, typically able to be visualized on plain radiographs.

252. **What is the role of discography in the evaluation of degenerative disc disease?**
Discography is a diagnostic procedure that involves introduction of a needle into the intervertebral disc with injection of radio-opaque contrast material to examine the pattern of contrast extravasation under fluoroscopy. Intradiscal pressure may also be measured

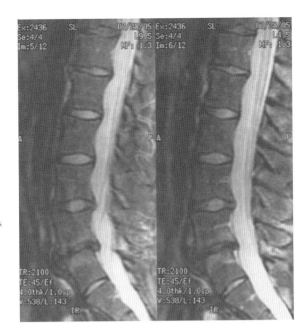

Figure 9.30. MRI demonstrates severe disc degeneration at L4–L5 with loss of disc hydration, collapse of the disc space, and anterior osteophyte formation. (*From Canale ST, Beaty JH [eds], Campbell's Operative Orthopaedics, 12th ed., Copyright © 2013, Mosby Elsevier Inc.*)

before and during injection. Provocative discography refers to the duplication of the patient's symptoms with increasing intradiscal pressure during injection, and is thought to confirm the presence of symptomatic degenerative disc disease. This procedure is controversial due to its invasive nature, and may possibly cause damage to the intervertebral disc further accelerating the degeneration process.

CASE 9-11 continued

The patient undergoes provocative discography which demonstrates extensive tearing of the annulus fibrosus and concordant pain during intradiscal injection at the degenerated level seen on MRI.

253. What are the therapeutic options at this point?

Degenerative disc disease remains a poorly understood and controversial clinical entity. While there are many patients whose symptoms are improved by surgical intervention aimed at eliminating the disc as a potential pain generator (such as interbody fusion or total disc replacement), it remains difficult to predict which patients will have a positive response despite seemingly consistent history, examination, and imaging findings. As a result, conservative treatment, including oral analgesia, activity modification, physical therapy, injections, and weight loss must be thoroughly exhausted prior to consideration of any surgical intervention. The presence of ongoing litigation or worker's compensation claims must also be considered when evaluating potential surgical candidates due to the relatively poorer outcomes observed in these populations. For axial back pain due to degenerative disc disease, the mainstay of surgical treatment is segmental fusion. While posterolateral fusion may be performed, interbody fusion has become increasingly popular, with or without posterior instrumentation, to ensure maximum stability of the anterior column.

254. What are the indications for lumbar fusion?

Lumbar fusion is indicated for unstable fractures, spondylolisthesis with progression or neurologic symptoms, recurrent disc herniations, and refractory degenerative disc disease.

Examples of unstable lumbar fractures include burst fractures with greater than 60% canal compromise, compression fractures with significant kyphosis (greater than 40°), or flexion–distraction injuries.

255. **What are the different available techniques for lumbar fusion?**
Lumbar fusion can be performed from a posterior approach with or without the simultaneous use of instrumentation. During a posterolateral fusion, bone graft is placed over the decorticated transverse processes, lateral facet joints, and sacral ala if applicable. During a posterior lumbar interbody fusion (PLIF), bone graft is placed into the disc space from a posterior approach. Spinal instrumentation increases fusion rates, especially if instability or spondylolisthesis is present. Posterior instrumentation usually involves placement of pedicle screws connected together with rods. Lumbar fusion can also be performed from an anterior (either trans- or retroperitoneal) approach. During an anterior lumbar interbody fusion (ALIF), bone graft is placed into the disc space anteriorly and is often accompanied by posterior instrumentation. A number of implants have been developed from titanium and other inert materials to serve as structural supports and aid in the delivery of bone graft to the disc space (so called "cages"). These may be placed into the disc space from either an anterior, posterior, or transforaminal approach (ALIF, PLIF, or TLIF, respectively). These may be performed with or without simultaneous pedicle screw instrumentation depending on the surgeon's assessment of stability.

256. **What are potential future alternatives to intervertebral fusion?**
While effective at eliminating mechanical pain from disc degeneration or spondylosis of the posterior elements, fusion does result in a loss of spinal range of motion. In the lumbar spine, this loss is not typically clinically significant in a 1 or 2 level fusion, but may be significant with longer constructs. There is also concern that, over the long term, fusion may result in accelerated wear of the adjacent motion segments, leading to progressive degeneration at these levels. This has not been conclusively proven in clinical studies. To address these concerns, the technology and materials of arthroplasty of other joints have been applied to the intervertebral disc, resulting in the development of metal and polyethylene total disc replacement implants. These are implanted via an anterior approach, and offer the advantages of not disrupting the posterior elements and not having to rely on bony fusion to prevent instrumentation failure. This technology is currently controversial, and its indications are continuing to be refined in both the cervical and lumbar spine. Additional injectable and tissue-engineered solutions for disc regeneration are currently under laboratory investigation, and may result in new therapeutic approaches that attempt to preserve the native biology and mechanics of the motion segment.

BIBLIOGRAPHY

1. Abbed KM, Coumans JV. Cervical radiculopathy: pathophysiology, presentation, and clinical evaluation. Neurosurgery 2007;60(1 Suppl 1):S28–34.
2. Agabegi SS, Asghar FA, Herkowitz HN. Spinal orthoses. J Am Acad Orthop Surg 2010;18:657–67.
3. Anderson PA, McCormick PC, Angevine PD. Randomized controlled trials of the treatment of lumbar disk herniation: 1983–2007. J Am Acad Orthop Surg 2008;16:566–73.
4. Askar Z, Wardlaw D, Koti M. Scott wiring for direct repair of lumbar spondylolysis. Spine 2003;15:354–7.
5. Bigos S, Bowyer O, Braen G. Acute Low Back Problems in Adults. Rockville (MD): Agency for Health Care Policy and Research (AHCPR); 1994 Dec. (AHCPR Clinical Practice Guidelines, No. 14.).
6. Biyani A, Andersson GB. Low back pain: pathophysiology and management. J Am Acad Orthop Surg 2004;12(2):106–15.
7. Bodner RJ, Heyman S, Drummond DS, et al. The use of single-photon emission computed tomography (SPECT) in the diagnosis of low-back pain in young patients. Spine 1988;13:1155–60.
8. Bracken MB. Steroids for acute spinal cord injury. Cochrane Database Syst Rev 2012;(2):CD001046.
9. Bridwell KH, DeWald RL, editors. The Textbook of Spinal Surgery. 3rd ed. Philadelphia: Lippincott, Williams, and Wilkins; 2011.
10. Carragee EJ, Hurwitz EL, Cheng I, et al. Treatment of neck pain: injections and surgical interventions: results of the Bone and Joint Decade 2000–2010 Task Force on Neck Pain and Its Associated Disorders. Spine 2008;33(Suppl. 4):S153–69.
11. Charbot JNC, Herkowitz HN. Spine tumors: Patient evaluation. Semin Spine Surg 1995;7:260.
12. Cunningham ME, Frelinghuysen PH, Roh JS, et al. Fusionless scoliosis surgery. Curr Opin Pediatr 2005;17(1):48–53.

13. Denaro V, Papalia R, Di Martino A, et al. The best surgical treatment for type II fractures of the dens is still controversial. Clin Orthop Relat Res 2011;469(3):742–50.
14. Denis F. The three column spine and its significance in the classification of acute thoracolumbar spinal injuries. Spine 1983;8(8):817–31.
15. Dubousset J. Treatment of spondylolysis and spondylolisthesis in children and adolescents. Clin Orthop 1997;337:77–85.
16. Esses SI, McGuire R, Jenkins J, et al. The treatment of symptomatic osteoporotic spinal compression fractures. J Am Acad Orthop Surg 2011;19(3):176–82.
17. Ginsburg GM, Bassett GS. Back pain in children and adolescents: Evaluation and differential diagnosis. J Am Acad Orthop 1997;5:67–78.
18. Herkowitz HN, Garfin SR, Eismont FJ, et al., editors. Rothman-Simeone: The Spine. 6th ed. Philadelphia: WB Saunders; 2011.
19. Herman MJ, Pizzutillo PD. Cervical spine disorders in children. Orthop Clin North Am 1999;30(3):457–66.
20. Hoppenfeld S. Orthopaedic Neurology: A Diagnostic Guide to Neurological Levels. Philadelphia: JB Lippincott; 1977.
21. Hurwitz EL, Carragee EJ, van der Velde G, et al. Treatment of neck pain: noninvasive interventions: results of the Bone and Joint Decade 2000–2010 Task Force on Neck Pain and Its Associated Disorders. Spine 2008;33(Suppl. 4):S123–52.
22. Klimo P Jr, Rao G, Brockmeyer D. Congenital anomalies of the cervical spine. Neurosurg Clin N Am 2007;18(3):463–78.
23. Lenke LG, Betz RR, Harms J, et al. Adolescent idiopathic scoliosis: A new classification to determine extent of spinal arthrodesis. J Bone Joint Surg 2001;83A:1169–81.
24. Looby S, Flanders A. Spine trauma. Radiol Clin North Am 2011;49:129–63.
25. McMaster MJ, Singh H. Natural history of congenital kyphosis and kyphoscoliosis: A study of 112 patients. J Bone Joint Surg 1999;81A:1367–83.
26. Petraco DM, Spivak JM, Cappadona JG, et al. An anatomic evaluation of nerve stretch in spondylolisthesis reduction. Spine 1996;21:1133–8.
27. Schouten R, Albert T, Kwon BK. The spine-injured patient: initial assessment and emergency treatment. J Am Acad Orthop Surg 2012;20:336–46.
28. Seitsalo S, Osterman K, Hyvarinen H, et al. Progression of spondylolisthesis in children and adolescents: A long-term follow-up of 272 patients. Spine 1991;16:417–21.
29. Skaf GS, Domloja NT, Fehlings MG, et al. Pyogenic spondylodiscitis: An overview. J Inf Pub Health 2010;3:5–16.
30. Skaf GS, Zeina A, Kanafanib GF, et al. Non-pyogenic infections of the spine. Int J Antimicrob Agents 2010;36:99–105.
31. Stevens JM, Rich PM, Dixon AK. The Spine. In: Adam A, Dixon AK, editors. Grainger & Allison's Diagnostic Radiology. 5th ed. Churchill Livingstone; 2007.
32. Sucato DJ. Management of severe spinal deformity: scoliosis and kyphosis. Spine 2010;35:2186–92.
33. Suh SW, Sarwark JF, Vora A, et al. Evaluating congenital spine deformities for intraspinal anomalies with magnetic resonance imaging. J Pediatr Orthop 2001;21:525–31.
34. Taher F, Essig D, Lebl DR. Lumbar degenerative disc disease: current and future concepts of diagnosis and management. Adv Orthop 2012;970752. [Epub 2012 Apr 2].
35. Tracy JA, Bartleson JD. Cervical spondylotic myelopathy. Neurologist 2010;16:176–87.
36. Weinstein JN, Lurie JD, Tosteson TD. Surgical versus nonsurgical treatment for lumbar degenerative spondylolisthesis. N Engl J Med 2007;356:2257–70.
37. Weinstein JN, Tosteson TD, Lurie JD. Surgical vs nonoperative treatment for lumbar disk herniation: the Spine Patient Outcomes Research Trial (SPORT): a randomized trial. JAMA 2006;296:2441–50.
38. Weinstein JN, Tosteson TD, Lurie JD. Surgical versus nonsurgical therapy for lumbar spinal stenosis. N Engl J Med 2008;358:794–810.

CHAPTER 10

SPORTS

Hassan Alosh, Kevin McHale, Laura Wiegand, Surena Namdari
and Fotios P. Tjoumakaris

KNEE

MENISCAL INJURIES

CASE 10-1

A 20-year-old college football player presents to your clinic 1 week after twisting his knee while at practice. His knee swelled overnight after the injury and he had to sit out of practice. He is able to bear weight and ambulate but reports his knee feels like it is catching and locking. He reports that his symptoms are worse with deep flexion activities such as climbing stairs. He also reports episodes where his knee feels that it "locks" and his pain is exacerbated. On examination, he ambulates with a slight limp. His knee has a moderate effusion. He has full motor strength. He has no ligamentous instability. He does have some point tenderness to deep palpation of his posterior medial joint line. He also has a positive McMurray test and a positive Apley grind test.

1. What is in the differential diagnosis for acute knee pain and effusion after trauma?
   - Ligamentous injury
   - Meniscus injury
   - Osteochondral fracture
   - Patella dislocation
   - Capsular tear.

2. The evaluation of the injured knee begins with a detailed history. What are the important aspects of the history?
   Mechanism of injury: the position of the knee at the time of injury, the weight-supporting status, varus or valgus load, contact versus non-contact injury
   Non-contact injury with an audible "pop": associated with anterior cruciate ligament (ACL) injury
   Contact injury with an audible "pop": more likely a collateral ligament injury, meniscal tear, or fracture
   Swelling: intra-articular swelling or effusion within the first 2 hours after trauma suggests hemarthrosis, whereas swelling that occurs overnight may be an indication of acute traumatic synovitis
   Pain: location, severity, type
   Instability: was there a sensation of the knee slipping out of joint, giving way, or deforming with weight bearing?
   Past history: previous injury or problems before current injury.

3. What is the most common injury to the knee requiring surgery?
   Meniscus tears.

4. Describe the shape of the medial and lateral menisci.
   The medial meniscus is semilunar in shape and has a larger antero-posterior dimension than width. It covers roughly two-thirds of the peripheral articular surface of the tibial plateau. It has a thick convex outer edge that tapers to a thin inner edge; this yields its familiar triangular cross-section. In contrast, the lateral meniscus is more circular in shape than the medial meniscus, with approximately the same antero-posterior dimension as width. It covers more tibial surface area than the medial meniscus and helps to give the lateral compartment of the knee a concavity that the joint surface otherwise doesn't provide.

5. **Describe the tibial attachments of the medial and lateral menisci.**
   The meniscal insertion into the bone is called the *enthesis*, and it represents a transition from uncalcified to calcified fibrocartilage. These attachments occur at the horns of the meniscus. They are commonly referred to as the "root" attachments of the meniscus. There are also meniscofemoral ligaments which help to stabilize the posterior meniscus to the distal end of the femur, further enhancing the structural support for the meniscus:
   Medial meniscus: The entire periphery of the medial meniscus is attached to the capsule by the coronary ligaments, which also serve as fibers of the deep medial collateral ligament. This accounts for the medial meniscus being less mobile than the lateral meniscus.
   Lateral meniscus: The lateral meniscus also has capsular attachments but is not as developed or organized as the medial meniscus. There is no fixation to the lateral collateral ligament.

6. **Describe the microstructure of the meniscus and its relation to injury.**
   The menisci are composed of dense, tightly woven collagen fibers arranged in a pattern that is highly elastic and able to withstand compression. The major orientation of collagen fibers in the meniscus is circumferential; radial and perforating fibers are also present. The arrangement of the collagen fibers determines to some extent the characteristic patterns of meniscal tears. Collagen fibers function primarily to resist tensile forces along the directions of the fibers. The normal tensile stresses on the menisci are in the longitudinal axis. Because the predominant fiber pattern is in this plane, tears are not unusual. The small number of peripheral radial collagen bundles is inadequate to prevent longitudinal tears when the force is substantial. Likewise, horizontal cleavage tears occur because of the paucity of vertically oriented fibers.

7. **Discuss the composition of the menisci.**
   Collagen makes up 60–70% of the dry weight of the meniscus. Type I collagen accounts for 90% of the collagen fibers. There are also small amounts of type II, III, IV, V, and VI.

8. **What is the role of proteoglycans in the menisci?**
   They have a high content of carbohydrates that are able to trap approximately 50 times their weight in water, which accounts for much of the physical properties of the menisci.

9. **What is the vascular supply to the meniscus?**
   Superior and inferior branches of the medial and lateral geniculate arteries arborize to form the perimeniscal capillary plexus. Approximately 10–30% of the periphery of the medial meniscus and 10–25% of the lateral meniscus are vascularized in adulthood. There are additional vessels from the middle geniculate artery that supply the horns of the menisci.

10. **Describe the three vascular zones of the menisci.**
    Red-red zone: This represents the outer or peripheral one-third of the meniscus. This is the vascular zone.
    Red-white zone: This is the middle one-third that represents a transitional zone between the vascular and avascular sections of the meniscus.
    White-white zone: This is the inner one-third of the meniscus which is completely avascular in adults (Fig. 10.1).

11. **What happens to load transmission and shock absorption if a meniscectomy is performed?**
    The menisci transmit approximately 50% of the load in extension and up to 85% of the load with the knee flexed 90°. With removal of the medial meniscus there is a 50–70% reduction in femoral contact area and a 100% increase in contact stress. With lateral meniscectomy, that contact stress can increase to 200–300% of normal.

12. **What is the usual mechanism of injury for meniscal tear?**
    The meniscus tears when it is excessively loaded. There is usually a rotational force applied to the meniscus as the knee is brought from flexion to extension. Traumatic tears

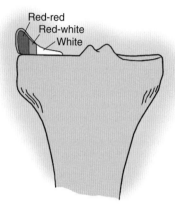

Figure 10.1. Zones of the meniscus. (*Redrawn from Miller MD, Warner JJP, Harner CD: Meniscal Repair. In: Fu FH, Harner CD, Vince KG, eds: Knee Surgery, Baltimore, 1994, Williams & Wilkins.*)

occur more frequently in younger individuals and are typically an acute event, whereas degenerative tears are more frequently found in those older than 60 and can be asymptomatic.

13. **Where is the most common meniscal tear located?**
The posterior horn of the medial meniscus is most commonly torn. This may be in part due to the difference in excursion between the medial and lateral meniscus. The average excursion of the medial meniscus is 5 mm and for the lateral it is 11 mm. However, recent investigations suggest medial and lateral meniscus tears may occur with almost equal frequency.

14. **What are the "mechanical symptoms" associated with a torn meniscus?**
Pain, swelling, catching, locking, popping, and giving way.

15. **Which meniscal tears are treated surgically?**
    - Younger patients with acute tears
    - Tears causing mechanical symptoms
    - Tears in older patients unresponsive to non-operative management.

16. **List common physical exam signs found in a meniscal tear.**
    - Joint line tenderness
    - Knee effusion
    - McMurray test
    - Apley grind test.

17. **What is the McMurray test?**
To test the medial meniscus, place the patient supine with the knee flexed. The medial hemi-joint is palpated. The leg is then slowly externally rotated and extended. The femur will pass over the tear and produce a click or pop. The lateral meniscus is checked by palpating the lateral margin of the joint, internally rotating the leg as far as possible, and slowly extending the knee while listening and feeling for a click. A negative McMurray test is not entirely sensitive for a tear (Fig. 10.2).

18. **What is the grinding test as described by Apley?**
The patient is positioned prone, and the anterior thigh is fixed against the examining table. The foot and leg are then pulled upward to distract the joint. Next, with the knee in the same position, the foot and leg are pressed downward and rotated as the joint is

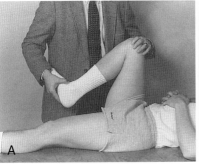
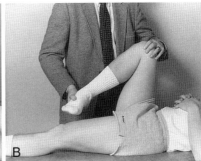
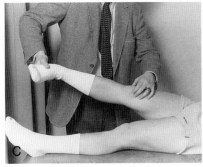

Figure 10.2. McMurray test. (A) Starting position for testing of the medial meniscus. The knee is acutely flexed, with the foot and tibia in external rotation. (B) Starting position for testing of the lateral meniscus. The knee is acutely flexed, and the foot and tibia are internally rotated. (C) Ending position for the lateral meniscus. The knee is brought into extension while rotation is maintained. Ending position for the medial meniscus is the same but with the external rotation. If pain or a "clunk" is elicited, the test result is considered positive. (*Reprinted with permission from Mellion MB. Office Sports Medicine, 2nd ed. Philadelphia, Hanley & Belfus, 1996, p. 28.*)

slowly flexed and extended; when a meniscus is torn, popping and pain localized to the joint line may be noted (Fig. 10.3).

19. **What is the Thessaly test?**
The examiner supports the patient by holding his or her outstretched hands while the patient stands flatfooted on the floor. The patient then rotates his or her knee and body, internally and externally, three times with the knee in slight flexion (5°). The same procedure is carried out with the knee flexed 20°. Patients with suspected meniscal tears experience medial or lateral joint-line discomfort and may have a sense of locking or catching. The test is always done on the normal knee first to teach the patient how to keep the knee in 5° and 20° of flexion and how to recognize a possible positive result in the symptomatic knee.

CASE 10-1   continued

You obtain an MRI to confirm your suspicion of a meniscus tear. The MRI (see Fig. 10.4) demonstrates a tear of the posterior horn of the medial meniscus. You discuss operative and non-operative treatment strategies. Given the patient's persistent pain, high-level athletic function, and desire to continue participating in sports, he decides to undergo knee arthroscopy with a meniscal debridement (partial meniscectomy) versus repair. You counsel the patient that your decision to repair or debride the meniscus will be an intraoperative decision based on the tear pattern, quality of the meniscal tissue, and the location of the tear.

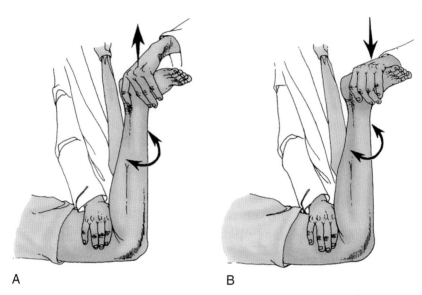

A   B

Figure 10.3. (A and B) Apley grind test for meniscal injury. (*From Tria AJ Jr: Clinical Examination of the Knee. In: Scott WN, ed: Insall & Scott Surgery of the Knee, 4th ed. Philadelphia, 2006, Churchill Livingstone.*)

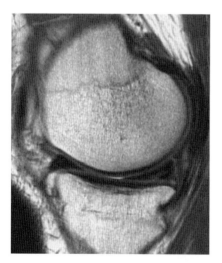

Figure 10.4. Posterior horn meniscus tear on T1 weighted MRI. (*From Beynnon BD, Johnson RJ, Brown L, Knee: DeLee JC (ed), DeLee and Drez's Orthopaedic Sports Medicine, 3rd ed. Saunders, 2010.*)

20. **Describe the appearance of the meniscus on MRI.**
    It is a uniformly low-signal structure on both T1 and T2 images.

21. **Which acute meniscal tears can be treated non-operatively?**
    An incomplete meniscal tear or a small, stable peripheral tear with no other pathologic condition, such as a torn anterior cruciate ligament, can be treated non-surgically with predictably good results. Meniscal tears that cause infrequent and minimal symptoms can be treated with rehabilitation and a period of restricted activity. Small, stable vertical tears found at the time of concomitant ACL reconstruction can be treated non-operatively with a high degree of success in most patients.

22. How can a meniscus tear be surgically managed?
   A partial meniscectomy is typically used to trim torn or frayed edges of the meniscus. This eliminates the mechanical symptoms caused by a meniscus tear.
   A meniscus tear that occurs in the peripheral third of the meniscus, the so-called "red-red zone" of the meniscus, should be treated by repair with suture. The reason for this is that the peripheral third of the meniscus is well-vascularized and capable of healing. Tears in the "red-white zone" may be treated with suture repair or augmented with fibrin clot to stimulate an enhanced healing response.

23. During medial meniscal repair, what structure is most commonly injured?
   The saphenous nerve and its branches are most at risk.

24. Describe the medial approach to the knee for meniscal repairs.
   A 3- to 4-cm incision is made with the knee flexed at 90° just posterior to the medial collateral ligament. The sartorial fascia is opened with care to protect the saphenous vein and nerve. These structures are retracted posteriorly and a plane is developed between the sartorius and capsule. Deep retractors are then placed to protect the posteromedial knee structures.

25. During lateral meniscal repair, what structures are at risk of injury?
   The peroneal nerve is at greatest risk, as well as the popliteal artery and vein and the tibial nerve.

26. Describe the lateral approach to the knee for meniscal repairs.
   A 3- to 4-cm incision is made posterior to the lateral collateral ligament with the knee flexed to 90° to relax the biceps femoris and peroneal nerve. The interval between the biceps femoris and iliotibial band is developed. The biceps tendon is retracted posteriorly to protect the peroneal nerve. The lateral head of the gastrocnemius must be swept off the capsule for visualization. Deep retractos can then be placed between the lateral head of the gastrocnemius and joint capsule to protect the neurovascular structures.

27. Describe the suture placement for meniscal repairs.
   Evenly spaced 2–3 mm apart in a vertical mattress fashion, which is stronger than a horizontal placement. Sutures can be placed in the traditional "inside-out" manner (where the sutures are passed from an intra-articular to an extra-articular position with the knots being placed on the capsule), an "outside-in" position (sutures passed from the capsule to the intra-articular portion of the joint with suture knots placed intra-articular, or an "all-inside" technique with newer fixation devices that rely on capsular fixation without the need for conventional knot tying.

28. What clinical factors may positively influence meniscal repairs?
   Repairs done in association with ACL surgery, tears with rim widths less than 3 mm, acute tears, and lateral meniscus tears.

29. What patient is a potential candidate for meniscal allograft transplantation?
   A patient who has previously undergone a total or near total meniscectomy and has joint line pain, early or minimal chondral changes, normal limb alignment, and a ligamentously stable knee. This clinical entity is commonly referred to as "overload pain."

30. What is a meniscus cyst?
   Degenerative cyst within the meniscus that is often found with horizontal cleavage tears of the lateral meniscus. These can often be treated by partial meniscectomy and decompression of the cyst (Fig. 10.5).

31. What is a Baker cyst?
   Collection of synovial fluid usually made in response to meniscal pathology or joint degeneration, palpable on the posterior aspect of the knee and also known as a popliteal cyst. Usually found between the semimembranosus and medial head of the gastrocnemius.

32. What is a discoid meniscus?
   A rare anatomic variant of meniscus that results in a "saucer" like meniscus with minimal amount of underlying exposed tibia and can cause symptoms such as popping, clicking, and catching. It usually affects the lateral meniscus and is often asymptomatic. There are

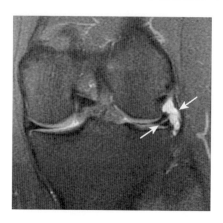

Figure 10.5. Meniscus cyst. (*From Miller TT: Magnetic Resonance Imaging of the Knee. In: Scott WN, ed: Insall & Scott Surgery of the Knee, 4th ed. Philadelphia, 2006, Churchill Livingstone.*)

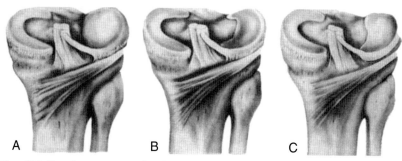

A   B   C

Figure 10.6. Discoid meniscus variant (from left to right): (A) Complete. (B) Partial. (C) Wrisberg – with stability of the meniscus only arising from attachment to the ligament of Wrisberg. (*From Kocher MS, Klingele K, Rassman SO: Meniscal disorders: Normal, discoid, and cysts. Orthop Clin North Am 34:329–340, 2003.*)

three variants described by Watanabe: I – complete variant where the meniscus most represents a thickened disk rather than a crescent, II – partial variant, and III – Wrisberg variant (lacing meniscofemoral attachment). The thickened meniscus is classically seen on three consecutive sagittal cuts of an MRI to make the diagnosis. It can be treated with meniscal "saucerization" if symptomatic or if found incidentally at arthroscopy (Fig. 10.6).

ACL INJURY

CASE 10-2

A 21-year-old college basketball player felt a loud "pop" in her knee after landing on a single leg after a jump shot. Her knee immediately swelled and she could not continue playing. She presented 1 week after her injury with a sore knee and a large effusion.

33. **Describe the anatomy and function of the ACL.**
    On average, the adult ACL is 33 mm in length and 11 mm in width. It has two bundles, the anteromedial bundle – tight in flexion – and the posterolateral bundle – tight in extension. Ninety percent of the ACL is composed of type I collagen. Its blood supply comes from the middle geniculate artery. It is primarily a stabilizer to anterior translation of the tibia and a secondary stabilizer of varus–valgus stress on the knee.

34. **Describe the mechanism of ACL injuries in non-contact sports.**
    Deceleration injuries with increased quadriceps contraction: Anterior force on the proximal tibia is caused by tremendous quadriceps contraction. Such injuries may be seen in basketball and football players who suddenly decelerate to change direction.

Hyperextension: Non-contact ACL injuries also are seen with hyperextension injury in basketball players (e.g., in rebounding) and in gymnasts during the dismount.

Skiing injuries: The classic cause of knee injury in downhill skiers is a forward fall in which the inside edge of the ski is caught in the snow, placing the knee in external rotation and valgus stress. A second injury mechanism is the so-called "boot-induced" injury, resulting from a backward fall. With the skier's center of gravity posterior to the boot, the back of the boot causes an anteriorly directed force onto the tibia. When coupled with significant quadriceps contraction (the skier attempts to right himself), the ACL undergoes tension failure.

35. **What percent of patients with acute knee injuries and hemarthrosis have an ACL tear?**
Seventy percent.

36. **What is the knee "unhappy triad"?**
Medial meniscus tear, anterior cruciate ligament (ACL) tear, medial collateral ligament (MCL) tear. It is caused by an excessive valgus force applied to the knee.

37. **What kind of meniscal tear is associated with ACL injuries?**
Acute lateral meniscus tears are more common in acute ACL injuries; medial meniscus tears are most common with chronic ACL deficiency.

38. **Describe the physical examination in a patient with a suspected ligamentous knee injury.**
The examination should start with evaluating the normal knee for comparison. Some patients have excessive hypermobility or generalized ligamentous laxity that must be taken into account in evaluating knee laxity. The knee should be inspected for areas of ecchymosis, swelling, effusion, or tenderness. Range of motion should be evaluated. Flexion and extension are frequently compromised because of the large amount of effusion following injury. Ligament stability testing is performed and should include a minimum of the Lachman test, anterior drawer, pivot shift, posterior drawer, external rotation measurement with dial test, and varus and valgus stability testing.

39. **What are the physical examination maneuvers that are meant to identify ACL injury?**
The Lachman test: The Lachman test is performed in approximately 30° of flexion. The femur is stabilized with the examiner's hand. The opposite hand is used to apply an anteriorly directed force to the posterior tibia while stabilizing the femur. The examiner senses any tibial displacement and compares it with the uninvolved knee. The endpoint may be graded as either firm, marginal, or soft. The Lachman test may be graded as negative, 1+ (3–5 mm displacement), 2+ (5–10 mm displacement), or 3+ (>10 mm displacement). Excessive anterior displacement compared with the normal side, especially when coupled with a marginal or soft endpoint, usually signifies a torn ACL.

The anterior drawer test: The anterior drawer test is performed with the patient's knee at 90° of flexion with muscular relaxation. The hip is flexed at 45°. A smooth, steady pull is placed in an anterior direction on the posterior portion of the tibia. In a positive test, increased anterior step-off occurs between the femoral condyle and tibial plateau.

The pivot shift test: The pivot shift describes the anterior subluxation of the lateral tibial plateau on the femoral condyle. With the patient in the supine position and relaxed, the knee is examined in full extension. The tibia is rotated internally, with one hand grasping the foot and the other hand applying a mild valgus stress at the level of the knee joint. Then, with flexion in the knee to approximately 20–30°, a jerk is suddenly experienced at the anterolateral corner of the proximal tibia. The patient also may feel the anterior subluxation and comment that it is the same feeling that occurred when the knee was injured or, in chronic cases, when it is continually injured. The jerk or "clunk" is the result of the extended, anteriorly subluxed tibia, reducing back into femorotibial alignment with knee flexion. The result is graded as 0 (absent), 1+ (mild), 2+ (moderate), or 3+ (severe) (Fig. 10.7).

40. **Which physical examination test is most sensitive for ACL injury?**
Lachman test.

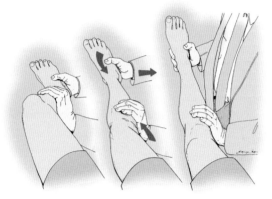

Figure 10.7. The pivot shift test. The knee examination starts in full extension, and a valgus/internal rotation force is applied as the knee is flexed. (*Courtesy of JC Hughston, MD, redrawn. In: Miller III RH, Azar FM, Knee Injuries: Canale ST, Beaty JH (eds), Campbell's Operative Orthopaedics, 11th ed. Mosby, 2008.*)

41. **Which physical examination test is most predictive of outcome after ACL reconstruction?**
    Pivot shift test.

42. **What is a Segund fracture?**
    Also known as a lateral capsule sign, it is an avulsed fragment off the lateral aspect of the lateral tibial plateau the capsule pulls off when the tibia shifts anteriorly during an ACL rupture (Fig. 10.8).

CASE 10-2   continued

You examine the patient's knee and note that she has an effusion. She has a positive Lachman test. You are unable to reliably perform a pivot shift test in the office due to muscle guarding by the patient during the maneuver. You order an MRI that demonstrates an ACL tear (Fig. 10.9). You discuss ligament reconstruction with the patient.

43. **What is the best diagnostic radiographic test for ACL tears?**
    Magnetic resonance imaging (MRI) is the best diagnostic test. The advantages of an MRI include its non-invasive nature, lack of radiation, and ability to image in any plane and to detect non-osseous injuries such as ligament, meniscal, or articular damage. A complete tear is visualized on both T1- and T2-weighted images as a discontinuity in the ligament, with fluid filling the defect. A lateral compartment bone bruise can help to confirm a diagnosis in questionable cases. MRI is also helpful in assessing fractures, medial and lateral collateral ligament injuries, PCL injuries, and meniscal injuries.

44. **What graft options are available for ACL reconstruction?**
    1. Hamstring autograft: Carries risk of weakness with knee flexion and potential iatrogenic injury to infrapatellar branch of saphenous nerve
    2. Bone-patella tendon-bone autograft: Demonstrates faster incorporation into bone tunnels, though it has a higher incidence of anterior knee pain, delayed quadriceps recovery, and loss of extension
    3. Quadriceps tendon autograft: Rarely used, not as strong as bone patella bone graft and carries the risk of prolonged quadriceps weakness
    4. Allograft: Used with older (>30 years old) patients. Associated with higher rupture rates in young adults, and it carries risk of disease transmission (less than 1:1 million for HIV).

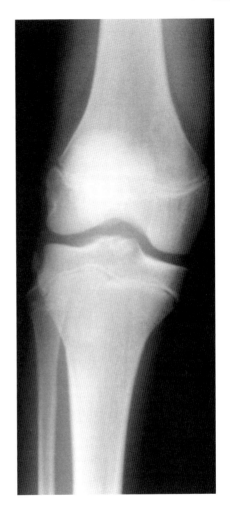

Figure 10.8. Segond fracture consistent with anterior cruciate ligament rupture. *(From Miller III RH, Azar FM, Knee injuries: Canale ST, Beaty JH (eds), Campbell's Operative Orthopaedics, 11th ed. Mosby, 2008.)*

45. Describe the procedure for an ACL reconstruction using the central one-third patellar tendon autograft.
    1. Diagnostic arthroscopy
    2. Meniscus repair or excision
    3. ACL stump excision
    4. Lateral superior expansion notchplasty
    5. Graft harvest and preparation (some surgeons prefer to perform this at the beginning of the procedure)
    6. Placement of appropriately sized tibial tunnel centered 7 mm in front of the posterior cruciate ligament. This center point is usually at, or slightly posterior to, the anterior horn of the lateral meniscus
    7. Placement of an appropriately sized femoral bone tunnel centered 6–7 mm in front of the "over-the-top" position within the intercondylar notch (this position would be at 2:00 in a left knee). The bifurcate ridge helps to identify the native insertion site of the ACL and serves as the anatomic landmark separating the AM and PL bundles.

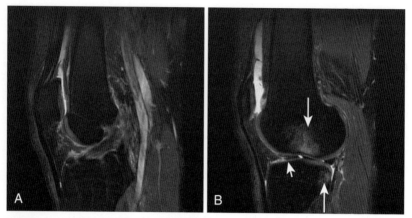

Figure 10.9. Anterior cruciate ligament tear with bone contusions and lateral meniscal tear. (A) Sagittal T2-weighted fat-saturated MR image demonstrates full-thickness tear of the anterior cruciate ligament. (B) More lateral image shows typical pivot shift bone contusions along the weight-bearing aspect of the lateral femoral condyle and the posterior rim of the tibial plateau (arrows). There is also a bucket handle tear of the body and posterior horn of the lateral meniscus with a fragment flipped anteriorly adjacent to the anterior horn of the lateral meniscus (small arrow). *(From Clement J, Basic Imaging Techniques: DeLee JC (ed), DeLee and Drez's Orthopaedic Sports Medicine, 3rd ed. Saunders, 2010.)*

8. Secure fixation of the graft in both bone tunnels. Usually performed with interference screw fixation. Acceptable alternatives include many other types of suspensory fixation methods
9. Careful evaluation of graft fixation, stability, and impingement-free range of motion
10. Standard wound closure over drains.

46. **Do all ACL ruptures need to be reconstructed?**
No, especially isolated ACL ruptures in patients older than age 40. For older patients with lower demand activities and a minimum of twisting and pivoting recreational sports, ACL ruptures can be managed non-operatively, with a focus on developing quadriceps and hamstring strength to help offset the knee instability.

47. **What exercises should be emphasized in the early rehabilitation of an ACL reconstruction?**
Closed chain exercises, particularly focusing on knee range of motion, are important in early rehabilitation. Exercises that should be avoided in early rehabilitation are open chain exercises where the foot is not fixed to surface as they place undue strain on the new graft and risk graft failure.

48. **What are the complications of ACL reconstruction?**
The most common problems include failure to regain full extension or flexion, patellofemoral complications (e.g., chondromalacia and fracture), graft impingement, and graft failure.

49. **What are the reasons for loss of full extension after cruciate surgery?**
- Lack of full preoperative extension. Patients should regain complete extension before reconstruction. This may be achieved with physical therapy or arthroscopic removal of mechanical blocks to extension.
- Anterior tibial placement of the graft causing roof impingement.
- Cyclops lesion. This nodular abundance of fibrous tissue lying anterior to the tibial portion of the graft impinges on the anterior notch, which may be caused by roof impingement.
- Infrapatellar contracture syndrome.

50. What is arthrofibrosis?

This syndrome involves contracture of the retropatellar fat pad and patellar tendon. Patients present with severe postoperative pain, diminished patellar mobility, and failure to gain extension and flexion. The best initial treatment is aggressive physical therapy.

PCL Injury

CASE 10-3

A 33-year-old male presents to your clinic 2 weeks after an automobile accident. He was a passenger and his knee struck the dashboard. He reports that at the time of the injury he developed a large knee effusion and his knee was aspirated, yielding 30 cc of hematoma. The plain films he presents with are negative for fracture.

51. What is the most common mechanism for a PCL rupture?

Also known as a "dashboard injury," the PCL is most commonly ruptured when a direct blow is applied to the anterior tibia with the knee flexed. It can also occur after a fall on a plantarflexed foot.

52. Describe the anatomy of the PCL.

The PCL is 38 mm in length and 13 mm in width. It has an anterolateral and posteromedial bundle. There are variable meniscofemoral ligaments that start from the lateral meniscus and attach to the PCL (ligaments of Humphrey and Wrisberg). It is predominantly a primary restraint to posterior translation of the tibia.

53. How do you examine for a PCL rupture?

The 90° posterior drawer test is the most sensitive. The patient is supine, the hip is flexed 45°, and the knee is flexed 90°. Force is applied from anterior to posterior on the proximal tibia. Excessive motion in an anterior to posterior direction is a positive test indicative of PCL injury. A grade I posterior drawer reflects 5 mm of movement. At maximal posterior displacement, the tibial condyles are still anterior to the femoral condyles. A grade II posterior drawer reflects 5- to 10-mm posterior displacement, in which the tibial condyles are flush with the femoral condyles. A grade III posterior drawer reflects a 10-mm posterior displacement. In a grade III posterior drawer, the tibial condyles are displaced posterior to the femoral condyles. This is usually accompanied with a posterolateral corner or ACL injury.

54. What is the posterior sag test?

The posterior sag test is similar to the posterior drawer test. It essentially detects the amount of posterior displacement caused by gravity when the knee and hip are flexed to 90°. When compared with the opposite side, the PCL-injured knee reveals a posterior sag of the tibial condyles relative to the femoral condyles. A positive test reflects absence of the PCL.

55. What is the treatment for grade I and II PCL injuries?

Usually non-operative management with physical therapy focusing on quadriceps strengthening and avoiding hamstring strengthening early after injury (to reduce the risk of further injury to the PCL with active flexion of the knee). Some authors advocate early immobilization in extension to allow for ligament healing before beginning range of motion.

56. Is a bony avulsion of the PCL a good prognostic factor?

Bony avulsions of the PCL typically have good outcomes when repaired primarily.

57. When should the isolated PCL-deficient knee be reconstructed?

Some clinicians believe that an acute knee injury with a grade III posterior drawer should be acutely reconstructed. Most, however, still recommend conservative treatment. If conservative treatment fails, resulting in persistent pain or functional instability, surgical reconstruction may still be performed (Fig. 10.10).

58. What are the two methods for reconstructing the PCL?

Transtibial or tibial inlay graft. The tibial inlay graft avoids a sharp change in angulation of the graft, also known as the "killer turn," and decreases stress on the graft, though the screws used for this technique are within 20 mm of the popliteal artery (Fig. 10.11).

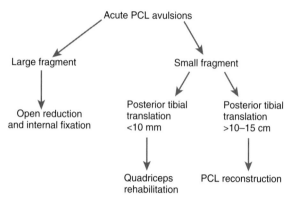

Figure 10.10. Algorithm for management of treating posterior cruciate ligament ruptures. (*From Veltri DM, Warren RF: Isolated and combined posterior cruciate ligament injuries, J Am Acad Orthop Surg 1:67, 1993.*)

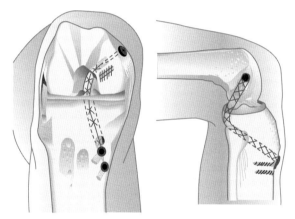

Figure 10.11. Figure demonstrating the transtibial technique for double bundle posterior cruciate ligament reconstruction. Note the sharp angle, i.e., "the killer turn", the graft must take. (*From Beynnon BD, Johnson RJ, Brown L, Knee: DeLee JC (ed), DeLee and Drez's Orthopaedic Sports Medicine, 3rd ed. Saunders, 2010.*)

MULTILIGAMENTOUS KNEE INJURY/PLC/MCL/LCL
CASE 10-4

A 40-year-old man presents to your office 1 week after dislocating his knee during a fall at a construction worksite. He reports that his knee was reduced in the Emergency Room and he was placed in a brace. He was subsequently admitted to the hospital for 24 hours of neurovascular monitoring. He was then discharged and told to follow-up with you for further surgical management.

59. **What combined ligamentous injury is usually found with knee dislocation?**
    Combined ACL/PCL injury.

60. **How is a knee dislocation classified?**
    Based on the position of the tibia relative to the femur. A knee dislocation can be classified as posterior, anterior, medial, and lateral.

61. **What is the acute treatment for a knee dislocation?**
    Closed reduction followed by confirmation of vascular sufficiency with further imaging studies, either in the form of an arteriogram or CT angiogram. Ligamentous reconstruction

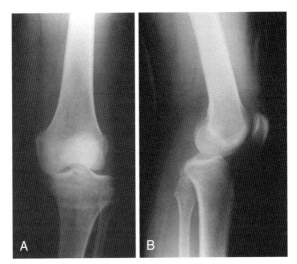

Figure 10.12. Posterior dislocation of the knee. *(From Miller III RH, Azar FM, Knee Injuries: Canale ST, Beaty JH (eds), Campbell's Operative Orthopaedics, 11th ed. Mosby, 2008.)*

often is delayed by 2 weeks to allow for soft-tissue swelling and to avoid precipitating compartment syndrome or other vascular injuries (Fig. 10.12).

62. **What injury is usually associated with grade III PCL injury?**
Posterolateral corner injury.

63. **What structures compose the posterolateral corner?**
   • Biceps femoris
   • Iliotibial band
   • Popliteus
   • Politeofibular ligament
   • Lateral capsule
   • Arcuate ligament
   • Fabellofibular ligament.

64. **What is the purpose of the PLC?**
To stabilize against external tibial rotation.

65. **What is the external rotation recurvatum test?**
The external rotation recurvatum test may reflect posterolateral rotatory instability. With the patient supine, the great toe is grasped and the foot is raised from the table. The test is positive if the knee falls into hyperextension, external rotation, and varus.

66. **What is the reverse pivot shift test?**
It can reflect injury to the posterolateral corner. With the patient supine, the flexed knee is brought into extension while the tibia is externally rotated and a valgus load is applied to the knee. A discernable clunk is suggestive of a posterolateral corner injury.

67. **How do you test for external rotation of the tibia? Why is such testing important?**
The patient is placed prone on the examining table with the hips and knees resting on the table. The knees are flexed at 30°, and the feet are rotated externally. If external rotation on the injured side is 10° more than on the normal side, the test is considered positive. A positive test is usually consistent with a tear of the posterolateral corner. This is considered the most specific test for posterolateral rotatory instability. A dial test that is positive at both 30° and 90° is indicative of a combined PCL/PLC injury.

68. **What is the treatment of combined PCL/posterolateral rotatory instability injuries?**

    Surgical repair and reconstruction are required. Patients generally are markedly symptomatic, with both pain and instability, if untreated. The rate of medial compartment arthritis is significant.

    If the patient has a varus knee or walks with a varus thrust gait, valgus high tibial osteotomy placing is performed first. Some patients are so dramatically improved by this procedure alone that later ligament reconstruction is not required. Most of the time, however, the PCL and posterolateral corner must be reconstructed. The posterolateral corner is reconstructed by either anatomic ligament repair or reconstruction of the posterolateral corner. Multiple techniques have been described, and the long-term prognosis of multiligamentous knee reconstruction is guarded.

69. **What are the lateral structures of the knee?**

    Layer I: IT band, biceps
    Layer II: Patellar retinaculum, patellofemoral ligament
    Layer III: Arcuate ligament, fabellofibular ligament, capsule, LCL.

70. **How does one test for varus instability of the knee? Why is such testing important?**

    With the patient relaxed and supine on the examination table, the distal femur is stabilized manually. The lower leg is grasped with the opposite hand, and varus stress is placed on the knee. The test should be performed at 0°, 30°, 60°, and 90° of knee flexion.

    Varus instability at 30° alone is diagnostic for isolated LCL injury. Isolated LCL injuries are rare and often do not require surgical intervention. When combined with posterolateral corner injury, the varus laxity is moderate to severe.

71. **What are the medial structures of the knee?**

    Layer I: Sartorius and fascia
    Layer II: Superficial MCL, semimembranosus, posterior oblique ligament
    Layer III: Deep MCL, capsule.

72. **How does one test for valgus instability of the knee?**

    Similar to testing for varus instability, this is done with the patient's knee flexed at 30°. A valgus load is used to open the medial compartment of the knee. The test should be done with the foot in the same degree of external rotation, because an extra grade of instability may be perceived if the examination allows the tibia to move externally. The test is considered positive when medial instability is present at 30° of flexion.

73. **How is an MCL tear treated?**

    Multiple studies have shown excellent results with bracing alone. A hinged knee brace has also been shown to be effective after ACL reconstruction for a combined ACL/MCL injury. Injuries on the tibial side of the joint may require repair or reconstruction if non-operative management fails.

74. **Which MCL injuries are at greater risk of not healing?**

    Distal MCL injuries do not heal as frequently.

75. **What is the Pellegrini–Stieda sign?**

    A calcification at the or adjacent to the insertion of the MCL on the medial femoral condyle indicative of a chronic MCL injury.

OSTEOCHONDRAL LESIONS

CASE 10-5

A 12-year-old tennis player reports persistent clicking in his right knee. He denies any specific injury or trauma. His knee now often swells and the knee pain is nearly constant. His knee has no joint line tenderness on exam and demonstrates firm endpoints on ligamentous examination. His MRI demonstrates subchondral edema of his medial femoral condyle in addition to separation of the overlying cartilage.

76. **What is osteochondritis dessicans?**
    Injury to the subchondral bone and a separation of the associated cartilage for unknown reasons, thought possibly due to occult trauma.

77. **What is the most common location of an OCD lesion?**
    Lateral aspect of medial femoral condyle.

78. **What is the treatment for OCD?**
    Children with open physis have the best prognosis and often improve with observation alone. Non-displaced lesions can be addressed with microfracture and retrograde drilling. Displaced lesions often require debridement followed by a reconstructive technique, as discussed below.

79. **What are the clinical results with microfracture?**
    In small defects, meaning less than $4\,cm^2$, good clinical results are reported in up to 80% of patients. The deficient cartilage is replaced by fibrin clot which eventually becomes fibrocartilagenous tissue (Fig. 10.13).

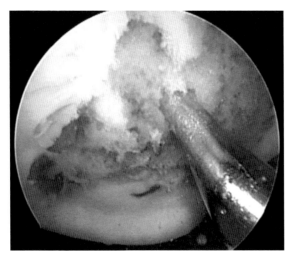

Figure 10.13. Microfracture technique employed in chondral defect. (*From Canale ST, Azar FM: Osteochondritis Dissecans. In: Jackson DW: Master Techniques in Orthopaedic Surgery: Reconstructive Knee Surgery, 3rd ed. Philadelphia, 2007, Lippincott Williams & Wilkins.*)

80. **What is autologous chondrocyte implantation?**
    This procedure involves harvesting autologous articular cartilage from the non-weight-bearing area of the knee, followed by expansion of the chondrocyte cell number in a sterile tissue culture. The chondrocyte cell suspension that results is then implanted into the defect area under a flap of periosteum or a porcine membrane. These cells are capable of adhering to the subchondral bone and forming the extracellular matrix, a process which occurs over the ensuing 12 months.

81. **What is osteochondral plug implantation?**
    Osteochondral plug implantation is referred to as as mosaicplasty or osteochondral autograft transfer system (OATS). These techniques differ basically in the size of plugs that are used, OATS using larger plugs. The technique involves excision of all damaged articular tissue and creating various sized cylindrical holes in the base of the defect. The holes are then filled with autologous matched cylinders of articular cartilage and its underlying bone. These techniques are suitable for confined defects of small to medium size. The limiting factor is the amount of autologous donor tissue available without excessive donor site morbidity. These techniques are sufficient for lesions around $3\,cm^2$ (Table 10.1).

Table 10.1. Operative Treatment Options for Chondral Defects

LESION SIZE	OPERATIVE TREATMENT
≤1 cm	Observation Abrasion chondroplasty Microfracture Osteochondral autograft transfer
1–2 cm	Abrasion chondroplasty Microfracture Osteochondral autograft transfer
2–3.5 cm	Fresh osteochondral allograft Autologous chondrocyte implantation
3.5–10 cm	Autologous chondrocyte implantation
Multiple (2 or 3)	Autologous chondrocyte implantation

(From Canale ST, Beaty JH. Campbell's Operative Orthopaedics, 11th ed. Philadelphia, Mosby, Elsevier, 2008.)

82. **What is the disadvantage of allograft plugs?**
    - Decreased chondrocyte viability
    - Limited supply
    - Risk of disease transmission.

PATELLOFEMORAL DISORDERS

CASE 10-6

A 21-year-old college student presents to your clinic 3 weeks after starting a long-distance running program. The pain is present in both knees and is primarily anterior. The patient also notes pain in both knees with deep squats or stair climbing. He denies previous injury to the knees. On examination, he has tight hamstrings and lateral tracking of the patellae on knee extension.

83. **What are the causes of anterior knee pain?**
    - Patellofemoral syndrome (also known as chondromalacia patellae)
    - Quadriceps or patella tendonitis
    - Quadriceps or patella tendon rupture
    - OCD lesion of patella
    - Patella instability/subluxation
    - Synovial plica.

84. **What is the common presentation of quadriceps and patella tendon ruptures?**
    Quad ruptures occur more frequently in patients older than 40 years old, whereas patella tendon ruptures occur in younger patients.

85. **What is patellar tendonitis?**
    Also known as jumper's knee, this entity is common to sports which require repeated jumping such as basketball. As with most patellofemoral disorders, the treatment comprises antiinflammatory medications, bracing, modifying the inciting activity, and directed physical therapy.

86. **What is housemaid's knee?**
    An inflammation of the prepatellar bursa, also known as prepatellar bursitis. This is most common in sports that require kneeling (such as wrestling) or among those with

professions that require kneeling (housekeepers, construction workers). Non-operative management is the standard approach to management of this condition.

87. **What is lateral patellar compression syndrome?**
Excessively tight lateral structures of the knee cause lateral tilt of the patella, causing compression and pain with knee motion.

   This is often remedied with antiinflammatory medication and directed physical therapy aimed at strengthening the VMO. Bracing and taping regimens have also been found to be effective in some studies.

   In some circumstances an arthroscopic lateral release can be performed when non-operative management has failed to release the tight lateral structures and promote better tracking of the patellofemoral joint.

88. **What is the first-line treatment for patella dislocation and instability?**
Non-operative management consisting of bracing and directed physical therapy. Distal realignment procedures, frequently tibial tubercle medialization osteotomies, are reserved for refractory cases. Medial patellofemoral ligament (MPFL) reconstruction has also gained increasing acceptance as a surgical technique for this disorder.

89. **Which cartilage is most frequently damaged in a patella dislocation?**
The medial patella facet.

90. **What maneuver reduces a patella dislocation?**
Knee extension.

91. **What anatomic factors can predispose to patella dislocation?**
A high Q-angle. The Q-angle is a line drawn from the anterior superior iliac spine to the patella, and a second line from the patella to the tibial tubercle. A high Q-angle predisposes to patella maltracking and patellofemoral syndrome or patella instability. Femoral anteversion and pronated feet, seen in some adolescents, also predisposes to this condition. A shallow trochlear groove or trochlear dysplasia can also be seen in a high percentage of patients with this disorder.

HIP

FEMOROACETABULAR IMPINGEMENT

CASE 10-7

A 16-year-old gymnast complains of worsening groin pain that is exacerbated during practice. The pain is localized to the groin area and does not radiate down her leg. She denies any back pain. She occasionally feels clicking when she ranges her hip. She presents concerned that her hip range of motion has decreased over the past 6 months.

92. **What is the differential diagnosis for an athlete with groin pain?**
   - Sports hernia
   - Inguinal hernia
   - Femoral neck stress fracture
   - Hip intra-articular loose bodies
   - Hip labral tears
   - Femoroacetabular impingement
   - Snapping hip syndrome
   - Osteitis pubis
   - Iliopsoas or ischial bursitis.

93. **What is femoroacetabular impingement?**
Impingement between proximal femur and acetabulum leading to cartilage injury and pain, thought due to an anomaly in hip development.

94. **What are the types of FAI?**
Cam impingement: Anomaly in femoral head or neck structure, with loss of femoral head sphericity and decreased femoral neck offset. Cam impingement is most commonly seen in young males. The acetabulum cannot accommodate an abnormally shaped femoral

head resulting in impingement. The impingement is worse with flexion. Impingement results in excess loads placed on the hip labrum and chondral surface, lesions are typically found on the anterosuperior aspect of acetabulum. Contrecoup lesions and posterior pain in the hip can also occur as the impingement progresses due to levering an excessive force transmission posteriorly.

Pincer impingement: Anomaly in acetabular structure, most commonly seen in athletic middle aged females, with common deformities being acetabular protrosio or inadequate acetabular anteversion. Often times the pathology is over-coverage of the femoral head, resulting in impingement of the femoral neck on the anterior acetabulum with flexion.

Combined: Both cam and pincer impingement. This is the most common form of FAI (Figs 10.14 and 10.15).

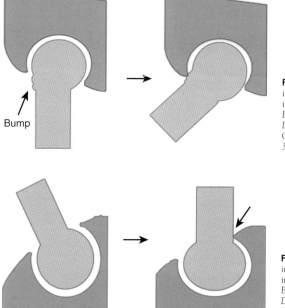

Figure 10.14. Femoral cam impingement in femoroacetabular impingement. (*From Shah A, Buschoni B, Hip, Pelvis, and Thigh: DeLee JC (ed), DeLee and Drez's Orthopaedic Sports Medicine, 3rd ed. Saunders, 2010.*)

Figure 10.15. Acetabular pincer impingement in femoroacetabular impingement. (*From Shah A, Buschoni B, Hip, Pelvis, and Thigh: DeLee JC (ed), DeLee and Drez's Orthopaedic Sports Medicine, 3rd ed. Saunders, 2010.*)

95. What are the acquired causes of FAI?
    Old slipped capital femoral epiphysis, retroversion of proximal femur resulting from fracture, decreased femoral head/neck ratio as a result of old trauma, Perthes disease.

96. What is the prevalence of FAI?
    Recent investigations have yielded a nearly 15% prevalence rate among asymptomatic volunteers based on MRI findings, with the majority found in males (80%).

97. What are the physical examination findings associated with FAI?
    Pain with hip range of motion classically localized to groin
    The anterior impingement test is performed by flexion of the hip followed by internally rotating and adducting the hip. Reproduction of the patient's symptoms confirms the diagnosis
    The posterior impingement test is the reverse, and is performed by extending and externally rotating the patient's hip.

98. What are the radiographic signs of a cam lesion?
A flattened femoral head or pistol grip deformity of the proximal femur.

99. What are the radiographic signs of a pincer lesion?
The "crossover" sign as evident on an AP radiograph of the hip. This is the intersection of the anterior acetabular wall superolaterally, intersecting with the posterior wall inferomedially.

100. What is the surgical treatment for FAI?
Arthroscopic management consists of arthroscopic debridement and shaving of impinging lesions. Arthroscopy of the hip can be done in the supine or lateral positions and it requires fluoroscopy and traction. A 70° arthroscope is usually used. Femoral head or neck resections for cam impingement or pincer lesions in the acetabulum can be debrided arthroscopically. Labral tears in the periphery of the hip joint have the potential to heal, though most are more central and debrided.

Open dislocation of the hip as described by Ganz and colleagues allows complete exposure of the hip, and permits resection of pincer lesions, repair of labral tears, and osteotomy of the pelvis in circumstances of acetabular retroversion. It carries the risk of avascular necrosis if the external rotators or medial femoral circumflex is compromised during the operation. This risk has been reported in some series to be approximately 1 : 1000.

Cases with end-stage arthritis require hip replacement.

101. What are the reported complications with hip arthroscopy?
Complications are associated with traction or iatrogenic injury with arthroscopy instruments; reported rates range from 0.5% to 5%. Posterior oriented portals can damage the sciatic nerve, anterolateral portals place the lateral femoral cutaneous nerve at risk; anterior portals have also been described to cause injury to the femoral nerve. Heterotopic ossification and avascular necrosis may also occur in some instances.

102. What is snapping hip syndrome?
Two entities exist for snapping hip syndrome. External snapping hip occurs when the iliotibial band gets caught on the greater trochanter and is worsened with hip flexion and adduction. It is more common in women. Running on slanted surfaces can exacerbate this condition.

The other snapping hip entity is internal snapping hip syndrome. This is less common and occurs when the iliopsoas hits against the hip capsule. The provocative maneuver for diagnosis of this condition consists of extending and internally rotating the hip from an externally rotated position.

103. What is the treatment for snapping hip syndrome?
The mainstay of management is non-operative. Physical therapy, NSAIDs, and modalities such as ultrasounds or occasionally ultrasound guided injections are effective in the management of snapping hip syndrome. Rarely, surgical release is required in refractory cases of snapping hip syndrome.

104. What is trochanteric bursitis?
Trochanteric bursitis is inflammation of the bursa overlying the greater trochanter. This occurs in any age group, but is more common in young female runners.

105. What physical exam findings are consistent with trochanteric bursitis?
Patients will often complain of pain directly over the greater trochanter. Deep palpation of the greater trochanter will reproduce the patient's pain.

106. What is the treatment for trochanteric bursitis?
Activity modification, NSAIDs, and directed physical therapy aimed at strengthening and stretching the hip abductors and IT band. Occasionally a steroid injection can be given for refractory cases, though repeat injections can place the abductors at risk of atrophy.

STRESS FRACTURES
CASE 10-8

A 15-year-old high school track athlete reports worsening right groin pain since they started the season. Her past medical history is significant for anorexia. The pain has become progressively worse and she now has pain with ambulation. She denies any mechanical symptoms in her hip and has no history of trauma.

107. **What condition should always be ruled out in the athlete with the insidious onset of groin pain and history of overuse?**
Femoral neck stress fracture.

108. **What other stress fractures in the leg are common in the athletic population?**
- Tibial shaft stress fractures
- Femoral shaft stress fractures.

109. **What is the "dreaded black line"?**
Seen on plain films of the tibia in the setting of stress fracture, this finding is indicative of a stress fracture in the tibia that may require surgical intervention. The presence of the "dreaded black line" in the tibia for over 6 months will often require intramedullary nailing of the tibia for healing.

110. **What physical examination findings should raise suspicion for a femoral neck fracture?**
Passive hip range of motion may be painless. Difficulty with performing a straight leg raise, abductor weakness or a Trendelenberg gait, and pain with hopping on one foot should raise suspicion of a femoral neck stress fracture.

111. **What imaging modalities can be used to diagnose a femoral neck stress fracture?**
Plain films, CT scan, and MRI are all useful in the diagnosis of a femoral neck stress fracture. MRI is the most sensitive modality for detecting a femoral neck stress fracture.

112. **What are the two broad categories of femoral neck stress fractures?**
Distraction type: Transverse fracture along the superolateral aspect of the femoral neck
Compression type: Fracture along the inferomedial aspect of the femoral neck.

113. **What is the management of a distraction type femoral neck stress fracture?**
This entity most often occurs in adults and occurs on the tension side of the femoral neck. Because it carries a risk of becoming displaced, it requires immediate surgical fixation, usually in the form of three cannulated screws with protected weight-bearing postoperatively.

114. **What is the management of a compression type femoral neck stress fracture?**
This usually occurs in younger athletes and can be treated non-operatively with protected weight-bearing until there is radiographic and clinical evidence of fracture healing (Fig. 10.16).

115. **What other studies should be considered in the setting of a femoral neck stress fracture?**
This condition may be caused by nutritional deficiencies, as suggested in the clinical vignette. Nutritional studies including serum calcium, vitamin D, and albumin studies may be useful. A DEXA scan should also be considered to rule out osteoporosis.

PELVIS – CONTUSIONS AND STRAINS
CASE 10-9

A high school hurdler complains of groin and lower abdominal pain that is worst when he is forced to flex his abdomen or perform crunches in practice. Physical examination does not demonstrate any evidence of an inguinal hernia. He reports they have been focusing heavily on abdominal strengthening exercises in practice for the last 4 weeks.

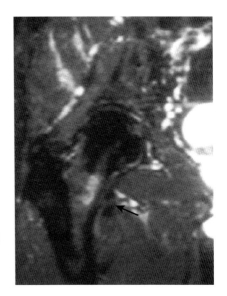

Figure 10.16. MRI of compression sided femoral neck stress fracture. *(From Shah A, Buschoni B, Hip, Pelvis, and Thigh: DeLee JC (ed), DeLee and Drez's Orthopaedic Sports Medicine, 3rd ed. Saunders, 2010.)*

116. **What are the common muscle strains around the athlete pelvis?**
   - Rectus strain: pain elicited with hip flexion
   - Hamstring strain: pain elicited with knee flexion, associated with sprinting activities
   - Lesser trochanter avulsion fracture
   - Athletic pubalgia.

117. **What is athletic pubalgia?**
   Also known as a sports hernia, this involves strain of the muscles in the abdominal wall or adductors. It presents as groin or abdominal pain but physical examination rules out an inguinal hernia.

118. **What is herniated in a sports hernia?**
   A sports hernia is not a true hernia, but derives its name from the fact that it elicits symptoms and patient complaints similar to an inguinal hernia.

119. **What is the prevalence of sports hernia?**
   Investigations of professional athletes suggest that it may be as high at 20% in some sports such as soccer.

120. **What sports and activities are associated with sports hernia?**
   Soccer and hockey players have a higher rate of sports hernia than other professional sports. Hurdling events require the athlete to hyperextend the abdomen and forcibly abduct the leg, resulting in microtears of the rectus abdominus or adductors.

121. **What anatomic structures are thought to be involved in a sports hernia?**
   The internal oblique aponeurosis, rectus abdominis, and adductor longus have all been described as playing a role in the pathogenesis of sports hernia. Attenuation of the transversalis fascia and conjoined tendon has also been described.

122. **What history and physical examination findings are consistent with sports hernia?**
   An insidious onset of unilateral groin pain that is worse with activity is typically reported. The pain may mimic a neuralgia, in that it can radiate to surrounding structures including the perineum, adductors, and testicles. Abrupt movements can exacerbate the condition and include coughing, kicking, or attempting abdominal curls.

Physical examination findings are generally non-specific, but can include point-tenderness to deep palpation of the inguinal canal, conjoined tendon, or pubic tubercle. Pain with abdominal curls or forced hip adduction can also reproduce symptoms.

123. **What is the role of imaging in sports hernia?**
Though no imaging modality is entirely sensitive or specific for sports hernia, nuclear medicine scans, ultrasound, and MRI have all been described in the evaluation of this condition. Bone scan may demonstrate increased uptake in the pubic region or adductor tendon origin. MRI is useful in that it can rule out other causes of groin pain, notably stress fracture. MRI may demonstrate a broadened pubic symphysis and high-intensity on T2 imaging.

124. **What is the management of sports hernia?**
Non-operative management is the first line of treatment. Activity modification, rest, and physical therapy should be attempted. Ultrasound therapy and exercises emphasizing balanced muscle strengthening have been successful in treating this condition.

When this fails, occasionally the anterior abdominal musculature must be reinforced surgically. This is the last line of treatment and should only be pursued when all other causes of groin or abdominal pain have been ruled out and non-operative management has failed. The general surgery literature describes both laparoscopic and open techniques for addressing this condition. Open repair can involve reinforcement of the oblique aponeurosis. Adductor tenotomy has also been described in the management of this condition.

SHOULDER INSTABILITY

CASE 10-10

A 19-year-old college football player is tackled and his right arm is torqued in abduction and external rotation. He feels a "pop" and has immediate right shoulder pain. He is seen by the training staff on the field and is thought to have dislocated his shoulder. The on-site physician promptly reduces the shoulder and he is placed in a sling.

125. **What are the primary stabilizers of the shoulder joint?**
Shoulder stability can be considered a static and a dynamic process. The static restraints include the glenoid labrum, articular version of the glenoid and the humerus, articular conformity, negative intra-articular pressure, capsule and rotator interval, and capsuloligamentous structures. The dynamic restraints include the joint concavity compression produced by synchronized movement of the rotator cuff acting to stabilize the humeral head within the glenoid; increased capsular tension produced by direct attachments of the rotator cuff to the capsule; the scapular stabilizers; and proprioception.

126. **What are the major capsular ligaments of the shoulder? What directional stability do they impart?**
The *inferior glenohumeral ligament* (IGHL) complex resists inferior, posterior, and anterior displacement with shoulder abduction (45° to 90°); with internal rotation it resists posterior translation; and with external rotation it resists anterior translation. The *middle glenohumeral ligament* limits external rotation of the adducted humerus, inferior translation of the adducted and externally rotated humerus, and anterior and posterior translation of the partly abducted (45°) and externally rotated arm. The *superior glenohumeral ligament* resists inferior translation with the arm in neutral position and external rotation at low-range of abduction. The *coracohumeral ligament* resists posterior–inferior humeral head translation. The superior glenohumeral ligament and coracohumeral ligament are reinforcing structures of the rotator interval (Fig. 10.17).

127. **During midrange of motion, which factors provide glenohumeral stability?**
During midrange of motion the capsular ligaments are lax and stability is created by the rotator cuff and biceps that maintain a *concavity-compression effect* around the joint. This is a dynamic action in which the rotator cuff compresses the humerus into the congruent

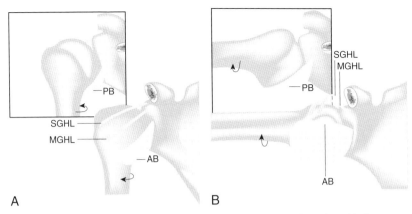

Figure 10.17. Function of the glenohumeral ligaments. The glenohumeral capsule is enhanced by ligamentous thickenings that provide static restraint at different functional positions. (A) With the shoulder in adduction, the superior glenohumeral ligament (SGHL) and middle glenohumeral ligament (MGHL) are tight, and the inferior glenohumeral ligament (IGHL) is lax. (B) With abduction and external rotation, the IGHL anterior band (AB) and posterior band (PB) tighten. (*From Warner JP; Boardman ND III: Anatomy, Biomechanics, and Pathophysiology of Glenohumeral Instability. In: Warren RF, Craig EV, Altcheck DW (eds): The Unstable Shoulder. Philadelphia, Lippincott-Raven, 1999, pp. 51–76.*)

glenoid cavity. Lesions that affect this congruency, such as a glenoid rim fracture or labrum detachment, result in a loss of this normal concavity compression.

128. **Is the glenohumeral joint a congruent or incongruent articulation?**
The glenohumeral joint articular surfaces are congruent, although the surface area of the humerus is much greater than that of the glenoid. The subchondral bone of the glenoid is less curved than the humerus, but the articular cartilage of the glenoid is thickest at the periphery. The thickness of the cartilage, along with the labrum, deepens the articulating portion of the glenoid and creates a highly conforming joint.

129. **What is the difference between laxity and instability?**
Laxity is a clinical exam finding and simply refers to the ability to translate the humeral head on the glenoid. A given amount of laxity is required for normal functioning of the shoulder and is affected by age, sex, activities and biologic factors. With certain activities, such as pitching and swimming, a given amount of laxity of the shoulder is beneficial.
Instability is a pathologic condition associated with *pain* and excessive translation of the joint. Due to the wide spectrum of what is considered normal, it is the inclusion of symptoms with the clinical finding of laxity that implies instability. The shoulder has extensive range of motion, is therefore at risk for developing instability, and is the most commonly dislocated joint in the body.

130. **What are the most common mechanisms for production of anterior shoulder dislocations?**
Anterior dislocation, which is the direction of 95% of all dislocations, is produced by an external rotation and/or hyperextension force applied to the shoulder that is already in approximately 90° of abduction.

131. **Describe some of the preferred methods for reducing an anterior dislocation.**
There are several described methods for reducing a shoulder dislocation. Several include:
• Apply gentle longitudinal traction to the injured arm with counter-traction in the axilla. Slow alternation between internal and external rotation is often required to achieve a reduction when performing this maneuver.

- Place the patient prone with the injured arm lying off the side of the bed. A wrist weight suspended from the unsupported, injured arm is used to apply traction on the arm anteriorly. Rotating the scapula toward the humeral head by application of pressure to the scapular spine is often helpful in achieving a reduction.

132. **How do you diagnose shoulder instability on physical examination?**
A thorough history and physical examination are essential for the diagnosis of shoulder instability. The patient may recall a specific traumatic instability event or numerous incomplete instability events, or may describe generalized laxity of both shoulders. The type of instability (subluxation versus dislocation), mechanism of injury (contact versus non-contact), and initial versus recurrent instability can be determined during the physical examination. Acute presentation of anterior shoulder dislocation is notable for a palpable prominence of the humeral head anterior and inferior to the shoulder, as well as a lack of shoulder contour over the deltoid. The arm is generally held in a position of adduction and internal rotation, and abduction of the arm is limited to <90°.

Active and passive range of motion (ROM) in both the injured and asymptomatic shoulder should be assessed to ensure reduction and to assess rotator cuff function. Neurovascular examination of the upper extremity must be performed before and after all reduction attempts, with specific evaluation of the axillary and radial nerves. In addition, ligamentous laxity has been linked with shoulder instability and has implications for treatment.

133. **What specific tests can be used to characterize instability patterns on physical examination?**
Specific tests, including the anterior load-shift test, sulcus sign, apprehension–relocation, can enable the physician to characterize the anterior shoulder instability pattern (Figs 10.18, 10.19, 10.20).

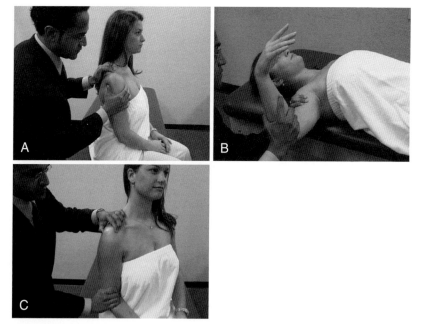

Figure 10.18. (A and B) The load-and-shift test is used to evaluate the degree of translation at different levels of glenohumeral abduction and can be performed with the patient seated or supine. (C) Longitudinal inferior traction is applied to the humerus, and the distance from the humerus to the acromion is evaluated. The degree of laxity is measured as the displacement of the humerus relative to the inferior border of the acromion. It is thought to be a test of the superior glenohumeral and coracohumeral ligaments. (*From DeLee JC, Drez D, Miller MD: Shoulder. In: DeLee, JC (ed), DeLee and Drez's Orthopaedic Sports Medicine, 3rd ed. Saunders, 2010.*)

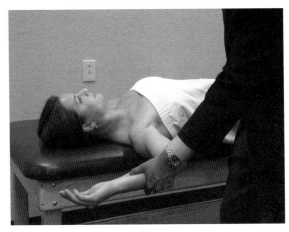

Figure 10.19. The apprehension test is a provocative exam in which the involved ligament structures are placed in the position of maximal tension, conceptually confirming end-range instability. For the classic apprehension test, the inferior glenohumeral ligament is tested by placing the arm in abduction, external rotation, and extension, also known as the provocative position. In a patient with anterior instability this will cause an abnormal anterior translation of the humeral head, thus producing a sense of impending subluxation. (*From DeLee JC, Drez D, Miller MD: Shoulder. In: DeLee JC (ed), DeLee and Drez's Orthopaedic Sports Medicine, 3rd ed. Saunders, 2010.*)

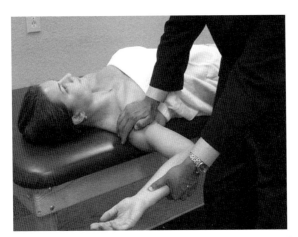

Figure 10.20. The relocation test is performed by applying a posteriorly directed pressure on the humeral head while performing the apprehension test. If this posterior pressure relieves the subluxation symptoms, it is considered a positive test and is suggestive of anterior instability. (*From DeLee JC, Drez D, Miller MD. Shoulder. In: DeLee JC (ed), DeLee and Drez's Orthopaedic Sports Medicine, 3rd ed. Saunders, 2010.*)

134. **What has been described as the "essential lesion" of a traumatic shoulder dislocation?**

The Bankart lesion is the most common lesion in traumatic anterior shoulder dislocations and is a detachment of the antero-inferior labrum from the bony glenoid rim. It also represents an avulsion of the glenoid attachment of the inferior glenohumeral ligament. It has been found that before failing at the glenoid insertion, a significant amount of midsubstance strain (plastic deformation) of the IGHL occurs, leading to the concomitant capsular laxity that often accompanies Bankart lesions. Variants include a bony or osseous

Bankart (associated with a rim fracture of the glenoid), a non-displaced labral tear with intact medial scapular periosteum, anterior labroligamentous periosteal sleeve avulsion (ALPSA), a reverse Bankart (postero-inferior labral tear associated with posterior instability), or a labral tear extending into the glenoid articular cartilage.

Variants include a bony or osseous Bankart lesion (glenoid rim fracture with functional labral detachment); Perthes lesion (nondisplaced labral tear with intact medial scapular periosteum); anterior labroligamentous periosteal sleeve avulsion (ALPSA, or "medialized Bankart" lesion: medial antero-inferior labral tear displaced medially by intact medial scapular periosteum); reverse Bankart lesion (posteroinferior labral tear); and glenolabral articular disruption (labral tear extending into glenoid cartilage).

135. **Are any other injuries associated with anterior shoulder dislocations?**
Rotator cuff tears are frequently noted in those patients over the age of 40. Fractures of the greater tuberosity, glenoid, and humeral head are common in the elderly. Major vascular injury to the axillary vessels has been reported in patients with atherosclerotic disease. Brachial plexus injuries, specifically to the axillary nerve, are uncommon but can occur.

136. **Which rotator cuff lesions are associated with chronic shoulder instability?**
Rotator cuff tendinitis and partial-thickness undersurface tears are very common in patients with chronic shoulder subluxation, whether traumatic or atraumatic. This is thought to be due to abnormal translation of the humeral head increasing the likelihood of rotator cuff impingement and by overworking the cuff in an attempt to keep the head in a reduced position. Shoulder subluxation often presents as an "impingement syndrome" and should be suspected in a young "overhead athlete" (e.g., tennis player, pitcher, swimmer) or a person with a history of traumatic instability who has what appears to be impingement pain.

CASE 10-10   continued

The football player is taken to the Emergency Department and x-rays are obtained that demonstrate a concentrically reduced glenohumeral joint. There is no evidence of fracture, but a flattening of the posterolateral humeral head is noted. The patient is scheduled for an MRI evaluation of the shoulder and a follow-up appointment with an orthopedic surgeon.

137. **Which radiographic views are useful in evaluating shoulder dislocations?**
Plain radiographs should be the first imaging study used to document a dislocation or to confirm reduction. Radiographs taken from perpendicular planes are required: a "true" AP radiograph (which demonstrates the inferior glenoid rim) and either an axillary or transcapular "Y" lateral view. The West Point view may be obtained if an inferior glenoid rim fracture is suspected (Fig. 10.21).

MRI can be beneficial for diagnosis of Bankart lesions as well as humeral avulsions of the inferior glenohumeral ligament. Hemarthrosis can improve imaging of labral pathology if obtained acutely after the injury, similar to injected contrast dye. The presence of a bone bruise in the region of a Hill–Sachs lesion can also be helpful for diagnosis. CT scan is reserved for patients with suspected bone loss, failed primary repair, or large bony Bankart lesions.

138. **What is a Hill–Sachs lesion? How does it contribute to recurrent shoulder instability?**
Caused by impaction of the dislocated humeral head on the glenoid rim, a Hill–Sachs lesion is an osteochondral depression in the posterior humeral head. It may play a causal role in cases of recurrent instability when the lesion is large enough to decrease the humeral head's contribution to passive stability. This is reported to require a depression of about 30% of the articular surface (Fig. 10.22).

139. **What is a humeral avulsion of the glenhumeral ligament (HAGL) lesion?**
The HAGL lesion occurs with a hyperabduction injury to the arm and is also associated with traumatic dislocations. Since this lesion is associated with continued instability, due to the disruption of an important static stabilizer, it is important to recognize and repair it anatomically. A HAGL has typically necessitated open repair in the past, because of its inferior location, but newer arthroscopic techniques are being developed (Fig. 10.23).

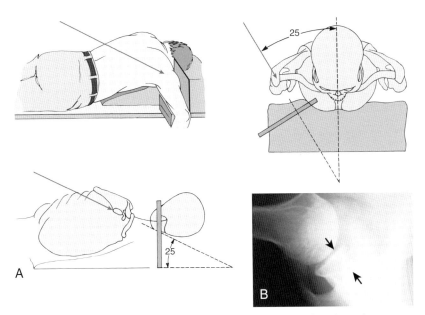

Figure 10.21. West Point axillary view to visualize the anteroinferior glenoid rim for evidence of a rim fracture. (A) Radiographic evaluation. (B) Anterioinferior rim fracture (arrows) after anterior dislocation. *(From Browner BD, et al. (eds), Skeletal Trauma, 4th ed, p.1633. Copyright © Saunders, 2008.)*

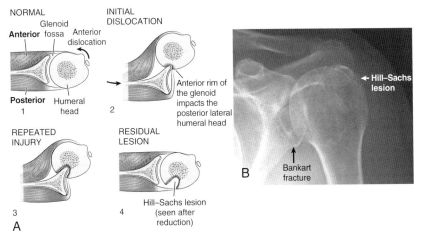

Figure 10.22. 1, Normal. With repeated anterior shoulder dislocations, a Hill–Sachs lesion may form. 2, During the dislocation, the humeral head is damaged by the sharp anterior rim of the glenoid. 3, With repeated dislocation, the lesion, called the "hatchet sign" develops. 4, On the reduction film, the lesion is apparent. *(From Horn AE, Ufberg JW. Roberts and Hedges' Clinical Procedures in Emergency Medicine, 6th ed., pp. 954–998. Saunders, Elsevier Inc.)*

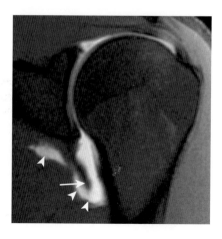

Figure 10.23. Humeral avulsion of the anterior glenohumeral ligament (HAGL) (arrow) on magnetic resonance arthrography. There is extravasation of contrast material (arrowheads) from the joint into the adjacent soft tissues. (*From DeLee JC, Drez D, Miller MD: Shoulder. In: DeLee JC (ed), DeLee and Drez's Orthopaedic Sports Medicine, 3rd ed. Saunders, 2010.*)

140. **What is the recurrence rate for patients who sustain an anterior shoulder dislocation?**
Studies of the recurrence rate for patients who sustain an anterior shoulder dislocation correlate recurrence with a patient's age and activity level. Hovelius et al. reported on 227 patients (229 shoulders) with primary anterior shoulder dislocations that were managed non-surgically. The authors found that the rate of recurrence was lower in patients older than 30 years (27%) than in those younger than 23 years (72%). Similarly, others have reported even higher recurrence rates (87–92%) in young patients. Importantly, the recurrence rate after treatment varies depending on the type of treatment and associated injuries.

141. **Do recurrent dislocations lead to an increased risk of glenohumeral joint arthritis?**
This is an area of research that is in need of more complete data. However, Hovelius and Saeboe found that shoulder arthritis occurred in up to 40% of patients with recurrent instability. Moreover, the number of recurrent events has been shown to correlate with development of osteoarthritis. These studies are concerning for a link between recurrent dislocation and glenohumeral joint arthritis.

142. **What is MDI?**
Though standardized diagnostic criteria do not exist, MDI is an abbreviation for multidirectional instability. It is a term that encompasses a variety of instability patterns. Most patients present with insidious onset and non-specific, activity-related pain in the second to third decade of life. Decreased strength and deteriorating athletic performance also may be reported. MDI is more common in patients involved in repetitive overhead activities, particularly in sports such as volleyball, swimming, or gymnastics. Collagen disorders can also be a contributing factor and should be considered in patients who present with MDI because surgical stabilization is less successful in patients with these disorders.
The acronyms TUBS (Traumatic, Unilateral, Bankart lesion, Surgery) and AMBRI (Atraumatic Multidirectional, Bilateral, Rehabilitation, and if surgery is needed, Inferior capsular shift) have been used to describe shoulder instability in etiological terms. Unfortunately, shoulder instability is often more complex and multifactorial than these acronyms would imply. More comprehensively, Gerber and Nyffeler have classified instability as unidirectional or multidirection with or without hyperlaxity (Table 10.2).

143. **Should patients with voluntary shoulder instability be operated upon?**
Many voluntary subluxators or dislocators have underlying psychiatric problems that an orthopedic surgeon cannot help. Patients who can dislocate voluntarily are considered

Table 10.2. Gerber and Nyffeler Classification of Dynamic Shoulder Instability

CLASSIFICATION	DESCRIPTION
Unidirectional without hyperlaxity	Symptoms elicited in a single direction Traumatic capsulolabral lesion frequently present
Unidirectional with hyperlaxity	Symptoms elicited in a single direction Patulous capsular tissue frequently present Presence of capsulolabral lesion less likely
Multidirectional without hyperlaxity	Symptoms elicited in two or more directions Anterior and posterior capsulolabral lesions frequently present
Multidirectional with hyerlaxity	Symptoms elicited in two or more directions Patulous capsular tissue frequently present Signs of generalized hyperlaxity frequently present Frequent recurrent subluxation

poor surgical candidates. Any patient with generalized laxity, scapulothoracic instability, or maltracking should be placed in an aggressive rehabilitation program for a minimum of 6–12 months before any procedure is considered.

There are other patients who are considered positional dislocators. These are patients who are able to voluntarily dislocate their shoulder when they place their arm in a provocative position, but are generally reluctant to do so. They often will prevent future dislocations by avoiding these positions in their daily activities. These patients are good surgical candidates with historically favorable outcomes.

CASE 10-10 continued

The patient is noted to have Bankart and Hill–Sachs lesions on his MRI. After 2 weeks the patient is feeling much improved and has regained full shoulder motion. He continues to have some strength limitation and soreness. You discuss operative and non-operative treatment strategies. He would like to try non-operative management at this time, and so, you initiate a course of physical therapy. He would like to return to play during this season.

144. **What are the criteria for return to play after a shoulder dislocation?**

Criteria for in-season return to play following an initial acute shoulder instability event include symmetric pain-free shoulder motion and strength, ability to perform sports specific skills, and the absence of subjective or objective instability. In general, non-surgical management often entails a brief period of shoulder immobilization (approximately 1 week) and early rehabilitation to achieve full pain-free motion. Motion-limiting braces that prevent extreme shoulder abduction, extension, and external rotation are sometimes used once the athlete has returned to sport. These braces limit overhead motion and are likely too restrictive for throwing athletes.

145. **Describe a typical non-operative treatment plan for a first-time traumatic shoulder anterior dislocation.**

Non-surgical management of an initial shoulder dislocation may include immobilization, physical therapy, and bracing, with a delayed return to activity. The position of immobilization and the duration of immobilization are controversial. Several studies indicate that immobilization in external rotation better approximates the torn labrum in an anatomic position and reduces the risk of recurrence; however, others have shown no difference between immobilization in internal or external rotation. Similarly, longer periods of immobilization (3–4 weeks) have been used after dislocation and some studies have demonstrated equivalent redislocation rates after initiation of early motion. In fact, age and activity level have been shown to be more predictive of redislocation than position and duration of immobilization.

Goals of rehabilitation are (1) restoration of a full painless range of motion, (2) avoidance of the "provocative" positions for 6 weeks, and (3) strengthening the cuff and scapulothoracic muscles. Patients start with isometric exercises and gradually progress to isotonic exercises. Scapular stabilizers are strengthened to provide a stable base for humeral rotation and to maintain the glenoid in a position that allows for maximal congruency. Patients greater than 45 years old should have motion restored as quickly as tolerated because their incidence of stiffness is higher, while their risk of recurrent dislocation is lower.

CASE 10-10   continued

The patient returns to football 4 weeks after his initial dislocation. He wears a shoulder brace to prevent "at risk" positions of the arm. During his first game, he again dislocates the shoulder. After reduction and repeat imaging, you discuss surgical treatment with him. After a long discussion regarding risks, benefits, and expectations of surgery, he agrees to undergo an arthroscopic Bankart repair.

146. **List the indications for surgery for traumatic shoulder instability.**
    - Failed or unstable closed reduction
    - Soft-tissue interposition by the rotator cuff, capsule, or biceps tendon
    - Greater tuberosity fractures that remain displaced greater than 0.5 cm after reduction
    - Large glenoid rim fractures.

147. **Discuss the incidence of bone loss after a shoulder dislocation.**
    Bone loss is more commonly seen after recurrent episodes of dislocation or subluxation and can occur on the glenoid, humerus, or both. This type of defect in the humeral head, when large enough, can drop over the glenoid rim when the arm is externally rotated and lever the head out of its articulation with the glenoid. Authors have found that 7–14% of patients with recurrent instability have an engaging Hill–Sachs lesion. An antero-inferior glenoid rim fracture lessens the stabilizing effect of concavity-compression and may lead to instability. It is also thought to release the negative pressure formed in the glenohumeral joint and makes the labrum an ineffective chock-block anteriorly. Studies have shown glenoid bone loss of >25% or an inverted pear-shape of the glenoid in up to 73% of patients with recurrent instability.

148. **Should shoulder stabilization (labral repair or capsular plication) be performed via open or arthroscopic approaches?**
    This is a controversial question and likely varies depending on the specific pathology, patient characteristics, and surgeon's comfort level with each technique. Historically, open techniques have been associated with lower rates of recurrence when compared to arthroscopic procedures. However, more recent studies of arthroscopic treatment of shoulder instability have demonstrated similar rates of recurrence to open techniques. In addition, arthroscopic procedures do not violate the subscapularis and are associated with less loss of external rotation.

149. **What are the commonly performed shoulder stabilization procedures?**
    The most common types of anterior reconstruction of the shoulder are bone block-type procedures (Bristow, Latarjet), subscapularis-shortening procedures (Putti–Platt, Magnuson–Stack), and capsular procedures. The Bankart repair and the various modifications to this surgery involve reattachment of the detached antero-inferior labrum to the glenoid, indirectly repairing the inferior glenohumeral ligament complex. When a shoulder develops chronic instability, the capsular ligaments may become incompetent due to interstitial damage. This secondary capsular laxity requires the ligament tension also be addressed with a capsulorrhaphy or capsular shift, in addition to the repair of the injured labrum. This can be achieved with a medially, inferiorly, or laterally based shift of the capsule. The capsular procedures, such as the Bankart repair, are directed toward restoring normal anatomy with direct repair of the capsulolabral structures. These procedures have been reported to have a high success rate combined with a low complication rate and are the most commonly used today.

    The subscapularis-shortening procedures work by limiting the shoulder's range of motion so that end-range laxity cannot be challenged. The concern with these procedures, as well as the bone-block procedures, is that a non-anatomic reconstruction can lead to altered glenohumeral joint mechanics, increased joint reactive forces, and degenerative joint disease.

150. **What are bone-block procedures (Bristow or Latarjet)?**

These procedures are often performed when there is bone loss from the anterior of the glenoid (as a result of a bony Bankart lesion or repeated dislocations). The procedure involves transfer of the coracoid with its attached muscles to the deficient area over the anterior rim of the glenoid. This replaces the missing bone and the transferred muscle also acts as an additional muscular sling preventing further dislocations. More specifically, the procedure is thought to be beneficial for three main reasons: (1) the bone block increases or restores the glenoid contact surface area; (2) the conjoint tendon stabilizes the joint when the arm is abducted and externally rotated, by reinforcing the inferior subscapularis and antero-inferior capsule; (3) repair of the capsule decreases the effective joint space. This is a non-anatomic reconstruction and is also associated with a possible risk of degenerative joint disease.

151. **What is remplissage?**

Remplissage is French for "to fill", and involves filling a Hill–Sachs defect with the infraspinatus tendon and posterior capsule. The remplissage technique has been reported to be effective in reducing the incidence of recurrent anterior shoulder instability, when used along with arthroscopic Bankart repair. This technique can be performed arthroscopically and is used when the Hill–Sachs lesion is very large and "engaging" the anterior glenoid with little overhead movement. This technique makes the Hill–Sachs defect extra-articular, thereby eliminating engagement of the defect with the anterior glenoid rim. Whether remplissage results in a clinically significant loss of motion is a topic of controversy.

152. **What is thermal capsular shrinkage?**

The procedure uses heat to shrink and tighten the shoulder capsule. Early short-term results with thermal capsulorrhaphy were encouraging, and the procedure rapidly gained in popularity. However, more recent results with patients over a longer follow-up period have shown a much higher failure rate than was first seen. Also, more complications, including axillary nerve injury and chondrolysis have been reported, and so, this procedure is not considered as a viable treatment option for instability.

153. **What is the most common mechanism for a posterior shoulder dislocation?**

Posterior dislocations can be caused by force applied to the arm when the shoulder is flexed, adducted, and internally rotated. The force is usually directed posteriorly along the axis of the arm. This position is often seen when patients fall from a height or grab the dashboard in a motor vehicle accident. Posterior dislocations are often also associated with seizures, electrocutions, and lightning strikes. Competitive athletes are among the most common patients owing to overuse or a single traumatic episode resulting in posterior subluxation or dislocation (Fig. 10.24).

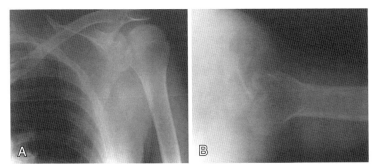

Figure 10.24. Posterior dislocation of shoulder. (A) Anteroposterior radiograph shows only subtle changes. (B) Axillary lateral radiograph shows posterior dislocation of humeral head with posterior rim of glenoid caught in humeral head defect. (*From Canale ST, Beaty JH [eds], Campbell's Operative Orthopaedics, 11th ed. Copyright © 2008, Mosby Elsevier Inc.*)

154. **What are the anatomic constraints to posterior instability?**

Static stabilization is provided by the articular cartilage surfaces, glenoid labrum, capsular ligaments, and intra-articular pressure. Glenohumeral joint stability is markedly reduced under tangential forces when the glenoid rim is partially resected. Glenoid version and humeral retroversion help contribute to static stability. The most important structure responsible for preventing posterior translation is the posterior capsule, between the intra-articular portion of the biceps tendon and the posterior band of the inferior glenohumeral ligament complex. The posterior capsule, posterior band of the inferior glenohumeral ligament, and posterior labrum provide the greatest support posteriorly. An isolated lesion in any one of these posterior structures often results in unidirectional posterior instability. Posterior translation is resisted dynamically, mostly by the subscapularis. Contraction of the rotator cuff across the joint increases joint stability through the concavity compression effect on the humeral head within the glenoid socket (Fig. 10.25).

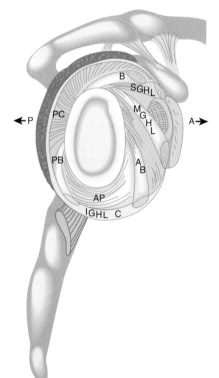

Figure 10.25. Schematic drawing of the shoulder capsule showing the glenohumeral ligaments, highlighting the inferior glenohumeral ligament. A, anterior; AB, anterior band; AP, axillary pouch; B, biceps tendon; IGHL C, IGHL complex; P, posterior; PB, posterior band; and PC, posterior capsule. (*From O'Brien SJ, Neves MC, Arnoczky SP, et al.: The anatomy and histology of the inferior glenohumeral ligament complex of the shoulder. Am J Sports Med 18[5]:449–456, 1990.*)

155. **What athletes are most at risk for posterior instability?**

Overhead throwers – volleyball, football, and tennis players; swimmers; and weight lifters – are among the athletes at highest risk for posterior instability. Linemen and defensive backs in football seem to also be at risk.

156. **What three physical examination maneuvers are typically used to evaluate posterior instability?**

Posterior drawer test: The examiner stabilizes the shoulder with one hand and holds the humeral head with the other hand. The examiner presses the humeral head medially into the center of the glenoid to evaluate the neutral position of the joint. Posterior stress is then applied and the degree of passive translation determined.

Kim test for postero-inferior instability: The arm is abducted to 90° while the patient is sitting. The examiner then passively elevates the arm an additional 45° while applying a downward and posterior force to the upper arm, with an axial load to the elbow. Posterior subluxation with pain indicates a positive test result.

Jerk test: The examiner grasps the scapular spine and the clavicle with one hand while holding the elbow with the other. With the arm flexed 90° and internally rotated with the elbow flexed 90°, the shoulder girdle is pressed anteriorly with one hand and the elbow pushed posteriorly with the other, causing posterior subluxation of the humeral head. The arm is then abducted as it is pushed posteriorly. If the patient experiences a sudden painful jerk as the humeral head relocates, this is considered a positive test result.

157. What physical findings are typical of an unreduced posterior dislocation?
The arm is usually positioned at the side with an inability to flex or externally rotate the shoulder. The anterior shoulder is flattened and the coracoid process may be prominent. The patient may be noted to have a posterior fullness of the shoulder as the head sits trapped behind the glenoid. This type of dislocation is often missed, usually because of inadequate physical and radiographic exams.

158. What is the treatment for posterior instability?
The treatment for symptomatic recurrent posterior instability is often non-operative. This includes not only a shoulder-strengthening routine, but also avoidance of provocative activities. The exercise protocol focuses on strengthening the rotator cuff and the scapular stabilizers through resisted external rotation exercises. Conservative treatment is less successful for instability that occurred after a single injury to the shoulder. If after prolonged, dedicated physical therapy the patient continues to have symptoms, surgery should be considered. Surgical options include arthroscopic and open soft tissue and osseous procedures. Common soft-tissue procedures include posterior labral repair and/or tightening of the posterior capsule (open posterior-inferior capsular shift or arthroscopic capsular plication). Posterior capsule redundancy is the most common pathologic lesion. The osseous procedures include the posterior bone block, posterior opening wedge osteotomy of the glenoid neck, posterior glenoid osteochondral allografting, or the McLaughlin procedure.

159. What is the McLaughlin procedure?
This procedure involves the transfer of the subscapularis tendon from the lesser tuberosity to the reverse Hill–Sachs defect. A modification involves transfer of the lesser tuberosity along with subscapularis. This procedure is conceptually similar to the remplissage procedure and functions to make the reverse Hill–Sachs lesion extra-articular (Fig. 10.26).

INJURIES OF THE THROWING ATHLETE
CASE 10-11

A 25-year-old minor league pitcher presents with a complaint of 2 weeks of shoulder pain on his dominant side. He notes that his velocity has decreased approximately 5–10 miles per hour and he has a feeling of a "dead arm." He has taken antiinflammatory medication and has tried to pitch through the pain, but has pitched poorly as a result.

160. Why is the shoulder so often injured in the throwing athlete?
The glenohumeral joint has more range of motion than any other joint in the human body. The forces generated in the throwing shoulder are much greater than the forces generated in the shoulder musculature alone, and, therefore, cause significant stresses around this joint, making it susceptible to acute and chronic inflammatory conditions.

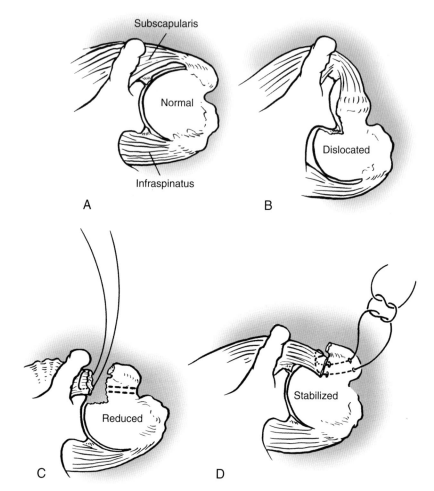

Figure 10.26. McLaughlin technique for posterior dislocation of shoulder. (A) Cross section of left shoulder viewed from above. (B) Deformity in posterior dislocation with engagement of posterior glenoid rim in defect of anterior aspect of humeral head. (C) Dislocation has been reduced but instability remains; redislocation occurs with internal rotation, flexion, adduction. (D) Stabilization by medial transposition of subscapularis insertion into defect. (*Redrawn from McLaughlin HL: Posterior dislocation of the shoulder, J Bone Joint Surg 34A:584, 1952.*)

161. List the five phases of pitching.
1. Wind-up: ends when the ball leaves the non-throwing glove hand
2. Early cocking, period of shoulder abduction and external rotation that begins as the ball is released from the non-dominant hand and terminates with contact of the forward foot on the ground
3. Late cocking: continues until maximal external rotation at the shoulder is obtained
4. Acceleration: short propulsive phase that starts with internal rotation of the humerus and ends with ball release
5. Follow through: starts with ball release and ends when all motion is complete (Fig. 10.27).

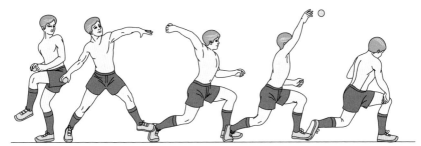

Figure 10.27. Schematic of the stages of overhead throwing. (*From DeLee JC, Drez D, Miller MD: Shoulder. In: DeLee JC (ed), DeLee and Drez's Orthopaedic Sports Medicine, 3rd ed. Saunders, 2010.*)

162. **What is the concept of kinetic chain? How does throwing form affect the incidence of shoulder injuries in the throwing athlete?**

     A kinetic chain is a coordinated sequencing of activation, mobilization, and stabilization of body segments to produce a dynamic activity. The majority of force required to propel the ball forward is developed in the legs and trunk and is funneled through the scapulohumeral complex. It is then transferred to the arm (baseball), racquet (tennis), or club head (golf). An effective athletic kinetic chain is characterized by three components: (1) optimized anatomy (strength, flexibility, and power generation); (2) well-developed, efficient task specific, motor patterns for muscle activation; and (3) sequential generation of forces appropriately distributed across motions that result in the desired athletic function.

     In general, shoulder injuries occur in one of two ways. Improper body mechanics during the wind-up and cocking phases place more dependence on the shoulder muscles to generate the required energy to propel the object, thus leading to fatigue of the shoulder muscles. After the thrown object is released, the retained energy in the throwing arm needs to be dissipated by reversing the initial process, i.e., using the large muscles in the lower limb and back to absorb this energy. An improper follow through results in retention of excessive energy in the soft tissues of the shoulder, subsequently causing tissue damage.

163. **What is the function of the scapular rotators?**

     Muscles included in the scapular rotator group are the trapezius, serratus anterior, and the rhomboids. Their main function in the throwing athlete is to aid in glenohumeral stability by placing the glenoid in an optimal position for the throwing event.

164. **What type of injuries may occur in the throwing athlete?**

     Acute overuse injuries, such as rotator cuff tendinitis and biceps tendinitis, are common. Chronic injuries include impingement syndrome, rotator cuff tears, glenoid labrum tears, and shoulder instability. Inflammation from repetitive stress may injure the acromioclavicular and the sternoclavicular joints. Uncommon causes of shoulder pain in the throwing athlete include quadrilateral space syndrome, suprascapular nerve entrapment, axillary artery occlusion, axillary vein thrombosis, posterior capsular laxity, and glenoid spurs.

165. **What are the common presenting symptoms of an athlete with shoulder pain?**

     The athlete generally reports anterior shoulder pain that becomes worse with increased throwing velocity in his or her throw, stating that he or she cannot obtain maximum velocity in workouts or in a game situation. Occasionally, posterior shoulder pain is present.

166. **How should the throwing athlete be evaluated for shoulder symptoms?**

     The physician should identify the primary symptom and attempt to correlate these symptoms with particular phases of the throwing motion. Observing the thrower's mechanics can be helpful. Any changes in the throwing routine, including changes in velocity or accuracy should be determined. Additionally, one should probe for signs of instability. With instability, the thrower may note a sensation of their "arm going dead" or the feeling of actual subluxation, which usually will correspond with the late cocking or early acceleration phase.

CASE 10-11   continued

On physical examination, the affected shoulder demonstrates 90° of external rotation compared to 70° on the contralateral side. There is a 25° decrease in internal rotation with the shoulder in abduction compared to the contralateral side. The patient has a positive O'Brien's test and a positive Mayo shear test (the examiner holds the standing patient's shoulder in maximal external rotation and moves the arm from 120° to 80° in order to elicit posterior shoulder pain). He has full rotator cuff strength.

167. **What are the important aspects of the physical examination?**
In terms of physical examination, one should begin by inspecting the shoulder girdle. While some throwers will have hypertrophy on the throwing side, evidence of atrophy in the infraspinatus fossa may indicate nerve compression as an etiology. Shoulder ROM should be assessed, specifically noting the often increased external rotation in the involved shoulder, with concomitant loss of internal rotation. Posterior capsular tightness, marked by a decrease in internal rotation is a significant finding in a thrower and can identify a shoulder that is at risk for injury. Additionally, the shoulder should be examined for impingement signs and provocative maneuvers to help delineate labral, biceps, acromioclavicular joint, or rotator cuff pathology.

168. **What is O'Brien's test?**
O'Brien's test is performed with the arm flexed to 90° with the elbow in extension and adducted 10° to 15° with maximal supination; it is then performed again in maximal pronation. Symptoms referred to the AC joint with either of these maneuvers or with the arm in supination indicate more of an AC joint disorder, whereas symptoms referred to the anterior glenohumeral joint that are increased in maximal pronation indicate more of a superior labral disorder (Fig. 10.28).

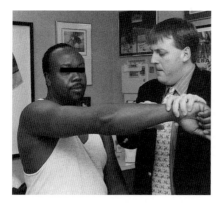

Figure 10.28. O'Brien's test with the arm in pronation. Pain should be decreased with the arm in maximal supination. (*From DeLee JC, Drez D, Miller MD: Elbow and Forearm. In: DeLee JC (ed), DeLee and Drez's Orthopaedic Sports Medicine, 3rd ed. Saunders, 2010.*)

169. **Are imaging studies helpful in the diagnosis of shoulder pain?**
Yes. Plain x-rays should be taken to rule out bony pathology such as fractures and osteoarthrosis. Special x-ray views such as the axillary view and the West Point view may demonstrate signs of instability (spurring or erosion of the anterior glenoid or a Hill–Sachs lesion).

170. Which imaging modality may be the most useful tool in diagnosing the cause of shoulder pain?

Recent studies indicate that MRI is superior to ultrasound and CT arthrography in evaluating shoulder pain due to rotator cuff tears, subacromial impingement, coracoacromial arch stenosis, and osteoarthritis of the glenohumeral or acromioclavicular joint. MR arthrography is best indicated for evaluation of the labrum.

171. How does anterior instability develop in the throwing athlete?

The pathoanatomy involved in shoulder instability stems from the abnormal shear stresses that occur around the center of glenohumeral rotation during throwing that contribute to microinstability and resultant pathologic anatomic findings. Anterior instability may develop after a high-energy trauma, but in the throwing athlete it more commonly starts as an overuse injury. Chronic overuse can stretch the static stabilizers of the shoulder, thus causing mild instability. Such instability leads to asynchrony in the firing of the scapular rotators and rotator cuff muscles, putting increased stress on the rotator cuff to contain the humerus in the center of the glenoid. As the rotator cuff muscles become weakened from the overload, the head of the humerus subluxes more anteriorly as the arm is abducted and externally rotated. Anterior subluxation can then cause secondary impingement of the rotator cuff on the acromion and the coracoacromial ligament. The current prevailing theories on shoulder instability, therefore, agree that an unstable shoulder in the throwing athlete is likely multifactorial and unlikely to be due to isolated injury of the anterior shoulder structures.

172. Describe the treatment for primary instability and secondary impingement.

Treatment of shoulder instability in the throwing athlete initially involves non-operative protocols focusing on dynamic rotator cuff strengthening and scapular stabilization exercises. After a brief period of rest, with cessation of overhead activity and throwing, and selective use of NSAIDs for pain relief. Stretching should be done carefully and only for muscle groups and capsular structures with obvious tightness. Strengthening exercises concentrating on the rotator cuff and scapular rotators should be performed. The athlete may be slowly returned to a throwing program consisting of long ball tossing with progression to more advanced throwing. Lack of improvement after an adequate period of rest and progressive throwing activities requires further investigation into the athlete's symptoms.

CASE 10-11 continued

The patient stops pitching and undertakes a rehabilitation program aimed at stretching the posterior capsule and strengthening the rotator cuff and scapular rotators. He subsequently begins a graduated throwing program. Unfortunately, he has reproduction of his symptoms after pitching in an exhibition game. He obtains an MR arthrogram that demonstrates a type II SLAP tear. He subsequently undergoes a shoulder arthroscopy and labral repair with debridement of an articular sided, partial-thickness rotator cuff tear.

173. Is surgery ever necessary?

Yes. If a throwing athlete with instability has faithfully completed 6–12 months of an aggressive supervised rehabilitation program and still cannot participate in throwing secondary to pain, a surgical procedure that addresses the anterior capsule and labrum should be performed. Athletes with documented rotator cuff tears, labrum lesions, or loose bodies should have such lesions repaired or excised. These decisions should be based on a complete picture of the patient's history, physical examination, imaging, failed non-operative treatment, and expectations for recovery.

174. What is a SLAP lesion?

A SLAP lesion is an entity originally described and classified by Snyder in 1990. SLAP (Superior Labrum Anterior and Posterior) involves the superior labrum, the biceps anchor, and a portion of the glenohumeral ligament attachment. Some authors have proposed that SLAP lesions are due to a "peel-back" phenomenon that occurs when the abducted, externally rotated arm of a thrower causes posterior rotation of the biceps anchor and peels the biceps from its attachment on the superior labrum. Despite this, SLAP tears can result from acute traumatic events or from repetitive microtrauma (Fig. 10.29).

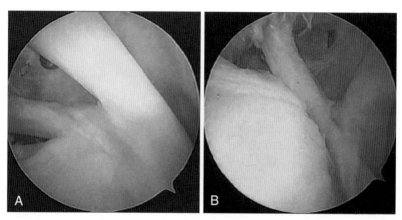

Figure 10.29. Dynamic peel-back test. (A and B) As arm is brought from resting position (A) into 90° abduction and 90° external rotation (B), biceps–superior labral complex displaces medially over the edge of the glenoid, confirming posterior SLAP lesion. *(From Burkhart SS, Morgan CD, Kibler WB: The disabled throwing shoulder: spectrum of pathology, part II: evaluation and treatment of SLAP lesions in throwers, Arthroscopy 19:531, 2003.)*

175. **Describe the four common types of SLAP lesions.**

SLAP lesions have been classified into four types by Snyder:

Type I: SLAP lesion involves degenerative fraying and tearing of the glenoid labrum at its superior attachment usually seen in degenerative or arthritic shoulders.

Type II: SLAP lesion, which is the most common, involves the biceps anchor. This anchor is unstable anteriorly and posterior from approximately the 10 o'clock to the 2 o'clock position. These lesions are usually treated by repair, whereas type I lesions are treated with debridement.

Type III: SLAP lesion involves a bucket-handle tear of the glenoid labrum. This is usually seen in a meniscoid type labrum. The biceps anchor is commonly stable and treatment usually is debridement of the bucket-handle fragments.

Type IV: SLAP lesion involves a bucket-handle tear of the labrum with a longitudinal tear extending into the biceps tendon. Treatment of this lesion is controversial and depends on the stability of the biceps anchor.

176. **How do these tears appear on MR arthrogram? (Fig. 10.30)**

177. **What is internal impingement? What are treatment options for internal impingement?**

Internal impingement is the process by which maximal shoulder abduction and internal rotation causes impingement of the rotator cuff between the greater tuberosity and postero-superior labrum. Symptoms may result from repetitive microtrauma and can lead to articular-sided rotator cuff pathology. A tight posterior capsule has been associated with internal impingement (Fig. 10.31).

Treatment of internal impingement has focused on rest, antiinflammatory drugs, normalizing range of motion, and stretching. Throwing programs to improve mechanics, core strengthening, and posterior capsular stretching should be instituted. When conservative treatment fails, operative treatment should focus on debridement of the partial-thickness rotator cuff tear and repair of the superior labrum if involved.

178. **What is GIRD? What are the treatment options?**

GIRD stands for Glenohumeral Internal Rotation Deficit and is a result of posterior capsular contracture. This posterior capsular contracture leads to obligate postero-superior translation of the humeral head. These patients often present with an increase in shoulder external rotation and limited shoulder internal rotation. It is believed that the changing

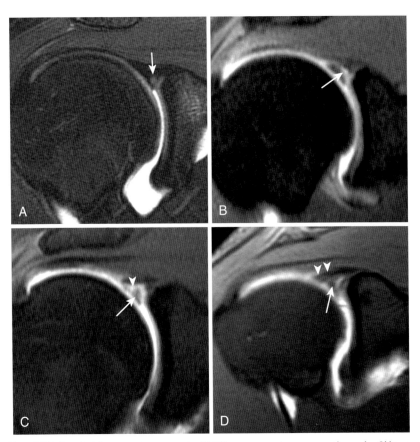

Figure 10.30. Superior labrum, anterior-to-posterior (SLAP) tears, magnetic resonance arthrography. Oblique coronal T1-weighted images reveal various types of SLAP lesions. (A) Type I SLAP tear. Abnormal signal is noted along the inferior margin of the superior labrum (arrow), indicating a degenerative pattern tear with no displaced or unstable fragment noted. (B) Type II SLAP tear. An abnormal collection of contrast material (arrow) extends into the substance of the superior labrum, indicating a partial avulsion. (C) Type III SLAP tear. A displaced bucket-handle fragment (arrow) is seen extending off the inferior aspect of the superior labrum. Contrast (arrowhead) completely surrounds the avulsed bucket-handle fragment. (D) Type IV SLAP tear. A bucket-handle fragment (arrow) is seen extending from the inferior aspect of the superior labrum, involving the biceps anchor (arrowhead). (*From DeLee JC, Drez D, Miller MD: Shoulder. In: DeLee JC (ed), DeLee and Drez's Orthopaedic Sports Medicine, 3rd ed. Saunders, 2010.*)

biomechanics of the shoulder (posterior capsular contracture, anterior capsular laxity, increased external rotation, postero-superior translation of the humeral head) that results from GIRD place a thrower at increased risk for SLAP tears and internal impingement. Throwers with internal rotation deficits of ≥25° compared with the non-throwing side and a total arc of motion of <180° are considered to have significant glenohumeral internal rotation deficit.

Physical therapy is the initial treatment with a regimen focusing on stretching the tight posterior capsule. Even once symptoms resolve, athletes should continue to perform stretching exercises to prevent recurrence. If non-operative treatment is unsuccessful, arthroscopic capsular release of the posterior inferior glenohumeral ligament may be a reasonable option in select patients (Fig. 10.32).

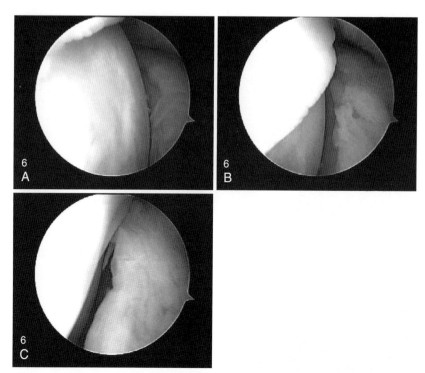

Figure 10.31. (A) Arthroscopic view of the glenohumeral joint from a posterior portal. The humeral head and cuff insertion is visualized along with the postero-superior aspect of the glenoid rim. (B) The arm is progressively brought into external rotation and abduction bringing the rotator cuff insertion closer to the glenoid rim and labrum. (C) Contact is seen between the rotator cuff insertion and the glenoid rim as the arm is brought further into abduction and external rotation. When the shoulder is subjected to repetitive, supraphysiologic stresses (as in throwers), this normal contact can develop into internal impingement. *(From DeLee JC, Drez D, Miller MD. Shoulder. In: DeLee JC (ed), DeLee and Drez's Orthopaedic Sports Medicine, 3rd ed. Saunders, 2010.)*

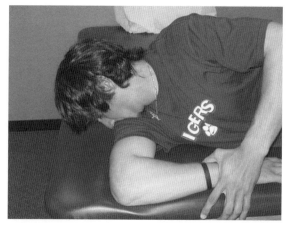

Figure 10.32. "Sleeper" stretch for stretching of the posterior capsule. *(From DeLee JC, Drez D, Miller MD. Shoulder. In: DeLee JC (ed), DeLee and Drez's Orthopaedic Sports Medicine, 3rd ed. Saunders, 2010.)*

ATHLETIC INJURIES OF THE ELBOW

CASE 10-12

A 22-year-old, right hand dominant, female volleyball player presents with complaint of right medial sided elbow pain that is exacerbated by spiking a volleyball. She notes that pain begins when she cocks her arm back and persists through her follow-through. These symptoms have been present for several months and she denies any specific trauma.

179. What are the static and dynamic restraints of the elbow?
   - Primary static constraints:
     - Bony = ulnohumeral articulation
     - Ligamentous = anterior bundle of the ulnar collateral ligament, lateral ulnar collateral ligament (UCL):
       - The UCL, specifically the anterior band, provides the most static stability at the elbow joint to oppose a valgus stress
   - Secondary static constraints: capsule, radiocapitellar articulation, common flexor and extensor tendon origins
   - Dynamic constraints: muscles that cross elbow joint (anconeus, triceps, brachialis) apply compressive forces (Fig. 10.33).

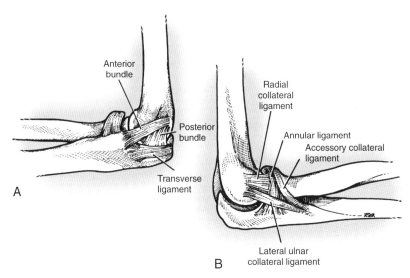

Figure 10.33. Collateral ligaments of the elbow. (A) Classic representation of medial collateral ligament complex consisting of anterior and posterior oblique bundle and transverse component. (B) Typical pattern of more variable radial collateral ligament complex consists of contribution from humerus to ulna, which Morrey termed lateral ulnar collateral ligament. (*Redrawn from Morrey BF, ed: The Elbow and Its Disorders, 2nd ed. Philadelphia, 2000, Saunders.*)

180. What is the mechanism of injury in the thrower's elbow?
   Those that partake in high-velocity overhead activity (throwers, volleyball players, javelin throwers, etc.) generate high levels of torque during the throwing or spiking motion. This positioning of the limb results in substantial valgus stress at the elbow. Injury is usually a result of repetitive microtrauma to the anterior band of the ulnar collateral ligament during the late cocking phase. Over time, the repetitive trauma can lead to stretch and attenuation of the ligament and resultant valgus instability. As the ulnar collateral ligament becomes attenuated, increased compressive forces can be transferred to the lateral (radial) side of the elbow (Fig. 10.34).

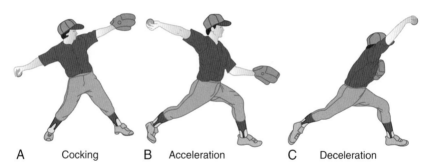

| A | Cocking | B | Acceleration | C | Deceleration |

Figure 10.34. Valgus compressive stresses of the elbow commonly occur during late cocking (A) and early acceleration (B) in the arm of the throwing athlete. (C) Deceleration of the arm. (*Modified from Miller MD, Cooper DE, Warner JJP: Review of Sports Medicine and Arthroscopy, p.123. Philadelphia, WB Saunders, 1995.*)

181. **What is the first step in diagnosing an elbow injury?**
    As always, evaluation should begin with a thorough history, including mechanism of injury, location of pain, activities that aggravate or relieve symptoms, and history of prior injuries or treatment.

182. **How should one perform the physical examination of the thrower with elbow pain?**
    Examination should begin with inspection for skin changes, swelling, shape, or carrying angle. Passive and active range of motion in flexion, extension, pronation, and supination should be evaluated and compared to the contralateral side. Strength should also be tested. Palpation of the anterior, posterior, medial, and lateral aspects of the elbow for tenderness, crepitus, or deformity can be important in localizing pathology. Finally, the neurovascular status of the limb should be determined with an examination of pulses and sensory/motor nerve function in the distal limb.

    It is important to remember that patients with ulnar-sided elbow pain often present with ulnar nerve symptoms. As was discussed with evaluation of the throwing shoulder, the concept of the kinetic chain is critical. Proper conditioning of the core musculature and lower extremities is integral to the transfer of energy from the lower extremity to the upper extremity during throwing. As a result, tightness of the muscles of the lower extremity, weakness of hip abductors and trunk stabilizers, and conditions affecting spinal alignment and mobility should be evaluated. Similarly, the shoulder should be carefully evaluated for evidence of scapular dyskinesia and GIRD. Any disturbances along the kinetic chain can manifest in elbow pathology.

183. **List the differential diagnosis for an athlete presenting with medial elbow pain.**
    - Medial epicondylitis/flexor-pronator strain (see Shoulder/Elbow chapter)
    - Ulnar collateral ligament sprain/rupture
    - Medial epicondyle fracture (see Pediatrics chapter)
    - Cubital tunnel syndrome
    - Little leaguer's elbow (see Pediatrics chapter).

CASE 10-12   continued

On examination, the patient has a 25° decrease in glenohumeral internal rotation compared to the contralateral side. At the elbow, she has tenderness at the sublime tubercle and ulnar-sided elbow pain with valgus stress and milking maneuver. Her examination is otherwise unremarkable. Plain radiographs of the elbow are obtained and noted to be normal. An MRI demonstrates evidence of a high-grade partial tear of the ulnar collateral ligament at the sublime tubercle. You initiate treatment with a temporary cessation of volleyball activities, antiinflammatory medication, and a physical therapy program.

184. What physical examination findings can be seen in a patient with ulnar
collateral ligament injury?
The pain is often localized to the course of the ligament from the medial epicondyle to
the sublime tubercle. Valgus instability is not always evident on physical examination
because it is a dynamic phenomenon involving the flexor digitorum superficialis and flexor
carpi ulnaris origin. Test for valgus stability should be performed with the patient supine
and the arm abducted and externally rotated in order to limit scapular motion. The elbow
is flexed 20°, and a valgus stress is applied. Pain in the region of the UCL or increased
laxity with a soft end point may be indicative of UCL disorder. Testing of the posterior
band of the anterior bundle can be accomplished by the milking maneuver, which is
performed by pulling on the patient's thumb with the patient's forearm supinated, shoulder
extended, and elbow flexed beyond 90°. This maneuver generates a valgus stress on the
flexed elbow; a subjective feeling of apprehension and instability, in addition to localized
medial-side elbow pain (Fig. 10.35).

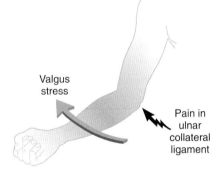

Figure 10.35. Medial joint-line pain elicited by
applying a valgus stress to the elbow identifies injury
to the ulnar collateral ligament. (*From Morrey BF:
The Elbow and Its Disorders. Philadelphia, WB
Saunders, 1985.*)

185. What imaging studies should be obtained to evaluate the throwing elbow?
Plain films should generally be the first imaging study ordered. Radiographs may show
changes consistent with chronic instability (calcification or ossification of the ligament,
heterotopic bone, etc.). Stress (valgus) radiographs that demonstrate greater than 3 mm of
medial joint opening can be used to confirm instability, MRI is useful in evaluating
ligamentous avulsions, partial ligamentous injuries, mid-substance tears, and the status of
the surrounding soft tissues (Fig. 10.36).

186. What are non-operative treatment strategies for a patient with ulnar-sided
ligament injury?
A brief period of rest (2–4 weeks), antiinflammatory medication, and physical therapy can
be effective treatment options. Physical therapy should focus on stretching and
strengthening of the flexor-pronator mass because these muscles serve as secondary
stabilizers of the elbow. Additionally, shoulder-related pathology, such as GIRD, and other
sites of weakness or contracture in the kinetic chain should be addressed. Sports-specific
training should be reintroduced in a graduated, pain-free manner.

187. When is surgical intervention recommended? What does operative treatment
entail?
Surgical intervention is indicated for competitive athletes with acute full-thickness
ruptures of the UCL or chronic symptoms secondary to instability that have not
significantly improved after at least 3 to 6 months of non-operative management.
Operative treatment consists of either repair or reconstruction of the
UCL. Reconstruction involves the use of allograft or autograft tendon to replace the
attenuated or torn UCL. Ligament reconstruction is more commonly performed given the

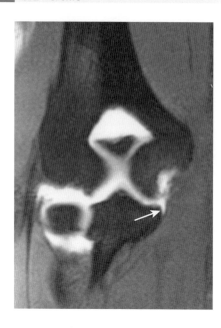

Figure 10.36. Partial ulnar collateral ligament tear at MRI arthrography of elbow. Coronal fat-suppressed, T1-weighted image reveals contrast tracking deep to ulnar attachment of ulnar collateral ligament (arrow). *(From Canale ST, Beaty JH [eds], Campbell's Operative Orthopaedics, 11th ed. Copyright © 2008, Mosby Elsevier Inc.)*

chronic nature of these injuries. Ulnar nerve transposition may accompany the procedure depending on the patient's preoperative symptoms. Studies demonstrate that nearly 75–80% of athletes return to sports at the same level or better at 1 year after reconstruction.

188. **What other injuries are associated with UCL instability?**
As the UCL becomes increasingly stretched, posteromedial osseous constraint is thought to play a greater role in elbow stability during the throwing motion and can lead to valgus extension overload. The typical spectrum of disease in the thrower's elbow also includes ulnar neuritis and ulnar nerve subluxation, radiocapitellar joint injury, and even stress fracture of the olecranon (Fig. 10.37).

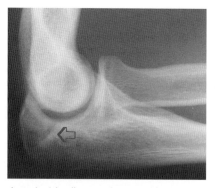

Figure 10.37. Plain lateral radiograph of the elbow in a throwing athlete with posterior elbow pain. The *arrow* indicates lucency through the proximal olecranon consistent with a stress fracture. Typically, these types of injury cause pain with rapid extension of the elbow, as seen in throwers. Also, pain on palpation of the stress fracture site is typically present. *(From DeLee JC, Drez D, Miller MD: Elbow and Forearm. In: DeLee JC (ed), DeLee and Drez's Orthopaedic Sports Medicine, 3rd ed. Saunders, 2010.)*

189. **What medial elbow problem may present with vague aching in the forearm and tingling in the fourth and fifth fingers?**

Such symptoms suggest cubital tunnel syndrome, an entrapment neuropathy of the ulnar nerve at or about the elbow. It may be the result of a cubitus valgus deformity, but in athletes it is more commonly due to trauma (contusion or subluxation of the ulnar nerve), muscle hypertrophy (especially of the flexor carpi ulnaris from excessive curls), or inflammation from adjacent tissue injury (UCL sprain).

190. **List the findings suggestive of cubital tunnel syndrome.**
   - Positive Tinel's sign at the cubital tunnel
   - Decreased sensation in the ulnar forearm and hand
   - Increased pain and numbness with forced elbow flexion
   - Weakness or atrophy of the first dorsal interosseous muscle (resisted index finger abduction)
   - Weakness in grip strength.

191. **What other conditions must be considered? Name a test for each.**
   - Cervical radiculopathy – foraminal compression (Spurling's sign)
   - Thoracic outlet syndrome (Adson's sign)
   - Ulnar nerve compression at the wrist (Tinel's sign at Guyon's canal).

192. **What diagnostic test may confirm cubital tunnel syndrome?**

Electromyography (EMG) and nerve conduction velocity (NCV) studies may demonstrate slowing of conduction velocity across the elbow.

193. **Is surgical decompression necessary?**

Surgical decompression may be necessary with a progressive neurologic deficit or with failure of non-surgical management. Initial treatment should consist of rest, NSAIDs, protective padding, and avoidance of extreme flexion. If symptoms warrant, acute episodes may be treated with splinting at 30–45° of flexion for a few days or at night to relieve compression.

194. **List the differential diagnosis for an athlete presenting with posterior elbow pain.**
   - Triceps tendinitis
   - Triceps rupture (or olecranon fracture) (see Shoulder/Elbow chapter)
   - Olecranon impingement syndrome
   - Olecranon bursitis.

195. **What are the common findings in athletes with triceps tendinitis?**
   - Posterior elbow pain
   - Tenderness at the triceps insertion or in the distal part of the tendon
   - Resisted elbow extension causes increased pain.

196. **Should radiographs be obtained?**

Yes. Degenerative calcifications or traction spurs may be present. Of greater importance, stress fracture of the olecranon should be excluded.

197. **Define valgus extension overload syndrome of the elbow.**

Also called olecranon impingement syndrome, posteromedial impingement syndrome, or boxer's elbow, this condition is an overuse syndrome caused by repetitive valgus extension overload of the elbow. It is common in the throwing motions, which cause the olecranon process to impinge against the medial wall of the olecranon fossa. Athletes commonly complain of pain during the extension phase of throwing and catching or locking in or near extension.

198. **How do you examine an elbow for valgus extension overload?**

Typical findings include posterior tenderness or swelling, and lack of full extension. The test for valgus extension overload is done by repeatedly forcing the elbow into hyperextension while a valgus force is applied. This test attempts to re-create the stress across the elbow with throwing. Pain in the posteromedial aspect of the elbow is considered a positive test and may indicate bony or soft tissue impingement in the area of the pain.

199. **What findings may be seen on radiographs?**
Yes. Anteroposterior, lateral, and axial radiographs may reveal spurring or fracture of the olecranon tip, loose bodies, or hypertrophy of the olecranon.

200. **What is the leading differential diagnosis for traumatic or chronic olecranon bursitis? How should it be ruled out?**
Septic olecranon bursitis is usually much more painful and more impressive on examination but may be confused with the non-septic conditions in the early stages. It can be ruled out by aspirating the bursa through a sterile field and checking a Gram stain and culture for bacteria.

201. **How does treatment of the two types of olecranon bursitis differ?**
Chronic bursitis, caused by repetitive trauma or irritation to the bursa, should be treated with NSAIDs and protective padding. Both chronic and acute traumatic bursitis can be decompressed by aspiration, compression, and splinting for a short period. Septic olecranon bursitis should be treated by surgical incision, drainage, and antibiotics.

202. **List the differential diagnosis for an athlete presenting with lateral elbow pain.**
- Lateral epicondylitis (see Shoulder/Elbow chapter)
- Radial head fracture (see Trauma chapter)
- Radiocapitellar chondromalacia/osteochondritis dissecans
- Posterior interosseous nerve compression syndrome
- Lateral plica
- Posterolateral instability (see Shoulder/Elbow chapter).

203. **A pitcher being treated for a UCL sprain also complains of lateral elbow pain. What other elbow problem should you suspect? Why?**
Tension overloading of the medial structures during throwing and in racquet sports is frequently accompanied by compression overloading of the radiocapitellar joint laterally. Repeated stresses may cause diffuse articular damage (chondromalacia) or more specific lesions, such as osteochondritis dissecans, osteochondral fractures, or loose bodies.

204. **What are the expected findings?**
Affected athletes frequently cannot achieve extension. Palpation reveals tenderness at the radiocapitellar joint and crepitus with pronation and supination. Radiographs should be evaluated for decreased radiocapitellar joint space, articular spurring, defects or irregularities in the radial head or the capitellum, and loose bodies. Such lesions may require computed tomography, MRI, or arthroscopy for complete evaluation.

205. **What diagnosis should be considered in an athlete complaining of lateral pain and clicking, snapping, or locking as the arm is extended and the forearm supinated?**
Both posterolateral instability and plica syndrome may cause these symptoms. Rotatory stress testing may confirm subtle posterolateral laxity. A palpable snapping band in the lateral gutter may indicate a fibrotic plica band.

206. **List the differential diagnosis for an athlete presenting with anterior elbow pain.**
- Biceps tendinitis
- Anterior capsular strain or tear
- Biceps rupture (see Shoulder/Elbow chapter)
- Median nerve compression syndrome.

207. **What specific elbow motion should be tested when biceps tendinitis or rupture is suspected?**
The biceps is an elbow flexor and forearm supinator. Both conditions can be expected to cause pain and weakness with resisted elbow flexion and supination.

208. **How is anterior capsule strain differentiated from biceps injury?**
Anterior capsule strain is usually related to hyperextension as opposed to flexion–supination. Ecchymosis and deep tenderness to palpation may be present, but tenderness is usually more diffuse rather than isolated around the biceps tendon.

209. **What more significant injury must be ruled out when anterior capsular strain is suspected?**
With a hyperextension mechanism the possibility of a spontaneously reduced elbow dislocation should be considered.

210. **Should radiographs be obtained in hyperextended elbow injuries?**
Yes. Fracture and/or dislocation should be ruled out. With an anterior strain, bony avulsion flecks from the capsular margins may be seen. Later radiographs may reveal heterotopic calcification in the anterior tissues.

211. **How long should the injury be splinted or immobilized? Why?**
Immobilization should be minimal – perhaps 1 day, if needed for comfort. Prolonged splinting greatly increases the likelihood of developing a flexion contracture at the elbow. Early active range-of-motion exercises are essential to regain full motion.

212. **Give another name for median nerve compression syndrome at the elbow.**
Pronator syndrome.

213. **How do the symptoms of pronator syndrome differ from those of other causes of anterior elbow pain?**
Pain is usually just distal to the elbow in the proximal forearm, may be associated with numbness in the volar forearm or median distribution in the hand, and is often aggravated by resisted pronation activities.

214. **What four structures may be responsible for pronator syndrome?**
- Ligament of Struthers/supracondylar process
- Lacertus fibrosus
- Pronator teres
- Flexor digitorum superficialis (FDS) arcade.

215. **What provocative tests may help to identify which structure is responsible?**
The following maneuvers should reproduce pain or numbness:
- Supracondylar process – elbow flexion of 120–135°
- Lacertus fibrosus – resisted forearm supination
- Pronator teres – resisted forearm pronation
- FDS arcade – resisted long finger flexion.

216. **How is pronator syndrome treated?**
Most cases respond to modification of activities and physical therapy modalities for stretching and strengthening. Surgical decompression may be required for recalcitrant cases.

MISCELLANEOUS CONDITIONS IN THE ATHLETE

CERVICAL SPINE/HEAD TRAUMA

CASE 10-13

A high school football player spear tackles another player who fails to get up after the tackle. He is not responsive to verbal commands and is not moving any extremities. He has audible breath sounds and a pulse.

217. **What is the initial management of the non-responsive athlete?**
As with any emergency scenario, the ABCs of resuscitation should be first:
- Airway
- Breathing
- Circulation.

218. **How should the patient in the above vignette be approached?**
Unlike a standard trauma in a hospital setting, the patient is not completely stripped of protective wear. The facemask is removed to secure an airway when necessary. The head should be stabilized and the helmet/shoulder pads should stay on to prevent further damage to the cervical spine. A backboard should be applied to

stabilize the cervical spine and the patient should be transported to the nearest Emergency Room.

219. **What is spear tackler's spine?**
Typically found in contact sports such as rugby and football, this often occurs in the setting of poor tackling form when playing. It is associated with narrowing of the cervical canal, and a decrease in cervical lordosis.

220. **What are the contraindications to allowing return to contact sports?**
Congenital abnormalities including odontoid hypoplasia or odontoid agenesis, spear tackler's spine, instability on flexion/extension films, and severe stenosis should preclude an athlete from contact sports.

221. **In what sports are lumbar spine injuries most prevalent?**
Sports which force the athlete's back into hyperextension are associated with spondylolysis and spondylolisthesis, such as football and gymnastics.

222. **What is post-concussive syndrome?**
Headache, confusion, and difficulty concentrating after blunt head trauma.

223. **When should a head CT be obtained after blunt head injury?**
For persistent concussive symptoms that do not resolve within 5 minutes of the initial injury.

224. **What are the NCAA rules for allowing return to play after blunt head injury?**
A player is not to return to play on the day of sustaining a concussion, and should abstain from playing for 1 week to 1 month following the injury.
After a second concussion, the player should be removed from play for the season.

CARDIOVASCULAR/MEDICAL

CASE 10-14

A 20-year-old college track athlete suddenly collapses at practice. He is unresponsive and on initial survey, has no pulse. Immediate cardiopulmonary resuscitation is initiated. An emergency response is called as resuscitative efforts are continued. Upon calling his family, his mother reports he had an uncle who had died at a young age from sudden cardiac arrest while playing soccer.

---

225. **What is the most common cause of cardiac death in athletes under the age of 35?**
Hypertrophic cardiomyopathy.

226. **What is the most common cause of cardiac death in athletes over the age of 35?**
Coronary artery disease.

227. **What is the prevalence of hypertrophic cardiomyopathy?**
It occurs in 1 out of every 500 adults. It has an autosomal dominant inheritance pattern.

228. **What screening methods can detect this condition?**
EKG has an approximately 50% sensitivity in detecting this condition.

229. **What are other causes of cardiac death in athletes?**
Commotio cordis: A contusion of the heart resulting from a direct blow to the chest – best treated with immediate defibrillation
Arrhythmogenic right ventricular cardiomyopathy
Congenital coronary artery anomalies.

230. **What sports should be avoided for 6 weeks after diagnosis with infectious mononucleosis? Why?**
Contact sports are contraindicated after this diagnosis given the risk of splenic rupture with contact injury.

BIBLIOGRAPHY

1. Armfield DR, Kim DH-M, Towers JD, et al. Sports-related muscle injury in the lower extremity. Clin Sports Med 2006;25:803–42.
2. Asif IM, Drezner JA. Sudden cardiac death and preparticipation screening: the debate continues-in support of electrocardiogram-inclusive preparticipation screening. Prog Cardiovasc Dis 2012;54: 445–50.
3. Boden BP, Jarvis CG. Spinal injuries in sports. Neurol Clin 2008;26:63–78, viii.
4. Boileau P, O'Shea K, Vargas P, et al. Anatomical and functional results after arthroscopic Hill–Sachs remplissage. J Bone Joint Surg Am 2012;94:618–26.
5. Bowman KF Jr, Sekiya JK. Anatomy and biomechanics of the posterior cruciate ligament, medial and lateral sides of the knee. Sports Med Arthrosc 2010;18:222–9.
6. Braun P, Jensen S. Hip pain – a focus on the sporting population. Aust Fam Physician 2007;36:406–8, 410–3.
7. Browner BD, Green NE. Skeletal Trauma. Edinburgh: Saunders; 2008.
8. Burkhart SS, Morgan CD. The peel-back mechanism: its role in producing and extending posterior type II SLAP lesions and its effect on SLAP repair rehabilitation. Arthroscopy 1998;14:637–40.
9. Burkhart SS, De Beer JF. Traumatic glenohumeral bone defects and their relationship to failure of arthroscopic Bankart repairs: significance of the inverted-pear glenoid and the humeral engaging Hill–Sachs lesion. Arthroscopy 2000;16:677–94.
10. Cain EL Jr, Andrews JR, Dugas JR, et al. Outcome of ulnar collateral ligament reconstruction of the elbow in 1281 athletes: Results in 743 athletes with minimum 2-year follow-up. Am J Sports Med 2010;38:2426–34.
11. Campbell WC, Canale ST, Beaty JH, et al. Campbell's operative orthopaedics. Philadelphia: Mosby Elsevier; 2008.
12. Caudill P, Nyland J, Smith C, et al. Sports hernias: a systematic literature review. Br J Sports Med 2008;42:954–64.
13. Chen FS, Rokito AS, Jobe FW. Medial elbow problems in the overhead-throwing athlete. J Am Acad Orthop Surg 2001;9:99–113.
14. Dai B, Herman D, Liu H, et al. Prevention of ACL injury, part II: effects of ACL injury prevention programs on neuromuscular risk factors and injury rate. Res Sports Med 2012;20:198–222.
15. DeLee J, Drez D, Miller MD. DeLee & Drez's Orthopaedic Sports Medicine: Principles and Practice. Philadelphia: Saunders/Elsevier; 2010.
16. Detterline AJ, Goldstein JL, Rue J-PH, et al. Evaluation and treatment of osteochondritis dissecans lesions of the knee. J Knee Surg 2008;21:106–15.
17. Dheerendra SK, Khan WS, Singhal R, et al. Anterior cruciate ligament graft choices: a review of current concepts. Open Orthop J 2012;6:281–6.
18. Diesen DL, Pappas TN. Sports hernias. Adv Surg 2007;41:177–87.
19. Dumont GD, Hogue GD, Padalecki JR, et al. Meniscal and chondral injuries associated with pediatric anterior cruciate ligament tears: relationship of treatment time and patient-specific factors. Am J Sports Med 2012;40:2128–33.
20. Farber AJ, Wilkens JH. Sports hernia: diagnosis and therapeutic approach. J Am Acad Orthop Surg 2007;15:507–14.
21. Flatow EL, Warner JI. Instability of the shoulder: complex problems and failed repairs: Part I. Relevant biomechanics, multidirectional instability, and severe glenoid loss. Instr Course Lect 1998;47:97–112.
22. Gerber C, Nyffeler RW. Classification of glenohumeral joint instability. Clin Orthop Relat Res 2002;400:65–76.
23. Gill TJ, Micheli LJ, Gebhard F, et al. Bankart repair for anterior instability of the shoulder. Long-term outcome. J Bone Joint Surg Am 1997;79:850–7.
24. Giuliani JR, Burns TC, Svoboda SJ, et al. Treatment of meniscal injuries in young athletes. J Knee Surg 2011;24:93–100.
25. Glousman R, Jobe F, Tibone J, et al. Dynamic electromyographic analysis of the throwing shoulder with glenohumeral instability. J Bone Joint Surg Am 1988;70:220–6.
26. Gnannt R, Chhabra A, Theodoropoulos JS, et al. MR imaging of the postoperative knee. J Magn Reson Imaging 2011;34:1007–21.
27. Goldman AB, Pavlov H, Rubenstein D. The Segond fracture of the proximal tibia: a small avulsion that reflects major ligamentous damage. AJR Am J Roentgenol 1988;151:1163–7.
28. Gomoll AH, Farr J, Gillogly SD, et al. Surgical management of articular cartilage defects of the knee. J Bone Joint Surg Am 2010;92:2470–90.
29. Gu Y, Wang Y. Treatment of meniscal injury: a current concept review. Chin J Traumatol 2010;13:370–6.
30. Gwathmey FW Jr, Golish SR, Diduch DR. Complications in brief: meniscus repair. Clin Orthop Relat Res 2012;470:2059–66.
31. Harris-Hayes M, Royer NK. Relationship of acetabular dysplasia and femoroacetabular impingement to hip osteoarthritis: a focused review. PM R 2011;3:1055–67.e1.

32. Hart ES, Kalra KP, Grottkau BE, et al. Discoid lateral meniscus in children. Orthop Nurs 2008;27:174–9, quiz 180–1.
33. Hensler D, Van Eck CF, Fu FH, et al. Anatomic anterior cruciate ligament reconstruction utilizing the double-bundle technique. J Orthop Sports Phys Ther 2012;42:184–95.
34. Hovelius L, Eriksson K, Fredin H, et al. Recurrences after initial dislocation of the shoulder: Results of a prospective study of treatment. J Bone Joint Surg Am 1983;65:343–9.
35. Hovelius L, Olofsson A, Sandström B, et al. Nonoperative treatment of primary anterior shoulder dislocation in patients forty years of age and younger: a prospective twenty-five-year follow-up. J Bone Joint Surg Am 2008;90:945–52.
36. Hovelius L, Saeboe M. Neer Award 2008: Arthropathy after primary anterior shoulder dislocation – 223 shoulders prospectively followed up for twenty-five years. J Shoulder Elbow Surg 2009;18:339–47.
37. Howells NR, Brunton LR, Robinson J, et al. Acute knee dislocation: an evidence based approach to the management of the multiligament injured knee. Injury 2011;42:1198–204.
38. Huang R, Diaz C, Parvizi J. Acetabular labral tears: focused review of anatomy, diagnosis, and current management. Phys Sportsmed 2012;40:87–93.
39. Hurley JA, Anderson TE. Shoulder arthroscopy: its role in evaluating shoulder disorders in the athlete. Am J Sports Med 1990;18:480–3.
40. Imam S, Khanduja V. Current concepts in the diagnosis and management of femoroacetabular impingement. Int Orthop 2011;35:1427–35.
41. Itoi E, Hatakeyama Y, Sato T, et al. Immobilization in external rotation after shoulder dislocation reduces the risk of recurrence. A randomized controlled trial. J Bone Joint Surg Am 2007;89:2124–31.
42. Itoi E, Sashi R, Minagawa H, et al. Position of immobilization after dislocation of the glenohumeral joint. A study with use of magnetic resonance imaging. J Bone Joint Surg Am 2001;83-A:661–7.
43. Kibler WB, Sciascia A, Wilkes T. Scapular dyskinesis and its relation to shoulder injury. J Am Acad Orthop Surg 2012;20:364–72.
44. Jancosko JJ, Kazanjian JE. Shoulder injuries in the throwing athlete. Phys Sportsmed 2012;40:84–90.
45. Jansson KS, Costello KE, O'Brien L, et al. A historical perspective of PCL bracing. Knee Surg Sports Traumatol Arthrosc 2013;21:1064–70.
46. Jarit GJ, Bosco JA 3rd. Meniscal repair and reconstruction. Bull NYU Hosp Jt Dis 2010;68:84–90.
47. Jerosch J, Castro WH. Shoulder instability in Ehlers–Danlos syndrome. An indication for surgical treatment? Acta Orthop Belg 1990;56:451–3.
48. Karachalios T, Hantes M, Zibis AH, et al. Diagnostic accuracy of a new clinical test (the Thessaly test) for early detection of meniscal tears. J Bone Joint Surg Am 2005;87:955–62.
49. Kalke RJ, Di Primio GA, Schweitzer ME. MR and CT arthrography of the knee. Semin Musculoskelet Radiol 2012;16:57–68.
50. Keener JD, Brophy RH. Superior labral tears of the shoulder: pathogenesis, evaluation, and treatment. J Am Acad Orthop Surg 2009;17:627–37.
51. Kim HM, Stannard JP. How I manage the multiple-ligament injured (dislocated) knee. Oper Tech Sports Med 2011;19:42–50.
52. Kodali P, Islam A, Andrish J. Anterior knee pain in the young athlete: diagnosis and treatment. Sports Med Arthrosc 2011;19:27–33.
53. Kovacevic D, Mariscalco M, Goodwin RC. Injuries about the hip in the adolescent athlete. Sports Med Arthrosc 2011;19:64–74.
54. Larrain MV, Montenegro HJ, Mauas DM, et al. Arthroscopic management of traumatic anterior shoulder instability in collision athletes: analysis of 204 cases with a 4- to 9-year follow-up and results with the suture anchor technique. Arthroscopy 2006;22:1283–9.
55. Levy BA, Dajani KA, Whelan DB, et al. Decision making in the multiligament-injured knee: an evidence-based systematic review. Arthroscopy 2009;25:430–8.
56. Levy BA, Fanelli GC, Whelan DB, et al. Controversies in the treatment of knee dislocations and multiligament reconstruction. J Am Acad Orthop Surg 2009;17:197–206.
57. Li S, Chen Y, Lin Z, et al. A systematic review of randomized controlled clinical trials comparing hamstring autografts versus bone-patellar tendon-bone autografts for the reconstruction of the anterior cruciate ligament. Arch Orthop Trauma Surg 2012;132:1287–97.
58. Liavaag S, Brox JI, Pripp AH, et al. Immobilization in external rotation after primary shoulder dislocation did not reduce the risk of recurrence: A randomized controlled trial. J Bone Joint Surg Am 2011;93:897–904. doi:10.2106/JBJS.J.00416. [Epub 2011 Apr 15].
59. Limpisvasti O, ElAttrache NS, Jobe FW. Understanding shoulder and elbow injuries in baseball. J Am Acad Orthop Surg 2007;15:139–47.
60. Lively MW, Feathers CC. Increasing prevalence of anterior cruciate ligament injuries in a collegiate population. W V Med J 2012;108:8–11.
61. Maak TG, Fabricant PD, Wickiewicz TL. Indications for meniscus repair. Clin Sports Med 2012;31:1–14.
62. Macintyre J, Johnson C, Schroeder EL. Groin pain in athletes. Curr Sports Med Rep 2006;5:293–9.
63. Madry H, Grün UW, Knutsen G. Cartilage repair and joint preservation: medical and surgical treatment options. Dtsch Arztebl Int 2011;108:669–77.
64. Magit D, Wolff A, Sutton K, et al. Arthrofibrosis of the knee. J Am Acad Orthop Surg 2007;15:682–94.

65. Makris EA, Hadidi P, Athanasiou KA. The knee meniscus: structure-function, pathophysiology, current repair techniques, and prospects for regeneration. Biomaterials 2011;32:7411–31.
66. Marchant MH Jr, Tibor LM, Sekiya JK, et al. Management of medial-sided knee injuries, part 1: medial collateral ligament. Am J Sports Med 2011;39:1102–13.
67. May JH, Gillette BP, Morgan JA, et al. Transtibial versus inlay posterior cruciate ligament reconstruction: an evidence-based systematic review. J Knee Surg 2010;23:73–9.
68. Miller MD. Review of Orthopaedics. 6th ed. Philadelphia: Elsevier/Saunders; 2012.
69. Moses B, Orchard J, Orchard J. Systematic review: Annual incidence of ACL injury and surgery in various populations. Res Sports Med 2012;20:157–79.
70. Nakamura N, Miyama T, Engebretsen L, et al. Cell-based therapy in articular cartilage lesions of the knee. Arthroscopy 2009;25:531–52.
71. Nelson MC, Leather GP, Nirschl RP, et al. Evaluation of the painful shoulder. A prospective comparison of magnetic resonance imaging, computerized tomographic arthrography, ultrasonography, and operative findings. J Bone Joint Surg Am 1991;73:707–16.
72. Nho SJ, Magennis EM, Singh CK, et al. Outcomes after the arthroscopic treatment of femoroacetabular impingement in a mixed group of high-level athletes. Am J Sports Med 2011;39(Suppl):14S–9S.
73. Noyes FR, Heckmann TP, Barber-Westin SD. Meniscus repair and transplantation: a comprehensive update. J Orthop Sports Phys Ther 2012;42:274–90.
74. Ogawa K, Yoshida A, Matsumoto H, et al. Outcome of the open Bankart procedure for shoulder instability and development of osteoarthritis: a 5- to 20-year follow-up study. Am J Sports Med 2010;38:1549–57.
75. Park MJ, Tjoumakaris FP, Garcia G, et al. Arthroscopic remplissage with Bankart repair for the treatment of glenohumeral instability with Hill–Sachs defects. Arthroscopy 2011;27: 1187–94.
76. Patel V, Elliott P. Sudden death in athletes. Clin Med 2012;12:253–6.
77. Peltola EK, Mustonen AO, Lindahl J, et al. Segond fracture combined with tibial plateau fracture. AJR Am J Roentgenol 2011;197:W1101–4.
78. Peskun CJ, Whelan DB. Outcomes of operative and nonoperative treatment of multiligament knee injuries: an evidence-based review. Sports Med Arthrosc 2011;19:167–73.
79. Polousky JD. Juvenile osteochondritis dissecans. Sports Med Arthrosc 2011;19:56–63.
80. Posner MA. Compressive neuropathies of the median and radial nerves at the elbow. Clin Sports Med 1990;9:343–63.
81. Quatman CE, Quatman-Yates CC, Schmitt LC, et al. The clinical utility and diagnostic performance of MRI for identification and classification of knee osteochondritis dissecans. J Bone Joint Surg Am 2012;94:1036–44.
82. Roberts JR, Hedges JR. Clinical procedures in emergency medicine. Philadelphia: Saunders/Elsevier; 2010.
83. Robinson CM, Howes J, Murdoch H, et al. Functional outcome and risk of recurrent instability after primary traumatic anterior shoulder dislocation in young patients. J Bone Joint Surg Am 2006;88:2326–36.
84. Safran M, Ahmad CS, Elattrache NS. Ulnar collateral ligament of the elbow. Arthroscopy 2005;21:1381–95.
85. Samora JB, Ng VY, Ellis TJ. Femoroacetabular impingement: a common cause of hip pain in young adults. Clin J Sport Med 2011;21:51–6.
86. Schreiber VM, van Eck CF, Fu FH. Anatomic double-bundle ACL reconstruction. Sports Med Arthrosc 2010;18:27–32.
87. Sciascia A, Thigpen C, Namdari S, et al. Kinetic chain abnormalities in the athletic shoulder. Sports Med Arthrosc 2012;20:16–21.
88. Shen W, Jordan S, Fu F. Review article: anatomic double bundle anterior cruciate ligament reconstruction. J Orthop Surg (Hong Kong) 2007;15:216–21.
89. Shortt CP, Zoga AC, Kavanagh EC, et al. Anatomy, pathology, and MRI findings in the sports hernia. Semin Musculoskelet Radiol 2008;12:54–61.
90. Skendzel JG, Sekiya JK, Wojtys EM. Diagnosis and management of the multiligament-injured knee. J Orthop Sports Phys Ther 2012;42:234–42.
91. Snyder SJ, Karzel RP, Del Pizzo W, et al. SLAP lesions of the shoulder. Arthroscopy 1990;6: 274–9.
92. Speer KP, Deng X, Borrero S, et al. Biomechanical evaluation of a simulated Bankart lesion. J Bone Joint Surg Am 1994;76:1819–26.
93. Stojanovic MD, Ostojic SM. Preventing ACL injuries in team-sport athletes: a systematic review of training interventions. Res Sports Med 2012;20:223–38.
94. Sun Y, Jiang Q. Review of discoid meniscus. Orthop Surg 2011;3:219–23.
95. Tannenbaum E, Sekiya JK. Evaluation and management of posterior shoulder instability. Sports Health 2011;3:253–63.
96. Tibor LM, Marchant MH Jr, Taylor DC, et al. Management of medial-sided knee injuries, part 2: posteromedial corner. Am J Sports Med 2011;39:1332–40.

97. Tjoumakaris FP, Abboud JA, Hasan SA, et al. Arthroscopic and open Bankart repairs provide similar outcomes. Clin Orthop Relat Res 2006;446:227–32.

98. Tjoumakaris FP, Bradley JP. The rationale for an arthroscopic approach to shoulder stabilization. Arthroscopy 2011;27:1422–33.

99. Turman KA, Diduch DR. Meniscal repair: indications and techniques. J Knee Surg 2008;21:154–62.

100. Versier G, Dubrana F. Treatment of knee cartilage defect in 2010. Orthop Traumatol Surg Res 2011;97:S140–53.

101. Wang RY, Arciero RA. Treating the athlete with anterior shoulder instability. Clin Sports Med 2008;27:631–48.

102. Waninger KN, Swartz EE. Cervical spine injury management in the helmeted athlete. Curr Sports Med Rep 2011;10:45–9.

103. Wheeler JH, Ryan JB, Arciero RA, et al. Arthroscopic versus nonoperative treatment of acute shoulder dislocations in young athletes. Arthroscopy 1989;5:213–17.

104. Wolf EM, Pollack M, Smalley C. Hill–Sachs "Remplissage:" An arthroscopic solution for the engaging Hill–Sachs lesion. Arthroscopy 2007;23:e1–2.

105. Wong JM-L, Khan T, Jayadev CS, et al. Anterior cruciate ligament rupture and osteoarthritis progression. Open Orthop J 2012;6:295–300.

106. Wright RW, Gill CS, Chen L, et al. Outcome of revision anterior cruciate ligament reconstruction: a systematic review. J Bone Joint Surg Am 2012;94:531–6.

107. Yiannakopoulos CK, Mataragas E, Antonogiannakis E. A comparison of the spectrum of intra-articular lesions in acute and chronic anterior shoulder instability. Arthroscopy 2007;23:985–90.

108. Yocum LA. The diagnosis and nonoperative treatment of elbow problems in the athlete. Clin Sports Med 1989;8:439–51.

CHAPTER 11

ORTHOPEDIC TRAUMA

John A. Scolaro and Ryan M. Taylor

BIOMECHANICS

1. **What is meant by an absolute stability construct? What is relative stability?**
Absolute stability refers to the fact that there is alignment and compression across a fracture resulting in no micromotion at physiological loads, which results in primary bone healing.
    Relative stability describes a situation where some degree of motion still exists at the fracture site which is reversible (elastic) and provides the mechanical stimulation for fracture healing. Relative stability results in fracture healing by secondary bone healing.

2. **What are the five different functions of a plate?**
Each time a plate is applied to bone the surgeon must define its function. Below are the different functions of a plate:
    Compression: A compression plate produces compression at the fracture site utilizing the oblique screw holes in the plate and placing the screws eccentrically. Primary bone healing is expected (e.g., transverse humeral fracture).
    Neutralization: A neutralization plate is used to "protect" lag screw fixation or another absolute stability construct. Usually screw fixation alone is not adequate in many settings and a plate is needed to allow for early motion (e.g., oblique fracture of distal fibula).
    Buttress: A buttress plate creates a stable shoulder with the intact bone to resist shear forces. These plates are usually found in peri-articular fractures and result in primary bone healing (e.g., simple split fracture of lateral tibial plateau).
    Tension band: A tension band construct converts distractive forces into compressive forces by its orientation. This will produce compression at the fracture site and primary bone healing (e.g., transverse fracture of proximal ulna).
    Bridge: A bridge plate is used to span an area of comminution and is a relative stability construct. The overall length, alignment and rotation of the bone needs to be restored (e.g., comminuted diaphyseal femur fracture) (Fig. 11.1).

3. **What does the term "modulus of elasticity" mean?**
Modulus of elasticity describes the deformation of a material to a certain amount of force. It is the slope of the stress–strain curve. Stiffer materials (stainless steel) have a higher modulus of elasticity while more flexible materials (titanium) have a lower modulus of elasticity. The modulus of elasticity is an important concept in orthopedics as implants must be strong enough to resist deformation, but also be flexible enough, in the desired setting, to allow for micromotion and stimulation of fracture healing.

FRACTURE HEALING

4. **What are the stages of fracture healing? How do each of these stages last?**
There are three stages of fracture healing: inflammation, repair, and remodeling. The inflammatory stage lasts from the time of initial injury and fracture hematoma formation to 2 weeks. By this point, a callus has started to develop. The repair stage lasts from 2 to 4 weeks as the fracture callus matures and ossifies. The remodeling stage begins during the repair phase and usually lasts between 4 and 12 weeks after the injury as woven bone is replaced by trabecular bone (Fig. 11.2).

5. **How do fractures heal? What is meant by primary and secondary bone formation?**
The first stage of fracture healing is inflammation. During this stage, a fracture hematoma forms which consists of hematopoietic cells and growth factors. The combination of certain growth factors leads to subsequent presence of fibroblasts, mesenchymal cells, and osteoprogenitor cells. Next, the hematoma develops into a callus as osteoblasts and

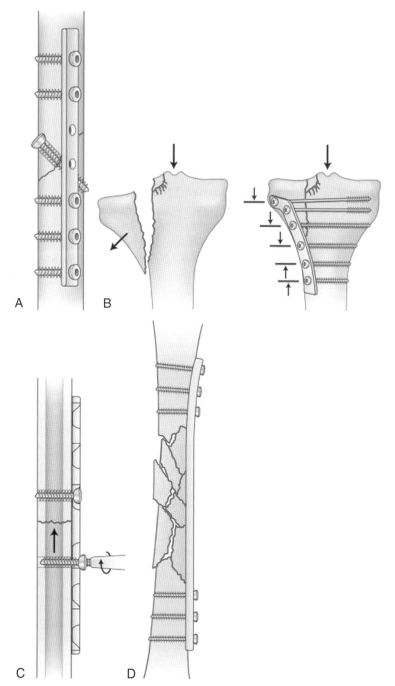

Figure 11.1. Plate functions. (A) Neutralization plate with interfragmentary lag screw outside of the plate. (B) Buttress plate fixation of proximal tibia. (C) Compression plating of a transverse fracture. (D) Bridge plating of an area of comminution. *(From Mazzocca AD, DeAngelis JD, Caputo AE, et al.: Principles of Internal Fixation. In: Browner BD, Levine AM, Jupiter JB, et al. [eds]: Skeletal Trauma: Basic Science, Management, and Reconstruction, 4th ed. Philadelphia, 2008, WB Saunders.)*

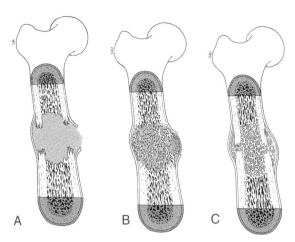

Figure 11.2. Normal fracture healing. (A) After the injury, bleeding is related to osseous and soft-tissue damage. A hematoma, followed by clot formation, develops within the medullary canal between the fracture ends and beneath the periosteal membrane, which may have been torn. (B) Callus formation takes place and consists of external bridging callus at the periosteal surface, intramedullary callus, and primary callus at the ends of the fracture fragments. (C) Callus envelops the bone ends rapidly and produces increasing stability at the fracture site. (*Modified from Resnick DL: Bone and Joint Imaging, 3rd ed, Copyright © 2005 Saunders, Elsevier.*)

fibroblasts proliferate and lay down matrix. If the bones are not apposed, a bridging callus will form, which eventually is ossified, forming a hard callus. This hard callus, also known as woven bone, will eventually be remodeled into normal appearing lamellar bone.

Primary bone formation is bone healing that occurs with no callus. The mechanism of repair is primary cortical healing through intramembranous ossification. This type of healing occurs in absolute stability constructs and mimics normal bone remodeling.

Secondary bone formation occurs through enchondral ossification of a periosteal bridging callus. This type of healing occurs in non-rigid constructs. The more stable a fracture is, the less callus will be formed.

6. **Is either healing type more desirable than the other in injuries involving an articular surface? In non-articular areas?**
Primary bone healing is more desirable in injuries involving the articular surface. When performing reduction and fixation of an intra-articular injury, quality of a reduction of the articular surface usually determines outcome. As a result, an absolute stability construct and primary bone healing is preferred to minimize displacement of the articular fragments. In non-articular areas, there is a less significant need for anatomic reduction, and the allowable deformities are much greater than those tolerated at the articular surface. As a result, secondary healing, with callus formation, is acceptable in extra-articular injuries.

COMPARTMENT SYNDROME
CASE 11-1

A 37-year-old female sustains a tibia fracture in a high-energy motor-vehicle collision. She is taken to the operating room for a reamed intramedullary tibial nail. Approximately 2 hours following surgery she reports pain that is not relieved by her intravenous pain medications and increasing anxiety.

7. **What is compartment syndrome?**
Compartment syndrome is increased tissue pressure due to swelling, edema, or bleeding within an enclosed anatomic space surrounded by the semi-rigid fascia of a muscular compartment. This increase in pressure leads to venous obstruction and collapse of the low-pressure arteriolar plexus, thereby reducing blood flow through the capillary network.

When not addressed in an expedient manner it can have disastrous sequelae including loss of limb and even death.

8. **What are the primary causes of acute compartment syndrome?**
The majority of cases of acute compartment syndrome are caused by severe trauma associated with a fracture or vascular reperfusion of a limb. Other causes are prolonged compression on an area by a tourniquet, dressing, or even a patient's own body weight. Burns, as well as extravasation of intravenous fluid or contrast material, can also cause a compartment syndrome. Exercise-induced compartment syndrome follows the same pathophysiology, but is almost always reversible with cessation of exercise and is usually not limb threatening like the compartment syndrome seen after extremity trauma or reperfusion injury.

9. **How is compartment syndrome diagnosed?**
In the setting of any high-energy injury, a high level of suspicion should exist of the presence of compartment syndrome. The diagnosis is made entirely based on the physical exam in an awake, cooperative patient. The primary finding is increasing *pain*. Pain is often out of proportion to the exam and is not responsive to medication. Additionally, pain is often present with passive stretch of the distal extremity. Other signs that have been cited are *paresthesias*, skin *pallor*, *paralysis*, arterial *pulselessness*, and *poikilothermia*, meaning that the skin is cool to touch. The latter are late findings, and when the process has progressed to this point, irreversible damage has likely occurred to the limb.

10. **How can compartment syndrome be measured?**
The pressure within a muscular compartment can be measured by the use of a needle attached to a manometer. These are portable units which are inexpensive, require little equipment, and can be used in any setting. In addition, slit catheters or wick catheters can be placed to provide continuous compartment measurements (Fig. 11.3).

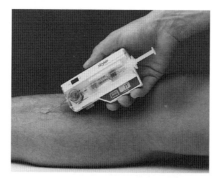

Figure 11.3. Hand based portable intracompartmental pressure monitor system. (*Courtesy of Stryker Instruments, Kalamazoo, Michigan.*)

11. **At what pressure does acute compartment syndrome exist?**
It can generally be agreed that compartment syndrome exists when the absolute pressure exceeds 30 mmHg or when the pressure is within 30 mmHg of the diastolic blood pressure. It is also important to know that factors such as general anesthesia can affect compartment pressure readings.

12. **Which compartments are most commonly involved in an acute compartment syndrome of the tibia?**
The deep posterior and anterior compartments are most frequently affected following a tibia fracture. This is related to the proximity of those muscular compartments to the tibia. The lateral and superficial posterior compartments can also be affected and should be released if a fasciotomy is performed.

13. Can compartment syndrome exist in the setting of an open fracture?
Yes. The fact that a fracture is open does not exclude the possibility that a compartment syndrome can develop. The open wound may help decompress one compartment but the other fascial compartments can still be affected.

14. Can compartment syndrome occur in the upper extremity?
Yes, acute compartment syndrome can occur in the hand, at the carpal tunnel, in the forearm, and in rare instances, in the upper arm.

15. What is the treatment of acute compartment syndrome?
Once the diagnosis of acute compartment syndrome is established or is suspected, the only treatment is emergent surgical decompression of all compartments of the limb. In the lower leg this can be accomplished through single- or double-incision fasciotomy. The skin wounds are then left open until they are closed or skin grafted at a later time.

16. What is an important aspect of the postoperative care of a patient who has developed compartment syndrome?
If muscle ischemia and/or death has occurred as a result of the compartment syndrome, myoglobinuria may result. Hydration and monitoring of renal function (BUN and creatinine) should be performed to ensure that any abnormalities are recognized and addressed.

17. What are the complications of an untreated acute compartment syndrome?
An unrecognized or untreated acute compartment syndrome will ultimately lead to the death and loss of function of the neuromuscular structures within the affected compartment. In the upper extremity, Volkmann's contractures, paralysis, and sensory loss are the end result once the necrotic tissue is replaced by scar. In the lower extremity, loss of sensation and motor control can occur with a plantar flexion contracture of the ankle usually resulting. In the foot, clawing of the toes is classic sequelae of untreated or missed compartment syndrome.

18. What is the proper initial management of a responsive patient who has a limb in which there is concern for compartment syndrome?
Initially, all constrictive dressings should be loosened or removed. If a cast exists, it should be bivalved and the cast padding should be split or loosened. The extremity should then receive a full neurovascular exam with a high index of suspicion for developing compartment syndrome with particular attention paid to the previously mentioned signs and symptoms. If the diagnosis requires pressure measurements to be performed they should be done immediately. As the sequelae of a missed compartment syndrome can be catastrophic to the limb, many would advocate for fasciotomy if there is clinical concern for this diagnosis.

19. What are the compartments in the lower leg?
The four compartments are the anterior, lateral, deep and superficial posterior compartments (Fig. 11.4).

20. What are the compartments in the forearm?
The three compartments in the forearm are the volar and dorsal compartments, as well as the mobile wad.

21. What are the compartments in the hand?
There are ten compartments in the hand: one for each of the four dorsal interosseous muscles, three for the volar interossei, and one each for the adductor pollicis, thenar muscles and hypothenar muscles.

22. What are the compartments in the foot?
The exact number of compartments in the foot is still debated (with some having described as many as nine compartments) but most would agree that there are four distinct compartments: an intrinsic, medial, central and lateral compartment.

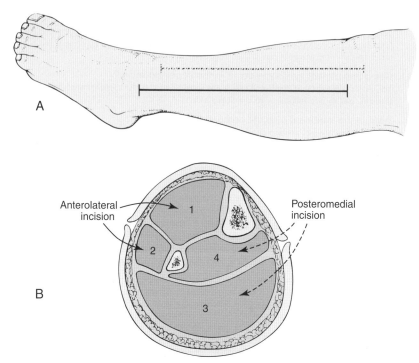

Figure 11.4. (A) The double-incision technique for performing fasciotomies of all four compartments of the lower extremity. (B) Cross section of lower extremity showing a position of anterolateral and posteromedial incisions that allows access to the anterior and lateral compartments (1 and 2) and the superficial and deep posterior compartments (3 and 4). (A, B, *Modified with permission from AAOS Instructional Course Lectures, Vol. 32. St Louis, CV Mosby, 1983, p. 110.*)

POLYTRAUMA

23. **How is the trauma patient initially evaluated?**
    All trauma patients should be evaluated using standard advanced trauma life support (ATLS) protocols, which include the ABCDE of initial evaluation: Airway, Breathing, Circulation, Disability (neurologic evaluation), and Exposure (undress the patient). The primary survey is followed by a secondary survey to identify non-life-threatening injuries.

24. **What is the standard radiographic "trauma series?"**
    A trauma series includes an antero-posterior view of the chest, an antero-posterior view of the pelvis, and a lateral view of the cervical spine that includes the top of the first thoracic vertebrae.

25. **What is the Injury Serverity Score? How is it measured?**
    The Injury Severity Score is a numerical, anatomically based, scoring system for patients with multiple injuries. Each of six body regions (head/neck, face, chest, abdomen, extremity, external) is given a numerical score. Then, the highest three scores are squared and summed to acquire the final score. The score ranges from 1 to 75. A score greater than 15 is used to define a polytrauma patient.

26. **What are some clinical markers that can be used to determine the severity of injury in a polytrauma patient?**
    Serum lactate is probably the best marker of initial injury and adequacy of resuscitation. Other values that can be used are heart rate, blood pressure, urine output, and the

Glasgow Coma Scale. There have been recent suggestions that other serum markers, such as IL-1 and IL-6, may also play a role in the assessment of trauma patients.

27. **What is meant by the "golden hour" in the management of a trauma patient?**
The care delivered to a trauma patient in the first minutes to hours following injury may prevent death or significant morbidity. The use of this term highlights the importance of prompt and aggressive treatment of the severely injured patient. It is important to recognize that treatment is first initiated in the field by emergency medical responders.

28. **What is damage control orthopedics?**
Damage control orthopedics refers to the temporary stabilization of skeletal fractures. Temporary stabilization is advocated in some patients because the initial insult of trauma has compromised the ability of the patient to undergo the physiologic stress of definitive treatment of their orthopedic injury. For example, the use of temporary external fixation of a long bone fracture or pelvic ring disruption in a patient with a closed head injury or pulmonary injury is an example of damage control orthopedics. In these situations, the fracture is definitively treated at a later date when the patient can physiologically tolerate such a procedure.

CLAVICLE
CASE 11-2

A 21-year-old male comes into the Emergency Room after falling from his bike. He reports right shoulder pain and has point tenderness just medial to the shoulder. A fracture of the clavicle is suspected and radiology wants to know what plain radiographs should be obtained.

29. **How is the clavicle best examined radiographically?**
Fractures of the clavicle can be identified on a regular AP chest film but a dedicated clavicle series will show the clavicle the best. This can be performed with the contralateral scapula bumped using a rolled towel and the involved side flat against the film plate. The beam is then angled 20° cephalad. A Zanca view, which is an AP of the acromioclavicular (AC) joint with a 15° cephalic tilt, is the best view for distal clavicle fractures. Medial fractures are best seen with a Serendipity view (40° cephalic tilt with the beam centered on the sternoclavicular (SC) joint) or CT scan (Fig. 11.5).

30. **What are the important anatomic relationships of the clavicle?**
The clavicle articulates with the sternum medially, the acromion laterally and is an "s-shaped" bone. It lies superior to the brachial plexus and the axillary artery. It serves as a strut between the axial skeleton and the shoulder girdle and as the origin and insertion of several large muscles, including the pectoralis major and trapezius, respectively.

31. **What is the classification of clavicle fractures?**
There are multiple classification schemata for clavicle fractures, but generally, fractures of the clavicle are divided up into three groups:
Group I – Middle third. These are the most common type.
Group II – Lateral third. These are the second most common type and have been further subdivided into five subtypes:
  Type I – coracoclavicular (CC) ligaments intact
  Type II – CC ligaments disrupted, trapezoid ligaments intact to distal segment
  Type III – fracture has intra-articular extension to acromioclavicular joint.
Group III – Medial third (Fig. 11.6).

32. **How are most clavicle fractures treated?**
The majority of closed clavicle fractures, where there is no skin or neurovascular compromise, are treated with a figure of eight harness or shoulder sling for comfort with progressive range of motion as fracture healing occurs.

33. **When are clavicle fractures treated with surgery?**
The operative indications for surgical fixation of clavicle fractures continue to evolve. Fractures that are open or put the overlying skin at risk and those that are associated with

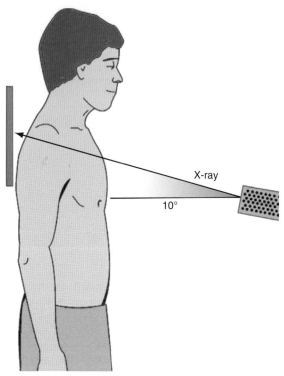

Figure 11.5. Zanca view of the acromioclavicular joint is obtained with a 10° cephalic tilt and 50% penetrance. *(From Rockwood CA Jr, Young DC: Disorders of the Acromioclavicular Joint. In: Rockwood CA Jr, Matsen TA III, eds: The Shoulder, Philadelphia, 1985, WB Saunders, pp. 413–476.)*

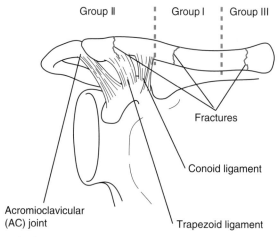

Figure 11.6. Allman classification groups clavicle fractures according to their anatomic location: middle (Group I), distal (Group II), or proximal (Group III). *(From Barei DP, et al., Fractures About the Shoulder: Trumble TE, et al., [eds], Core Knowledge in Orthopaedics – Hand, Elbow, and Shoulder, 1st ed. Copyright © 2006, Mosby, Elsevier.)*

neurovascular injury are often treated with surgery. In addition, some distal third clavicle fractures, fractures that demonstrate a "zed" or "z" pattern, those that are shortened by >2 cm or displaced >100%, and some fractures in young active individuals or polytraumatized patients are frequently stabilized with operative fixation.

34. **How are clavicle fractures fixed and what are the potential complications?**
Clavicle fractures can be treated with plates and screws, intramedullary implants such as pins, screws or flexible rods or in some instances, suture and/or soft-tissue repair. Potential complications with fixation include iatrogenic injury to nearby neurovascular structures during fixation, prominent hardware or wound healing problems, migration of hardware and nonunion, malunion and refracture.

SCAPULA/GLENOID

35. **How are fractures of the scapula described?**
Although there are classification systems described, most fractures of the scapula are described by anatomic location. This includes: body, spine, glenoid neck, glenoid (intra-articular), coracoid or acromion. Fractures of the body and neck are the most common.

CASE 11-3

A 40-year-old female sustains multiple injuries following a motor-vehicle collision. She was noted to be the restrained driver in the vehicle that careened off the road and struck a pole. She was intubated on arrival to the hospital because of respiratory distress. Initial antero-posterior chest radiograph noted severe lung opacities and bilateral rib fractures. On CT scan the following day, a comminuted scapula fracture is noted. You are called to consult on the patient and determine if surgery is needed (Fig. 11.7).

36. **What other injuries are associated with fractures of the scapula?**
Fractures of the scapula are often the result of a high-energy mechanism of injury and over 95% are associated with other injuries. Injuries to the ribs, lungs and torso are frequently identified and oftentimes carry a greater morbidity than the scapula fracture.

37. **How are fractures of the scapula and glenoid best imaged?**
The glenoid and glenoid neck can be seen well on a true antero-posterior view of the glenohumeral joint. An axillary lateral, Stryker notch or West Point view can also be used to evaluate the glenoid and glenoid rim. For the scapula, a lateral radiograph of the scapular body can be of some utility. Computed tomographic scans, including 3-D reconstructions, are frequently used to evaluate these fractures. This imaging modality helps determine fracture displacement and intra-articular extension.

38. **What are the indications for surgery for fractures of scapula and glenoid?**
The overwhelming majority of scapular and glenoid fractures are treated non-operatively. Indications for surgical fixation of extra-articular scapula fractures include glenoid neck fractures that are medialized more than 1 cm or angulated >40°. In addition, if there is a fracture of the acromion that creates impingement in the subacromial space or a fracture of the scapular body that impinges on the thoracic cage, these may also be treated with surgery. Intra-articular glenoid fractures are treated surgically if there is resultant shoulder instability (usually when >25% of articular surface involved), >5 mm displacement within the fossa, or >10 mm displacement of the rim.

39. **What are the surgical approaches to the scapula and glenoid?**
Posteriorly, the scapular body and both the posterior and inferior glenoid neck can be accessed through the modified Judet approach between the infraspinatus and teres minor. The overlying deltoid is reflected to improve exposure and access. For anterior rim fractures of the glenoid or fractures that cannot be reached from a posterior approach, a deltopectoral approach is utilized with take down (full or partial) or split of the subscapularis.

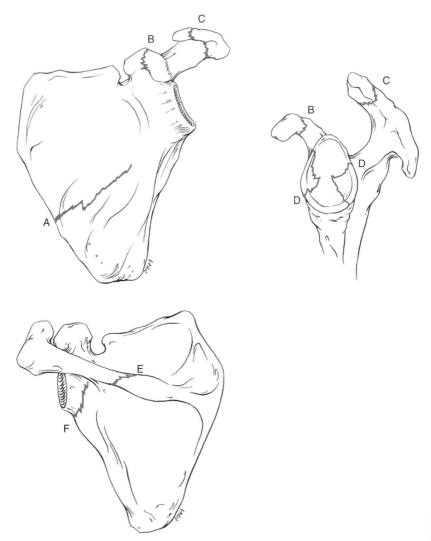

Figure 11.7. Fractures of the scapula as described by anatomic location: body (A), coracoid process (B), acromion (C), glenoid fossa (E), spine (F), and glenoid neck (F). (*From Eiff MP, Hatch R, [eds], Fracture Management for Primary Care, 3rd ed, Copyright © 2012, Saunders, Elsevier Inc.*)

40. **What is scapulothoracic dissociation and what is a "floating shoulder?"**
    Scapulothoracic dissociation is the result of a very high-energy injury where there is lateral displacement of the scapula away from the posterior thoracic wall and often an associated fracture of the clavicle or disruption of the acromioclavicular (AC) or sternoclavicular (SC) joint. There may be severe injury to the muscular attachments around the shoulder and disruption to the axillary artery or brachial plexus should be considered. A "floating shoulder" refers to an injury where there is a scapular fracture associated with a clavicular fracture (or AC joint disruption) or proximal humerus fracture. In this situation, usually one of the injuries is treated surgically to stabilize the shoulder.

HUMERUS

PROXIMAL HUMERUS FRACTURES

CASE 11-4

A 45-year-old female presents to the Emergency Room reporting left shoulder pain after falling from a painting ladder. She reports numbness and tingling over the lateral aspect of the upper arm and inability to raise her arm. Radiographs show a displaced fracture dislocation of the proximal humerus. What nerve is responsible for the patients presenting symptom?

41. **What radiographs are necessary for evaluation of the glenohumeral (GH) joint?**
Two orthogonal views of the shoulder must always be obtained; this includes an antero-posterior and axillary lateral radiograph. If the patient cannot tolerate an axillary film, a Velpeau view can be obtained. The position of the humeral head in relation to the glenoid must be evaluated so a dislocation (anterior or posterior) is not missed. In some instances, a CT scan can be used in addition to plain radiographs to evaluate the glenoid or proximal humerus (Fig. 11.8).

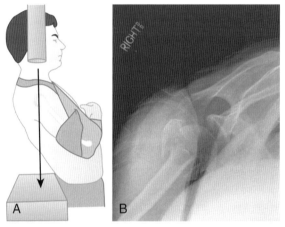

Figure 11.8. (A) Velpeau axillary view may be taken; this allows the patient to keep the arm immobilized in the sling. The patient leans back and over the plate while the beam is directed from superior to inferior. (B) Velpeau axillary radiograph showing proximal humerus fracture. Note that the head is located and the greater tuberosity is displaced posteriorly. *(From Cuomo F, Zuckerman JD: Proximal Humerus Fracture. In: Browner BD [ed]: Techniques in Orthopaedics, vol 9. New York, Raven Press, 1994, p. 143.)*

42. **What are the important muscular attachments around the shoulder?**
The supraspinatus and infraspinatus attach to the greater tuberosity. The subscapularis attaches to the lesser tuberosity. The teres major, pectoralis major, and latissimus dorsi attach to the proximal humeral shaft. The long head of the biceps tendon runs from the superior aspect of the glenoid, between the greater and lesser tuberosity in the bicipital groove.

43. **What is the blood supply to the proximal humerus?**
The blood supply to the humeral head is from the anterior humeral circumflex artery. The ascending branch of the anterior circumflex courses just lateral to the bicipital groove and forms the arcuate artery which enters the bone and perfuses the majority of the humeral head. The posterior circumflex artery also contributes to the blood supply of the proximal humerus and may have a more significant contribution than originally believed.

44. **Which nerve injuries are commonly associated with fractures about the shoulder?**
The axillary nerve, which arises from the posterior cord of the brachial plexus and passes through the quadrangular space of the shoulder along with the posterior circumflex

humeral artery, is the nerve most often affected by glenohumeral dislocations and proximal humerus fractures. It innervates the deltoid, teres minor, and long head of the triceps and its dermatome is a patch of skin over the lateral aspect of the shoulder. The musculocutaneous nerve is also susceptible to injury, especially if there is dislocation or displacement of the proximal humerus near the coracoid.

45. **How are proximal humerus fractures classified?**
Codman was the first to define the four "parts" of the proximal humerus. These are the humeral head, the lesser tuberosity, the greater tuberosity, and the humeral shaft. The Neer classification system elaborated on this and defines a "part" as a fragment that is displaced >1 cm or has >45° of angulation (Fig. 11.9).

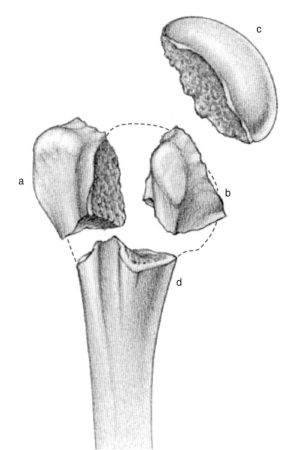

Figure 11.9. Codman divided the proximal humerus into four distinct fragments that occur along anatomic lines of epiphyseal union. He differentiated the four major fragments as (a) greater tuberosity, (b) lesser tuberosity, (c) head, and (d) shaft. (*Modified from Codman EA: The Shoulder: Rupture of the Supraspinatus Tendon and Other Lesions in or About the Subacromial Bursa. Boston: Thomas Todd, 1934. Rockwood: The Shoulder, 4th ed.*)

46. **How are proximal humerus fractures treated?**
Proximal humerus fractures can be treated non-operatively, with closed reduction and percutaneous pinning, open reduction and internal fixation or with arthroplasty. The decision is made taking into account the patient's age, bone quality and functional demand as well as the pattern and displacement of the fracture. The majority of all proximal humerus fractures are still treated non-operatively with early progression to functional exercises.

47. What are some instances in which operative treatment is favored over non-operative management for proximal humerus fractures?

Any instance where there is a fracture–dislocation of the proximal humerus, where the humeral head cannot be reduced within the glenoid, is an indication for surgery. In addition, if there is a vascular injury to the upper extremity because of a displaced fracture fragment, this must be addressed with surgery.

Displaced proximal humerus fractures in younger patients are often treated more aggressively. In addition, two-part fractures, where there is isolated displacement of the greater tuberosity (>5 mm) that may cause later impingement underneath the acromion or loss of function, are often reduced and fixed. Likewise, displaced lesser tuberosity fractures, which cause subscapularis insufficiency and possible glenohumeral instability, are more likely to be treated with surgery.

The quality of the patient's bone and severity of fracture also dictate treatment. Fracture fixation in severely osteoporotic bone can be difficult and lead to hardware complications or nonunion. In severe three or four part fractures, especially where the humeral head is split, replacement of the proximal humerus with a hemiarthroplasty or reverse prosthesis may be performed. This is done because with such fractures, the vascular supply to the humeral head has been disrupted to such a degree that fixation often yields poor results (Fig. 11.10).

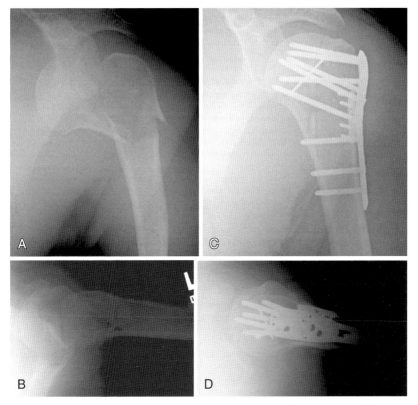

Figure 11.10. (A and B) Antero-posterior and axillary lateral images show a three-part fracture–dislocation of the proximal humerus. (C and D) Postoperative antero-posterior and lateral radiographs show satisfactory reduction and fixation with a screw/plate construct using a lateral locking plate. (*Modified from Trumble TE: Core Knowledge in Orthopaedics – Hand, Elbow, and Shoulder, 1st ed, p. 618. Copyright © 2006, Mosby.*)

48. **What is the surgical approach to the proximal humerus?**

    The deltopectoral approach is the primary exposure used to treat fractures of the proximal humerus. The exposure is between the deltoid laterally and the pectoralis major medially. The cephalic vein lies superficially over this muscular interval and is often taken laterally with the deltoid. The clavipectoral fascia is then encountered and incised, allowing access to the tuberosities and shoulder joint.

    An alternative approach sometimes used is the deltoid split. In this approach, the skin incision is carried from the anterolateral aspect to the acromion to approximately 5 cm distally. The raphe (or demarcation) between the anterior and middle thirds of the deltoid is identified and split. This allows immediate access to the greater tuberosity. Great care must be taken to identify and protect the axillary nerve during this approach.

HUMERAL SHAFT

49. **What nerve is most commonly injured with a fracture of the humeral shaft?**

    The radial nerve runs along the posterior aspect of the humerus within the spiral groove. It is therefore highly susceptible to injury both at the time of injury and during operative treatment. A specific type of humeral shaft fracture, named the Holstein–Lewis fracture, is a spiral oblique fracture of the distal third of the humerus which is notorious for its association with radial nerve involvement.

50. **Is paralysis of the radial nerve following humeral shaft fracture an absolute indication for surgical exploration and/or operative fixation?**

    No, oftentimes the radial nerve is stretched or contused at the time of injury and will recover if treated with observation alone. If the fracture is open or open surgery will be undertaken for another reason, exploration of the nerve should take place. Surgical exploration may also be warranted if closed reduction of the humerus causes an immediate palsy, which would suggest that the nerve is trapped between fracture fragments, although this is controversial.

51. **How are humeral shaft fractures immobilized and treated non-operatively?**

    Initially, most humeral shaft fractures are treated with a coaptation (or "sugar-tong") splint made from plaster that runs from the axilla, along the medial aspect of the arm, distally around the elbow and then over the lateral aspect of the arm, ending over the acromion. After a short period of time this splint is transitioned to a functional brace. This device resembles a plastic clamshell and is removable, usually with Velcro straps. It allows motion at the shoulder and elbow while relying on the muscular envelope around the humerus to provide and maintain bony alignment.

    Other means of non-operative treatment include hanging arm casts, long arm casts, shoulder spica casts and olecranon traction. Each of these methods carries its own morbidity and is not used nearly as frequently as functional bracing (Fig. 11.11).

52. **What are the recommended parameters for operative treatment of humeral shaft fractures?**

    Fractures that cannot be maintained in a state of closed reduction and exhibit shortening >3 cm, rotation >30°, antero-posterior angulation >20°, or varus–valgus angulation >30° are often treated operatively. In addition, fractures that are segmental or highly comminuted, involve pathologic lesions, or have intra-articular extension either proximally or distally are usually treated operatively.

53. **In what other instances may a patient with a humeral shaft fracture not be an ideal candidate for non-operative management?**

    Patients who cannot tolerate a splint or brace because of skin condition or body habitus may be good candidates for operative intervention. In addition, those with bilateral humeral fractures, ipsilateral upper extremity injuries, victims of polytrauma, or who may not be compliant with non-operative restrictions are considered for surgical stabilization.

54. **How are humeral shaft fractures operatively treated?**

    The two most common methods of treating humeral shaft fractures are with a plate and screw device or with an intramedullary nail. The intramedullary nail can be inserted proximally or distally through the greater tuberosity or olecranon fossa, respectively. Either surgical treatment requires attention, and protection, of the radial nerve to avoid iatrogenic injury (Fig. 11.12).

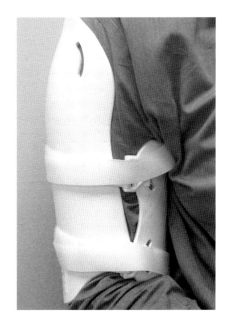

Figure 11.11. Functional humerus brace (Sarmiento humeral fracture brace).

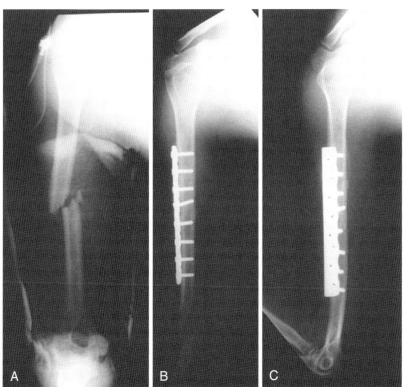

Figure 11.12. (A) Displaced diaphyseal humeral shaft fracture in a polytrauma patient. (B and C) Anteroposterior and lateral radiographs demonstrating open reduction and internal fixation with a limited-contact dynamic compression plate. (*Modified from Browner BD, et al. [eds], Skeletal Trauma, 4th ed, p. 1608. Copyright © 2009, Saunders, Elsevier Inc.*)

DISTAL HUMERUS
CASE 11-5

A 30-year-old right-hand-dominant male sustains an intra-articular distal humerus fracture after falling off his motorcycle. He is treated with open reduction and internal fixation and has an uncomplicated postoperative course. He is seen in follow up 2 weeks following surgery and his wounds are well healed but after starting immediate range of motion following surgery, he states he is starting to feel stiff. He does not make his next two follow-up appointments, but is seen at 3 months following surgery. He now reports that he is unable to move the elbow despite his best efforts.

55. **How can fractures of the distal humerus be generally classified?**
    Distal humerus fractures can be generally classified as extra articular, partial articular, or complete articular (as described in the AO classification system). When the fracture involves the articular segment, the management and surgical approach differs from those fractures that do not extend distally into the articular block. The Jupiter classification system is also used frequently and is based upon the morphology of the fracture and the stability of the elbow.

56. **What radiographic technique is useful in assessing fractures of the distal humerus?**
    In addition to a standard antero-posterior and lateral radiograph of the elbow (including any relevant imaging of the joint above and below the fracture), a traction antero-posterior view can be used. This is performed in the same manner as a standard antero-posterior with stabilization of the humerus proximal to the fractured segment and traction on the forearm or wrist distally. This view is especially useful with highly comminuted and intra-articular injuries. Recently, CT evaluation, especially 3-D reconstructions have proven to be useful in the evaluation of these fractures.

57. **What are isolated articular surface fractures?**
    In some instances, a fracture can occur through the articular surface of the distal humerus, usually through the capitellum. There are two described types. In Type I (Hahn–Steinthal) fractures, the capitellar surface and a part of the trochlea (with subchondral bone) is fractured from the lateral condyle. In Type II (Kocher–Lorenz) fractures, the fractured articular fragment is sheared off, leaving little subchondral bone attached to it. Type III fractures exhibit a comminuted pattern (Fig. 11.13).

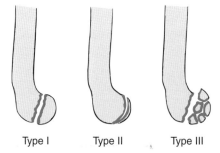

Type I   Type II   Type III

Figure 11.13. Fractures of the capitellum can be divided into Type I (Hahn–Steinthal), a complete capitellar fracture; Type II (Kocher–Lorenz), a coronal shear; Type III, a comminuted capitellar fracture. (*Modified from Browner BD, et al. [eds], Skeletal Trauma, 4th ed, p. 1577. Copyright © 2009, Saunders, Elsevier Inc.*)

58. **What are the principles of distal humerus fracture fixation?**
    The articular surface must be reconstructed in an anatomic and stable manner. The medial and lateral column must be stabilized with parallel or orthogonal plates. The overall construct should be stable enough to allow for early postoperative motion.

59. **What surgical technique is utilized to increase visualization of the distal humeral articular surface?**
    An olecranon (chevron) osteotomy is commonly used to access the distal humeral articular segment. The proximal olecranon's attachments to the triceps tendon is maintained and reflected proximally. At the end of the procedure the osteotomy is fixed with a plate or tension band construct.

60. **What are some common complications of distal humeral fractures?**

The specific complications vary with the fracture type and treatment but stiffness and loss of motion occur commonly following treatment of many of these fractures. Heterotopic ossification can be a cause of loss of motion and complicate any fracture around the elbow.

Limited soft-tissue envelope around the elbow makes wound healing problems and hardware prominence other common issues. Finally, along these lines, ulnar nerve irritation because of scar tissue or hardware placement is something that warrants discussion with every patient (Fig. 11.14).

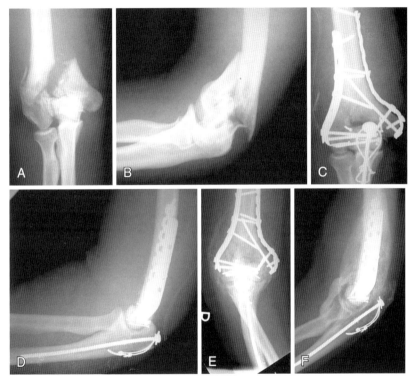

Figure 11.14. (A and B) Antero-posterior and lateral radiographs demonstrating an intra-articular distal humerus fracture. (C and D) Immediate postoperative radiographs following open reduction and internal fixation of the humeral fracture utilizing an olecranon osteotomy. (E and F) Follow-up radiographs showing maintenance of reduction and union of fracture, but development of massive heterotopic ossification around the elbow resulting in complete ankylosis of the joint. (*Modified from Wolfe SW, et al. [eds]: Green's Operative Hand Surgery, 6th ed, p. 779. Copyright © 2011, Churchill Livingstone, Elsevier Inc.*)

61. **What is the role of total elbow arthroplasty in treating distal humeral fractures?**

The use of total elbow arthroplasty to primarily treat fractures of the distal humerus is limited primarily to elderly, low-demand, patients who sustain highly comminuted fractures of the distal humerus. Oftentimes, these patients have other medical co-morbidities (e.g., Alzheimer's, rheumatoid arthritis) that make a complex reconstruction of their fracture less likely to yield a successful result. The limitations in weight bearing associated with total elbow prosthesis make its routine use undesirable in an active patient of any age.

ELBOW

PROXIMAL RADIUS

62. **What is the most common mechanism of radial head fracture?**
    The most common mechanism is a fall on the outstretched arm. This
    imparts an axial load as the radial head impacts the capitellum. Associated
    injuries can occur anywhere along the path of force, from the distal radius through
    the proximal humerus.

63. **What is the most commonly used classification system of radial
    head fractures?**
    Mason classification system (as modified by Morrey) is the most widely used:
    Type I: Non-displaced fracture
    Type II: Displaced, partial articular fractures
    Type III: Comminuted or significantly displaced radial head fracture
    Type IV: Radial head fracture associated with an elbow dislocation.
        Morrey defined "displacement" as a fracture fragment that involves >30% of the
    articular surface and is displaced >2 mm) (Fig. 11.15).

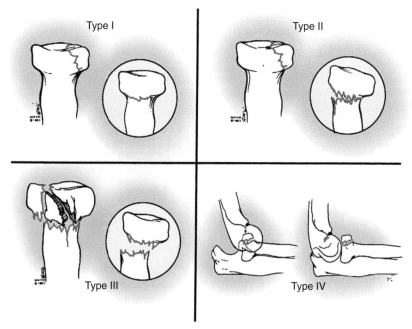

Figure 11.15. Mason classification of radial head and neck fractures. (*By permission of Mayo Foundation for Medical Education and Research. All rights reserved.*)

64. **What is the treatment for a radial head fracture?**
    Type I fractures are treated with a short period of immobilization and then gentle range
    of motion.
    Type II fractures can be treated, in some instances, like Type I fractures. Type II
    fractures where there is block to forearm rotation or where there is greater than 2 mm
    of displacement without a block to rotation are considered a relative operative
    indication.
    Type III fractures are treated with prosthetic replacement or excision. These fractures are
    unable to be reconstructed.

65. **What is the "safe zone" of the proximal radius?**
The safe zone of the proximal radius (as described by Caputo) is the surface area of the radial head where hardware can be placed without concern for impingement. This area lies between the radial styloid and Lister's tubercle (Fig. 11.16).

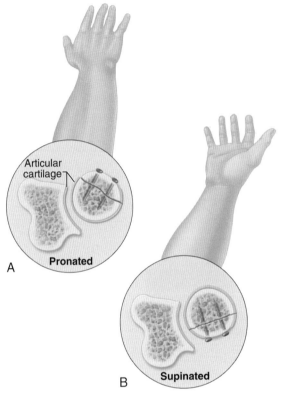

Figure 11.16. "Safe zone" (area of radial head that does not articulate with the ulna) for placement of fixation. *(From Perez EA, Fractures of the Shoulder, Arm, and Forearm: Canale ST, Beaty JH (eds), Campbell's Operative Orthopaedics, 12th ed. Mosby, 2013.)*

66. **What is the Essex-Lopresti lesion?**
The Essex-Lopresti lesion is a comminuted fracture of the radial head, with disruption of the interosseous membrane and distal radioulnar joint. Excision of the radial head in this situation can lead to disastrous results, because of proximal migration of the radius. Treatment therefore involves open reduction and internal fixation or arthroplasty of the radial head followed by reduction and fixation of the distal radioulnar joint (Fig. 11.17).

67. **When should the radial head be replaced and when should it be excised?**
The radial head should be replaced, with a metallic implant, in instances where the radial head cannot be reconstructed. Excision is still a viable option in older patients who are lower demand or in the setting of a painful malunited radial head fracture without any concurrent instability; it should not be performed in the acute setting or when there is radioulnar joint instability or an incompetent medial collateral ligament (MCL).

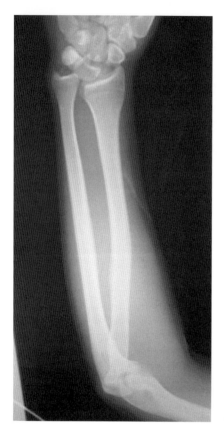

Figure 11.17. Antero-posterior radiograph demonstrating an Essex-Lopresti lesion. Shown is a fracture of the radial head associated with injury to the triangular fibrocartilage complex and the interosseous ligament. This patient also has a transscaphoid perilunate fracture dislocation. *(From Trumble TE, et al., [eds], Core Knowledge in Orthopaedics – Hand, Elbow, and Shoulder, 1st ed. Copyright © 2006, Mosby, Elsevier.)*

PROXIMAL ULNA

68. **What is the mechanism of olecranon fractures?**
   Olecranon fractures usually result from a fall directly onto the olecranon or can result from the sudden pull of the triceps mechanism

69. **How are olecranon fractures classified?**
   There are many different classification schemes. The Mayo classification for olecranon fractures separates these injuries up into three major types: Type I is undisplaced, Type II is displaced but the ulnohumeral joint is stable, and Type III has an unstable ulnohumeral joint. Within each type, "A" fractures are non-comminuted while "B" fractures are comminuted (Fig. 11.18).

70. **Describe the treatment recommendations for olecranon fractures.**
   A short period of splinting or casting is recommended for Type I fractures that are stable with elbow flexion to 90°.
   Type II and III fractures are treated with open reduction and internal fixation. Two techniques are commonly used: tension band construct or plate fixation. A tension band construct with longitudinal wires or screw and figure-of-eight tension wiring is advocated for non-comminuted transverse fracture patterns. Plate fixation can also be used for non-comminuted transverse fracture pattern. Plate fixation is generally preferred for oblique fractures distal to the midpoint of the trochlear notch or comminuted fractures.

Type I
Undisplaced

Type II
Displaced–
stable

Type III
Unstable

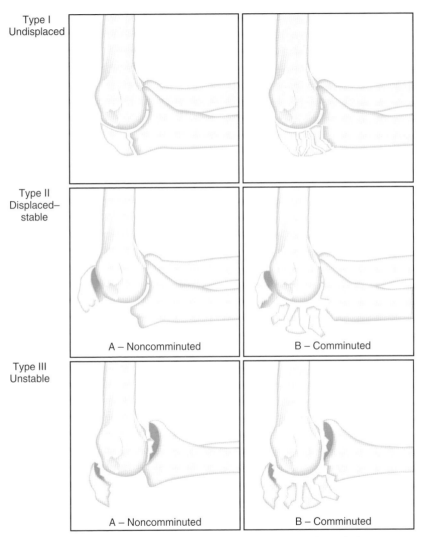

A – Noncomminuted

B – Comminuted

A – Noncomminuted

B – Comminuted

Figure 11.18. The Mayo classification of olecranon fractures divided fractures according to displacement, comminution, and subluxation–dislocation. (*From Morrey BF, Elbow and forearm: DeLee JC (ed), DeLee and Drez's Orthopaedic Sports Medicine, 3rd ed. Saunders, 2010.*)

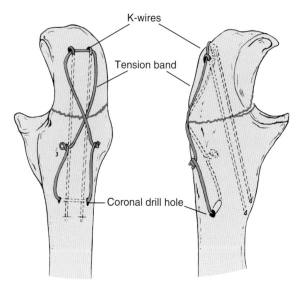

Figure 11.19. Illustration of a transverse olecranon fracture treated using a tension band wire technique. Note the placement of the two parallel K-wires and tension band wire placed through a drill hole in distal fragment. *(From Browner BD, et al. [eds], Skeletal Trauma, 4th ed, Copyright © 2009, Saunders, Elsevier Inc.)*

Excision of the proximal fragment and triceps advancement and repair is reserved for low demand or osteoporotic patients when this fragment involves less than 50% of the articular surface (Figs 11.19–11.20).

FOREARM

71. **What are the common mechanisms of injury for diaphyseal fractures of the radius and ulna?**
Fractures of the radial and ulnar shafts are commonly known as "both bone" forearm fractures and occur following a fall on the outstretched hand or a direct blow to the forearm.

72. **What is the treatment of radial and ulnar shaft fractures in adults?**
The treatment of most non-displaced, as well as displaced, radial shaft fractures is open reduction and internal fixation. This is also the treatment of choice for proximal third as well as mid-diaphyseal ulnar shaft fractures. Some isolated distal third ulnar shaft fractures can be treated non-operatively with cast or splint immobilization.

73. **Why are fractures of the radius and ulna so frequently operated on?**
Anatomic reduction and fixation of the radius and ulna are important because cadaveric studies have shown that small amounts of malalignment or displacement in either bone have a significant effect on clinical range of motion of the forearm. Working together, the bowed radius rotates around the straight ulna to allow for supination and pronation. Disruption of as little as 10° of either bone can cause a 20° loss of pronation or supination in the forearm. Restoration of the radial bow is essential.

74. **What are the common surgical approaches to the radial shaft?**
The anterior approach (Henry) allows exposure to the whole anterior aspect of the radius and is extensile both proximally and distally. It is used primarily for fractures of the distal two-thirds of the radius. The initial interval is between the brachioradialis and the flexor

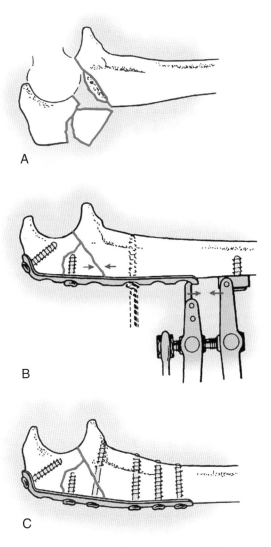

Figure 11.20. (A) Illustration showing a comminuted olecranon fracture. (B) Illustration showing fixation of distal fracture fragments and utilization of a tensioning device to achieve interfragmentary compression. (C) Final fixation construction demonstrating anatomical reduction and fixation. (*Modified from Heim U, Pfeiffer KM: Internal Fixation of Small Fractures, 3rd ed, Berlin, 1988, Springer-Verlag.*)

carpi radialis. Deep, the supinator must be detached to gain access to the proximal third of the radius, whereas the pronator teres, flexor pollicis longus and pronator quadratus may need to be detached to gain access to the distal two-thirds of the radial shaft.

The dorsal approach (Thompson) allows exposure to the posterior aspect of the radius. It is used primarily for middle third radial shaft fractures. The interval between the extensor carpi radialis brevis and extensor digitorum communis is developed. Deep, the abductor pollicis longus and extensor pollicis brevis must be detached and mobilized proximally to gain access to the radius.

75. How are fractures of the radial and ulnar shaft fixed?
Although other fixation devices have been described, plate fixation is the primary means of treating these fractures. Specifically, compression plating of simple fracture patterns, neutralization plating of fractures with anatomic reduction and fixation, and bridge plating of highly comminuted fractures allows a simple plate and screw construct to be used in a variety of ways depending on the morphology of the fracture.

76. What is a night-stick fracture?
A night-stick fracture is an isolated fracture of the ulnar diaphysis, typically in the distal one-third of the shaft. These fractures often result from a direct blow to the ulna. Non-operative treatment of an isolated distal third ulnar shaft fracture consists of cast immobilization or functional bracing as long as displacement does not exceed 50% or 10° of angulation. If these parameters are exceeded, internal fixation is recommended.

77. What is a Monteggia fracture?
A Monteggia fracture is a fracture of the ulna between the proximal third and the base of the olecranon with a concomitant dislocation of the radiocapitellar joint.

78. What are the four types of Monteggia fractures?
Bado classified these fractures based on the direction of the radial head. In Type I lesions, the radial head is dislocated anteriorly, in Type II lesions, the radial head is dislocated posteriorly, in Type III lesions, the radial head is dislocated laterally, and in Type IV lesions there is a dislocation of the radial head associated with a fracture of both the radius and ulna (Fig. 11.21).

79. What is a Galeazzi fracture?
A Galeazzi fracture occurs when a fracture of the radial diaphysis is accompanied by a disruption to the distal radioulnar joint. This can be identified by the presence of an ulnar styloid fracture, shortening of the distal radius or displacement of the distal ulna on the antero-posterior or lateral radiograph of the wrist.

80. When can compartment syndrome occur with fractures of the forearm?
Compartment syndrome can occur any time after the initial injury as well as after surgery because of the swelling and bleeding that can accompany a fracture or surgical intervention. This orthopedic emergency must be monitored closely because of the potentially disastrous sequelae.

DISTAL RADIUS
CASE 11-6

A 70-year-old, left-hand-dominant female falls on an outstretched left hand outside her home. She comes into the office with significant bruising and swelling around the wrist. Radiographs are obtained and show an extra-articular fracture of the distal radius with dorsal displacement.

81. What are the important articular portions (or facets) of the distal radius?
The three weight-bearing articular surfaces of the radius are scaphoid facet, the lunate facet, and sigmoid notch. They articulate with the scaphoid, lunate, and distal ulna, respectively (Fig. 11.22).

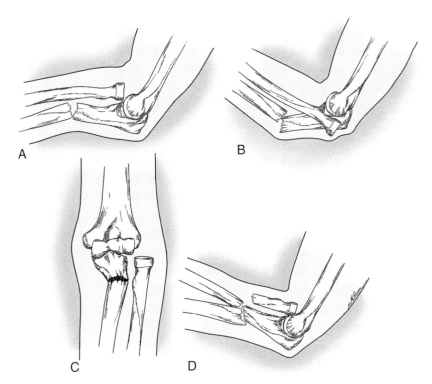

Figure 11.21. Classification of Monteggia fracture–dislocations. (A) Type I, anterior radial head dislocation. (B) Type II, posterior radial head dislocation. (C) Type III, lateral radial head dislocation. (D) Type IV, fracture of both proximal radius and ulna. (*Modified from Crenshaw AH: Adult Fractures and Complex Joint Injuries of the Elbow. In: Stanley D, Kay NRM, eds: Surgery of the Elbow: Practical and Scientific Aspects, London, 1998, Arnold.*)

82. What are the three columns of the wrist and why are these important in the fixation of distal radius fractures?

The three columns of the wrist are: the radial column, the intermediate column, and the ulnar column. The radial column contains the radial styloid and scaphoid facet. This column usually contains relatively dense bone and should be adequately buttressed and be a target for screw placement when plate fixation is used.

The intermediate column contains the lunate facet and sigmoid notch. This column is important, as failure to maintain articular congruity and reduction can lead to altered radiocarpal force transmission, especially through the lunate.

The ulnar column is composed of the distal ulna and ulnar styloid (and its associated soft-tissue attachments).

83. What radiographic parameters must be maintained in the non-operative treatment of distal radius fractures?

Palmar tilt: The normal palmar tilt is approximately 11°. Following reduction, no more than neutral alignment is tolerated.

Radial length: Radial length varies between individuals but shortening greater than 2–3 mm as compared to the contralateral side (if uninjured) is associated with loss of grip strength and pain.

Radial inclination: The normal radial inclination is approximately 22°. Loss of radial inclination greater than 5° is associated with poorer outcomes.

Intra-articular step-off: Articular displacement greater than 2 mm has also been associated with poor clinical outcomes.

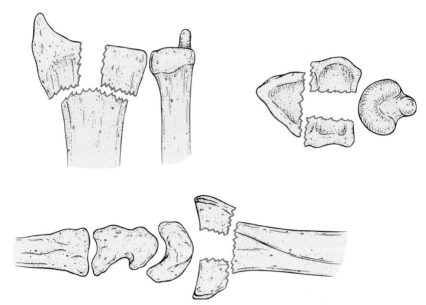

Figure 11.22. Illustration demonstrating the facets of the distal radius. (*From McMurtry RY, Jupiter JB: Fractures of the distal radius. In: Browner BD, Jupiter JB, Levine AM, et al. [eds]: Skeletal Trauma: Fractures, Dislocations, Ligamentous Injuries. Philadelphia, WB Saunders, 1992, p. 1070.*)

84. **What is the dorsal approach to the radius? What is the volar approach to the radius?**
    The dorsal approach to the radius is centered over Lister's tubercle. The extensor retinaculum is incised and the extensor pollicis longus tendon is elevated and retracted medially. The tendons in the fourth dorsal compartment (extensor digitorum communis) are retracted medially, exposing the dorsal aspect of the radius.
    The skin incision for the volar approach is centered over the flexor carpi ulnaris tendon. The tendon sheath is incised and the tendon is retracted ulnarly. This is followed by incision through the dorsal aspect of the same tendon sheath and protection of the radial artery laterally. The pronator quadratus is incised from its radial origin and reflected, exposing the volar surface of the distal radius.

85. **What are surgical treatment options for distal radius fractures?**
    Many different fixation devices are used to treat distal radius fractures. These include: dorsal plates, volar plates, external fixation systems, wires, intramedullary systems, and combinations of these techniques. The preferred approach is based on surgeon preference and fracture morphology. Each has its own benefits and drawbacks.

86. **What is the diagnosis if a patient cannot flex his thumb after volar plating of a distal radius fracture? What is the diagnosis if a patient cannot extend their thumb after non-operative treatment of a distal radius fracture?**
    Rupture of the flexor pollicis longus can occur following volar plating of the distal radius. Rupture of the extensor pollicis longus can occur following non-operative treatment of a minimally displaced distal radius fracture.

87. **What is a chauffeur's fracture?**
    This eponym refers to a fracture of the radial styloid.

88. **What is a Colles' fracture?**
    A Colles' fracture is a dorsally displaced extra-articular fracture of the distal radius.

89. **What is a Smith's fracture?**
A Smith's fracture is a volarly displaced extra- or intra-articular fracture of the distal radius. It is also called a reverse Colles' fracture.

90. **What is a Barton's fracture?**
A Barton's fracture is a fracture–dislocation of the distal radius. It may be displaced either dorsally or volarly, in which case it is called a reverse Barton's.

91. **What structure can be injured in fractures or fracture–dislocations of the distal radioulnar joint?**
The triangular fibrocartilage complex (TFCC) may be damaged in injuries to the distal ulna or ulnar styloid. The complex consists of a triangular fibrocartilaginous structure and the ulnocarpal ligament. Its base is along the sigmoid notch of the radius, and its apex is attached to the ulnar styloid process.

92. **What is the most frequent neurologic complication of distal radius fractures treated both non-operatively and with surgery?**
Acute carpal tunnel syndrome can occur after the initial injury (especially if high energy), reduction and immobilization (especially if multiple attempts are performed or wrist is immobilized in extreme flexion or extension), and surgical fixation (if the carpal tunnel is not released intraoperatively). Patients should be vigilantly monitored for signs and symptoms of median nerve compression.

PELVIS/ACETABULUM/SACRUM

CASE 11-7

A 27-year-old male is brought into the trauma bay after a motor-vehicle collision in which he was an unrestrained passenger. The patient has a variety of injuries to multiple organ systems. As part of his initial trauma workup, an antero-posterior pelvis radiograph is performed which reveals a fracture of the pelvic ring.

93. **What is the Young–Burgess classification of pelvic fractures?**
The Young–Burgess classification describes four different types of pelvic fractures: lateral compression (LC), antero-posterior compression (APC), vertical shear (VS), and combined mechanism. Each mechanism is further broken down into subtypes. An LC1 is an anterior sacral impaction and a horizontal pubic ramus fracture. An LC2 is an anterior sacral impaction with either a posterior iliac wing fracture or posterior sacroiliac ligament disruption. An LC3 is an LC2 with external rotation of the opposite hemipelvis. An APC1 is a pubic diastasis less than 2.5 cm or an isolated pubic rami fracture. An APC2 is a pubic diastasis greater than 2.5 cm with widening of the anterior sacroiliac joint. An APC3 is a pubic diastasis greater than 2.5 cm with complete sacroiliac joint disruption. A vertical shear injury is one with vertical displacement of one side of the pelvis. A combined mechanism of injury is made up of injury patterns from each of the different classes (Fig. 11.23).

94. **What is the Tile classification of pelvic fractures?**
The Tile classification divides fractures into Type A (stable), Type B (rotationally unstable), and Type C (rotationally and vertically unstable). Type A fractures include those fractures not involving the pelvic ring, avulsion fractures, iliac wing fractures, and transverse sacral fractures. Type B fractures consist of isolated anterior pelvic ring disruptions and anterior pelvic disruptions combined with anterior sacroiliac ligament disruption. Type C fractures are those in which the anterior pelvis is disrupted in combination with both anterior and posterior sacroiliac ligament disruption or sacral and posterior ilium fractures (Fig. 11.24).

95. **What additional radiographic views are helpful in evaluating a pelvic fracture?**
Other radiographic views that are helpful in evaluating fractures of the pelvis are pelvic inlet/outlet views. An outlet view is taken with the x-ray beam tilted 45° towards the head of a supine patient. An outlet view helps to determine vertical displacement of the pelvis. It also helps to better evaluate the sacroiliac joints, non-displaced fractures of

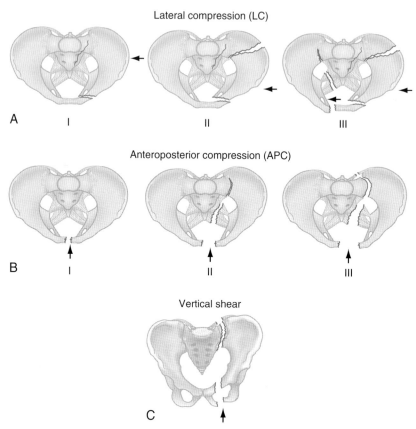

Figure 11.23. Young–Burgess classification. (A) Lateral compression: Types I, II, and III. (B) Antero-posterior (AP) compression: Types I, II, and III. Arrow indicates the direction of force. (*Redrawn from Young JWR, Burgess AR: Radiologic Management of Pelvic Ring Fractures. Baltimore, Munich, Urban & Schwarzenberg, 1987.*)

the sacrum, or sacral foraminal disruption. An inlet view is taken with the x-ray beam tilted 60° towards the feet. The inlet view helps to determine anterior and posterior displacement of the sacroiliac joint, the sacrum, or the iliac wing. It also helps to identify sacral impaction injuries which may otherwise be missed on an antero-posterior view of the pelvis (Fig. 11.25).

96. **What are common non-orthopedic injuries associated with pelvic fractures?**
    Head injuries, thoracic injuries, abdominal injuries, and genitourinary injuries are all commonly present in the setting of a pelvic fracture. Given the high-energy mechanism that is the cause of most pelvic ring injuries, this is not at all surprising.

97. **What is the initial step in stabilization of a patient with an open book pelvic fracture and hypotension?**
    Massive hemorrhage into the pelvis can lead to hypotension, hemorrhagic shock, and ultimately death. This is most common in Young–Burgess APC2, APC3, and LC3 injury patterns. Immediate measures should be taken to decrease the volume of the pelvis and provisionally stabilize it. Immediate interventions include a sheet tied around the greater trochanters or a pelvic binder. Emergent external fixation, application of a C-clamp, or open reduction and internal fixation are options; however, more rapid interventions such

as those listed above should be employed in the interim. If hemorrhage or hypotension continues despite closing down the pelvic volume, one should consider other sources of bleeding and/or angiography for possible arterial embolization.

98. What is the most common injury mechanism responsible for pelvis and acetabular fractures?
Both pelvic and acetabular fractures can be the result of high- or low-energy mechanisms. Low-energy mechanisms are more common in the elderly or those with poor bone quality and often result from a fall from standing. Younger populations are more likely to sustain a pelvic or acetabular injury secondary to a high-energy mechanism such as a motor-vehicle collision.

CASE 11-7 continued

After closer analysis of the AP pelvis radiograph, it is revealed that the patient has an acetabular fracture in addition to the pelvic ring disruption.

99. What are the six radiographic lines identified in reading an antero-posterior radiograph of the pelvis?
The six radiographic lines identified in reading an anterior-posterior pelvis x-ray are: (1) the iliopectineal line, representing the anterior column, (2) the ilioischial line, representing the posterior column, (3) the posterior wall, which is the more lateral of the acetabular walls on the antero-posterior view, (4) the anterior wall, which is the more medial of the acetabular walls on the antero-posterior view, (5) the sourcil or weight-bearing portion of the acetabulum, and (6) the teardrop (Fig. 11.26).

100. What is the most common system used to classify acetabular fractures? Name the different fracture patterns in this classification system.
The Judet–Letournel classification is the most commonly used classification system to describe acetabular fractures. Acetabular fractures are divided into two groups, elementary

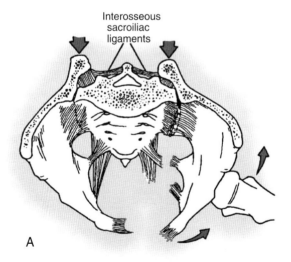

Interosseous
sacroiliac
ligaments

A

Figure 11.24. Tile classification of pelvic fractures based on forces acting on the pelvis. (A) Type B1: external rotation or antero-posterior compression. (B) Type B2-1: lateral compression (internal rotation) force implodes hemipelvis. (C) Type C: shearing (translational) force disrupts symphysis, pelvic floor, and posterior structures. (*From Tile M: Acute pelvic fractures. I. Causation and classification, J Am Assoc Orthop Surg 4:143, 1996.*)

Continued

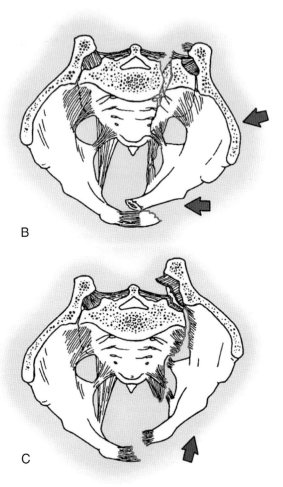

B

C

Figure 11.24, continued

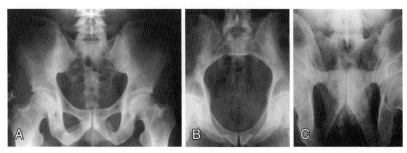

Figure 11.25. Normal views of the pelvis. AP (A), outlet (B) and inlet (C) views of the pelvis. (*Modified from Adam A, et al., [eds], Grainger & Allison's Diagnostic Radiology: A Textbook of Medical Imaging, 5th ed, Copyright © 2008, Elsevier Ltd.*)

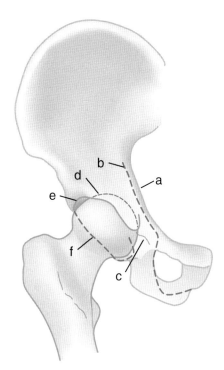

Figure 11.26. Radiographic lines evaluated on the AP pelvis view: (a) iliopectineal line, (b) ilioischial line, (c) teardrop, (d) acetabular roof, (e) anterior wall, and (f) posterior wall. (*Redrawn from Rogers LF, Novy SB, Harris NF: Occult central fractures of the acetabulum. AJR Am J Roentgenol 124:98, 1975.*)

fracture patterns and associated fracture patterns. Elementary fracture patterns are the result of a single fracture line, while associated fracture patterns have more than one fracture line.

101. What are the Judet–Letournel elementary fracture patterns?
     The elementary fracture patterns are posterior wall, posterior column, anterior wall, anterior column, and transverse (Fig. 11.27).

102. What are the Judet–Letournel associated fracture patterns?
     The associated fracture patterns are t-type, posterior column and posterior wall, transverse and posterior wall, anterior column and posterior hemi-transverse, and associated both columns (Fig. 11.27).

103. What additional radiographic views are indicated to evaluate acetabular fractures?
     Judet views are extremely helpful in characterizing acetabular fractures. The two Judet views are called the iliac oblique and the obturator oblique. The obturator oblique view is taken with the affected hip elevated 45° off the bed and the x-ray beam directed through the hip joint. The iliac oblique view is taken with the affected hip down and the uninjured side elevated 45° off the bed and the x-ray beam directed through the hip joint (Fig. 11.28).

104. What does CT add to the diagnosis of acetabular fractures?
     Most acetabular fractures can be characterized by an antero-posterior pelvis and Judet views. A CT is helpful in determining the number of fracture fragments, orientation of the fracture lines, displacement of the fracture, direction and rotation of fracture displacement, presence of marginal impaction, or presence of incarcerated fragments in the hip joint. A CT is absolutely essential to preoperative planning.

Elementary fracture types

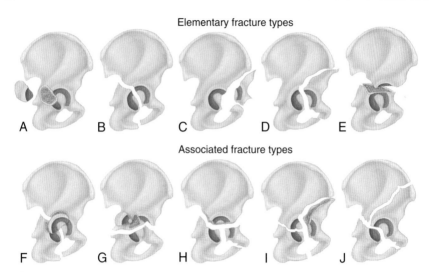

Associated fracture types

Figure 11.27. Letournel and Judet classification of acetabular fractures. (A) Posterior wall fracture. (B) Posterior column fracture. (C) Anterior wall fracture. (D) Anterior column fracture. (E) Transverse fracture. (F) Posterior column and posterior wall fracture. (G) Transverse and posterior wall fracture. (H) T-shaped fracture. (I) Anterior column and posterior hemitransverse fracture. (J) Complete both-column fracture. (*Redrawn from Letournel E, Judet R: Fractures of the Acetabulum, New York, 1981, Springer-Verlag.*)

105. **What are long-term sequelae of acetabular fractures?**
Long-term sequelae of acetabular fractures include avascular necrosis of the femoral head, post-traumatic arthritis, heterotopic ossification, and persistent pain. Quality of reduction is thought to correlate with outcomes, meaning the more anatomic the reduction is, the better the patient's final outcome.

106. **What is the goal in surgical fixation of acetabular fractures?**
The goals of surgical fixation of acetabular fractures are stabilization of the various fracture fragments, anatomic reduction of the articular surface, and recreation of a stable, concentric hip joint.

107. **What nerves are most commonly injured in acetabular fracture fixation?**
Nerve injuries vary based on the fracture pattern and the surgical approach used for fixation. The sciatic nerve is most at risk with posterior approaches such as the Kocher–Langenbeck approach. The peroneal branch of the sciatic nerve is more commonly involved than the tibial branch. The femoral nerve and lateral femoral cutaneous nerve of the thigh are both at risk with anterior approaches such as the ilioinguinal approach.

108. **What is the classification of sacral fractures?**
The most common classification used for sacral fractures is the Denis classification which divides the sacrum into three zones. Zone I fractures occur lateral to the sacral foramina. Zone II fractures are transforaminal, meaning the fracture line goes through the foramen. Zone III fractures are medial to the foramina and extend into the spinal canal. The classification is based on the location of the most medial part of the fracture (Fig. 11.29).

109. **What sacral fracture pattern is associated with the highest rate of neurologic injury?**
Denis Zone III sacral fractures have the highest associated incidence of neurologic injury.

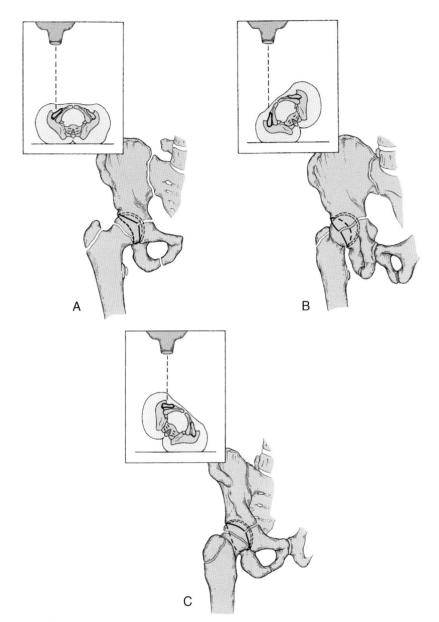

Figure 11.28. Schematics of three radiographic views necessary for assessment of acetabular fractures. (A) The antero-posterior pelvis (or hip) view allows assessment of the iliopectineal line, the ilium, the anterior and posterior walls, and the pubis. (B) The iliac oblique view of Judet allows optimal assessment of the ischial spine and the posterior column and wall, as well as the iliac fossae. (C) The obturator oblique view of Judet allows optimal assessment of the iliac wing, anterior column, and anterior wall. (*From Swiontkowski MF, Fractures and Dislocations About the Hip and Pelvis: Green NE, Swiontkowski MF (eds), Skeletal Trauma in Children, 4th ed, Saunders, 2009.*)

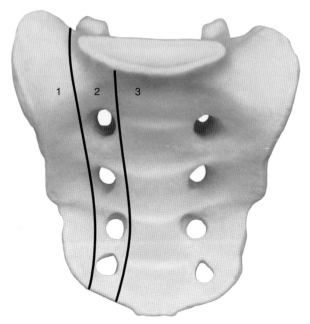

Figure 11.29. Denis classification of sacral fractures. (*From Bellabarba C, Schildhauer TA, Chapman JR. Management of Sacral Fractures. In: Quiñones-Hinojosa A (ed), Schmidek and Sweet Operative Neurosurgical Techniques, 6th ed. Philadelphia, WB Saunders.*)

HIP DISLOCATIONS

CASE 11-8

A 28-year-old female is brought in by fire rescue after being a restrained front seat passenger in a motor-vehicle collision. She was non-ambulatory at the scene and is currently on a stretcher. You notice her right leg appears slightly shorter than her left leg and that her foot is also internally rotated. The patient recalls her knees hitting the front of the dashboard during the collision.

110. **What is the most common type of hip dislocation?**
Posterior hip dislocations are the most common and make up about 90% of hip dislocations with anterior dislocations being the next most common.

111. **What is the mechanism of injury for a posterior hip dislocation?**
Posterior hip dislocations most often result from an axially directed force on a flexed knee. This often occurs when a passenger's knee strikes the dashboard in a motor-vehicle collision. Other common mechanisms of injury include a fall from a height, industrial accident, or motorcycle collision.

112. **What are the different types of anterior hip dislocation? What are their mechanisms?**
Anterior hip dislocations can be further broken up into inferior or obturator dislocations and superior or pubic/iliac dislocations. Inferior dislocations are the result of abduction, external rotation, and hip flexion. Superior dislocations are the result of abduction, external rotation, and hip extension.

113. **Why is dislocation of a native hip an orthopedic emergency?**
Native hip dislocations are an orthopedic emergency because the rate of avascular necrosis following hip dislocation is related to the amount of time the hip remains dislocated. The longer the time interval from injury to reduction, the higher the risk is of developing

subsequent avascular necrosis. The goal should be to have a dislocated native hip reduced within 6 hours of the injury.

114. What is the maneuver for reduction of a posterior hip dislocation?
The most commonly used maneuver for posterior hip dislocation is the Allis method. The person responsible for the reduction will be standing/kneeling above the patient on the stretcher while an assistant stabilizes the pelvis. Axial traction is applied to the affected limb as the hip is flexed to 90°. The leg is then internally rotated and adducted to allow the femoral head to clear the posterior lip of the acetabulum. An audible clunk can often be heard as the femoral head reduces into the acetabulum. After reduction is achieved, the affected limb should be externally rotated and abducted to prevent repeat dislocation of an unstable hip (Fig. 11.30).

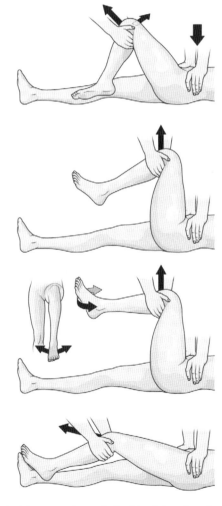

Figure 11.30. Allis method for reducing posterior hip dislocation. (*From DeLee JC: Fractures and Dislocations of the Hip. In: Rockwood CA, Green DP [eds]: Fractures in Adults, vol 2. Philadelphia, JB Lippincott, 1991, p. 1594. Reproduced by permission.*)

115. What is the most common neurologic injury seen in posterior hip dislocations?
The most common neurologic injury seen in posterior hip dislocations is sciatic nerve injury. This is the result of impingement of the nerve by the posteriorly

dislocated femoral head and is more common in fracture–dislocations than in pure dislocations.

116. **What injury must be ruled out before attempting to reduce a dislocated hip?**
Before attempting to reduce a dislocated hip, one must be certain to rule out a non-displaced femoral neck fracture, as manipulation may lead to displacement of the fracture and increased risk of development of avascular necrosis.

117. **What other injuries should be looked for in posterior hip dislocations?**
Most hip dislocations are the result of high-energy trauma and a full trauma workup should be completed to rule out head injuries, thoracic injuries, abdominal injuries, and genitourinary injuries, as well as other orthopedic injuries.

118. **In what position would you observe a patient's leg after a posterior hip dislocation? Anterior hip dislocation?**
After sustaining a posterior hip dislocation, the affected leg will be shortened, adducted, and internally rotated. After sustaining an anterior hip dislocation, the affected leg will be abducted, externally rotated, and either flexed (inferior dislocation) or extended (superior dislocation).

119. **What is avascular necrosis?**
Avascular necrosis is the death of bone and bone marrow cells in the femoral head that results from ischemia. The final common pathway is decreased perfusion to the femoral head which can be the result of several different processes including mechanical disruption secondary to trauma, thrombosis secondary to hypercoagulable state, embolic event secondary to arterial or fat emboli, or idiopathic. Other causes of avascular necrosis of the femoral head include alcohol abuse, systemic chemotherapy, Caisson's disease, and anabolic steroids.

120. **What is the classification of avascular necrosis of the hip?**
Both the Ficat classification and the Steinberg classification are used for classifying avascular necrosis of the hip. The Steinberg classification is a modification of the Ficat classification.
    Ficat classification:
0: Normal x-ray, normal MRI/bone scan
I: Normal x-ray, abnormal MRI/bone scan
II: X-ray with sclerosis but no collapse
III: X-ray with subchondral collapse
IV: X-ray with flattening of femoral head
V: X-ray showing narrowing of joint
VI: X-ray showing advanced degenerative changes.
    Steinberg classification:
I: Normal x-ray, abnormal MRI/bone scan
II: X-ray with sclerosis but no collapse
III: X-ray with subchondral collapse
IV: X-ray with flattening of femoral head.
    Stages I–IV of the Steinberg are the same as the Ficat system with the addition of a modifier:
A: <15% involvement of the femoral head
B: 15–30% involvement of the femoral head
C: >30% involvement in the femoral head.
    Stage V is an x-ray showing narrowing of the joint with the addition of a modifier:
A: Mild joint space narrowing with or without acetabular changes
B: Moderate joint space narrowing with or without acetabular changes
C: Severe joint space narrowing with or without acetabular changes.

FEMUR

PROXIMAL FEMUR

CASE 11-9

A 34-year-old male fell three stories off scaffolding while washing windows at work. He does not recall how he landed, but was unable to ambulate following the accident. He outwardly appears to have no significant injuries; however, on exam he complains of severe pain in his right hip with minimal range of motion in any direction. Radiographs of the right hip reveal a fracture of the right femoral neck.

121. What is the blood supply to the femoral head and neck?

The blood supply to the femoral neck is comprised of three main vessels. The medial femoral circumflex artery by way of the lateral epiphyseal artery supplies most of the superior weight bearing portion of the femoral head. The lateral femoral circumflex artery supplies a portion of the anterior and inferior femoral head. The ligamentum teres supplies a small portion of the femoral head that is not sufficient to maintain perfusion in the setting of a displaced femoral neck fracture.

122. What initial imaging studies should be obtained when a femoral neck fracture is suspected?

An antero-posterior and lateral radiograph of the affected hip should be obtained as well as an antero-posterior pelvis radiograph. An antero-posterior pelvis can be helpful in evaluating native hip morphology and for preoperative templating. If the x-rays are non-diagnostic and the concern for fracture is still high, a CT scan of the affected hip can be helpful. In the setting of normal x-rays and CT scan, an MRI can help in identifying stress reactions and non-displaced stress fractures.

123. What is the classification of femoral neck fractures?

There are several systems used to classify femoral neck fractures based on location, displacement, and angle of the fracture line.

An anatomic classification system divides femoral neck fractures into subcapital (just proximal to the femoral head), transcervical (through the midportion of the femoral neck), and basicervical (just distal to the junction of the femoral neck and intertrochanteric region).

The Garden classification is based on the amount of valgus displacement of the fracture:

Type I: Incomplete fracture with valgus impaction

Type II: Complete fracture but non-displaced

Type III: Complete fracture with partial displacement, discontinuity of the femoral head and neck trabeculae on x-ray

Type IV: Complete fracture with total displacement, trabeculae of femoral head become parallel to trabeculae in acetabulum.

Types I and II are considered non-displaced. Types III and IV are considered displaced.

The Pauwel classification is based on the angle of the fracture line from the horizontal:

Type I: 30°

Type II: 50°

Type III: 70° (Fig. 11.31).

124. What is the most common complication following femoral neck fracture?

The most common complication following femoral neck fracture is avascular necrosis of the femoral head. Other complications include varus collapse, nonunion, and hardware failure following fixation.

125. Why is a femoral neck fracture in an adolescent a surgical emergency?

A femoral neck fracture in an adolescent is considered a surgical emergency in order to reduce the risk of avascular necrosis of the femoral head. Anatomic reduction, either open or closed with internal fixation must take place as soon as possible. The greater the time from initial injury and the greater the displacement of the fracture, the greater the chance of subsequent development of avascular necrosis.

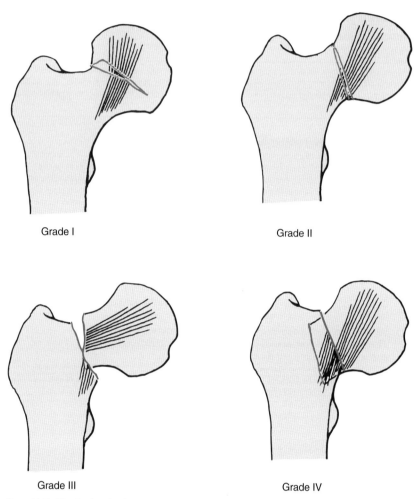

Grade I

Grade II

Grade III

Grade IV

Figure 11.31. The Garden classification of femoral neck fractures. (*Modified from Browner BD, et al. [eds], Skeletal Trauma, 4th ed, p. 1855. Copyright © 2009, Saunders, Elsevier Inc.*)

126. **What surgical interventions are most commonly used for femoral neck fractures?**

There are multiple options for surgical fixation in femoral neck fractures. The reduction can be achieved either open or closed based on the fracture pattern and degree of displacement. Screw fixation in an inverted triangular configuration is a commonly used method, as are the dynamic hip screw and cephalomedullary femoral nails. In elderly populations, hemiarthroplasty or total hip arthroplasty is also an option when fractures are displaced or there is pre-existing hip arthritis.

127. **What is the classification of femoral head fractures?**

The most commonly used classification system for femoral head fractures is the Pipkin classification. The Pipkin classification assumes that the femoral head fracture is the result of a hip dislocation, as hip dislocations are almost always present in the setting of femoral head fractures.

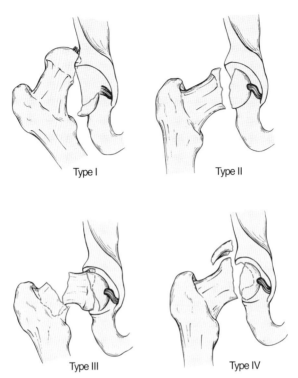

Figure 11.32. Pipkin classification system of femoral head fractures. (*Modified from Browner BD, et al. [eds], Skeletal Trauma, 4th ed, Copyright © 2009, Saunders, Elsevier Inc.*)

Pipkin classification:
Type I: Fracture inferior to the fovea capitas femoris/ligamentum
Type II: Fracture superior to fovea capitis femoris/ligamentum
Type III: Type I or II with associated femoral neck fracture
Type IV: Type I or II with any acetabular rim fracture (Fig. 11.32).

CASE 11-10

A 73-year-old lady presents to the Emergency Room after falling in her bathroom earlier in the evening. She reports that she slipped on some water and fell directly onto her left side. Since that time she has not been able to ambulate and complains of severe pain in her left hip. Radiographs of the left hip show a fracture line running between the greater trochanter and the lesser trochanter.

128. **What is the difference between an intertrochanteric fracture and a pertrochanteric fracture?**
Intertrochanteric and pertrochanteric fractures are not the same thing. A true intertrochanteric fracture has a fracture line that passes between the two trochanters, meaning above the lesser trochanter medially and below the crest of the vastus lateralis laterally. A pertrochanteric fracture starts laterally anywhere on the greater trochanter and exits the medial cortex either proximal or distal to the lesser trochanter.

129. **What is the Evan's classification of intertrochanteric femur fractures?**
The Evan's classification divides intertrochanteric fractures into stable and unstable patterns. In stable patterns, the posteromedial cortex remains relatively intact with either no or minimal comminution. Unstable patterns have significant comminution in the

posteromedial cortex, are reverse obliquity, or have extension into the subtrochanteric region.

130. **What surgical interventions are most commonly used for intertrochanteric femur fractures?**

Intertrochanteric femur fractures are most commonly stabilized with either a dynamic hip scew or a cephalomedullary femoral nail. Stable fracture patterns are amenable to fixation with either a dynamic hip screw or a cephalomedullary nail, while unstable fractures patterns that are either reverse obliquity or have subtrochanteric extension are better stabilized with a cephalomedullary nail. Other options include a calcar replacing hip prosthesis or a proximal femoral replacement for severe fractures or those that have failed prior fixation.

131. **What is the tip apex distance?**

The tip–apex distance is the sum of the distance between the apex of the femoral head and the distal extent of the cephalomedullary lag screw in both the antero-posterior and lateral views. To reduce the risk of screw cutout, the sum of these distances should be less than 25 mm (Fig. 11.33).

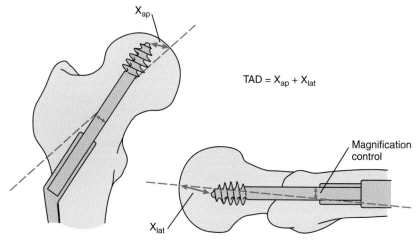

$$TAD = X_{ap} + X_{lat}$$

Figure 11.33. Measurement of the tip-apex distance (TAD). (*Redrawn from Baumgaertner MR, Curtin SL, Lindskog DM, et al. J Bone Joint Surg Am 77:1058–1064, 1995.*)

132. **What are common complications following internal fixation of intertrochanteric femur fractures?**

Loss of fixation is one of the most common complications following stabilization of intertrochanteric femur fractures. This often presents with varus collapse of the proximal fragment and lag screw cutout from the femoral head. This is most commonly caused by poor placement of the lag screw, unstable reduction, excessive fracture collapse, or extremely poor bone quality. Other complications include nonunion, malrotation, lag screw migration into the pelvis and, rarely, avascular necrosis of the femoral head.

CASE 11-11

A 17-year-old male is brought into the trauma bay after being struck by a car while riding his bike. The boy complains of severe pain in his left thigh and has a visible deformity in his proximal thigh. Radiographs reveal a displaced fracture of the proximal femur just distal to the lesser trochanter.

133. **What is a subtrochanteric femur fracture?**

A subtrochanteric femur fracture is a fracture of the femur within 5 cm of the distal extent of the lesser trochanter.

134. **What are the deforming forces on the proximal segment of a subtrochanteric femur fracture?**
The deforming forces on the proximal segment of a subtrochanteric femur fracture lead to a deformity consisting of flexion, external rotation, and abduction. The iliopsoas causes the proximal segment to go into flexion and external rotation. The hip abductors cause the proximal segment to go into abduction. The short external rotators also contribute to the external rotation of the proximal fragment.

135. **What is the most common treatment for subtrochanteric femur fractures?**
The most common treatment for subtrochanteric femur fractures is intramedullary nailing. Fixed angle blade plates are also used, but not as frequently.

FEMORAL SHAFT

CASE 11-12

A 25-year-old male is brought into the trauma bay by fire rescue after being struck by a car while crossing a street near the hospital. The patient has a gross deformity of his right thigh with a significant amount of swelling. A femur fracture is suspected; however, radiographs have not yet been obtained.

136. **What is the most common mechanism of injury in a femoral shaft fracture?**
Femoral shaft fractures are most commonly the result of high-energy trauma, often from motor-vehicle accidents, motorcycle accidents, fall from extreme heights, or pedestrians struck by vehicles. Femoral shaft fractures can also result from a fall from standing, especially in the elderly population. Stress fractures of the femoral shaft from overuse are not common, but do occur. Finally, femoral shaft fractures can result from a pathologic fracture as a result of a primary bone tumor or bony metastases.

137. **What is one common classification system for femoral shaft fractures?**
The Winquist and Hansen classification of femoral shaft fractures uses amount of comminution to define femoral shaft fractures:
Type 0: No comminution
Type I: Minimal comminution
Type II: At least 50% of cortical contact with butterfly fragment
Type III: Less than 50% cortical contact
Type IV: Circumferential comminution with no cortical contact.
    More commonly, femoral shaft fractures are defined by whether they are open or closed, fracture location (proximal, middle, or distal third), the fracture pattern (spiral, oblique, or transverse), cortical comminution, and angulation (Fig. 11.34).

138. **Which is the compression and which is the tension side of the femur?**
The medial cortex of the femur experiences compressive forces while the lateral cortex experiences tensile forces.

139. **What must be ruled out before traction is applied to a femoral shaft fracture?**
Similar to a closed reduction attempt in a dislocated hip, a femoral neck fracture should always be ruled out before traction is applied.

140. **How often do ipsilateral femoral neck and femoral shaft fractures occur?**
Simultaneous ipsilateral femoral neck fractures occur anywhere from 3% to 10% of the time with femoral shaft fractures. Concomitant femoral neck fractures must always be looked for and ruled out in the setting of a femoral shaft fracture. The femoral neck fracture is often non-displaced and is often vertically oriented.

141. **What are the different types of traction that can be employed to help reduce a femoral shaft fracture?**
Different types of traction include skin traction, Bucks traction, Hare traction, and skeletal traction. Skin traction should not usually exceed 10 pounds to avoid soft-tissue complications. Bucks traction employs a soft splint or dressing about the lower extremity with an attached weight; however, weight should not exceed 10 pounds. Hare traction involves a harness around the ankle and a lever fit against the ischial tuberosity with a ratchet system to sequentially increase the amount of traction. This is often applied in the

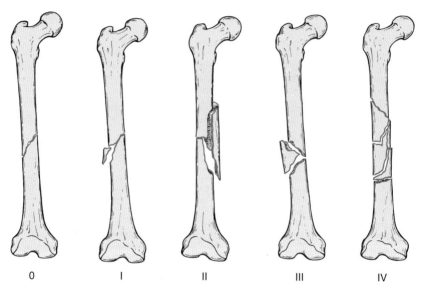

Figure 11.34. Winquist–Hansen classification of femoral shaft comminution. (*Modified from Browner BD, et al. [eds], Skeletal Trauma, 4th ed, Copyright © 2009, Saunders, Elsevier Inc.*)

field and commercially available traction splints are available to first responders. These are often used as a temporizing measure until a skeletal traction pin can be placed. Skeletal traction can accommodate more weight and is the preferred choice for long bone, acetabulum, and pelvic fractures prior to operative fixation. Skeletal traction requires the placement of a transosseous pin to accommodate a traction bow and subsequent weight.

CASE 11-12   continued

After discussing the case with the attending physician, the orthopedic resident on call places a traction pin to help reduce the fracture prior to surgical fixation.

142. Where should a distal femoral traction pin be placed? Where should a proximal tibial traction pin be placed?
A distal femoral traction pin should be placed from medial to lateral in order to protect the medial neurovascular bundle at Hunter's canal. The starting point should be at the adductor tubercle, just proximal to the medial epicondyle. The trajectory should be parallel to the joint line.
    A proximal tibial traction pin should be placed from lateral to medial in order to protect the common peroneal nerve. The starting point should be 2 cm distal and 1 cm posterior to the tibial tubercle with a trajectory parallel to the joint line.
    Radiographs on the knee should be obtained prior to traction pin placement to rule out fractures of the distal femur or proximal tibia.

143. What are the surgical options for femoral shaft fractures?
Surgical options include intramedullary nailing, external fixation, and plate fixation.

144. What are the advantages of intramedullary nailing over plate fixation?
Intramedullary nails can be inserted percutaneously and have the advantage of a less extensive exposure and dissection and lower infection rates. Intramedullary nailing also

does not disrupt the fracture hematoma and reaming can lead to deposition of biologic growth factors at the fracture site.

145. **What are the different types of intramedullary femoral nails?**
Intramedullary femoral nails can be either antegrade or retrograde. Antegrade intramedullary nails are divided further into trochanteric and piriformis nails based on their starting point.

146. **What are the indications for retrograde intramedullary nailing?**
Retrograde intramedullary femoral nails (placed through the knee joint) have the advantage of easy identification of the starting point and the disadvantage of violating the often uninvolved knee joint. Relative indications for retrograde nails include ipsilateral proximal femur, tibia, or acetabular injuries, bilateral femoral shaft fractures, obese patients, and periprosthetic fracture above a total knee arthroplasty.

DISTAL FEMUR
CASE 11-13

A 64-year-old man presents to the Emergency Room after falling 12 feet off a ladder. He reports having severe pain upon landing on his feet. Over the last several hours his knee has become increasingly more swollen and he is unable to bear any weight on his left lower extremity. A radiograph of the knee reveals a comminuted fracture of the distal femur.

147. **What is the classification of distal femur fractures?**
There is no widely used classification system to describe distal femur fractures, and most fractures are classified by location (supracondylar, intercondylar, or condylar), pattern (spiral, oblique, or transverse), comminution, articular involvement, displacement, and angulation.

148. **Where does a supracondylar femur fracture occur?**
A supracondylar femur fracture occurs between the femoral condyles and the junction of the femoral diaphysis and distal metaphysis. This region is usually between 10 cm and 15 cm in length.

149. **What is a Hoffa fracture?**
A Hoffa fracture is a fracture in the coronal plane through the femoral condyle. Hoffa fractures are often missed on plain radiographs and are indicative of a high-energy mechanism. A CT is necessary for complete fracture characterization and preoperative planning.

CASE 11-14

A 15-year-old male football player is brought to the Emergency Room after sustaining an injury to his left lower extremity during a football game earlier in the evening. He reports that his foot was planted in the turf when an opposing player delivered a blow with his helmet to the anterior aspect of his leg. The patient's knee looks deformed with the tibia sagging more posteriorly than normal. Emergent radiographs reveal a posteriorly dislocated knee.

150. **What is the most common type of knee dislocation?**
The most common type of knee dislocation is posterior dislocation of the tibia in relationship to the femur. Anterior dislocations as well as lateral, medial, and posterolateral dislocations also occur (Fig. 11.35).

151. **What is the initial management of a knee dislocation?**
Initial management of knee dislocation should include immediate closed reduction followed by stabilization with a knee immobilizer or an external fixator.

152. **What is crucial to examination of the patient with a knee dislocation?**
Thorough and serial vascular examinations should be performed on any patient with a knee dislocation. Frequent pulse checks should be performed as well as Ankle–Brachial Index (ABI) measurements. An ABI <0.9 is often used as the threshold for further workup to evaluate for vascular injury.

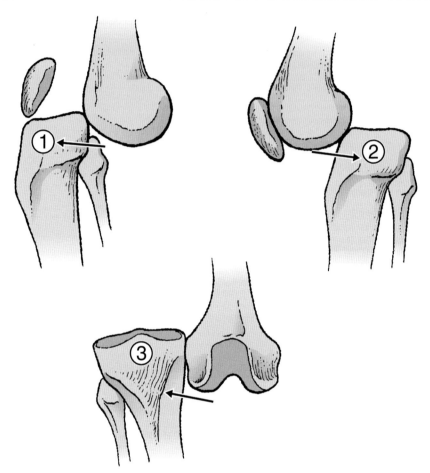

Figure 11.35. Three most common types of knee dislocations. Anterior (1), posterior (2), and lateral (3). (*From DePalma AF: Management of Fractures and Dislocations: An Atlas. Philadelphia, WB Saunders, 1970, p. 1621. Reproduced by permission.*)

The rate of associated vascular injury is high, and there should be a low threshold for additional imaging including angiography, CT angiography, or MR angiography. Arterial thrombosis resulting from an intimal injury can present up to 24–72 hours after the initial injury.

TIBIA/ANKLE

PROXIMAL TIBIA/TIBIAL SHAFT

CASE 11-15

A 37-year-old female presents to the Emergency Room after being struck by a car while riding her bicycle to work. She reports some pain in her left knee and has been unable to bear any weight on her left lower extremity since the accident. On exam she has extreme tenderness to palpation over her lateral joint line. A radiograph of her left knee reveals a tibial plateau fracture.

153. What is the classification for tibial plateau fractures?

The Schatzker classification is the most commonly used classification system to describe tibial plateau fractures:

Type I: Lateral tibial plateau split fracture

Type II: Lateral tibial plateau split depression fracture

Type III: Lateral tibial plateau depression fracture

Type IV: Medial tibial plateau split and/or depression

Type V: Bicondylar tibial plateau fracture

Type VI: Bicondylar tibial plateau fracture with dissociation of the metaphysis from the diaphysis (Fig. 11.36).

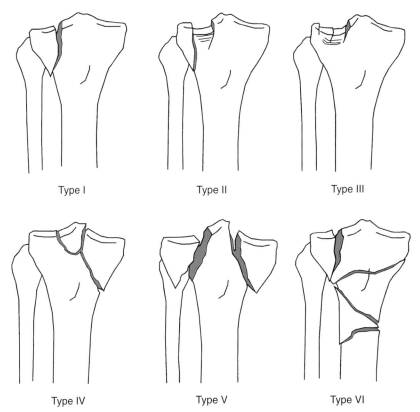

Figure 11.36. Schatzker classification of tibial plateau fractures. (*From Virkus WW, Helfet DL: Tibial Plateau Fractures. In: JN Insall, WN Scott [eds]: Surgery of the Knee, 3rd ed. New York, Churchill Livingstone, 2001, p. 1268.*)

154. Which tibial plateau patterns are considered high-energy injuries and which patterns are considered low-energy mechanisms?

Schatzker Types I–III are considered low-energy injuries. Schatzker Types IV–VI are considered high-energy injuries.

155. In addition to a routine neurovascular exam, what other diagnosis is important to consider in a patient with a tibial plateau fracture?

All patients who sustain a tibial plateau fracture should be ruled out for compartment syndrome. Evaluation should include serial neurovascular exams as well as serial evaluations for compartment syndrome. The classic Ps of compartment syndrome are pain out of proportion to exam, pain with passive stretch, pallor, pulselessness, increased pressure, and paresthesias/paresis. Importantly, increased complaint of pain and pain with passive stretch of the extremity are the early warning signs of compartment syndrome and should be used to make the diagnosis prior to the occurrence of the other "Ps". Patients who are obtunded or sedated may need further evaluation with intracompartmental pressure measurements.

156. **What is the treatment for acute compartment syndrome?**
Emergent four compartment decompressive fasciotomy.

157. **What is initial management of a severely comminuted, shortened, or deformed tibial plateau fracture?**
Initial management of a severely comminuted, shortened, or deformed tibial plateau fracture is application of an external fixator. When length is restored, fracture pattern can be better defined and ligamentotaxis can aide in fracture reduction. Acute open reduction and internal fixation in severe tibial plateau fractures often leads to soft-tissue complications and should be avoided.

158. **When should a CT scan be obtained in the workup of a tibial plateau fracture?**
Plain radiographs should be the first imaging study obtained when evaluating a suspected tibial plateau fracture. In instances when plain radiography is either non-diagnostic or there is a minimally displaced fracture, a CT scan can be obtained immediately to guide definitive treatment and for preoperative planning. In the case of a highly comminuted, displaced tibial plateau fracture, an external fixator should be applied prior to obtaining a CT.

159. **What are radiographic signs that could indicate ligamentous injury in a tibial plateau fracture?**
Fibular head avulsion, the Segond sign (capsular avulsion off the lateral proximal tibia), and a Pellegrini–Stieda lesion (calcification at the insertion of the MCL at the medial femoral epicondyle) are all signs of ligamentous injury. Fibular avulsion is indicative of posterolateral corner injury, Segond sign of an ACL injury, and a Pellegrini–Stieda lesion of an MCL injury.

160. **What are the indications for surgical fixation of a tibial plateau fracture?**
Indications for fixation of a tibial plateau fracture are articular incongruity of greater than 2 mm, instability greater than 10° in an extended knee, open fractures, fractures with an associated compartment syndrome, and fractures with an associated vascular injury.

161. **What dictates when tibial plateau fractures should be definitely fixed?**
Local soft-tissue condition should dictate when a tibial plateau fracture can be definitely fixed. Operating through a suboptimal soft-tissue envelope can lead to wound complications, deep infections, and osteomyelitis.

162. **When is non-operative management indicated in a tibial plateau fracture?**
Non-operative treatment of tibial plateau fractures is indicated in non-displaced or minimally displaced fractures in patients with severe osteoporosis and low functional status.

CASE 11-16

A 25-year-old male college student presents to the Emergency Room complaining of severe pain in his left leg. The patient reportedly jumped 8 feet from a rooftop to the ground. On exam, he has a marked deformity of the left leg with skin tenting over the anterior aspect of tibia. You assume there is a tibial shaft fracture based on your initial assessment.

163. **What is the most common mechanism for a tibial shaft fracture?**
Tibia fractures are most commonly the result of direct high-energy trauma such as that sustained in a motor-vehicle accident, motorcycle accident, or pedestrian versus automobile accident. Other mechanisms of injury include penetrating injuries such as

gunshot wounds and twisting injuries similar to those that cause severe ankle injuries. Falls from extreme heights can also result in tibial shaft fractures.

164. **What deformity is seen in a proximal third tibial shaft fracture?**
In a proximal third tibial shaft fracture, the deformity is varus alignment with apex anterior angulation. If these deformities are not adequately addressed, the fracture will go on to malunion.

165. **What treatment options exist for tibial shaft fracture?**
Non-operative management is always an option for any fracture. Long leg casting with the knee in slight flexion can lead to high rates of union if an acceptable and stable reduction is achieved. Operative interventions include intramedullary nailing, external fixation, and plate fixation.

166. **In spiral fractures of the middle or distal tibia shaft, what must be evaluated prior to surgical intervention?**
The ankle joint should always be evaluated prior to operative fixation in spiral fractures of the distal tibia. It must be insured that the fracture line does not extend into the ankle mortise. If this fracture is missed, intramedullary nailing could lead to further displacement and possible malreduction.

167. **What is the most common postoperative complication associated with intramedullary tibial nailing?**
Knee pain is the most common complication associated with intramedullary tibial nailing.

168. **What should be ruled out in all tibial shaft fractures both preoperatively and postoperatively?**
Similarly to tibial plateau fractures, all patients who sustain a tibial shaft fracture should be ruled out for compartment syndrome. Evaluation should include serial neurovascular exams as well as serial evaluations for compartment syndrome.

ANKLE/DISTAL TIBIA
CASE 11-17

A 45-year-old female presents to the Emergency Department after twisting her left ankle while walking down the stairs in her home yesterday evening. She reports that she heard and felt a pop in her ankle and that it started to swell almost immediately after the injury. She has been using an old set of crutches since the injury because she has been unable to bear weight on her left foot.

169. **What initial radiographic views are necessary to work up a suspected ankle fracture? How is a mortise view obtained?**
An antero-posterior, lateral, and mortise view of the ankle should be obtained. The mortise view is an antero-posterior radiograph taken with the foot in 15° to 20° of internal rotation.

170. **What is the Lauge–Hansen classification for ankle fractures?**
The Lauge–Hansen classification is based on the mechanism of injury and the position of the foot at the time of injury:
Supination adduction (SAD):
    I: Transverse distal fibula avulsion fracture or rupture of talofibular ligaments
    II: Vertical medial malleolus fracture with a transverse distal fibula fracture and possible medial plafond impaction
Supination external rotation (SER):
    I: Anterior inferior tibiofibular ligament sprain
    II: Short oblique fracture of the distal fibula (Weber B)
    III: Type II with a posterior malleolus fracture or disruption of the posterior tibiofibular ligament
    IV: Type III with medial malleolus fracture or deltoid ligament disruption
Pronation external rotation (PER):
    I: Medial malleolus fracture or disruption of the deltoid ligament
    II: Anterior tibiofibular ligament disruption or fracture of Chaput's tubercle
    III: Type I with associated high fibula fracture (Weber C)
    IV: Type III with a posterior malleolus fracture or posterior tibiofibular ligament disruption

Pronation abduction (PAB):
I: Medial malleolus fracture or deltoid ligament disruption
II: Anterior tibiofibular ligament disruption or fracture of Chaput's tubercle
III: Type I with associated transverse or comminuted fibula fracture.

171. **What is the Danis–Weber classification for fibula fractures?**
The Danis–Weber fibular fracture classification system is based on the location of the fracture relative to the syndesmosis. The more proximal on the fibula the fracture is located, the more likely that there is a syndesmotic injury and instability:
Type A: Fibula avulsion fracture below the level of the syndesmosis
Type B: Oblique or spiral fibula fracture occurring at the level of the syndesmosis
Type C: Fibula fracture above the level of the syndesmosis (Fig. 11.37).

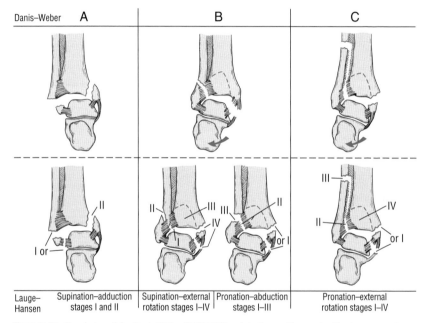

Figure 11.37. Correlation of the Danis–Weber (AO/ASIF) and the Lauge–Hansen classification systems for malleolar fractures. (*Modified from Browner BD, et al., eds: Skeletal Trauma, 3rd ed, Philadelphia, 2002, Elsevier.*)

172. **What is a Maisonneuve fracture? What structure is most likely disrupted?**
A Maisonneuve fracture is a spiral or oblique fracture of the proximal fibula that occurs with external rotation injuries. This fracture is associated with medial sided injuries, including medial malleolus fracture, deltoid ligament injury, and/or fractures of the posterior malleolus. There is also a high rate of syndesmosis disruption with this injury.

173. **What is the medial clear space? What is the definition of medial clear space widening? What does medial clear space widening indicate?**
The medial clear space is the distance between the medial aspect of the talus and the medial malleolus on an ankle mortise view. A medial clear space greater than 4 mm is considered abnormal. A widened medial clear space indicates lateral talar shift secondary to medial sided pathology, commonly deltoid ligament disruption (Fig. 11.38).

174. **When is a stress view of the ankle indicated?**
A stress view of the ankle is indicated in the presence of an isolated fibula fracture and suspicion for medial sided involvement, for example, a Weber B fibula fracture. The ankle

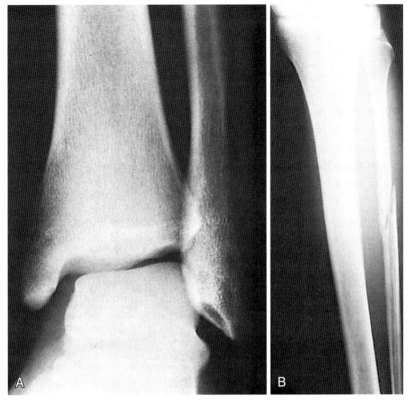

Figure 11.38. Maisonneuve fracture. (A) Anteroposterior view shows a slight widening of the ankle mortise and the medial clear space. (B) Lateral view shows an oblique fracture at the proximal shaft of the fibula. *(A and B, From Nicholas JA, Hershman EB [eds]: The Lower Extremity and Spine in Sports Medicine, 2nd ed. St Louis, Mosby, 1994.)*

is dorsiflexed and the foot is externally rotated to obtain a stress view. If there is medial clear space widening at the time of a stress view this indicates deltoid ligament disruption.

CASE 11-18

A 48-year-old construction worker is brought to the Emergency Department after falling 10 feet off of a ladder while working on the outside of a house. He is still wearing his work boots and socks, but it is clear that the patient has a significant deformity at his ankle. Radiographs of the ankle show a comminuted fracture of the distal tibia involving the articular surface.

175. **What is a pilon fracture?**
     A pilon fracture or tibial plafond fracture is a fracture of the distal tibia with intra-articular extension.

176. **What is the most commonly used classification system for pilon fractures?**
     The Ruedi and Allgower classification system is most commonly used to describe pilon fractures. It is based on the severity of articular comminution and displacement of the articular surface. Poor prognosis correlates with higher classification type:
     Type 1: Non-displaced cleavage fracture of the ankle joint
     Type 2: Displaced fracture with minimal impaction or comminution
     Type 3: Displaced fracture with significant articular comminution and metaphyseal impaction (Fig. 11.39).

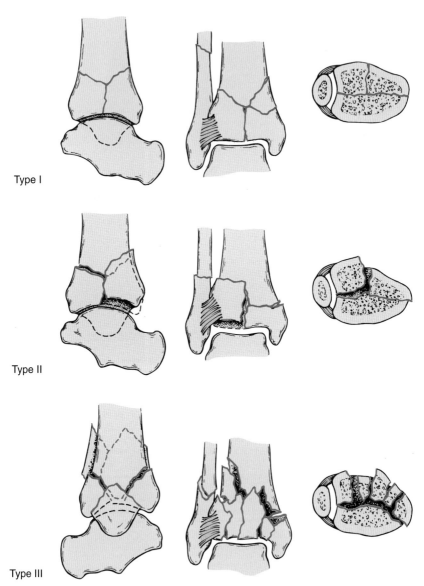

Type I

Type II

Type III

Figure 11.39. Ruedi and Allgower's classification of pilon fractures. (*Redrawn from Ruedi TP; Allgower M. The operative treatment of intra-articular fractures of the lower end of the tibia. Clin Orthop 138:105–110, 1979.*)

177. What is the most common mechanism of injury in a pilon fracture?
Pilon fractures are the result of either axial compression or shear stress that results from torsion and either a varus or valgus stress. Axial compression injuries most commonly result from motor-vehicle collisions or a fall from a height. Shear stress injuries are often the result of skiing accidents.

178. What associated orthopedic injuries are commonly seen with pilon fractures?
Other associated orthopedic injuries include fractures of the calcaneus, tibial plateau, pelvis, and spinal column.

179. Why is definitive fixation of a pilon fracture often delayed?
The soft-tissue envelope at the ankle is extremely precarious especially following high-energy trauma. To prevent wound complications in the postoperative period, waiting for swelling, fracture blisters, or other soft-tissue compromise to resolve is imperative to lowering the complication rate. Patients are often placed in an external fixator while soft-tissue swelling resolves.

TALUS

CASE 11-19

A 34-year-old male is brought into the trauma bay after being involved in a single person motorcycle crash. On secondary examination, he complains of severe tenderness to palpation over the anterior aspect of his left ankle and is in extreme pain with attempted dorsiflexion or plantar flexion of the ankle. Radiographs of the left foot and ankle reveal a talar neck fracture.

180. What is the classification of talar neck fractures?
Fractures of the talar neck are described using the Hawkins classification:
Type I: Non-displaced talar neck fracture
Type II: Displaced talar neck fracture with subtalar subluxation or dislocation
Type III: Displaced talar neck fracture associated subtalar and tibiotalar dislocation
Type IV: Displaced talar neck fracture with subtalar, tibiotalar, and talonavicular
dislocation (Fig. 11.40).

181. How does talus fracture classification correlate with avascular necrosis?
Increased rates of avascular necrosis of the talus correlate with increasing Hawkins type. Greater initial fracture displacement is associated with a higher risk of eventual avascular necrosis. Type I fractures are associated with 0–15% progression to avascular necrosis, Type II progress 20–50% of the time, Type III progress 20–100% of the time, and Type IV progress 100% of the time.

182. What radiographic sign is indicative of revascularization of the talar body? What radiographic finding indicates avascular necrosis?
The Hawkins sign, or progressive osteoporosis of the talar body, indicates revascularization of the talus. This usually becomes evident 6–8 weeks after the injury. Sclerosis of the talus indicates avascular necrosis. This may be evident as early as 3–6 months and can be better characterized by an MRI (Fig. 11.41).

HEEL/FOOT

CALCANEUS

CASE 11-20

A 54-year-old man is brought into the Emergency Room by his wife after sustaining an injury to his left foot. The gentleman was watering plants on a ledge in his house when he decided to jump down. He landed directly on his feet and experienced immediate, severe pain in his left heel. On exam he has swelling and ecchymosis over the medial and lateral aspect of his heel with severe tenderness to palpation in the same distribution. You suspect there is a fracture of the calcaneus.

183. What radiographic studies should be obtained to evaluate a potential fracture of the calcaneus?
All patients suspected of having a fracture of the calcaneus should have antero-posterior, lateral, and oblique radiographs of the foot performed. A CT scan of the foot should also

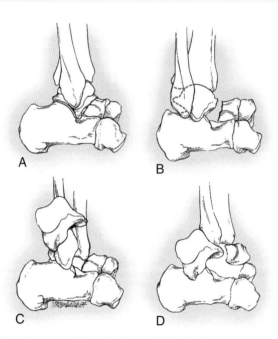

Figure 11.40. Hawkin's classification of talar neck fractures (A) Type I. (B) Type II. (C) Type III. (D) Type IV. *(From Canale ST, Kelly FB Jr: Fractures of the neck of the talus: long-term evaluation of 71 cases, J Bone Joint Surg 60A:143, 1978.)*

be performed with the axis shifted 30° in the coronal and sagittal planes in order to best visualize the posterior facet. The Harris view may also be helpful. This is taken with the beam angled cephalad 45° with the foot in dorsiflexion. This view helps characterize calcaneal widening, shortening, and varus deformity.

184. **What are the classic deformities seen in a fracture of the calcaneus?**
Classic deformities associated with calcaneus fractures include calcaneal widening, lateral wall blow-out, shortening, varus angulation, and loss of height.

185. **What are the most common classification systems used to describe calcaneus fractures?**
There are two common classification systems used to describe calcaneus fractures, the Essex–Lopresti classification and the Sanders classification.

The Essex–Lopresti classification divides calcaneus fractures into primary and secondary fracture lines. The primary fracture line usually traverses from plantar-medial to dorsal-lateral and divides the calcaneus into an antero-medial sustentacular piece and a postero-lateral tuberosity piece. Secondary fracture lines include those exiting posteriorly through the tuberosity, creating a tongue type fracture, and those exiting just posterior to the posterior facet, creating a joint depression fracture.

The Sanders classification of calcaneus fractures is based on coronal CT images of the posterior facet. The posterior facet is divided into lateral, middle, and medial segments by fracture lines labeled A, B, and C:
Type I: Non-displaced fracture regardless of the number of fracture lines
Type II: Two part fracture (subclassified into IIA, IIB, or IIC depending on where the fracture line traverses the posterior facet)
Type III: Three part fracture, (IIIAB, IIIAC, and IIIBC)
Type IV: Four part fracture, comminuted fracture (Figs 11.42 and 11.43).

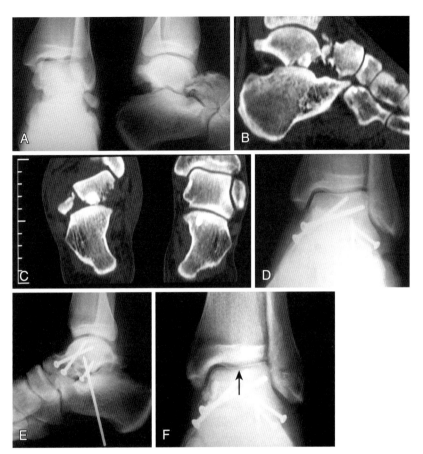

Figure 11.41. (A) Displaced type II talar fracture. (B and C) CT scans show comminution of medial aspect of talar neck and additional fracture of lateral process. (D and E) After open reduction through anteromedial and lateral Ollier approaches, fixation of talar neck with non-lagging fragment screw and lateral process with mini-fragment screws. (F) Positive Hawkins sign at 6 weeks. *(From Rammelt S, Zwipp H: Talar neck and body fractures, Injury 40:120, 2009.)*

186. **What are risk factors for poor outcomes in open reduction and internal fixation (ORIF) of the calcaneus?**
     Risk factors that lead to worse outcomes after ORIF of calcaneal fractures include age greater than 50, workers compensation cases, smokers, men, and manual laborers.

187. **What is a tongue-type fracture of the calcaneus?**
     A tongue-type calcaneal fracture is one that consists of the Essex–Lopresti primary fracture line separating the postero-lateral tuberosity fragment and the anteromedial sustentacular fragment with a secondary fracture line exiting posteriorly and inferiorly to the calcaneal tuberosity. A tongue-type fracture is extra-articular.

188. **What is a calcaneal avulsion fracture?**
     A calcaneal avulsion fracture is an extra-articular fracture through the calcaneal tuberosity caused by forced dorsiflexion. It is most commonly seen in elderly female patients with

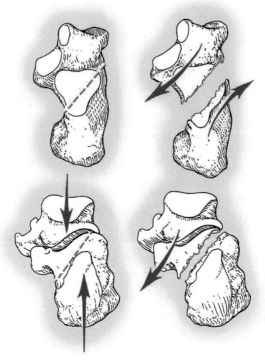

Figure 11.42. Primary fracture line in calcaneal fractures. (*From Lowery RBW, Calhoun JH. Fractures of the calcaneus, I: anatomy, injury, mechanism, and classification, Foot Ankle 17:230, 1996.*)

poor bone quality. They can also occur in younger adults with the mechanism being a direct blow to the calcaneus. Surgical indications include impending open fracture secondary to skin tenting and open fractures (Fig. 11.44).

189. **What is Bohler's angle?**
Bohler's angle is the angle formed between a line drawn from the highest point of the anterior process of the calcaneus to the highest point of the posterior facet and a line from the posterior facet to the most superior edge of the calcaneal tuberosity. The angle usually measures 20–40°. A decrease in this angle indicates depression of the posterior facet.

190. **What is the angle of Gissane?**
The angle of Gissane is the angle formed between the lateral margin of the posterior facet of the calcaneus and the anterior process of the calcaneus. The angle usually measures 95–105°. When the angle is increased, it indicates depression and flattening of the posterior facet (Figs 11.45A and B).

MIDFOOT

CASE 11-21

A 23-year-old college football player presents to your clinic complaining of left foot pain. He was recently seen in the local Emergency Room where he was diagnosed with a foot sprain. Today on exam he has severe tenderness to palpation over his midfoot, centered over his 1st tarsometatarsal joint and ecchymosis over the plantar aspect of his midfoot. You are suspicious that he has sustained a Lisfranc injury.

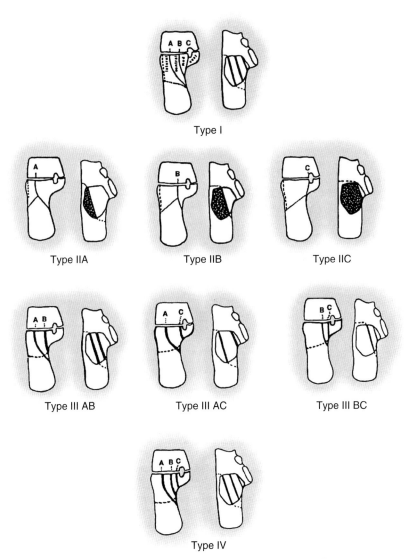

Figure 11.43. Sanders CT classification of intra-articular calcaneal fractures. (*From Sanders R, Fortin P, DiPasquale T, et al.: Operative treatment in 120 displaced intra-articular calcaneal fractures: results using a prognostic computed tomography scan classification. Clin Orthop Relat Res 290:87, 1993.*)

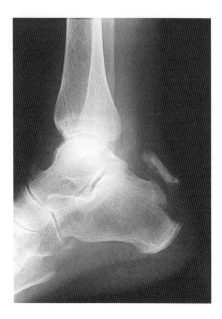

Figure 11.44. Calcaneal avulsion fracture. *(Modified from Eiff MP, Hatch R, [eds], Fracture Management for Primary Care, 3rd ed, Copyright © 2012, Saunders, Elsevier Inc.)*

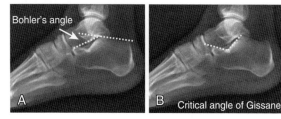

Figure 11.45. Bohler's angle and the critical angle of Gissane. *(From Banerjee R, Nickisch F. Calcaneus fractures. In: DiGiovanni CW, Greisberg J, eds. Core Knowledge in Orthopaedics: Foot and Ankle, Elsevier, New York, 2007.)*

191. **What is a Lisfranc injury?**
     A Lisfranc injury is an injury to the Lisfranc joint complex which includes the tarsometatarsal, intermetatarsal, and intertarsal articulations. A Lisfranc injury can range in severity from a mild soft-tissue injury to a tarsometatarsal fracture dislocation.

192. **What is the mechanism of injury in a Lisfranc injury?**
     The mechanism of injury is usually either a direct blow to the midfoot or an axial loading force applied to a plantarflexed foot (Fig. 11.46).

193. **What findings on clinical exam should make you suspicious for a Lisfranc injury?**
     Patients with Lisfranc injuries usually have tenderness to palpation and swelling over the midfoot. In addition, there is sometimes plantar ecchymosis. Patients are often unable to bear weight secondary to pain.

194. **What important technique should be used when obtaining radiographs of the foot in a patient suspected of a having a Lisfranc injury?**
     All radiographs of a patient with a suspected Lisfranc injury should be weight-bearing films to reveal widening between the 1st and 2nd metatarsals. Oftentimes a "fleck sign" can be

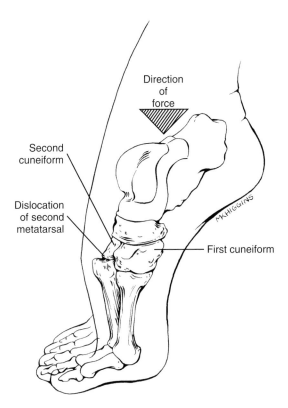

Direction
of
force

Second
cuneiform

Dislocation
of second
metatarsal

First cuneiform

M.K.HIGGINS

Figure 11.46. Common injury
mechanism in a Lisfranc injury.
*(Modified from Eiff MP, Hatch R,
[eds], Fracture Management for
Primary Care, 3rd ed, Copyright ©
2012, Saunders, Elsevier Inc.)*

seen which indicates an avulsion of the Lisfranc ligament from its insertion on the 2nd
metatarsal (Fig. 11.47).

195. What is the Lisfranc ligament?
The Lisfranc ligament is the ligament that extends from the plantar surface of medial
cuneiform to the base of the 2nd metatarsal.

196. What are the different types Lisfranc fracture–dislocations?
Using the Ouenu and Kuss classification system, Lisfranc injuries can be divided into three
types: homolateral, isolated, and divergent. Homolateral Lisfranc injuries occur when all
five metatarsals are displaced in the same direction. Isolated Lisfranc injuries occur when
only one or two metatarsals are displaced from the others. Finally, divergent Lisfranc
injuries occur when there is displacement of the metatarsals in both the coronal and
sagittal plane (Fig. 11.48).

197. What is the management of patients with Lisfranc injuries?
Management can involve either non-operative or operative treatment.
Non-operative treatments consist of non-weight bearing in a cast for up to
8 weeks. Operative treatment can consist of open reduction internal fixation, primary
arthrodesis of the 1st, 2nd, and 3rd tarsometatarsal joints, and midfoot fusion for advanced
disease.

198. What is the most common long-term complication of a Lisfranc injury?
Midfoot arthritis is the most common long-term complication in Lisfranc injuries.
Midfoot arthrodesis is the most common treatment for this complication.

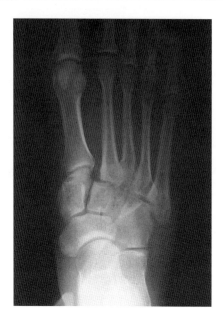

Figure 11.47. The fleck sign is an often subtle indication of underlying midfoot instability through the Lisfranc articulations. It is located between the first and second metatarsal bases on an antero-posterior view of the foot, and represents a bony avulsion off the base of the second metatarsal base from pull of the plantar Lisfranc's ligament, originating from the medial cuneiform. Even if the radiographs look otherwise normal, these patients should undergo stress examination of the midfoot to rule out occult midfoot instability. (*From Banerjee R, et al., Foot Injuries: Browner BD, et al. (eds), Skeletal Trauma, 4th ed, Saunders, 2009.*)

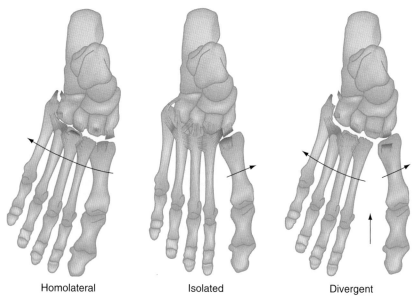

Homolateral   Isolated   Divergent

Figure 11.48. Classification of Lisfranc injuries. (*From Quenu E, Kuss G. Etude sur les luxation du metatarse (luxations metatarsotarsiennes) du diastasis entre le 2e metatarsien. Rev Chir 1909;39:281–336, 720–91, 1093–134.*)

OPEN FRACTURES

CASE 11-22

A 25-year-old male is airlifted by helicopter to the trauma bay after falling from approximately 20 feet while rock climbing. He has a grossly deformed lower extremity with a 10 cm laceration over the antero-medial aspect of the tibia. His distal pulses are intact, and he has a normal neurological examination. Radiographs show a comminuted tibia fracture.

199. How are open fractures classified?

Open fractures are classified by the Gustilo–Anderson classification system. This system describes open fractures both by the size of the superficial skin wound but also the degree of fracture comminution and soft-tissue injury:

Type I: <1-cm wound, low-energy fracture

Type II: 1–10-cm wound, higher energy fracture

Type III: >10-cm wound, high-energy fracture:

A: Moderate periosteal stripping, wound closure not requiring soft-tissue flap

B: Marked periosteal stripping, wound closure requires soft-tissue flap

C: Any open fracture with a vascular injury that requires repair.

200. Following presentation, when is the most appropriate time for a fracture to be classified?

The fracture should be classified at the time of initial debridement. This is the most appropriate time to fully evaluate the size of the soft-tissue lesion, and, more importantly, the degree of comminution and soft-tissue swelling beneath the surface of the skin.

201. What type of antibiotics should be administered for each fracture type?

A first-generation cephalosporin (cefazolin) should be given for all open fractures. Addition of an aminoglycoside (gentamicin) should occur for Type III injuries, and penicillin should be added for barnyard or heavily contaminated wounds. Tetanus status should be assessed and updated or treated as indicated.

202. How soon should antibiotics be initiated after the time of injury? How long should patients be treated with antibiotics after the time of injury?

Antibiotics should be administered as soon as possible. In some instances, paramedics or first responders give antibiotics in the field. The duration of antibiotic therapy is highly controversial and based largely on each individual patient. Evidence suggests that 48 hours of treatment is adequate, but if a patient requires serial operative debridements or has wounds that remain open, therapy may be extended.

203. What is the initial treatment for patients with open fractures?

Open fractures are associated with high-energy trauma such as motor-vehicle accidents and falls. Advanced trauma life support protocols should take place first and are the priority. An examination of the patient's neurologic status, head, spine, abdomen, and pelvis should be completed before turning attention to the open fracture.

Specific protocols with regards to treatment of open fractures differ by hospital system, but in general, the wound should be covered with a sterile dressing, with or without irrigation with a sterile solution beforehand. The facture should then be reduced and immobilized. Antibiotics and the appropriate tetanus treatment are administered and arrangements for a formal surgical debridement should be made.

204. What is the goal of surgical debridement?

The objective of surgical debridement is to remove all contamination from the wound and fracture site. In general, low flow normal saline is used to irrigate open fractures. The open wound should be extended and all foreign material must be removed. The bone ends should be brought into direct visualization and evaluated. Necrotic muscle, devitalized bone, and debris are removed from the zone of injury.

205. In the open fracture, how can you differentiate viable from non-viable muscle tissue?

The four Cs – color, contractility, consistency, and capacity to bleed – help the surgeon to decide which muscles to debride. Pale muscle that does not (1) bleed when cut or (2) contract when touched should be excised.

206. **What is the difference in treatment of open fractures between low-velocity and high-velocity gunshot wounds?**
High-velocity gunshot wounds (e.g., military rifle) or close-range gunshot wounds result in more disruption and destruction of soft tissue than low-velocity projectiles. High-velocity injuries may require multiple debridements to ensure that all non-viable tissue is excised. Low-velocity wounds may require only local irrigation, debridement of the entry and exit wounds, and supportive oral antibiotic treatment.

207. **When can open wounds be closed?**
If the wound is not grossly contaminated or there is little soft-tissue damage, the surgeon may decide to primarily close the open wound. This rarely occurs outside of Type I, and some Type II, wounds. If there is any concern that another debridement may be needed or that the skin cannot be closed in a tension free manner, then a sterile dressing may be temporarily applied until the patient returns to the operating room. Definitive closure or soft-tissue coverage is ideally performed within 5–7 days.

208. **How is the limb stabilized if a wound is grossly contaminated or soft tissue does not allow for placement of an internal fixation device?**
In many cases of open fractures and closed fractures where there is significant soft-tissue injury, external fixation is used to restore relative stability, length, alignment, and rotation to the limb.

LIMB SALVAGE

209. **How is the decision made to attempt limb salvage or amputation?**
The decision to attempt limb salvage or primarily amputate a severely injured limb is a difficult one; both for the surgeon as well as for the patient and/or their family. Each injury, from both a soft tissue and bony perspective, is different. Likewise each patient, from an age, comorbidity, and functional demand perspective is different and must be considered on a case-by-case basis. There have been attempts to help guide physicians and patients in making this decision (MESS) and some studies (LEAP) have attempted to look at the long-term outcomes of both treatment options.

210. **What are some potential pros and cons of primary amputation? Of limb salvage?**
Amputation can be a life-saving procedure in the setting of a severe injury to an extremity. The obvious disadvantage is loss of limb and dependence on a prosthetic limb. This can be psychologically difficult. In addition, prostheses can be quite expensive. Advantages include: fewer operations, shorter hospitalizations, immediate mobilization of the patient, and decreased risk of later complications such as infection, nonunion, delayed or malaligned bone healing, and hardware failure.
  Salvage of the leg has the primary advantage of saving the patient's own limb. This effort may result in multiple procedures, long stays in the hospital, and result in significant medical costs. Infection, non-healing bones or soft tissues, and prolonged immobilization are common. In addition, the end result of a prolonged, failed limb salvage effort is often an amputation.

211. **When there is an arterial injury and a fracture, which should be addressed first?**
Generally, the skeletal injury should be stabilized first, usually with temporary external fixation. This allows the vascular surgeons to perform a vascular repair or reconstruction on a stable limb. In addition, proper length alignment and rotation can be achieved so that when definitive fixation of the limb takes place, the vascular repair or graft is not stretched or disrupted.

212. **What is the Mangled Extremity Severity Score? How is it measured?**
The Mangled Extremity Severity Score is a numerical assessment of a severe, acute extremity injury. It takes into account age, severity of soft tissue and skeletal injury, presence and severity of shock, as well as peripheral perfusion to the limb. The scores from each group are added. A score greater than 7 is considered a relative indication for amputation over limb salvage. This score is meant only to help guide the treatment decision and should not be used to dictate treatment.

PERIPROSTHETIC FRACTURES

213. What is a periprosthetic fracture?

A periprosthetic fracture is any fracture around a total joint prosthesis. This occurs primarily in the femur around a total knee or total hip, but can also occur in any bone where a joint arthroplasty has been performed (humerus, tibia, ulna, etc.)

214. What is a critical point when planning treatment of periprosthetic fracture?

When evaluating treatment options for any periprosthetic fracture, the stability of the arthroplasty implant will dictate whether the fracture can be treated in isolation or whether the arthroplasty component needs to be revised and treated in conjunction with the fracture. Prosthesis stability is primarily related to the location of the fracture, but factors such as the age of the prosthesis, means of original prosthesis fixation, and pre-injury state of the implant should also be considered.

215. What types of orthopedic implants are used to fix fractures around total joint prostheses?

In general, around a stable total knee or hip prosthesis, lateral locking plates are used on the femur to fix periprosthetic fractures. Cerclage wires, unicortical screws, or screws directed around the prosthesis are used in the area of the bone where the prosthesis may prevent usual, bicortical screw placement. Another option to consider in some periprosthetic fractures around a total knee arthroplasty is a retrograde femoral nail through the intercondylar "box" of the femoral component of the knee arthroplasty. This is not always possible because of the fracture type or restrictions created by the design of the femoral component (Fig. 11.49).

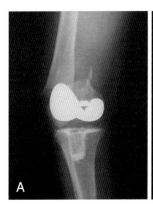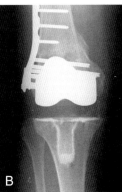

Figure 11.49. (A) Antero-posterior radiograph of a distal femoral periprosthetic fracture above a total knee arthroplasty. (B) Radiograph 7 months after internal fixation of fracture with a lateral locking plate. The fracture healed uneventfully. (*From Browner BD, et al. [eds], Skeletal Trauma, 4th ed, Copyright © 2009, Saunders, Elsevier Inc.*)

FRACTURES IN THE ELDERLY

216. What is the definition of osteoporosis? Of osteopenia?

Osteoporosis is defined as a decrease in bone mass by at least 2.5 standard deviations from the peak bone mass of young individuals of the same race and sex as measured by DEXA scan. The measurement is taken between the L2 and L4 vertebral levels. Osteoporosis can further be broken down into Type I and Type II. Type I includes postmenopausal osteoporosis, which mostly affects trabecular bone. Type II osteoporosis is age-related osteoporosis seen in patients older than 75 years of age and affects both trabecular and cortical bone. Osteopenia is defined as a decrease in bone mass between 1 and 2.5 standard deviations from the peak bone mass of a young individual of the same race and sex as measured by DEXA scan.

217. What is meant by the term "fragility fracture?"

A fragility fracture, also referred to as an insufficiency fracture or pathologic fracture, is a fracture that results from a mechanism that would not normally cause a fracture. This is usually the result of decreased bone mineral density.

218. **What are the locations of common fragility fractures?**

Locations of common fragility fractures include the proximal femur, the pelvis, the sacrum, the spine, the wrist, and the proximal humerus.

219. **What are some laboratory values that are important to obtain in the workup of osteoporosis and osteopenia?**

Laboratory workup of osteopenia and osteoporosis should include a complete blood count, erythrocyte sedimentation rate, a full chemistry panel including calcium and phosphate, albumin, liver function tests, alkaline phosphatase, serum protein electrophoresis, urine protein electrophoresis, urinalysis, and 25-hydroxyvitamin D.

220. **How can osteoporosis and osteopenia be addressed?**

Osteopenia and osteoporosis can be addressed through several interventions including vitamin D and calcium supplementation, bisphosphonate therapy, estrogen and progestin hormone therapy, calcitonin, selective estrogen receptor modulators, and recombinant parathyroid hormone.

221. **What is a serious musculoskeletal complication of bisphosphonate therapy?**

A serious musculoskeletal complication of bisphosphonate therapy is atypical fractures of the proximal femur and femoral shaft. Bisphosphonates disrupt the normal equilibrium of bone formation and resorption by inhibiting osteoclast attachment and resorption of bone. This leads to an environment in which bone remodeling is limited. As a result, the body is unable to adequately address repetitive microtrauma that can ultimately lead to a fracture.

BIBLIOGRAPHY

1. Baker SP, O'Neill B, Haddon W Jr, et al. The injury severity score: a method for describing patients with multiple injuries and evaluating emergency care. J Trauma 1974;14:187–96.
2. Bosse MJ, MacKenzie EJ, Kellam JF, et al. An analysis of outcomes of reconstruction or amputation after leg-threatening injuries. N Engl J Med 2002;347:1924–31.
3. Browner B, Levine A, Jupiter J, et al. Skeletal Trauma. 4th ed. Philadelphia: Saunders Elsevier; 2009.
4. Bucholz R, Heckman J, Court-Brown C, et al. Rockwood and Green's Fractures in Adults. 6th ed. Philadelphia: Lippincott, Williams, and Wilkins; 2006.
5. Johansen K, Daines M, Howey T, et al. Objective criteria accurately predict amputation following lower extremity trauma. J Trauma 1990;30:568–72.
6. Koval K, Zuckerman J. Handbook of Fractures. 3rd ed. Philadelphia: Lippincott, Williams, and Wilkins; 2006.
7. Lieberman J. AAOS Comprehensive Orthopaedic Review. American Academy of Orthopaedic Surgeons; 2009.
8. Miller M. Review of Orthopaedics. 5th ed. Philadelphia: Saunders Elsevier; 2008.
9. Stannard J, Schmidt A, Kreger P. Surgical Treatment of Orthopaedic Trauma. New York: Thieme Medical Publishers; 2007.

INDEX

Page numbers followed by "f" indicate figures, "t" indicate tables, and "b" indicate boxes.

A

A1 pulley, 93
Abducted thumb, 195
Abduction shoulder deformity, spastic, 232
Abductor digiti minimi (ADM) muscle, 87t
Abductor pollicis brevis (APB) muscle, 86t
Absent thumb, 195
Absolute stability, 381
Acetabular fractures
  injury mechanism of, 409
  long-term sequelae, 412
  radiographic views in, 411, 413f
  surgical fixation of, 412
Acetabular screws
  location for placement of, 16
  quadrant system for, 16f
  structures at risk with, 16t
Acetabulum, 407–416
  case study in, 407b, 409b
  fractures of. see Acetabular fractures
Achilles tendon
  tear/rupture of, 61, 61b, 62f
    casting/splinting of, 61
    physical examination for, 61
    surgical repair for, 61
  tendonitis/paratenonitis of, 61–62
Achondroplasia, 320
Acromial morphology, different types of,
      245, 245f
Acromioclavicular (AC) joints
  anatomy of, 251, 251f
  classification of, 252t
  mechanism of injury in, 251
  pain in, 253
  physical examination of, 251
  radiographic views of, 252
  separations of, treatment of, 253
  stability of, 251
Acromioclavicular injuries, 251–255
  acute type I or type II, treatment of, 252
  acute type III, 252
  acute type IV, 252
  acute type V, 252
  case of, 251b–254b, 253f
Acute carpal tunnel syndrome, 407
Acute hematogenous infection, 12
Acute subscapularis tears, mechanism of
      injury in, 249
Adamantinoma, 135
Adducted thumb, 195
Adductor muscle, 85t

Adductor pollicis muscle, 85t
Adhesive capsulitis, 255
  arthroscopic stages of, 256
  clinical stages of, 255
  treatment of, 256
  variables of, 255
Adolescent idiopathic scoliosis (AIS), 178–181,
      178b, 178f, 311
  braces used for, 313
  classification of, 180
  curve progression, risk factors for, 179
  diagnosis of, 180
  incidence of, 311
  risk factors for, 313
  spinal cord injury in, 181
  surgical approach for, 181
  treatment of, 180, 313
  untreated, symptoms of, 179
Adults
  amputation in, 235
  reconstruction in, 1–22
AEIOU mnemonic, 125
Age/aging
  bone metabolism and, 26–27
  rotator cuff tear and, 247
Allen's test, 90–91, 92f
Allis method, for reducing posterior hip dislocation,
      415f
Allograft, for ACL reconstruction,
      336
Allograft plugs, disadvantage of, 344
Alpha error, 48
American Academy of Orthopedic Surgeons
      (AAOS), treatment recommendations for
      knee, 3–4, 3t
Aminoglycosides, 42t
Amputation
  case of, 235b
  complications of, 236–238
  of diabetic foot, 70–71, 70b, 70f
  energy requirements for, 238
  indications of, 235
  primary, pros and cons of, 440
  and prosthetics, 235–238
  trans femoral, 236, 237f
  trans metatarsal, 236
  trans tibial, 236, 237f
Aneurysmal bone cyst, vs. unicameral bone cyst,
      160–161, 161f
Angiolipoma, 139
Angle of Gissane, 434, 436f

Ankle, 51–80, 424–431
  arthritis of, 72, 72b
    etiology of, 72
    radiograph for, 72, 72b
    symptoms of, 72
    treatment for, 72
  arthroscopy of, 58–61, 59b–60b
    portal placement for, 59–60, 60f
    surgical indication for, 59
  aspiration, 148
  fractures of, treatment options for, in children, 171–172
  instability of, 73–76
    lateral, 74, 74b
  neurologic disorder of, 76–80
  rehabilitation, principles of, 223
  sprain of, 73–76, 73b–74b
    acute, treatment for, 74
    classification of, 73, 73t
    eversion type, 75
    examination of, 73
    magnetic resonance imaging for, 74
    x-ray for, Ottawa rules in, 73–74, 74b
  stress view of, 428–429
Ankle-brachial index (ABI), 68–69
Ankle dorsiflexion, 225
Ankle foot orthoses (AFO), 229, 230f
  indications of, 229–230
Ankle plantar flexion, 225
Ankle (tibiotalar) joint, range of motion of, 221f
Annulus fibrosus, 33
Anterior approach (Henry), in radial shaft, 402–404
Anterior capsule strain, vs. biceps injury, 374
Anterior cruciate ligament (ACL)
  injury to, 334–339
    anatomy and function of, 334
    case study in, 334b, 336b, 338f
    complications of, 338
    mechanism of, 334–335
    meniscal tear associated with, 335
    test for, 335
  reconstruction rehabilitation of, principles of, 223
  tears, 217
Anterior drawer test, 73, 335
Anterior elbow pain, differential diagnosis of, 374
Anterior knee pain, 222
  see also Chondromalacia patella
  causes of, 344
Anterior talofibular ligament (ATFL), 73
Anterior tibial tendon rupture, 65b
  etiology of, 65
  treatment for, 65, 65b
Antero-posterior compression (APC), 407, 408f
Antoni A area, 140
Antoni B area, 140
Apert syndrome, 194
Apprehension test, 353f
Aquatherapy, 221
Arnold-Chiari malformation, 191
Arthralgias, of Lyme disease, 151
Arthritic disorders, 108–109
Arthritis
  acromioclavicular joint
    indication of treatment, 253

    management of, 253
    operative treatment of, 253
  of ankle, 72, 72b
  degenerative, 104
  of elbow, 272–276
    history of, 272
    types of, 272
  glenohumeral joint, 256–264, 356
  of hand, 102–104
    sites of, 103f
  of hip, 12
  juvenile idiopathic, 155–156, 155b
  of Lyme disease, 151
  septic, 146–148, 146b
  of wrist, 102–104
Arthritis mutilans, 108
Arthrodesis
  for ankle arthritis, 72
    smokers/non-smokers and, 72, 72b
  of shoulder, 263
Arthrofibrosis, 339
Arthropathy
  capsulorrhaphy, 259
  Charcot, 71
  cuff tear, 262
  Jaccoud's, 108
Arthroplasty
  see also Total elbow arthroplasty; Total hip
    arthroplasty (THA); Total knee
    arthroplasty (TKA); Total wrist arthroplasty
  of elbow, interposition/distraction, 273
  of hand, 102–104
  of knee, unicompartmental, 5f
  for metacarpophalangeal joint, 104
  proximal interphalangeal joint, 104
  resection, 264
  of shoulder, 260
    deltopectoral approach, 261
    overstuffing in, 261
  of wrist, 102–104
Arthroscopy
  of ankle, 58–61, 59b
  for osteoarthritis, 273
Articular cartilage, 30–33, 32b
  composition of, 31
  layers of, 31
  zone of, 32f
Aseptic glenoid loosening, revision shoulder
    arthroplasty and, 261
ASIA classification, 240
Aspirin, 40
Athetosis, 201–202
Athletes
  cardiovascular conditions in, 376, 376b
  miscellaneous conditions in, 375–376
Athletic pubalgia, 349
Atlantoaxial instability, 187
  congenital conditions associated with, 188
  symptoms of, 187
  treatment of, 188
Atlantoaxial joints, unstable, 281, 283f
Atlantodens interval (ADI), 188, 188f
Atrophic nonunion, 30
Autologous chondrocyte implantation, 343

Autonomic neuropathy, 67
Avascular necrosis, 416
  classification of, 416
Axial loading, 301
Axillary crutches, 227
Axillary nerves, 391–392
Axonotmesis, 34, 198

B

Bado classification, of Monteggia fracture,
    176–177, 177f
Baker cyst, 333
Bankart lesion, 353–354
Barlow maneuver, 210–211
Barton's fracture, 407
Basal joint arthritis, 102
  thumb, radiographic findings and anatomic
      considerations in, 102
Base of support, 223
Basic science, 23–50
Basilar invagination, 191
Becker's muscular dystrophy, 210
Belly-press test, 249, 250f
Bennett fracture, 117, 117b
  treatment for, 117, 117f
Beta error, 48
Beta-lactamase inhibitors, 42t
Biceps injury, *vs.* anterior capsule strain, 374
Biceps tendon, distal ruptures of
  imaging of, 277, 277f
  mechanism of injury in, 276
  physical examination of, 276–277
  treatment of, 277
"Biconcave glenoid", 259
Biologic glenoid resurfacing, 260
  hemiarthroplasty with, 260
Biomaterials, 43–46
Biomechanics, 43–46, 381
Biopsy
  excisional, 129
  incisional, 129
  for musculoskeletal tumors, 129
  needle, 129
Biostatistics, 46–50, 46b
Birth, brachial plexus palsy, 198
Bisphosphonates
  indications for, 40
  serious musculoskeletal complication of,
      442
Blunt head injury, head CT after, 376
Bohler's angle, 434, 436f
Bone
  anatomy of, 23, 24f
  function of, 23–30
  healing, novel modalities to enhance, 30
  homeostasis of, 23–24, 25f
  metabolism, with parathyroid dysfunction, 25
  miscellaneous lesions of, 142
  modulus of elasticity of, 44
  pisiform, 83
  primary formation of, 381–383
  types of, 23
Bone-block procedures, for shoulder stabilization,
    359

Bone cyst
  aneurysmal, 142, 143f
  unicameral, 142, 143f
Bone disease, metastatic, 142
Bone graft, characteristics of, 31t
Bone lesions, benign, 130–135, 130b–131b
Bone loss, after shoulder dislocation, 358
Bone-patella tendon-bone autograft, for ACL
    reconstruction, 336
Bone resorption, molecular mechanisms of, 24
Bone scans, 290
  radionuclide, for septic arthritis, 147
Bone tumors, malignant, 135–138
Bony avulsions, of PCL injury, 339
Borrelia burgdorferi, as cause of Lyme disease,
    151–152
"Both bone" forearm fractures, 402–404
Botulinum toxin, for cerebral palsy, 202
Bouchard's nodes, 104
Boutonnière deformity, 101–102, 101b, 101f
  in rheumatoid arthritis, 107, 107f
Bowstring test, 285
Bowstringing, prevention of, pulleys for, 93
Boxer's elbow, 373
"Boxer's fracture", 114b, 115, 115f
Brachial plexus palsy, 197–199, 197b
  birth, 198
    natural history of persistent, 199
    risk factors for, 198
    treatment for, 199
Brachymetacarpia, 196
Brain injury, heterotopic ossification in, 239
Brewerton view, 104–105
Bridge plate, 381, 382f
Brodie's abscess, 157
Brown-Séquard syndrome, 297
Bucks traction, for femoral shaft fracture, 421–422
Bulbocavernosus reflex, 296
"Bunion", 51
Bunionette, 55, 55b, 55f
  classification and imaging for, 55
  surgery for, 55, 55f
  type II/type III, 56
Bursitis
  chronic, 374
  prepatellar, 344–345
  septic olecranon, 374
  trochanteric, 347
Buttress plate, 381, 382f

C

C-reactive protein (CRP) tests, 50t
  sensitivity of, 50
  specificity of, 50
C4 quadriplegia, 298
C5-C6 disc herniation, 304
C5 quadriplegia, 298
C6 quadriplegia, 298
C7 abnormality, 304
C7 quadriplegia, 298
C8 nerve abnormality, 304
Cadence, 224
Calcaneal avulsion fractures, 436f
Calcaneofibular ligament (CFL), 73

Calcaneus, 431–434
case study in, 431b
fracture of, 431–432
classic deformities in, 432
classification system of, 432
Calcific tendonitis, 256
Calcium, to promote bone health, 25
Cam impingement, 215, 215f, 345–346, 346f
radiographic signs of lesion, 347
Camptodactyly, 196, 196f
Canadian/Lofstrand crutches, 227
Cancellous bone, 23
Cane, weak hip abductors and, 46
Capsular (sternoclavicular) ligaments, 254
Capsulorrhaphy arthropathy, 259
Caput ulnae syndrome, 105, 106f
Carcinoma
metastatic, 130
vs. sarcoma, 125
Cardiac death, cause of, in athletes, 376, 376b
Cardiomyopathy
in Friedrich's ataxia, 208–210
hypertrophic, 376
Carpal bone, 82
fractures and ligament injuries of, 120–121
proximal and distal rows of, 82–83
Carpal canal, 92
Carpal tunnel
borders of, 92
contents of, 93–102, 94f
Carpal tunnel syndrome (CTS)
causes of, 93
diagnosis and treatment of, 93
Carpometacarpal (CMC) joints
of hand, 82
osteoarthritis of, 102
thumb, arthritis of, 102–103, 102b, 102f
treatment options for, 103
Carpus, fractures and dislocations of, 109–121
Cartilage
injuries, 31–32
types of, 30–33
Case manager, 221
Categorical data, 47
Cauda equina syndrome
findings associated with, 310
pathophysiology of, 309
red flags in, 291
treatment of, 310
Cefepime, 37–38
Celecoxib, 40
Cement preparation technique, generations of, 15, 15t
Cementless stem, advantages of, 15
Center of gravity (mass), location of, 224–225
Central muscles, in hand, 87t–88t
Central one-third patellar tendon autograft, in ACL injury, 337–338
Cephalosporins, 42t
Ceramic-on-ceramic, 45
Cerebral palsy, 201–207, 201b–202b
foot deformities in, 205
gait disorders in, 205–206
geographic classification in, 202
hip instability in, 203–204, 204f

hip problems encountered in, 203
spastic, non-orthopedic surgical treatment options for, 202
upper extremity problems in, 206–207
Cervical burst fracture, mechanism of, 296
Cervical disc, herniated
age for, 303
pain pattern for, 303
Cervical lordosis, 281, 282f
Cervical nerve root compression, 287, 288t
Cervical radiculopathy, 303
affected levels with, 303
due to C5-C6 disc herniation, 304
due to herniated cervical intervertebral disk, 303
Cervical spine, 186–191, 186b, 293–307
case study in, 293b, 293f, 295b–296b, 295f, 303b, 305b
elements for mobility of, 281
flexion-extension, 281
fractures of, 295
radiographs for, 290
injuries to, 375–376, 375b
quadriplegia and, 301
lateral radiograph of, 295
level of, for neck rotation, 281
tests for, 284
vertebrae of, 281
vertebral arches of, 283
Cervical spondylosis, 306
arthritic changes in, 306, 307f
diagnosis of, 306
radiological test for, 306
risk factors for, 306
symptoms of, 306
treatment of, 306
Cervical vertebrae, 281
Cervicothoracic brace, 300, 300f
Chance fracture, 299
Charcot arthropathy, 71
classification of, 71, 71t
surgical correction for, 72
Charcot-Marie-Tooth disease, 78, 78b, 208, 209f
characteristics of deformity in, 78, 79f
treatment of, 80
Chauffeur's fracture, 406
Children
amputation in, 235
ankle fracture treatment for, 171–172
lower extremity septic arthritis in, 147, 150
Lyme disease in, 151
non-accidental trauma in, 163
osteomyelitis in, 150
pathologic fractures in, 162
recommendations for seating, in vehicles, 162–163
septic arthritis in, 150
tibia fracture treatment for, 171
Chondroblastoma, 132–133, 159, 159f
Chondromalacia, 374
Chondromalacia patella, 222
Chondromyxoid fibroma, 133
Chondrosarcoma, 137
Chordoma, 137
Chronic bursitis, 374

Chronic lateral ankle instability, 74b
　symptoms of, 74
　treatment for, 74
Chronic renal disease, bone pathology of, 26
Circumduction, 225
Clasped thumb, 195
Claudication
　neurogenic vs. vascular, 320
　in spine, pain cause by, 319
Clavicle, 387–389
　anatomic relationships of, 387
　case study in, 387b
　fractures of, 173b, 173f–174f
　　classification of, 387, 388f
　　complications of, 389
　　treatment of, 387
Clavicle physeal separation, treatment of,
　　　173
Clavicle shaft, fractures of, operative indications
　　　for, 173
Claw toe deformity, 56t
Cleft hand, 193
Clinodactyly, 196, 196f
Clostridium perfringens, 37
Coaptation splint, in humeral shaft fractures, 394
Cobalt alloy, 44
Cobb angle, 180, 311
Coccyx, vertebrae of, 281
Codman triangle, 157
Cold, as physical therapy modality, 221
Coleman block test, 78–80, 79f
Colles' fracture, 406
Compartments
　dorsal wrist, 85, 85t
　of foot, 385
　of forearm, 385
　of hand, 85, 385
　of lower leg, 385, 386f
Compartment syndrome, 83b, 85, 383–385
　acute
　　causes of, 384
　　complications of, 385
　　of tibia, 384
　　treatment for, 426
　associated with tibial tubercle fractures, 170
　case study in, 383b
　classic sign of, 171
　as complication of crush injury to foot, 172
　diagnosis of, 384
　forearm fracture and, 404
　initial management of, 385
　measuring of, 384, 384f
　in open fracture, 385
　postoperative care of patient with, 385
　pressure existence of, 384
　treatment of, 385
　in upper extremity, 385
Component malposition, as complications of
　　　shoulder arthroplasty, 261
Compression plate, 381, 382f
　in fracture healing, 29
Computed tomography (CT), 289
　in diagnosis of acetabular fractures, 411
　for elbow dislocation, 270
　of fatty degeneration of rotator cuff, 247, 247f

of glenohumeral arthritis, 258
　for orthopedic tumors, 128
Concavity compression, 262
Concentric action, of muscles, 220
Concussion, 216, 216b
Confounders, as variables, 47
Congenital basilar invagination, 191
Congenital overlapping fifth toe, 56
Congenital trigger digit, 197
Constriction band syndrome, congenital, 197
Continuous data, 47
Contralateral straight-leg raise, 285, 285f
Coracohumeral ligament, 350
Cord syndrome
　anterior, 297
　central, 297
　posterior, 297
Coronoid fractures, 268
Corrosion, occur in plates, 45, 45b
Cortical bone, 23
　modulus of elasticity of, 44
Corticosteroid injection, intra-articular, as treatment
　　　for polyarticular juvenile idiopathic
　　　arthritis, 156
Costoclavicular ligaments, 254
COX-1 inhibitors, 40, 40b
COX-2 inhibitors, 40, 40b
Coxa vara, as complication of pediatric hip fractures,
　　　165
Crankshaft phenomenon, 313–314, 314f
Creep, 44
"Crescent sign," of Legg-Calve-Perthes disease,
　　　152–153
CREST syndrome, 109
Crevice corrosion, 45
Crouch gait, 205b, 205f–206f, 206, 226
Cruess classification, of shoulder avascular necrosis,
　　　257
Crutches, 227
Cubital tunnel syndrome, 373
Cubitus varus, in untreated supracondylar humerus
　　　fractures, 176
Cuff tear arthropathy, 262
　non-operative treatment for, 262
　operative treatment for, 262
　radiographic hallmarks of, 262
Curettage, of orthopedic tumors, 129
Cyst
　see also Bone cyst
　Baker, 333
　meniscus, 333, 334f

D
Damage control orthopedics, 387
Danis-Weber classification, for fibula fractures, 428,
　　　428f
Dashboard injury. see Posterior cruciate ligament
　　　(PCL) injury
De Quervain's tenosynovitis, 85, 102b
　pathognomonic of, 102
Deafness, in Klippel-Feil syndrome, 302
Deep palmar arch, 90
Deep venous thrombosis (DVT), prophylaxis,
　　　40–41

Delbet classification, for hip fractures in children, 164, 165f
Delta phalanx, 196
Dens. *see* Odontoid process
Dependent variables, in biostatistics, 46–47
Desmoid tumor, 140
Developmental basilar invagination, 191
Developmental dysplasia of the hip (DDH), 210–212, 210b
  imaging for, 211, 211f
  in newborn, treatment of, 212
  in older children, treatment of, 212
Diabetes mellitus, conditions associated with, 66–67
Diabetic foot, 66–72, 66b–67b
  amputation of, 70–71, 70b, 70f
  Brodsky classification of, 67, 68t
  imaging studies for, 69, 69b
  infections of, 68
    antibiotics for, 68
  physical examination for, 67
  studies of, 68–69
  surgical debridement of, 69, 69b
  ulceration of, 67f
  vascularity of, 69, 69b
  Wagner classification of wound in, 68t
Disc herniation
  anatomic zones of, 289f
  diagnosis of, 304
  foraminal, 288
  sites for, 288
  tension signs in, 322
  treatment of, 304
  types of, 304
  unilateral paracentral
    at L3-L4, 322
    at L4-L5 disc, 322
    at L5-S1 disc, 322
Discography, for degenerative disc disease evaluation, 324–325
Discoid meniscus, 333–334, 334f
Dislocations
  see also under specific joints
  complex, operative treatment for, 271
Distal femoral traction pin, 422
Distal interphalangeal joints
  arthritis of, 102f
    surgical intervention in, 104
  inability to extend, 98b, 100f
  osteoarthritis of, 103b, 104
Distal phalanges
  crush injuries of, 111
  fractures of, 109–111
    categories of, 111
    intra-articular, 111
    treatment for, 111
    tuft, 111
Distal tibia, 427–431
  case study in, 427b, 429b
Distraction test, 284
Dorsal approach (Thompson), in radial shaft, 402–404
Dorsal interossei muscle, 87t–88t, 89f
Dorsal wrist ganglion, 83
Double-incision technique, 386f
Double-row rotator cuff repairs, 249

"Dreaded black line", 348
Duchenne muscular dystrophy (DMD), 210
Dupuytren's contracture, of fingers, 81
Dynamic peel-back test, 366f

E
Eccentric action, of muscles, 220
Ectrodactyly, 193
Eden-Lange procedure, 266
Elastic materials, *vs.* viscoelastic materials, 44
Elbow, 398–402
  acute biceps rupture of, 276
  arthritis/stiffness of, 272–276
  athletic injuries of, 369–375
    case study in, 369b–370b
  boxer's, 373
  case of, 267b, 270b–272b
  collateral ligaments of, 369f
  dislocations of, 267–271
    common, 267
    complications of, 271
    description of, 267
    mechanism of injury, 267
    neurovascular function in, 269
    neurovascular injuries in, 269
    physical findings of, 269
    procedure for, 270
    reducing of, 270
    surgical fixation of, 271
    treatment for, 271
  dynamic restraints of, 369
  heterotopic bone in, resection of, 240
  injuries to, in young athletes, 216–217, 216b
  instability of, 267–271
  osteoarthritis of, 272
  osteoarthrosis of, 272
  pain, physical examination of thrower with, 370
  rheumatoid arthritis of, 273
  spastic extended, treatment of, 232
  spastic flexed, treatment of, 232
  static restraints of, 369
  tennis. *see* Tennis elbow
  of thrower, mechanism of injury in, 369
  trauma to, 174–177, 174b, 175f
  valgus compressive stresses of, 370f
  valgus extension overload syndrome of, 373
Elderly patients
  acetabular fractures in, 409
  bone in, 26–27
  fractures in, 441–442
  Milwaukee shoulder in, 266
  pelvic fractures in, 409
  total elbow arthroplasty in, 275
Electrical stimulation, 221
Electrocardiography (EKG), in hypertrophic cardiomyopathy, 376
Electromyography (EMG), 290
  in cubital tunnel syndrome, 373
  in lumbar disc disease, 323
ELISA, for Lyme disease, 151
Enchondroma, 132, 132b, 132f
Endoneurium, 34–37
Enneking system, for orthopedic tumors, 125, 126t
Enthesis, 329

Eosinophilic granuloma (EG), and Langerhans cell histiocytosis, 161
Equinovarus foot, 205
Erb's palsy, 198
Erythema migrans rash, of Lyme disease, 151
Essex-Lopresti classification, of calcaneus fracture, 432, 434f
Essex-Lopresti lesion, 399, 400f
Evan's classification, of intertrochanteric fracture, 419–420
Ewing's sarcoma, 127f, 137, 162
    and neuroblastoma, 138
Exercises, 221
    in early rehabilitation of ACL reconstruction, 338
Extended shank, as shoe modification, 228–229
Extensor pollicis longus (EPL) tendon, rupture of, 101, 101b
Extensor tendon
    anatomy of, 99f
    injury of, zones of, 97, 98f
    laceration, 96b, 97f
        repair of, 97
    mechanism of, 97–98
External fixation, complications of, of femur fractures, 167
External rotation recurvatum test, 341
Extra depth shoe, as shoe modification, 228
"Extra-octave" fracture, 201
Extracellular matrix, components of, 23
Extrinsic flexor tendons, in hand, 88

F

FABER test, 286
Familial hypophosphatemic rickets, 26
Fanconi anemia, associated with radial clubhand, 193
Fasciotomy, treatment for compartment syndrome of hand, 85
Fat pad sign, 174
Fatigue strength, of biomechanics, 45
Fatty degeneration, of rotator cuff, 247
Fatty infiltration of muscle, rotator cuff repair and, 248–249
Femoral acetabular impingement (FAI), 214–215, 214b, 214f
Femoral component, rotation of, 9
Femoral condyles
    distal, 9
        normal alignment of, 9
    Hoffa fracture and, 423
    medial, osteochondritis dessicans lesion in, 343
Femoral fractures
    diaphyseal, 166b, 166f
    distal, 423–424
        case study in, 423b
        classification of, 423
        physeal, 168
    intraoperative, factors of, 16–17
    periprosthetic, classification and treatment of, 21, 21t
    proximal, 417–421
        case study in, 417b, 419b–420b

subtrochanteric, 420
        deforming forces on the proximal segment of, 421
        treatment for, 421
Femoral head
    blood supply to, 164
    fractures of, classification of, 418–419
Femoral neck
    blood supply to, 417
    fractures of, 164–168
        classification of, 417
        complication following, 417
        ipsilateral, 421
        stress-type, 348, 349f
        surgical interventions used for, 418
Femoral shaft, 421–423
    case study in, 421b–422b
    fractures of, 421
        classification system for, 421
        diaphyseal, treatment options for pediatric, 167
        surgical options for, 422
        traction to, 421
Femoral stem, cement mantle surrounding, 15
Femoral stretch test, 286
Femoroacetabular impingement (FAI), 345–347
    case study in, 345b
    causes of, 346
    findings associated with, 346
    prevalence of, 346
    treatment for, 347
    types of, 345–346
Femur, 417–424
    fractures of. *see* Femoral fractures
    lateral cortex of, 421
    medial cortex of, 421
Fibro-osseous flexor pulley system, for fingers, 93
Fibrocartilage, 30–33
Fibroma, non-ossifying, 134, 134f, 159, 159f
Fibrous dysplasia, 140, 160, 160f
Fibrous histiocytoma, malignant, 141
Ficat classification, for avascular necrosis, 416
"Fight bite", 81b, 82
Fingers
    hyperextended and compressed, 113b, 113f
    "resting cascade", 95
    rotational deformity of, 201
    rotational malalignment of, 116, 116f
    supination deformity of, 113, 113f
    trigger, treatment for, 93
Finkelstein's test, positive, 85
1st dorsal compartment tenosynovitis, 85
Flare, as shoe modification, 228
Fleck sign, indication of an avulsion of Lisfranc ligament, 436–437, 438f
Flexible nails, as femur fracture internal fixation complication, 167
Flexion-distraction injury, 299
Flexion teardrop fracture, 296
    management of, 296
Flexor digiti minimi (FDM) muscle, 87t
Flexor digitorum profundus (FDP), 94–95
    injury of, 93b, 94
    laceration of, 95, 95f
Flexor digitorum superficialis (FDS), 94–95
    injury of, 93b, 94
    laceration of, 95, 95f

Flexor pollicis brevis (FPB) muscle, 86t
Flexor pollicis longus (FPL) tendon, rupture of, in
    rheumatoid arthritis, 107
Flexor tendons, 93–102
    injury of, 90, 90b
        methods for diagnosing, 95
        zones of, 95, 96f
    repair of
        complications after, 96
        strength of, 95
"Floating shoulder", 390
Floating thumb, 195
Fluoroquinolones, 42t
Foot, 51–80, 431–437
    compartments of, 385
    diabetic, 66–72
    disorders, in Charcot-Marie-Tooth, 208
    neurologic disorder of, 76–80
    problems, in spina bifida, 208
    spastic equinovarus in, 233–234
Foot slap, 226
Forearm, 402–407
    compartments of, 385
    fracture of, compartment syndrome and, 404
    rotational forces on, 177–178
    spastic pronated, treatment of, 232
Four point gait, 228
Fracture-dislocation, 299
Fractures, 28
    see also specific types of fractures
    ankle, treatment options for, in children, 171–172
    Barton's, 407
    Bennett, 117, 117b
    "boxer's", 114b, 115, 115f
    of cervical spine. see Cervical spine, fractures of
    Chance, 299
    chauffeur's, 406
    "extra-octave", 201
    fragility, 441
    healing of, 381–383, 383f
        stages of, 381–383
        types of, 28–29, 29f
    of hip
        mechanism of injury of, 164–168
        treatment of choice for, 165
    of knee, 168–171, 168b, 168f
    lateral epicondyle, 176
    medial epicondyle, 176
    metacarpal, amounts of angulation in, 201
    Monteggia, Bado classification of, 176–177, 177f
    pathologic
        in children, 162
        management of, 162
    periprosthetic, 441
        treatment of, 441
    of radial head/neck, treatment options for, 176
    Segund, 336, 337f
    of shoulder, 172–174
    Smith's, 407
    of tibia, 168–171, 168b, 168f
    Tillaux, 171
    toddler's, 145b
    triplane, 171
Fragility fracture, 441
    locations of, 442

Frame walker, 227
Fretting corrosion, 45
"Friar Tuck" sign, 257–258
Friedrich's ataxia, 208–210
Functional humerus brace, 394, 395f
Functional range of motion, of elbow, 272

G
Gaenslen maneuver, 286
Gage sign, 153–154
Gait
    aids of, 226–231
        types of, 227–228
    "antalgic", 225
    components of, 223–226
    determinants of, 225
    normal and pathologic, 223–226
    painful, 225
    patterns of, 228
    Trendelenburg, 225
Gait cycle, 223
Galeazzi fracture, 404
Galvanic corrosion, 45
"Gamekeeper's thumb", 118, 118b
Garden classification, of femoral neck fractures, 417,
    418f
Gaussian distribution, 47f
Giant cell tumor, 126f, 134–135, 134b, 135f
Gill procedure
    in spondylolisthesis, 318
    in spondylolysis, 318
Glenohumeral instability, in young athletes,
    215–216
Glenohumeral internal rotation deficit, 222
    treatment of, 222
Glenohumeral internal rotation deficit (GIRD),
    366–367, 368f
Glenohumeral joints
    arthritis of, 256–264, 356
        anatomic variable for, 259
        case of, 256b, 259b
        etiologies of, 256
        hemiarthroplasty in, 260
        history and physical examination of, 257
        non-operative treatments of, 259
        non-prosthetic surgical intervention for,
            259
        prosthetic options for treatment of, 259
        radiographic appearance of, secondary to
            rheumatologic disease, 257, 257f
        total shoulder arthroplasty in, 260
    distinguish pain to AC joint, 251
    evaluation of, 391, 391f
    hemiarthroplasty of, 260
Glenohumeral osteoarthritis, radiographic
    appearance of, 257–258, 258f
Glenoid, 389–390
    case study in, 389b, 390f
    fractures of
        indications for, 389
        surgical approaches to, 389
Glenoid deformity, classification system for, in
    osteoarthritis, 258
Glenoid version, normal, 258

Glycopeptides, 42t
Golden hour, in trauma patient, 387
Golfer's elbow, 278
  symptoms and findings of, 279
  tendon origin of, 279
  treatment for, 279
Gout, hip arthritis and, 13t
Goutallier classification, 247
Gower's sign, 210
Great toe, disorder of, 51–55
Grinding test, 330–331, 332f
Gripping, motor function of, 81
Groin pain, differential diagnosis for an athlete with, 345
Gross Motor Function Classification system, for cerebral palsy, 202
Growth plate fractures, Salter-Harris classification for, 163
"Gunstock deformity." *see* Cubitus varus
Gustilo-Anderson classification, of open fractures, 439
Guyon's canal, 90

H

Haemophilus influenza, as pathogen of septic arthritis, 146
Hahn-Steinthal fractures, 396, 396f
Hallux rigidus, 51b, 52, 54f
  etiology of, 52
  surgery for, 54t
  symptoms of, 52
Hallux valgus, 51, 51b, 52f
  anatomical deformities in, 51
  causes of, 51
  nonsurgical treatment for, 51
  radiographic measurement for severity of, 52t
  surgical treatment for, 53f
  vector forces acting on, 51
Halo vest, 299, 299f
Hammer toe deformity, 56, 56b
  differentiated from mallet toe/claw toe deformities, 56, 56t
Hamstring autograft, for ACL reconstruction, 336
Hand, 81–124
  anatomy of, 81–102
    osseous structures, 81–83, 82f
  arthritis and arthroplasty of, 102–104
  blood supply of, 90, 91f
  bones and joints in, 81–83
  compartments of, 85, 385
  congenital abnormalities, 191–197
    categories of, 191–197
  fractures and dislocations of, 109–121
  functions of, 81
  injuries to, 199–201, 199b, 199f
  intrinsic muscles of, 85, 86f
  lupus, 108
  "opera glass", 108, 110f
  rheumatoid arthritis of, 104–107, 104b, 105f
  "safe" position of, 89f
  Salter Harris type II fractures of, 200
  sensory nerve distributions of, 91
  surface of, 81
Hand-Schuller-Christian disease, 161

Hangman's fracture, 301
  signs and symptoms of, 301
Hare traction, for femoral shaft fracture, 421–422
Hawkin's classification, of talar neck fractures, 431, 432f
Hawkins impingement test, 244
Head trauma, 375–376, 375b
Heat, as physical therapy modality, 221
Heberden's nodes, 104
Heel, 431–437
Heel pain, 56–58, 56b–57b, 57f
  central, 58
  diagnosis of, 57b
  etiology of, 57
Hemangioma, 140
Hemi-walker. *see* Frame walker
Hemiarthroplasty
  with biologic glenoid resurfacing, 260
  for cuff tear arthropathy, 262
  for glenohumeral arthritis, 260
  shoulder, 260
Hemipelvectomy, features of, 236
Hemophilia, associated with septic arthritis, 147
Heparin, mechanism of, 41f
Herring lateral pillar radiographic classification, of Legg-Calve-Perthes disease, 154, 154f
Heterotopic bone prophylaxis, utility of, 239
Heterotopic ossification (HO), 18
  case of, 238b
  clinical signs of, 239
  diagnostic tests of, 239
  etiologies of, 238
High ankle sprain, 74, 74b
Highly cross-linked polyethylene, 45
Hill-Sachs lesion, 354, 355f
Hip, 12–21, 12b, 13f
  arthritis, 13t
    initial treatment options for, 14, 14b
    radiographic findings with, 13t
    surgical treatment for, 14
  arthroscopy of, complications with, 347
  aspiration, 148
  disarticulation, 236
  disorders, pediatric, 210–215
  flexion contractures of, 233
  formation of heterotopic bone in, 239, 240f
  fractures of
    mechanism of injury of, 164–168
    treatment of choice for, 165
  injury to, 345–375
  periprosthetic infection of, 19
    radiographic appearance of, 19
  prosthesis, dislocation of, 17, 17b, 18f
  spastic adduction contractures of, 232
  surgical approaches to, 14
  transient synovitis, 148–149
Hip dislocations, 414–416
  anterior, type of, 414
  case study in, 414b
  mechanism of injury in, 166
  native, 414–415
  posterior, 414
    maneuver for, 415, 415f
    neurologic injury in, 415–416
  type of, 414

Hip hiking, 225
HKAFO orthosis, 231
Hoffa fracture, 423
Hoffman's sign, 284
Holt-Oram syndrome, associated with radial
    clubhand, 193
Hornblower test, 250
Horner's syndrome, 199
Housemaid's knee, 344–345
Humeral avulsion of the glenohumeral ligament
    (HAGL) lesion, 354, 356f
Humeral fractures
  distal
    classification of, 396
    complications of, 397, 397f
    fixation principles in, 396
    radiographic technique in, 396
    total elbow arthroplasty in, 397
  proximal, 391–394
    case study in, 391b
    classification of, 392, 392f
    operative indications for, in pediatric patient,
      173–174
    surgical approach to, 394
    treatment of, 392, 393f
  supracondylar
    medial pin in, 175
    neurovascular exam for, 174–175
Humeral shaft, 394
  fractures of
    displaced diaphyseal, 395f
    nerve injured with, 394
    treatment of, 174, 394, 395f
Humeral version, normal, 258
Humerus, 391–397
  distal, 396–397
    case study in, 396b
  fractures of. see Humeral fractures
  proximal, blood supply to, 391
Hyaline cartilage, 30–33
Hyperkyphosis, 181–182
Hypertrophic cardiomyopathy, 376
Hypoparathyroidism, 25
Hypoplastic thumb, types of, 195
Hypotension, patient stabilization in,
    408–409
Hypothenar muscles, of hand, 87t
Hypovolemic shock, vs. neurogenic shock, 299
Hysteresis, 44

I

Ibuprofen, mechanism of action for, 40
Idiopathic osteoarthritis, associated full-thickness
    rotator cuff tear, 259
Immobilization, in injury, 375
Impingement test, 215
Implantation
  autologous chondrocyte, 343
  osteochondral plug, 343
  silicone, silicone synovitis due to, 107
Implants
  linked, 275
  type of, 47
  unlinked, 275

Independent variables, in biostatistics, 46–47
Infections
  as complications of shoulder arthroplasty, 261
  in diabetic foot, 68
  musculoskeletal, 37–38, 37b
  periprosthetic, total knee arthroplasty and, 11
  prosthetic joint, categories of, 12, 20–21
  in spine, 291–292
Infectious arthritis, hip arthritis and, 13t
Inferior glenohumeral ligament (IGHL), 350, 351f
Inferior shoulder subluxation, treatment of, 231–232
Inflammatory arthritis (RA), of elbow, 273
  non-operative treatments for, 274
Initial contact, muscles acting during, 224
Initial swing, muscles acting during, 224
Injury Severity Score, 386
Inpatient setting, to outpatient setting, flow of
    surgical patients from, 221–222
Instability
  as complications of shoulder arthroplasty, 261
  in glenohumeral joint, 351
    vs. laxity, 351
Interclavicular ligament, 254
Interdigital neuritis, 76
Intermediate column, of wrist, 405
Internal fixation
  of femoral neck fractures, 417
  of femur fractures, complications of, 167
  shoulder arthrodesis and, 263
Internal impingement, 366, 368f
Interosseous nerve, anterior, 174–175
Interphalangeal joints
  distal. see Distal interphalangeal joints
  proximal. see Proximal interphalangeal (PIP)
    joints
Interspinous ligaments, 283
Intertrochanteric fracture, 419
  complications of, 420
  Evan's classification of, 419–420
  surgical interventions used for, 420
Intervertebral disc, 33
  biomarkers, 33
  composition of, 33
  structure and function of, 33
Intra-articular disc ligament, 254
Intramedullary nails
  advantages of, 422–423
  antegrade, of femoral fractures, 423
  bending stiffness and, 44
  in fracture healing, 29
  retrograde, of femoral fractures, 423
  rigid, as femur fracture internal fixation
    complication, 167
  tibial, complication associated with,
    427
Intrathecal Baclofen, for cerebral palsy, 202
Intrinsic minus position, of hand, 88
Intrinsic plus position, of hand, 88, 89f
Involucrum, in chronic osteomyelitis, 150
Isokinetic action, of muscles, 220
Isokinetic contraction, 36
Isolated articular surface fractures, 396, 396f
Isometric action, of muscles, 220
Isotonic action, of muscles, 220
Isotonic contraction, 36

J

Jaccoud's arthropathy, 108
Jefferson fracture, 301
  treatment of, 301
Jerk test, 361
Jersey finger, 96, 96b, 97f
Joints
  acromioclavicular. *see* Acromioclavicular (AC)
    joints
  ankle (tibiotalar), range of motion of, 221f
  atlantoaxial, unstable, 281, 283f
  bacteria gain access to, 146
  carpometacarpal. *see* Carpometacarpal (CMC)
    joints
  damage of, 148
  distal interphalangeal. *see* Distal interphalangeal
    joints
  glenohumeral. *see* Glenohumeral joints
  metacarpophalangeal. *see* Metacarpophalangeal
    (MCPs) joints
  metatarsal. *see* Metatarsal joints
  proximal interphalangeal. *see* Proximal
    interphalangeal (PIP) joints
Jones fracture, 65
  treatment for, 66
Judet-Letournel classification, of acetabular fractures,
  409–411, 412f
Jumper's knee, 344
Juvenile idiopathic arthritis, 155–156, 155b
  polyarticular, 156
Juvenile rheumatoid arthritis. *see* Juvenile idiopathic
  arthritis

K

Kim test, for postero-inferior instability, 361
Kinetic chain, 363
King classification, of adolescent idiopathic scoliosis,
  180
Klippel-Feil syndrome, 189, 190f, 302, 303f
  classic triad of, 189
  treatment for, 190, 303
Klumpke palsies, 198
Knee, 1–12, 1b, 328–345
  aspiration, 148
  degenerative joint disease of, 6
  differential diagnosis for, 1, 1b, 2f
  disarticulations, 236
  dislocations of
    classification of, 340
    examination of patient with, 423–424
    initial management of, 423
    treatment for, 340–341, 341f
    type of, 423, 424f
  housemaid's, 344–345
  injuries, in young athletes, 217, 217b
    treatment options for, 217–218
  isolated PCL-deficient, 339, 340f
  jumper's, 344
  lateral structures of, 342
  mechanical axis of, 9
  medial structures of, 342
  osteoarthritis of, 1, 4b
    AAOS recommendations for, 3t
    treatment for, 3–4

  posterolateral corner of, 341
  resection of heterotopic bone and, 239
  spastic flexion deformity of, 233
  unhappy triad, 335
  unicompartmental arthroplasty of, 5f
  valgus instability of, 342
  varus instability of, 342
  x-ray of, 32
Knee-ankle-foot orthoses (KAFOs)
  different types of, 230–231
  indications of, 231
Knee scooters, 228
Kocher criteria, 149
Kocher-Lorenz fractures, 396, 396f
Kruskal-Wallis test, 47–48, 48t
Kyphoplasty, 309
Kyphosis, 181–182, 314

L

Lachman test, 335
Lamellar bone, 23
Langerhan's cell histiocytosis, 142, 143f
  and eosinophilic granuloma, 161
Lasegue sign, 285, 285f
Lateral compression, 407, 408f
Lateral elbow pain, differential diagnosis of, 374
Lateral epicondyle fractures, treatment options for,
  176
Lateral epicondylitis. *see* Tennis elbow
Lateral patellar compression syndrome, 345
Lateral pivot shift test, of posterolateral instability of
  elbow, 268
Lateral trunk lean, 225
Lauge-Hansen classification, for ankle fractures,
  427–428
Laxity, in glenohumeral joint, 351
  vs. instability, 351
Leg, lower, compartments of, 385, 386f
Leg-length inequality, 225
Legg-Calve-Perthes disease, 152–155, 152b, 152f
  classification of, 154
  femoral head affected by, 152–153
  goals of treatment in, 154–155
  imaging for, 153–154
  osteotomy for
    acetabular, 155
    femoral, 155
  pathogenesis of, 152
  peak age of incidence of, 153
  physical exam findings of, 153
  prognosis of, 153
Lenke classification, of adolescent idiopathic
  scoliosis, 180
Lesser toe disorder, 55–56
  treatment for, 56
Letterer-Siwe disease, 161
Level of evidence, of study, 48, 49t, 50b
Lever arm dysfunction, 226
Lhermitte's sign, 284, 284f
Lift-off test, 249, 250f
Ligament Reconstruction Tendon Interposition
  (LRTI) procedure, for thumb CMC
  arthritis, 103
Ligamentous knee injury, 335

Ligaments, 33–34
injury to
healing, 34
mechanism of, 33
interspinous, 283
Lisfranc, 437
in sternoclavicular joint, 254
structure and function of, 33
supraspinous, 283
transverse, 283
wrist stabilization and, 83
Ligamentum flavum, 283
Limb salvage, 440
decision to attempt, 440
pros and cons of, 440
Lincosamides, 42t
Lipoma, 139, 139f
atypical, 139
Liposarcoma, 141
Lisfranc injury, 436
clinical exam for, 436
complication of, 437
management of patients with, 437
mechanism of injury in, 436, 437f
types of, 437, 438f
Lisfranc ligament, 437
List, in disc herniations, 322
Lite gait. *see* Partial weight bearing systems
"Little leaguer's shoulder", 215–216
Load-and-shift test, 352f
Loading response, muscles acting during, 224
Lobster claw deformity. *see* Cleft hand
Long bones, giant cell tumors of, 134–135
Longitudinal deficiency, of hand, 192
radial. *see* Radial clubhand
Low-molecular-weight heparin (LMWH), 40–41, 41f
Lower back rehabilitation, principles of, 222–223
Lower extremity amputation, level of, 236
Lumbar disc disease, 321
tests for, 322
Lumbar discectomy, 323
Lumbar fusion, 325–326
techniques for, 326
Lumbar lordosis, 281, 282f
Lumbar/sacral nerve root compression, 287, 288t
Lumbar spine
disease, 291
injuries to, 376
tests for, 285
vertebrae of, 281
Lumbrical muscles, 87t–88t, 89
Lupus hand, 108
Lyme disease, 151–152
Lymphoma, effect of, on bone, 138

M

Macrodactyly, 195
Macrophage activation syndrome (MAS), 156
Madelung deformity, 197, 198f
Maffucci disease, 132
Magnetic resonance imaging (MRI), 289–290
of ACL injury, 336
of Bankart lesion, 354
of cervical spondylosis, 306

of fatty degeneration of rotator cuff, 247, 247f
of glenohumeral arthritis, 258
of herniated discs, 304, 305f
of lumbar disc disease, 322, 323f
of lumbar spine, 320f
of orthopedic tumors, 128
of osteomyelitis, 149–150
of septic arthritis, 147
of spinal stenosis, 290
of ulnar collateral ligament injury, 371, 372f
Maisonneuve fracture, 428, 429f
Mallet finger, 100–101, 100f
injury of, 100
treatment of, 100–101
Mallet toe deformity, 56t
Mangled Extremity Severity Score, 440
Mannerfelt syndrome, 107
Manual muscle testing, strength graded by, 220
Manual therapy, 221
MARCO mnemonic, 126
Marginal excision, of orthopedic tumors, 129
Mason classification, of radial head fractures, 268, 269f
McCune-Albright syndrome, 160
McLaughlin procedure, 361, 362f
McMurray test, 330, 331f
Medial clear space, 428
Medial collateral ligament (MCL) tear, treatment of, 342
Medial elbow pain, 370
Medial epicondyle fractures, 176
Medial parapatellar capsular arthrotomy, in total knee arthroplasty, 7
Median nerve compression syndrome, 375
Meniscal allograft transplantation, 333
Meniscal injuries, 328–334
case study in, 328b, 331b, 332f
healing potential for, 33
Meniscal repairs
clinical factors in, 333
lateral approach to knee for, 333
medial approach to knee for, 333
suture placement for, 333
Meniscal tear, 329–330, 331b, 332f
acute, 332
associated with ACL injuries, 335
location of, 330
managing of, 333
mechanical symptoms of, 330
physical exam signs in, 330
Meniscectomy, 329
Menisci, 30–33
composition of, 329
cyst of, 333, 334f
discoid, 333–334, 334f
injuries to. *see* Meniscal injuries
lateral, 328
attachments of, 329
medial, 328
microstructure of, 329
MRI appearance of, 332
proteoglycans in, 329
structure and function of, 32–33
vascular supply to, 329
vascular zones of, 329, 330f

Metabolic bone disease, laboratory findings in, 27t
Metacarpals
    dislocations of, 114–116
    fracture of, 109
        classification of, 114–116
        dorsal angulation of, 115
Metacarpal fractures, amounts of angulation in, 201
Metacarpal neck fracture, 115
    tolerated degree of angulation in, 116
Metacarpophalangeal (MCPs) joints
    arthritis, surgical intervention in, 104
    arthroplasty for, 104
    deformity of, in advanced rheumatoid arthritis,
        105
    dislocations of, 114–116
        complex, 116, 117f
        simple vs. complex, 116, 117f
    fractures of, 114–116
Metal-on-metal, 45
Metatarsal joints
    5th, fracture zones of, 65, 65b, 66f
        Jones fracture, 65
        treatment for, 66
Metatarsophalangeal (MTP) joints, synovitis of,
        differentiated from interdigital neuroma, 77
Methicillin resistant Staphylococcus aureus, 38
Methotrexate, as treatment for polyarticular juvenile
        idiopathic arthritis, 156
Metizeau technique, 176
Meyerding classification, 185
Meyers and McKeever classification, of tibial
        eminence fractures, 168
"Micro-motion pain," in septic arthritis, 147
Microdiscectomy, lumbar, 323
Microfracture technique, 343, 343f
Mid-stance, muscles acting during, 224
Mid swing, muscles acting during, 224
Middle glenohumeral ligament (MGHL), 350, 351f
Midfoot, 434–437
    case study of, 434b
Milwaukee shoulder, 266
Modic changes, 324
Modulus of elasticity, 381
Mononucleosis, 376
Monteggia fracture, 404
    types of, 404, 405f
Monteggia fracture dislocation, definition of,
        176–177
Mortise view, 427
Morton's neuroma, 76, 76b, 76f
    after excision of, 77
    diagnostic/radiographic tests for, 76
    non-surgical management of, 77
    symptoms of, 76
Mosaicplasty, 343
Motion-limiting braces, in shoulder dislocations, 357
Motor neuropathy, 67
Mulder's sign, 76
Multidirectional instability (MDI), 356, 357t
Multiligamentous knee injury, 340–342, 340b
Multiple myeloma, 138, 138f
Muscle, 34–37
    actions of, 220–222
    contraction of, 35
    disorders of, 264–266

Muscle strains, in athlete pelvis, 349
Musculoskeletal infections, 37–38, 37b
Musculoskeletal tissue, 23–37
Musculoskeletal tumors, principles of diagnosis and
        treatment of, 128–130, 128b
Musculotendinous injury, 37
    differential diagnosis for, 37
Myelodysplasia, 207
Myelography, 289
Myelopathy, 304
Myositis ossificans, 140
Myxoma, 140

N

Nailbed injuries, pediatric, treatment of, 200
Nails, normal growth rate of, 111
Narakas classification, for brachial plexus birth palsy,
        198
NCAA rules, return to play, after blunt head injury,
        376
Necrotizing fasciitis, 37
Neer impingement test, 244
Negative predictive value (NPV), 50
Neonates, lower extremity septic arthritis in, 147
Nerot classification, of progressive scapular notching,
        263f
Nerves, 34–37
    axillary, 391–392
    disorders of, 264–266
    lesions of, categories of, 198
    median, in hand, 91
    peripheral
        anatomy of, 34–37, 35f
        injuries, classification and prognosis of, 34
        mechanism for, 34
    suprascapular. see Suprascapular nerves
    ulna, in hand, 91
Nerve conduction velocity (NCV), in cubital tunnel
        syndrome, 373
Nerve injuries
    in acetabular fracture fixation, 412
    operative treatment for, 34
Neurapraxia, 198
Neuro-orthopedic surgery
    case of, 231b
    general principles of, 220–222, 231
    rehabilitation and, 220–243
Neurofibroma. see Schwannoma
Neurofibrosarcoma, 140
Neurogenic shock, 298–299
    vs. hypovolemic shock, 299
Neurologic injury, direct trauma and, 239
Neurological examination, 286
Neuropathy
    autonomic, 67
    motor, 67
    peripheral, 66–67
    sensory, 66–67
Neuropraxia, 34
Neurotmesis, 34, 198
Neurovascular injuries, in elbow dislocations,
        269–270
Neutralization plate, 381, 382f
Night-stick fracture, 404

"No man's land" area, in flexor tendon and, 95
Non-accidental trauma, in children, 163
Non-parametric data, 47
Non-random systematic error, of design, 48–50
Non-steroidal antiinflammatory drugs (NSAIDs), 40
  mechanism of aspirin from, 40
  in osteoid osteomas, 157
Nonunion
  atrophic, 30
  as complication of pediatric hip fractures, 165
  oligotrophic, 30
  treatment of, 30
Null hypothesis, 48

O

O'Brien's test, 364, 364f
Occult fracture, 290
Occupational therapist (OT), 220
Odontoid fracture, 293
  classification of, 293–294, 294f
  diagnosis of, 293
  mechanism of, 293
  neurologic involvement in, 293
  treatment of, 294–295
  type I, 293
  type II, 294
    complication with, 294
    risk factors for, 294
  type III, 294
Odontoid process, 283
Olecranon
  fractures
    classification of, 400, 401f
    mechanism of, 400–402
    treatment for, 400–402, 402f–403f
  impingement syndrome, 373
  sleeve fracture, 176
Oligoarticular juvenile idiopathic arthritis, 155
Oligotrophic nonunion, 30
Ollier disease, 132
Open fractures, 439–440
  case study in, 439b
  classification of, 439
  treatment of, 439
    in high-velocity gunshot wounds vs.
      low-velocity gunshot wounds, 440
  type of antibiotics for, 439
"Opera glass hand", 108, 110f
Operative fixation, of complex elbow dislocations, 271
Opponens digiti minimi (ODM) muscle, 87t
Opponens pollicis (OP) muscle, 86t
Oral Baclofen, for cerebral palsy, 202
Ordinal data, 47
Orthopedic oncology, 125–144
  general, 125–128, 125b
Orthopedic pharmacology, 38–41, 38b
Orthopedic surgery, of rehabilitation, 231
Orthosis, 229
  purposes of, 231
Orthotics, 226–231
  case of, 226b
Ortolani maneuver, 210–211, 211f
Ortolani sign, 210–211

Os odontoideum, 188–189, 301–302, 302f
  surgical stabilization of, 189
  treatment of, 302
Osseous tissue, 23–30
Osteoarthritic articular cartilage, 32
Osteoarthritis, 1, 13t
  cartilage/ joints in, 1
  classification system for glenoid deformity in, 258
  differential diagnosis of, 1
  of elbow
    contraindications to arthroscopic treatment of, 273
    non-operative treatments for, 272
    physical examination of, 272
    surgical treatment of, 272
  joint pain, sources of, 1–2
  pathoanatomy of, 32
  pathogenesis of, 1
  risk factors associated with, 2
  total knee arthroplasty for, 4
Osteoarthrosis, of elbow, 272
Osteoblastoma, 158, 158f
  vs. osteoid sarcoma, 131
Osteoblasts, function in bone homeostasis, 23–24
Osteocalcin, 23
Osteochondral autograft transfer system (OATS), 343
Osteochondral lesions, 342–344, 342b
Osteochondral plug implantation, 343, 344t
Osteochondritis dessicans (OCD), 343
Osteochondroma, 133, 133b, 133f, 158, 158f
Osteoclasts, function in bone homeostasis, 23–24
Osteocytes, function in bone homeostasis, 23–24
Osteogenesis imperfecta
  associated with developmental basilar
    invagination, 191
  vs. non-accidental injury, 163
Osteogenic bone graft, 30
Osteoid osteoma, 130–131, 130f, 157
  treatment of, 131
Osteoinductive graft materials, 30
Osteomyelitis, 38, 39f, 149–151
  organisms causing, 39t
  septic arthritis and, 151
  surgical intervention for, 150
  treatment of, 150
Osteonecrosis
  as complication of lateral condyle fractures, 176
  as complication of pediatric hip fractures, 165
Osteopenia, 441–442
  laboratory workup of, 442
Osteopetrosis, 24–25, 28
  mechanism compare with, 28b
Osteophytes, 1
  excision of, 273
Osteoporosis, 441–442
  laboratory workup of, 442
  pathophysiology of, 27, 27f
  risk factors for, 28
  therapies available to treat, 28, 28b
Osteoprotegerin (OPG), 24
Osteosarcoma, 127f, 136, 136b
  parosteal, 137
  periosteal, 137

sunburst pattern of, 136f
telangiectatic, 136–137
Osteotomy, 155
  acetabular, 155
    for Legg-Calve-Perthes disease, 155
  Chiari, 212, 213f
  distal femoral, 4, 5f
    for degenerative joint disease of knee, 6
  femoral
    in Legg-Calve-Perthes disease, 155
  high tibial, 4–6, 4f
  olecranon, in distal humeral articular segment,
    396
  pelvic, 212
    redirectional, 212
    reshaping, 212
    salvage, 212
Outpatient setting, flow of surgical patients from
    inpatient to, 221–222
"Overstuffing," in shoulder arthroplasty, 261

P

Paget's disease, 28, 28b, 135
Pain
  back
    evaluating of, 283
    red flags in, 291
  localized, 283
  mechanical, 283
  neck, red flags in, 291
  night, 283
  in osteoarthritis, 1
  radicular, 283
Pain relief, and restoration of function, 260
Palmar interossei, 87t–88t, 89f
Palmar plate, 81
Palmaris brevis (PB) muscle, 87t
Palmaris longus tendon, 88
Paracentral herniation, 288
Parallel bars, 228
Parametric data, 47
Parapodiums, 228, 231
Partial weight bearing systems, 228
Patella tendon ruptures, 344
Patellar instability, treatment of, 217–218
Patellar sleeve fracture, 170
Patellar tendonitis, 344
  non-operative treatment of, 222
Patellofemoral arthroplasty (PFA), 4, 6f
Patellofemoral disorders, 344–345
  case study in, 344b
Patellofemoral pain syndrome. see Chondromalacia
  patella
Patellofemoral tracking, facilitation of, 10, 10b, 11f
Pathologic fractures, management of, in children,
  162
Pavlik harness, for developmental dysplasia of the
  hip, 212
Pediatric orthopedics, 145–219
  neuromuscular disorders in, 201–210
Pellegrini-Stieda sign, 342
Pelvic fracture
  injuries associated with, 408
  inlet view of, 407–408, 410f

mechanism of, 409
  outlet view of, 407–408, 410f
  patient stabilization in, 408–409
Pelvic rotation, 225
Pelvic tilt, 225
Pelvis, 407–416
  case study in, 407b, 409b
  contusions and strains, 348–350, 348b
  radiographic lines in, 409, 411f
Penicillinase, resistant, 42t
Penicillins, 42t
Perineurium, 34–37
Peripheral neuropathy, 66–67
Peroneal tendons
  function of, 64
  injury mechanism for, 64
  subluxation/dislocation/rupture, 64–65, 64f
Pertrochanteric fracture, 419
Phalanges
  distal. see Distal phalanges
  fractures of, 109
    "clinical healing" of, 112
    closed proximal spiral, 112b, 113, 113f
      treatment of, 113
    complications of, 112
    fixation used for, 112
    middle, 111–114
      surgery for, 111–114
    proximal, 111–114, 112b, 112f
      surgery for, 111–114
    treatment of, 112
Phalen-Dickson sign, 184
Philadelphia collar, 300, 300f
Phocomelia, 193–194
Physical exam, spinal column inspection and, 284
Physical medicine and rehabilitation physician
    (physiatrist /PM & R), 220
Physical therapist (PT), 220
Physical therapy
  for adult spinal problems, 222–223
  modalities/purposes of, 221
Pilon fracture, 429
  classification system for, 429, 430f
  definitive fixation of, 431
  mechanism of injury in, 431
  orthopedic injuries with, 431
Pincer impingement, 215, 215f, 346, 346f
  and cam impingement, 346
  radiographic signs of lesion, 347
Pipkin classification, of femoral head fractures,
    418–419, 419f
Pitching, phases of, 362, 363f
Pitting corrosion, 45
Pivot shift test, 335, 336f
Plain radiograph, of chronic rotator cuff pathology,
    247
Plane of motion, in adhesive capsulitis, 255
Planovalgus, 205
Plantar fasciitis, 57, 58b
  corticosteroid for, risk of, 58
  differentiated with central heel pain, 58
  first branch of lateral plantar nerve in, 58
  pain in, 57
  treatment for, 58
Plasmacytoma, 138

Plate, functions of, 381, 382f
Plate fixation
   in radial shaft fracture, 404
   in ulnar shaft fracture, 404
Poland syndrome, 194
Polyarthritis, 104
Polyarticular juvenile idiopathic arthritis,
   156
Polydactyly, 195
Polyethylene, metal on, 45
Polymerase chain reaction (PCR), 20
Polymorphonuclear (PMNs), 38
Polytrauma, 386–387
   golden hour in management of, 387
   patient evaluation in, 386–387
   pediatric, 162
   severity of injury in, 386–387
Positive predictive value (PPV), 50
Post-concussive syndrome, 376
Post-traumatic elbow stiffness, 276
Postaxial polydactyly, types of, 195
Posterior cruciate ligament (PCL) injury, 339,
   340f
   bony avulsions of, 339
   case study in, 339b
Posterior drawer test, in posterior instability,
   360–361
Posterior sag test, 339
Posterior tibial tendon, function of, 63
Posterior tibial tendon insufficiency (PTTI),
   62b, 63, 63f
   staging of, 63–64, 63t
Posterolateral rotatory instability, 267
   lateral pivot shift test of, 268
Posteromedial impingement syndrome. see Valgus
       extension overload syndrome
Posteromedial rotatory instability, 268
Power, 48
Pre-swing, muscles acting during, 224
Preaxial polydactyly, 195
Prepatellar bursitis, 344–345
Pronator syndrome, 375
Prosthesis
   components of, 238
   terminal device of, 238
Proteoglycans, in menisci, 329
Proximal interphalangeal (PIP) joints
   arthritis of, 102f
      surgical intervention in, 104
   arthroplasty for, 104
   dislocations of
      direction of, 113
      dorsal fracture, 114, 114b, 114f
         surgery and treatment for, 114
Proximal tibial traction pin, 422
Pseudo-Scheuermann disease, 183
Pseudogout, hip arthritis with, 13t
Pseudoparalysis, 262
Pseudowinging, 265
Psoriatic arthritis, of hand
   manifestations of, 108
   pathophysiology of, 108
   radiographic evaluation of, 108,
      109f
PT/OT assistants (PTA/OTA), 220

Q
Q-angle, in patella dislocation, 345
Quad cane, 227
Quadriceps rupture, 344
Quadriceps tendon autograft, in ACL injury,
   336
Quadrilateral space, 264, 265f
Quadrilateral space syndrome, 264

R
Radial clubhand, 192–193, 192b, 192f
   associated with Fanconi anemia, 193
   vs. ulnar clubhand, 193
Radial column, of wrist, 405
Radial head
   excision, after dislocation, 271
   fractures of, 268
      classification system of, 398, 398f
      mechanism of, 398–399
      treatment for, 398
   replacement of, 399
   resection of, 274
Radial nerve, 91, 394
Radial shaft, fractures of
   surgical approaches to, 402–404
   treatment of, 402
Radiation therapy, preoperative, 129
Radical excision, of orthopedic tumors, 129
Radiography
   in hyperextended elbow injuries, 375
   in shoulder dislocations, 354, 355f
Radius
   distal, 104, 178
      articular portions of, 404, 406f
   dorsal approach to, 406
   fractures of. see Radius fractures
   proximal, safe zone of, 399, 399f
   volar approach to, 406
Radius fractures
   distal, 404–407
      case study in, 404b
      treatment of, radiographic parameters in,
         405
   proximal, 398–399
Range of motion, testing of, 220, 221f
Reagan and Morrey classification, of coronoid
   fractures, 268
Reciprocating gait orthosis (RGO), 231
"Red-red zone," of meniscus, 333
Relative stability, 381
Relocation test, 353f
REMO mnemonic, 129
Remplissage technique, 359
Restraints, static and dynamic, to elbow dislocation,
   267
Retraction, rotator cuff tear with,
   248f
Reverse pivot shift test, 341
Reverse shoulder arthroplasty
   complication rate of, 262
   for cuff tear arthropathy, 262
Reverse shoulder prosthesis, components of,
   262f
Rhabdomyosarcoma, 142

Rheumatoid arthritis
  Boutonnière deformity in, 107, 107f
  of elbow, 273
    natural history of, 274
    surgical options for treatment of, 274
  of hand, 104–107, 105f
    advanced, metacarpophalangeal joint, 105
    non-surgical perioperative considerations, 105
    pathophysiology, 104
  hip arthritis with, 13t
Rheumatoid factor (RF), in polyarticular juvenile
    idiopathic arthritis, 156
Rhizotomy, 202
  for cerebral palsy, 202
RICE principle, 222
Rickets
  different forms of, 26
  vs. non-accidental trauma, 163
Risser classification, 179, 179f
Rocker bottom, as shoe modification, 229
Rocking horse phenomenon, 260
Rockwood classification, of acromioclavicular joint
    injuries, 252t
Rolando fractures, 118, 118f–119f
Rollators/rolling walkers, 227–228
Rotator cuff
  anatomy of, 245
  fatty degeneration of, 247
  intact, 259
  muscles of, 245, 246f, 246t
  operative approach to, 249
  repair, 248–249
  spectrum of, 245–246
  tears
    age and, 247
    bilateral, 247
    history and physical examination of, 246–247
    partial-thickness of, 248
    retraction with, 248f
    and subacromial impingement syndrome, 245
    tear progression in, 248
    treatment of, 250
  tendinitis, 354
  variables associated with, 249
Round cell tumors, pediatric and adult, 139t
Ruedi and Allgower's classification, of pilon fracture,
    429, 430f

s
"Saber shins", 151
Sacral fractures
  classification of, 412, 414f
  pattern, 412
Sacral kyphosis, 281, 282f
Sacral sparing, 296
Sacroiliitis, tests for, 286
Sacrum, 407–416
  case study in, 407b, 409b
Sacrum, vertebrae of, 281
Salter-Harris classification, for growth plate fractures,
    163, 164f
"SALTR" mnemonic, 163
Sanders classification, of calcaneus fracture, 432,
    435f

Sarcoma
  Ewing's, 127f, 137
  soft-tissue, 125, 141
  synovial, 141
  vs. carcinoma, 125
Scalloping, of cartilage forming tumors, 131–132,
    131f
Scaphoid bone
  anatomy of, 83
  blood supply of, 83
  complications of, 121
  fracture of, 83, 121
    healing rate of, 121
    treatment for, 121
Scaphoid nonunion advanced collapse (SNAC)
    wrist, 121, 122f
Scapholunate advanced collapse (SLAC) wrist, 121,
    122f
Scapula, 389–390
  case study in, 389b, 390f
  fractures of, 389–390
    indications for, 389
    injuries associated with, 389
  surgical approaches to, 389
Scapular notching, 263, 263f
Scapular rotators, function of, 363
Scapular winging, 265–266
  causes of, 266
  treatment of, 266
Scapulothoracic articulation, 265
Scapulothoracic crepitus. see "Snapping scapular
    syndrome"
Scapulothoracic dissociation, 390
Schatzker classification, of tibial plateau fractures,
    425, 425f
Scheuermann disease, 181–183, 181b, 182f
  lumbar. see Pseudo-Scheuermann disease
  management options for, 183
  surgical options for, 183
  symptoms associated with, 182
Scheuermann's kyphosis, 314, 315f
  bracing for, 315
  prevalence of, 314
  surgery for, 315
  symptoms of, 314
  treatment of, 315
Schmorl's nodes, 182
Schwannoma, 140
Scleroderma, of hand, 108b, 109, 110f–111f
Scoliosis
  in cerebral palsy, 202–203, 203f
  disorders associated with, 311
  in Duchenne muscular dystrophy, 210
  and Klippel-Feil syndrome, 190
  in Klippel-Feil syndrome, 302
  Risser classification for, 179f
  in spina bifida, 207
Scotty dog sign, 316, 317f
Secondary bone formation, 381–383
Segund fracture, 336, 337f
Sensation, in hand, 81
Sensory levels, 286, 286t, 287f
Sensory neuropathy, 66–67
Septic arthritis, 146–148, 146b
  in children, 150

definitive diagnosis of, 147
in immunocompromised patients, 147
osteomyelitis and, 151
treatment of, 148
Septic olecranon bursitis, 374
Sequestrum, in chronic osteomyelitis, 150
Serum lactate, marker of initial injury, 386–387
Seymour's fracture, 200
"Shepherd's crook" deformity, 160
Shoe, modifications and usage of, 228–229
Short thumb, 195
Shoulder
abduction relief test in, 284
arthrodesis of, 263
position of, 264
arthroplasty of, anterosuperior approach of, 261
avascular necrosis of, 257
difference between hemiarthroplasty and total
shoulder arthroplasty, 260
dislocations of, 172–174
anterior, 351
bone loss after, 358
fractures of, nerve injuries associated with,
391–392
hemiarthroplasty of, 260
injuries to, 215–216, 215b
incidence of, in throwing athlete, 363
instability, 350–361, 359f–360f
case study in, 350b, 354b, 357b–358b
muscular attachments in, 391
pain of
etiologies of, 244
exertional, 244
spastic adducted internally rotated, 232
stiffness, 255–256
case of, 255b
causes of, 255
Silicone elastomer based resection arthroplasty, 104
Silicone synovitis, due to silicone implantation, 107
Single photon emission computed tomography
(SPECT), in spondylolysis, 317–318
Single point cane, 227, 227f
Single-row rotator cuff repairs, 249
Skeletal maturity, Risser classification of, 311, 312f
Skeletal muscle
gross anatomy of, 35
sequence of, 36f
types of, 35–36
contraction, 36
Skeletal traction, for femoral shaft fracture,
421–422
"Skier's thumb", 118, 118b
Skin traction, for femoral shaft fracture, 421–422
"Sleeper" stretch, 368f
Slip angle, 185, 318, 318f
Slip percentage, 318, 318f
Slip reduction, methods for, 319
Slipped capital femoral epiphysis (SCFE), 212–214,
212b
diagnosis of, 212–214, 213f
knee pain in, 214
treatment of, 214
Smith's fracture, 407
Smoking, in fracture healing, 29–30, 30b
Snapping hip syndrome, 347

"Snapping scapular syndrome", 264
imaging of, 265
physical examination and treatment for, 265
"Snuff box", 83, 121
Social worker, 221
Soft-tissue tumors
benign, and reactive lesions, 139–141, 139b
malignant, 141–142, 141b
Space of Poirier, 83
Spasticity, 201–202
heterotopic ossification and, 239
Spear tackler's spine, 376
Speech therapist, 220
Spica casting, complications of, for diaphyseal femur
fractures, 167
Spina bifida (myelomeningocele), 207–208, 207b
Spinal cord injury, 240–241, 291
case of, 240b
complete, 296
functional levels of, 241
heterotopic ossification in, 239
incomplete, 296–297
orthopedic surgery in, 241
Spinal Cord Injury WithOut Radiologic Abnormality
(SCIWORA), 301
Spinal deformity
complications with, 313
goals of, 313
types of surgical intervention for, 313
Spinal muscular atrophy (SMA), 209
Spinal shock, 240, 296
level of, 240
Spinal stenosis
degenerative, pathology of, 320
disorders associated with, 320
epidemiology of, 321
surgery for, 321
treatment of, 321
Spine, 281–327
anatomy and examination of, 281–292
diagnostic tests for, 288
imaging techniques for, 288
infections in, 291–292
metastatic lesions to, 292
normal curves of, 281, 282f
pediatric, 178–191
regions of, 281, 282f
three-column concept of, 297
tumor in, 292, 292t
Spirochete, of Lyme disease, 151
Spondylolisthesis, 183, 183b, 183f–184f, 316
classification of, 316
dysplastic (type I), 184
incidence of, 317
indications for, 319
isthmic (type II), 184
non-operative treatment of pediatric, 185
radiographic views for, 185
surgical options for, 185
treatment for, 318–319
types of, 316
Spondylolysis, 184, 316
non-operative treatment of pediatric, 185
surgical options for, 185
treatment for, 318

Sports
  participation in, and elbow dislocations, 267
  pediatric, 215–218
Sports hernia. *see* Athletic pubalgia
Sports rehab, 222–223
  case of, 222b, 225b
Sports-related injury, 328–380
Sprain
  of ankle, eversion type, 75
  sternoclavicular, acute, treatment of, 254–255
Sprengel's deformity, 189, 189f
Spurling's test, 284, 284f
Squeeze test, 75, 75f
Stainless steel plates, 44, 44b
Stance, components of, 224
Stance phase knee flexion, 225
Standard medial parapatellar approach, in total knee
    arthroplasty, 8
Standard walkers, 227–228
Standers, 228, 231
Staphylococcus aureus, 19
  as pathogen of septic arthritis, 146
Staphylococcus epidermidis, 19
Steinberg classification, for avascular necrosis, 416
Stener lesion, 120, 120f
Step
  length, 223
  stride differentiated from, 223
Steppage gait, 225
Sternoclavicular dislocation, pediatric equivalent of,
    172–174
Sternoclavicular injuries, 251–255
  case of, 251b–254b, 253f
Sternoclavicular joint, 253
  dislocation of, 255
    treatment of, 254–255
  mechanism of injury in, 254
  physical examination of, 254
  radiographic evaluation of, 254
Sternoclavicular sprains, acute, treatment of,
    254–255
Steroids, in acute spinal cord injury, 297–298
Stiff knee gait, 206, 226
  spastic, 233
Stiffness
  as complications of shoulder arthroplasty, 261
  of elbow, 272–276
    causes of, 276
    non-operative treatments of, 276
    operative treatments of, 276
Straight posterior herniation, 288
Strain, 43–46
Streeter's dysplasia. *see* Constriction band syndrome,
    congenital
Strength, graded by manual muscle testing,
    220
Stress, 43–46
Stress corrosion, 45
Stress fractures, 348, 348b
Stress reaction, in spondylolysis, 317
Stress relaxation, 44
Stress-strain curve, 43, 43b, 43f
Stride, 223
  length, 223
  step differentiated from, 223

Subacromial impingement syndrome, 244
  physical examination for, 244
  treatment of, 244
Subacromial syndromes, 244–250
  case of, 244b, 248b
  causes of, 244
Submuscular plating, complications of, 167
Subscapularis, management during shoulder
    arthroplasty, 261
Subscapularis-shortening procedures, for shoulder
    stabilization, 358
Subvastus approach, in total knee arthroplasty, 7
"Sugar-tong" splint, in humeral shaft fractures, 394
Sulfonamides, 42t
Superior glenohumeral ligament (SGHL), 350, 351f
Superior labrum anterior and posterior (SLAP)
    lesion, 365
  in magnetic resonance arthrogram, 367f
Supracondylar femur fracture, 423
Suprascapular nerves
  anatomy of, 250
  entrapment of, 250
    treatment of, 250
Supraspinous ligaments, 283
Surgical debridement, goal of, 439
Surgical fixation
  of acetabular fractures, 412
  of elbow dislocation, 271
  of tibial plateau fractures, 426
Swan neck deformity, 107
Swing, components of, 224
Swing through gait pattern, 228
Swing to gait pattern, 228
Symptoms, systemic, 283
Syndactyly, 194, 194f
Syndesmotic ligaments, 75
Synovectomy, contraindications of, 105
Synovial facet joints, 283
Synovial fluid, in osteoarthritis, 20
Synovial sarcoma, 141
Synovium, structure and function of, 32
Syphilis, 151
Systemic lupus erythematosus (SLE), 108, 108b
  surgical concern for, 108
Systemic sclerosis, surgery indicated for, 109

T
"Tailor's bunion", 55
Talar neck fractures, classification of, 431, 432f
Talar tilt test, 73
Talus
  fractures of, 431
    case study in, 431b
  osteochondral lesions of
    Berndt and Hardy classification of, 60
    etiology and treatment of, 60
    Ferkel and Sgaglione CT staging system for, 61
  revascularization of, 431, 433f
Tarsal tunnel, 77, 78f
Tarsal tunnel syndrome, 77, 77b–78b
  diagnosis of, 77–78
  symptoms of, 77
  treatment of, 78
Technetium bone scans, 128, 317

Tendinitis
  rotator cuff, 354
  triceps, 373
Tendons, 33–34
  disorders of, 61–66
  injuries to, 276–279
    case of, 276b
    healing and repair, 34
    mechanism of, 33
  retraction of, 247
  structure and function of, 33–34
  surgery and, 232
Tendon atrophy, rotator cuff repair and, 248–249
Tendonitis
  Achilles tendon, 61–62
  calcific, 256
  patellar, 344
Tennis elbow, 278
  imaging of, 278
  nonsurgical treatment of, 278
  surgery for, 278
  tendon origin of, 278
Tennis players, tennis elbow and, 278
Tenodesis effect, 95
Tension band, 381, 382f
Tension band wire technique, in olecranon fractures,
    402f
Terminal stance, muscles acting during, 224
Terminal swing, muscles acting during, 224
Terrible triad injury, 267–268, 268f
"Terry Thomas" sign, 121
Thalidomide, as cause of phocomelia, 193–194
Thenar muscles, in hand, 86t
Thermal capsular shrinkage, 359
Thessaly test, 331
Thoracic kyphosis, 281, 282f
Thoracic outlet space, 264–266
Thoracic outlet syndrome, 264–266
  radiographs of, 264
  surgical treatment of, 264
Thoracic spine, vertebrae of, 281
Thoracolumbar compression fracture, 307–308
Thoracolumbar spine, 307–326
  case study, 307b, 308f, 309b–310b, 310f, 312f,
    315b, 316f, 319b, 321b, 324b, 325f
Thoracolumbosacral orthosis (TLSO), or adolescent
    idiopathic scoliosis, 180
Three point gait, 228
Thrombocytopenia-absent radius (TAR) syndrome,
    associated with radial clubhand, 193
Thrombophlebitis, incidence of, 17, 17b, 18f
Throwing athlete, injuries of, 361–367
  case study in, 361b, 364b–365b
  types of, 363
Thumb, fractures and dislocations of, 117–120
Thyroid cancer, metastatic to bone, 142
Ti-6Al-4V titanium-based alloy, orthopedic implants,
    44
Tibia
  external rotation of, test for, 341
  fractures of. *see* Tibial fractures
  proximal
    normal alignment of, 9
    tibial axis and, 9
Tibial alignment jigs, extramedullary, 9

Tibial axis, 9
  proximal tibia, 9
Tibial eminence fractures, 168, 169f
Tibial fractures, 424–431
  proximal, 424–427
    physeal, 170, 170f
  treatment of, in children, 171
Tibial plateau, 9
  fractures of
    classification of, 425, 425f
    CT scan for, 426
    diagnosis in patient with, 425–426
    indications for surgical fixation of, 426
    initial management of, 426
    ligamentous injury in, 426
Tibial shaft, 424–427
  case study in, 424b, 426b
  fractures of, 426–427
    pediatric, classic deformities with, 171
    proximal third, deformity in, 427
    treatment for, 427
Tibial tubercle avulsions, treatment of,
    217–218
Tibial tubercle fracture, 169
Tibiofibular diastasis, 75–76
Tibiotalar impingement, 58, 58b, 59f
  anterior, arthroscopy of, 60
  radiographic classification of, 58–59, 59f
Tile classification, 407, 409f–410f
Tillaux fracture, 171, 172f
Timed up and go test, 224
Tip-apex distance (TAP), 420, 420f
Titanium plate, 44, 44b
Toddler's fracture, 145–146, 145b, 146f
Toe drag, 226
Toe walking, 205–206
Torticollis, congenital muscular, 186, 186f
  etiology of, 186
  treatment of, 187
Total ankle arthroplasty, indications/
    contraindications to, 72
Total contact cast (TCC), 69–70
Total elbow arthroplasty, 274–275
  complications of, 275
  contraindications of, 275
  in distal humeral fractures, 397
  for elbow osteoarthritis, 273
  indications of, 275
  results of, 275
  for rheumatoid arthritis, 274f
  technical considerations of, 275
Total hip arthroplasty (THA), 14
  CBC, ESR, and CRP in patients with,
    19–20
  Charnley's original, biomechanical concept of,
    46, 46f
  diagnostic studies for, 20
  dislocation after, 17
  hip stability after, 17
    soft-tissue considerations, 17
  infected, signs/symptoms of, 19
  long-term complication after, 18
  nerve injuries during, 17
  prosthetic components in, 15
  structures at risk in, 14t

Total joint prostheses, 441, 441f
Total knee arthroplasty (TKA)
  causes of, 10–11
  diagnosis for patient, 11
  flexion and extension gap correction in, 10t
  goals of, 7, 7b, 9
  implant choices for revision, 12
  joint fluid analysis results for, 11
  lateral parapatellar approach of, 8
  major goals of revision, 12
  medial parapatellar capsular arthrotomy, 7
  midline skin incision for, 8f
  periprosthetic infection, 11
  standard medial parapatellar approach, 8
  subvastus approach, 7
  trivector approach, 8
Total shoulder arthroplasty, 260
  complications of, 261
  contraindications of, 261
  for glenohumeral arthritis, 260
  outcomes of, 261
  surgical approaches for, 261
Total wrist arthroplasty, 105–106, 106f
  complications of, 106–107
  contraindications for, 106
  indications for, 105–106
Trabecular bone, 23
Traction, 221
Transient synovitis, 148–149, 148b, 148f
Transosseous rotator cuff repairs, 249
Transverse deficiency, of hand, 192
Transverse ligament, 283
Trauma, 381–442
  adult, vs. pediatric orthopedic trauma, 162–164
  direct, neurologic injury and, 239
  elbow, 174–177, 174b, 175f
  foot and ankle, 171–172, 171b, 172f
  golden hour in, 387
  hip and femur, 164–168
  pediatric, 162–178, 163b, 163f
    vs. adult orthopedic trauma, 162–164
  radiographic series in, 386
  septic arthritis associated with, 147
Trendelenburg gait, 225
  bilateral, 225
Treponema pallidum, as cause of syphilis, 151
Triangular fibrocartilage complex (TFCC), 407
Triceps rupture, 277–278
  mechanism of injury in, 278
  physical examination of, 278
  treatment of, 278
Triceps tendinitis, 373
Trigger digit, 197
Triplane fracture, 171
Trochanteric bursitis, 347
Tumors
  orthopedic
    benign lesions, 125
    bone forming, 128
    cartilage forming, 128
    Enneking system for, 125, 126t
    malignant lesions, 125
  pediatric, 156–162, 156b, 157f
  round cell, 139t

Turf toe, 54, 54b
  radiographic findings for, 54
  treatment for, 54–55
Two point gait, 228
Type I errors, 48
Type II errors, 48

U

Ulcer, classification of, 67
Ulna fractures, proximal, 400–402
Ulnar artery, in hand, injury of, 90, 90b
Ulnar clubhand, vs. radial clubhand, 193
Ulnar collateral ligament injury, 371, 371f–372f, 374
  surgical intervention in, 371–372
  treatment for, 118–120, 120f
Ulnar column, of wrist, 405
Ulnar nerve, in hand, 91
  injury of, 90, 90b
Ulnar shaft, fractures, treatment of, 402
Ulnar-sided ligament injury, 371
Ulnar tunnel syndrome, symptoms of, 90
Ultrasound
  of developmental dysplasia of the hip, 211, 211f
  of septic arthritis, 147
Unicameral bone cyst, vs. aneurysmal bone cyst, 160–161, 161f
Unicompartmental knee arthroplasty (UKA), 4, 5f
  differentiated from total knee arthroplasty, 7
  indications/contraindications for, 7
Unilateral facet dislocation, 299
  treatment of, 299
University of California Biomechanics Lab (UCBL) brace, 229, 229f

V

VACTERL syndrome, 193
Valgus deformity, associated with proximal tibial metaphyseal (Cozen) fractures, 171
Valgus extension overload syndrome, 373
Vancomycin, 37–38
Varus deformity, correction of, 9
Vastus medialis splitting approach, 8
Vaulting gait, 225
Vertebra plana, 161
Vertebral artery, 283
Vertebroplasty, 309
Viable muscle tissue, vs. non-viable muscle tissue, 439
Vinculae tendinum, 93
Viscoelastic materials, vs. elastic materials, 44
Vitamin D
  deficiency, 25, 26f
  to promote bone health, 25
Volar plate, 81
  ruptured, in dorsal PIP dislocation, 113

W

Waddell signs, 286
"Waddling" gait. see Trendelenburg gait
Walch classification, of glenoid deformity, 258, 258f
Waldenstrom stages, of Perthes disease, 154t

Walking, 223–226
  base, 223
    causes of, 225–226
  measuring performance of, 224
Western blot, for Lyme disease, 151
Wheelchairs
  components of, 234, 235f
  different weights of, 234
  features of, 234–235
  prescription for, 234–235
    case of, 234b
    considerations of, 235
    purpose of, 234
"Whitesides line," of femur, 9
Wide excision, of orthopedic tumors, 129
Winquist-Hansen classification, of femoral shaft
      fractures, 421, 422f
Wolff's law, 29
Woven bone, 23
"Wrinkle test", 200

Wrist, 177–178
  anatomy of, 81–102
  arthritis and arthroplasty of, 102–104
  columns of, 405
  flexion contracture of, spastic, treatment of, 232
  ganglion on, 83
  hyperextension of, 83b
  ligaments of, 84f

Y

Young-Burgess classification, 407, 408f
Young's modulus, 43

Z

Z-plasty method, for congenital constriction band
      syndrome, 387
Zanca view, of acromioclavicular joint,
      387, 388f